Surgery

Christian de Virgilio • Areg Grigorian
Editors

Surgery

A Case-Based Clinical Review

Third Edition

Springer

Editors
Christian de Virgilio
Department of Surgery
Harbor–UCLA Medical Center
Torrance, CA, USA

Areg Grigorian
Department of Surgery
University of California
Irvine, CA, USA

ISBN 978-3-032-09798-9 ISBN 978-3-032-09799-6 (eBook)
https://doi.org/10.1007/978-3-032-09799-6

Cover and other illustrations by Meghan Lark, MD (mlarkillustrations.com)

This Springer imprint is published by the registered company Springer Nature Switzerland AG
The registered company address is: Gewerbestrasse 11, 6330 Cham, Switzerland

To my wonderful wife and fellow surgeon, Kelly, who has always supported me; to my five children, Nick, Michael, Emery, Sophia, and Andrew, who have always made coming home a pleasure; and to all the students over the last two decades who have inspired me to teach.

Christian de Virgilio

To my wife and best friend, Rebecca, who puts up with me every time I come home with a new idea or project! And to my two amazing daughters—Ella and Ava—I hope you become surgeons but if not I hope you find something that excites you as much as surgery and education excites me!

Areg Grigorian

Foreword

I am delighted to write the foreword for the third edition of *Surgery: A Case-Based Clinical Review* edited by Christian de Virgilio and Areg Grigorian.

I was honored to write the first and second one, and the book has had such impact since its initial publication in 2015—it has been adopted by several medical schools, and it is in the top five of Springer's medical books and among the top seven on Amazon! The book is meant for short chapter reads organized into sections with shelf questions at the end of each section to quickly assess one's understanding of the important content. One of my students who served as my Presidential intern at Wake Forest University who now is a medical student at the University of Pennsylvania texted me my second foreword as he was using the book and loved it.

Dr. de Virgilio was a third-year medical student on a pediatric surgical rotation when I was the senior resident. He was a fabulous student and went on to be a vascular surgeon—just like I did! He is a fabulous teacher and role model. Now, he is Professor of Surgery, UCLA School of Medicine, chair of the Department of Surgery at Harbor-UCLA Medical Center, as well as co-chair of the College of Applied Anatomy.

This medical school textbook is such a treasure for medical students. The chapters begin with a patient story followed by the pertinent facts needed on the history and physical examination—then the student can learn to design the work-up, make the diagnosis, and manage the surgical problem. The preparation is essential to be able to answer the shelf examination questions which follow—all of this getting the medical student ready to master the information and do well on their examination in surgery.

As a Chief Executive Officer and Chief Academic Officer at Atrium Health Wake Forest Baptist, Chief Academic Officer and Executive Vice President at Advocate Health, and Executive Vice President of Health Affairs at Wake Forest University, I still teach students in the clinic and the operating room as I still practice vascular surgery. I am delighted that this book has served medical students so well. Someone taught us—therefore, we should teach as well!

"Success isn't about just what you accomplish in your life, it's about what you inspire others to do."

Anonymous

Teaching makes the world a better place. Go do that!

Julie Ann Freischlag
Winston-Salem, NC, USA

Preface

We are delighted to have the opportunity to create a 3rd edition of our book. We are especially grateful to have heard from students around the country that our book continues to be valuable for their surgery clerkship, and for preparing for the Surgery shelf examination.

Over 10 years ago, my co-editor Dr. Areg Grigorian was a 4th year medical student rotating on my vascular surgery service at Harbor-UCLA. He showed great promise, so I asked him if he would want to help with a new book, *Surgery: A Case-Based Clinical Review*. He approached the project with incredible fervor, passion, and determination, and importantly, brought the perspective of a medical student to the book. As a result of his immense contributions, I offered him to be an Assistant Editor. Today, Dr. Grigorian is a trauma/acute care surgery faculty at UC Irvine!

Continuing the trend of getting important input from medical students, for this edition we have recruited another surgical star, Dr. James McDermott, who I similarly met while he was a medical student. His focus and drive have led him to being named an Assistant Editor of this new edition. Dr. McDermott is currently a 2nd year surgery resident at Stanford.

For this third edition, we've added key new content as well as new illustrations. As with prior editions, we've assembled a team of collaborators that include numerous surgery program directors, surgery clerkship directors, and various award-winning surgical educators. We've also included several medical students who were handpicked for their outstanding performance.

The goal of our book is to help you learn the essentials of surgery in the most efficient way possible. We feel our book will help you excel on the shelf exam, shine on the wards, think through the most commonly tested clinical vignettes, and develop your own deductive reasoning so that you make a great impression on your surgery clerkship. Additionally, each section is followed by a series of questions that are intended to mimic the style of questions you will find on the actual NBME shelf exam.

The start of the third year of medical school is terrifying. You're suddenly thrust into a hospital, where you meet a new team of residents and faculty, meet patients, learn a new language (medical abbreviations), learn an electronic health system, and are expected to somehow shine even though you're the least experienced and least knowledgeable. Once you finally get acclimated, you might get moved to another rotation in another specialty (sometimes even to another hospital), forced to start the orientation once again. At the same time, you're required to attend lectures and prepare for a final examination that may influence your ability to get a future residency. It is no doubt an extremely stressful time, but, at the end of the year, you will marvel at your professional growth and realize that being in the hospital with real patients is far better than being in a classroom all day. We hope our book gives you all the high-yield, test-relevant facts in an efficient and easy-to-understand manner so you can focus on what is important—how to be a great doctor!

Before discussing how to use our book, we want to share a few pearls about the surgery clerkship. First the "dos." Surgery is a team-based discipline. Always look for ways to help your team. Take an active role. Strive to make yourself irreplaceable, but do so with humility. Treat others like you would your family (assuming you get along with them). Be an effective communicator. Ask a lot of questions (but make it clear from your questions that you've been reading). Ask how you can help. Now the "don'ts." Don't be arrogant. Don't try to upstage your co-student or intern. And finally, don't worry! If you work hard, display enthusiasm, and take an active role, people will notice! You'll also be surprised to discover that most surgeons enjoy teaching (and aren't as mean as portrayed on TV). And you may even get bitten by the surgery bug (we hope)!

Now let's move on to how to use this book. The book is case-based and is in a short question-and-answer format. A risk of a case-based book is that you only learn that one specific case. To prevent falling into such a pitfall, we've also included pertinent differential diagnoses for each case and discuss how to distinguish them. We've tried to limit anatomy and pathophysiology to those that are clinically relevant. We've tried to exclude most cancer staging systems, as these constantly change, are hard to memorize, and are infrequently tested. We've tried to arrange the management in a "what's the next step" format, as such questions are frequently asked. We've purposely avoided too many details about specific aspects of surgical procedures as those are beyond the scope of a student. For those that want a bit more, we've added "areas where you can get in trouble," which are pitfalls in the diagnosis or management, and "areas of controversy." At the end of each chapter, there is a Summary of Essentials that permits a quick review. Finally, we've created questions and answers to follow each section (with an emphasis on why the wrong answers are wrong). It's important to realize that the questions are *not* intended to test your understanding of the reading. Rather, many of the questions are meant to supplement the reading by testing important topics that couldn't be covered (so don't be discouraged if you miss a lot of them!).

Our advice is to strive to read the whole book during your rotation. Read all the chapters in one section, and then do the supplement questions for that section. We've purposely made each chapter relatively short, so that you should be able to read each one in 20–30 min (or less). And, you should be able to read four to five chapters per week.

We're confident our book will help you during your surgery clerkship as well as for the shelf exam. We also realize that no single resource can do it all (including this book).

We hope you enjoy our book as much as we enjoyed writing it! We'd love to get your feedback. Feel free to email us on cdevirgilio@lundquist.org and agrigori@uci.edu or follow on Twitter @drdevirgilio. Best of luck on your rotation and in your (surgical) career!

Christian de Virgilio
Torrance, CA, USA

Areg Grigorian
Orange, CA, USA

Contents

I Acute Care Surgery

II Breast and Skin

III Cardiothoracic

IV Endocrine

IV Endocrine

V Head and Neck

V Head and Neck

VI Hepatopancreaticobiliary

VI Hepatopancreaticobiliary

VII Lower Gastrointestinal

VII Lower Gastrointestinal

VIII Neurosurgery

VIII Neurosurgery

IX Orthopedic

IX Orthopedic

X Pediatric

X Pediatric

XI Surgical Complications

XII Surgical Complications

XII Trauma

XV Vascular

Supplementary Information

Contributors

Tracey D. Arnell Department of Surgery, New York Presbyterian Columbia, New York, NY, USA

D'Ann E. Arthur Department of Orthopedics, Billings Clinic, Billings, MT, USA

Peyman Benharash Division of Cardiac Surgery, University of California at Los Angeles, Los Angeles, CA, USA

Jeremy M. Blumberg Department of Surgery, Division of Urology, Harbor-UCLA Medical Center, Torrance, CA, USA

Nina M. Bowens MemorialCare, Long Beach, CA, USA

David C. Chen Department of Surgery, Lichtenstein Amid Hernia Clinic, University of California, Los Angeles, Santa Monica, Los Angeles, CA, USA

Jon Mallen-St. Clair Department of Surgery, Cedars-Sinai, Ear, Nose & Throat, Los Angeles, CA, USA

Chantal Creighton Department of Surgery, Harbor-UCLA Medical Center, David Geffen School of Medicine at UCLA, Torrance, CA, USA

Joanna Curry Cardiovascular Outcomes Research Laboratories (CORELAB), University of California Los Angeles, Los Angeles, CA, USA

Patrick T. Delaplain Department of Pediatric Surgery, Texas Children's Hospital and Baylor College of Medicine, Houston, TX, USA

Christian de Virgilio Department of Surgery, Harbor-UCLA Medical Center, Torrance, CA, USA

Michael de Virgilio Department of Surgery, University of California, Irvine, Irvine, CA, USA

Jill Q. Dworsky Department of Colon and Rectal Surgery, Kaiser Permanente Baldwin Park Medical Center, UCLA School of Medicine, Los Angeles, CA, Baldwin Park, CA, USA

Fuad F. Elkhoury Department of Urology, University of California, Los Angeles, Santa Monica, CA, USA

Richard G. Everson Department of Neurosurgery, David Geffen School of Medicine of the University of California, Los Angeles, Los Angeles, CA, USA

Aaron J. Feinstein Department of Head and Neck Surgery, University of California Los Angeles Medical Center, Los Angeles, CA, USA

John F. Fleming III Department of Orthopedic Surgery, Cedars-Sinai Medical Group, Torrance, CA, USA

Cameron Gerhold Florida State University College of Medicine, Tallahassee, FL, USA

Kiran Gollapudi Department of Surgery, Division of Urology, Harbor-UCLA Medical Center, David Geffen School of Medicine at UCLA, Torrance, CA, USA

Areg Grigorian Department of Surgery, University of California, Irvine, CA, USA

McKensie Hammons David Geffen School of Medicine at UCLA, Torrance, CA, USA

Danielle M. Hari Department of Surgery, Division of Surgical Oncology, Harbor-UCLA Medical Center, Torrance, CA, USA

Dennis Y. Kim Department of Surgery, Harbor-UCLA Medical Center, Torrance, CA, USA

Irene A. Kim Department of Head and Neck Surgery, University of California, Los Angeles, Santa Monica, CA, USA

Edward C. Kuan Department of Otolaryngology-Head and Neck Surgery, University of California, Irvine Medical Center, Orange, CA, USA

Steven L. Lee Department of Pediatric Surgery, Seattle Children's Hospital and University of Washington Department of Surgery, Seattle, WA, USA

Matthew Y. C. Lin Department of Clinical Surgery, University of California, San Francisco, San Francisco, CA, USA

Masha J. Livhits Department of Endocrine Surgery, David Geffen School of Medicine, University of California, Los Angeles, Los Angeles, CA, USA

James McDermott Department of Surgery, Stanford University School of Medicine, Stanford, CA, USA

Vishad Nabili Department of Head and Neck Surgery, UCLA Medical Center, David Geffen School of Medicine at UCLA, Los Angeles, CA, USA

Cooper Nagaki Department of Surgery, Harbor-UCLA Medical Center, Torrance, CA, USA

Jeffry Nahmias Department of Surgery, University of California, Irvine, Irvine, CA, USA

Jessica Beth O'Connell Department of Surgery, University of California Los Angeles, Vascular Surgery, Greater Los Angeles VA Healthcare System, Los Angeles, CA, USA

Junko Ozao-Choy Division of Surgical Oncology, Harbor-UCLA Medical Center, Torrance, CA, USA

Eugene J. Park David Geffen School of Medicine, University of California, Los Angeles, Torrance, CA, USA

Flora Park Department of General Surgery, Harbor-UCLA Medical Center, Torrance, CA, USA

Kevin A. Peng Department of Neurotology and Otolaryngology, House Clinic / PIH Health, Los Angeles, CA, USA

Beverley A. Petrie Department of Surgery, Division of Colon and Rectal Surgery, Harbor-UCLA Medical Center, Torrance, CA, USA

Kevin W. Rolfe Department of Orthopedic Surgery, Harbor-UCLA Medical Center and Rancho Los Amigos Rehabilitation Center, Torrance, CA, USA

Jose Manuel Sarmiento Department of Neurosurgery, Cleveland Clinic Florida, Weston, FL, USA

Sebastian D. Schubl Department of Trauma and Critical Care Surgery, University of California Irvine Health, Orange, CA, USA

Manan P. Shah David Geffen School of Medicine, University of California, Los Angeles, Torrance, CA, USA

Jordan Shin Department of Surgery, University of California Irvine Medical Center, Orange, CA, USA

Brian R. Smith Department of Surgery and General Surgery Residency Program, University of California Irvine Medical Center, Orange, CA, USA

Veronica F. Sullins Department of Pediatric Surgery, UCLA Mattel Children's Hospital, Los Angeles, CA, USA

Amulya Vadlakonda David Geffen School of Medicine, University of California, Los Angeles, Torrance, CA, USA

Andrew M. Vahabzadeh-Hagh Department of Head and Neck Surgery, UC San Diego Health, San Diego, CA, USA

Justin P. Wagner Department of Pediatric Surgery, UCLA Health, Los Angeles, CA, USA

James X. Wu Department of Endocrine Surgery, UCLA Health, Los Angeles, CA, USA

Arezou Yaghoubian Department of Plastic Surgery, UCLA Medical Center, Los Angeles, CA, USA

Isaac Yang Department of Neurosurgery, David Geffen School of Medicine at UCLA, Los Angeles, CA, USA

Michael W. Yeh Department of Endocrine Surgery, UCLA David Geffen School of Medicine, Los Angeles, CA, USA

Acute Care Surgery

David C. Chen

Contents

Fever and Hypotension in the Intensive Care Unit

Areg Grigorian and Christian de Virgilio

Contents

C. de Virgilio, A. Grigorian (eds.), *Surgery*, https://doi.org/10.1007/978-3-032-09799-6_1

Case Study

A 57-year-old male patient develops confusion and lethargy in the intensive care unit. He is 4 days status post emergent surgery for a perforated gastric ulcer that developed as a result of daily nonsteroidal anti-inflammatory drug (NSAID) use for chronic lower back pain. He was treated with an exploratory laparotomy and an omental (Graham) patch closure of the ulcer. On physical examination, his temperature is 39.2 °C, heart rate is 96 beats per minute, respiratory rate is 24/min, and blood pressure is 82/62 mmHg. Oxygen saturation is 92% on room air. The surgical incisions appear clean and intact, and the abdomen is nontender. There are diminished breath sounds on the right. His urine output has been 10 cc/h for the last 6 h, and the urine appears dark. Laboratory values reveal a white blood cell count of 18 × 10^3/μL (normal 4.1–10.9 × 10^3/μL), serum creatinine of 3.2 mg/dL (from a baseline of 1.1 3 days earlier), and a blood pH of 7.1. Chest x-ray demonstrates a large area of consolidation in the right lower lobe. Given his lethargy, tachypnea, and low oxygen saturation, he is intubated by way of rapid sequence intubation. He is given several IV fluid boluses; however, the blood pressure does not improve. A vasopressor is initiated. Blood cultures are sent.

Diagnosis

What Is the Differential Diagnosis for a Postoperative Patient with Fever? (▫ Table 1.1)

▫ Table 1.1 Differential diagnosis for postoperative fever

Diagnosis	Comments
Aspiration pneumonia	Inhalation of gastric microbes causing infection, onset within days to weeks, symptoms may consist of cough, wheezing, and shortness of breath
Aspiration pneumonitis	Inhalation of gastric acid causing injury of epithelial cells, onset within minutes to hours, symptoms may consist of cough, wheezing, and shortness of breath
Atelectasis	Partial or complete collapse of a lung, often bibasilar, from obstruction or extrathoracic restriction (including pain); causes shortness of breath and hypoxemia; debatable whether it actually causes fever (may be coincidental as opposed to causal)
Drug reaction	Usually a diagnosis of exclusion if no other symptoms are present; may have a rash
Ventilator-associated pneumonia	Fever, leukocytosis, and consolidation on imaging in a patient that is requiring or required mechanical ventilation
Surgical site infection	Tenderness, erythema, swelling, warmth, delayed healing, purulent discharge
Urinary tract infection	Minimize catheter use and duration (less than 2 days, if possible)
Venous thromboembolism	Includes deep vein thrombosis and pulmonary embolism; prevented with chemical prophylaxis, sequential compression, and ambulation
Adrenal insufficiency	Hypotensive despite fluid resuscitation and vasopressors; may have fever, hyponatremia, hyperkalemia, hypoglycemia

What Is the Classic Timing for the Different Causes of Postoperative Fever (the Five Ws)? (Table 1.2)

Table 1.2 Classic timing of postoperative fever (The Five Ws)

W	Comment	Occurs
Wind	Atelectasis Pneumonia	POD 1 POD 2–4
Water	Urinary tract infection	POD 3
Walk	Venous thromboembolism	POD 5
Wound	Infection	POD 7
Wonder drugs	Drug reaction	Anytime

POD postoperative day

Watch Out

Necrotizing postoperative wound infections (due to *Clostridia* or *beta-hemolytic Streptococcus*) can rarely occur within 12 h of surgery. Such infections need prompt broad-spectrum IV antibiotics and return to the operating room for debridement.

What Is the Most Likely Diagnosis in This Patient?

The combination of fever and leukocytosis strongly suggests a diagnosis of sepsis. Given the diminished breath sounds and chest x-ray findings, the sepsis is most likely due to pneumonia. The addition of hypotension indicates that the patient is in shock. Although the differential of shock is broad (see below), with these findings, sepsis is the most likely cause. In addition, a rising creatinine, decreased urine output, and mental status changes indicate that there is end-organ damage.

What Other Diagnoses Should Be Considered in a Postoperative Patient with Fever and Hypotension?

Pulmonary embolism can also cause fever and hypotension (although the chest x-ray will generally be negative). Rarely, acute adrenal insufficiency can develop postoperatively (most often in patients with a history of steroid use), with a classic combination of fever, hyponatremia, hyperkalemia, hypoglycemia, and hypotension that is refractory to fluids and pressors.

History and Physical

What Clues Are Expected on History and Physical for a Patient in Sepsis?

The history and physical examination should provide clinical clues to guide a targeted approach to work up a septic patient. Always examine surgical wounds. Inspect the skin at the port of entry of all indwelling catheters (IVs, central lines) for evidence of infection. Look for other indwelling catheters (such as a bladder catheter) that might be a source of sepsis. If the patient progresses to shock, inflammatory mediators can lead to organ damage, which can present as oliguria, increased BUN and creatinine, and mental status changes. The skin is often warm and flushed from the increased peripheral vasodilation as total systemic vascular resistance drops similar to neurogenic shock, whereas other types of shock lead to cold, clammy skin. Confusion, disorientation, agitation, and anxiety are common in septic patients (septic encephalopathy). While fever is a common presentation for infection, an afebrile patient does not exclude sepsis. Patient populations who may not present with fevers include the very young, the elderly, those with dialysis-dependent renal failure, and the immunocompromised.

How Is Sepsis Defined and Evaluated?

Sepsis is defined as life-threatening organ dysfunction resulting from a dysregulated host response to infection. Various tools are used to screen for sepsis and predict prognosis, including the Sepsis-Related Organ Failure Assessment (SOFA), the quick SOFA (qSOFA), and the systemic inflammatory response syndrome (SIRS) criteria. The qSOFA, a bedside screening tool, predicts poor outcomes from infections by checking three criteria: respiratory rate ≥22/min, altered mental status, and systolic blood pressure ≤100 mmHg. A patient meeting two of these criteria is considered at higher risk for sepsis-related mortality. However, the latest Surviving Sepsis Campaign guidelines (2021) highlight qSOFA's poor sensitivity as a screening tool. While scoring systems are useful, they should not be the sole method for screening due to their variable diagnostic performance.

What Physical Exam Findings Suggest That a Patient Is Unable to Protect Their Airway?

A patient who is obtunded, has a Glasgow Coma Scale (GCS) score of 8 or less, has an absent gag reflex, or has an inability to swallow is unable to protect his or her airway.

Watch Out

If the GCS is 8 or less, intubate.

Compare and Contrast Aspiration Pneumonia and Pneumonitis

Aspiration pneumonia is an *infection* that develops several days after the inhalation of gastric microbes and/or oral secretions, requiring antibiotic treatment. In contrast, aspiration pneumonitis is an *immediate inflammatory reaction* to gastric acid that usually resolves on its own within 24–48 h with supportive care. They can sometimes be difficult to distinguish. Risk factors for both include altered mental status and neurological disorders such as dementia. Both commonly present with shortness of breath, cough, fever, wheezing, tachycardia, and abnormalities on chest radiographs. However, aspiration pneumonitis typically requires a large amount of aspiration, and as such is more often witnessed, and results in immediate symptoms within hours. The location of lung infiltrates in aspiration pneumonia tends to appear in more dependent positions such as the posterior segments of the upper lobes and superior segments of the lower lobes, and more likely on the right side, but may depend on the patient's position: infiltrates appear in the superior segment of the right lower lobe when supine, and in the posterior segment when upright. The primary diagnostic method to distinguish between them is bronchoalveolar lavage which requires bronchoscopy; the presence of bacteria suggests aspiration pneumonia.

Pathophysiology

What Are the Different Types of Shock? (Table 1.3)

Table 1.3 Hemodynamic profiles of the different types of shock

Type of shock	Causes	Preload (PCWP)	Cardiac output	Afterload (SVR)
Cardiogenic	MI, cardiac injury, arrhythmias, myocarditis	↑	↓	↑
Distributive	Anaphylaxis, sepsis	↓	↑	↓
Hypovolemic	Hemorrhage, dehydration, burns	↓	↓	↑
Neurogenic	Spinal cord injury, spinal anesthesia	↓	↓	↓
Obstructive	Cardiac tamponade, tension pneumothorax, PE	↑	↓	↑

PCWP pulmonary capillary wedge pressure, *SVR* systemic vascular resistance, *PE* pulmonary embolism

What Is the Pathophysiology of Septic Shock?

Sepsis is an inflammatory cascade that attempts to control a noxious stimulus (such as bacterial invasion). The core problem of septic shock is not poor perfusion but the poor *utilization* of oxygen. Therefore, hypotension is a sequelae and marker of the inflammation, and not a contributing factor to the pathophysiology of sepsis. Inflammatory mediators chiefly impair mitochondrial oxidation by inhibiting pyruvate dehydrogenase and cytochrome oxidase, and thus destroy the cell's ability to produce adenosine triphosphate (ATP). Additionally, inflammatory mediators induce production of nitric oxide resulting in systemic vascular dilation and high cardiac output (from increased heart rate). As stroke volume continues to decrease and stress on the cardiovascular system increases in untreated sepsis, compensatory tachycardia is unable to maintain cardiac output. The systemic venodilation sequesters the majority of the intravascular volume in the venous system, which is the basis of why fluid resuscitation is essential early in septic shock. However, to avoid the mortality associated with a large positive fluid balance, fluids should be titrated to an end-marker of resuscitation such as an adequate urine output. Lastly, although there is systemic vascular dilation, there is relative splanchnic vasoconstriction resulting in gut ischemia and mucosal injury. This allows for enteric pathogen translocation and additional subsequent inflammation; this self-sustaining process of continued inflammation is known as the "motor" of multi-organ failure.

What Is Acute Respiratory Distress Syndrome (ARDS)?

ARDS is an acute, diffuse inflammatory lung injury that was redefined in 2012 under the Berlin definition into a three-tiered grading system. Severity is based on the ratio of the arterial oxygen partial pressure (PaO_2) to fractional inspired oxygen (FiO_2) (known as the P/F ratio) and categorized as mild (200–300), moderate (100–199), and severe ARDS (<100). For example, if a patient has a PaO_2 of 92 mmHg while receiving 80% oxygen, the P/F ratio is 115 (92/0.8), suggestive of moderate ARDS. Patients with ARDS have an acute onset of respiratory symptoms and bilateral radiographic opacities not fully explained by heart failure. Trauma, sepsis, infection, or an inflammatory trigger leads to the release of pro-inflammatory cytokines which recruit and activate neutrophils, causing diffuse alveolar epithelial and endothelial damage. The resulting vascular leakage leads to diffuse pulmonary edema with fibrin secretion, hyaline membrane formation, loss of aerated lung tissue, and remodeling. There is resulting hypoxemia, increased physiological dead space, and decreased lung compliance.

If the Patient Were to Become Pulseless, What Are the Hs and Ts to Consider? (Table 1.4)

Table 1.4 Reversible causes of cardiac arrest (Hs and Ts)

H	**H**ypovolemia, **h**ypoxia, **h**ydrogen ion (acidosis), **h**ypokalemia, **h**yperkalemia, **h**ypothermia
T	**T**oxins (cocaine, tricyclics, digitoxin, beta blockers, calcium channel blockers), **t**amponade, **t**ension pneumothorax, **t**hrombosis (MI or PE)

Workup

What Are the Initial Laboratory Studies to Order for a Patient in Septic Shock?

Order a complete blood count (CBC) with differential, comprehensive metabolic panel (CMP), coagulation studies, serum lactate, arterial blood gas (ABG), peripheral blood cultures, and a urinalysis. If the patient has an indwelling central venous catheter, obtain a culture from that site as well. The peripheral blood should be cultured for aerobes and anaerobes from at least two different sites. Fungal cultures should be obtained in patients with central venous catheters or immunocompromised status, as these risk factors are often associated with candidemia.

What Is the Significance of Increased Serum Creatinine and Oliguria?

A patient with increased serum creatinine and oliguria has impaired kidney function and is at risk for acute kidney injury (AKI). The resulting metabolic acidosis may lead to worsening hypotension. Indications for acute renal replacement therapy are acidosis, hyperkalemia, uremia, and fluid overload. Such renal replacement should be considered early on in patients with septic shock and AKI.

What Is the Difference Between the Two Types of Renal Replacement Therapy: Hemodialysis (HD) and Continuous Renal Replacement Therapy (CRRT)?

CRRT is a slower type of dialysis that can be used as continuous therapy, whereas HD occurs over 3–6 h 2–3×/week. As such, the hourly rate of fluid and solute removal with CRRT is lower than with intermittent HD. This makes CRRT better tolerated by hypotensive patients. Both CRRT and HD provide fluid or solute removal through diffusion (dialysis), convection (filtration), or a combination of both. Because CRRT is continuous, this can allow for larger net solute and fluid removal over time. For the above patient in septic shock with AKI, the preferred option is CRRT.

What Are the Initial Imaging Studies to Order for a Postoperative Patient Believed to Be in Septic Shock?

A chest x-ray should be ordered, as well as sputum cultures if pneumonia is suspected in patients with productive cough, respiratory distress, and prolonged ICU stay. Obtain abdominal plain films if there is suspicion for bowel compromise or perforation (keep in mind that a small amount of free air may persist for a few days after laparotomy). If there is clinical suspicion for an intra-abdominal source of infection, obtain a CT scan of the abdomen and pelvis. Ultrasound can be used to detect acute cholecystitis.

> **Watch Out**
> Continuous bacteremia is usually seen in a persistent endovascular infection such as endocarditis or those with an infected central venous catheter. An echocardiogram should be ordered if a patient is found to have persistent bacteremia.

Management

What Are the Initial Management Goals for a Patient in Septic Shock?

The essential management of the septic patient includes early recognition, intravenous fluid (IVF) resuscitation, blood cultures, broad-spectrum IV antibiotics, and vasopressors (norepinephrine first; then vasopressin). Send cultures from the suspected source of infection before starting antibiotics if it will not delay treatment. If the source is not known, obtain aerobic and anaerobic blood cultures from two venipuncture sites. Start broad-spectrum IV antibiotics, and consider adding antifungal coverage if the patient is immunocompromised. After placing a central venous catheter, be sure to obtain a chest X-ray to confirm absence of a pneumothorax and to ensure proper placement prior to delivering medications. Urine output can be a surrogate for targeted fluid resuscitation with a goal of 0.5–1.0 mL/kg/h for adults. Blood products are only indicated if hemoglobin is <7.0 g/dL or if the patient is actively bleeding.

1

Watch Out

Resuscitating a patient in shock necessitates close monitoring of key resuscitation markers. While urine output is a primary indicator, other critical markers of under-resuscitation include a high lactate level (>2.0 mmol/L), a significant base deficit on arterial blood gases (a more negative value indicates under-resuscitation), low central venous pressure (<5 mmHg), and a flat or under-distended inferior vena cava observed on bedside ultrasound.

What Is Rapid Sequence Intubation (RSI)?

RSI is used to rapidly secure tracheal intubation in patients who have not fasted and, as such, are at high risk of vomiting and aspiration. The patient is medicated with weight-based, full-dose (rather than titrated) sedative and neuromuscular agents to allow intubation within several minutes. The patient should be pre-oxygenated with a face mask for a minimum of 3 min prior to the administration of an induction agent (such as ketamine or etomidate). Following induction, with normal intubation, the patient is then bag-valve masked. But with RSI, induction is followed immediately by a neuromuscular blocking agent (such as rocuronium or succinylcholine). Bag-valve-mask ventilation is typically avoided between the administration of induction agents and the placement of the endotracheal tube to reduce the risk of gastric insufflation and subsequent aspiration.

Watch Out

Etomidate can rarely lead to Addisonian crisis within 24 h after administration and result in refractory hypotension and fever.

Watch Out

Succinylcholine is a depolarizing agent that may lead to life-threatening hyperkalemia and should not be used acutely in patients with crush injury, burns, multiple trauma, or baseline hyperkalemia.

What Drugs Are Ideal to Use for Sedation in a Critically Ill and Intubated Patient?

Propofol (gamma-aminobutyric acid agonist) is commonly used for sedation because it has a rapid onset and is short acting (effects continue for only 5–8 min). It is also useful in patients with head injury because it reduces intracranial pressure. Dexmedetomidine (alpha-2 agonist) is also commonly used as it allows for cooperative sedation and has a mild analgesic effect. It has also been demonstrated to reduce ICU delirium. Both propofol and dexmedetomidine can have potential side effects of hypotension and bradycardia. Benzodiazepines can also be used for sedation but have largely been replaced because they seep into adipose tissue, which can lead to prolonged effect even after discontinuation of the drug and make weaning from the ventilator difficult. Propofol and benzodiazepines have no analgesic effect.

What Drugs Are Ideal to Use for Analgesia in a Critically Ill and Intubated Patient?

Opioids are the most widely used medications for analgesia in the hospital. Of the available opioid drugs, fentanyl is the most commonly used in critically ill patients because it has a fast onset (highly lipid soluble) and low risk of hypotension (not associated with histamine release) and does not have highly active metabolites (does not need to be renally dosed). Two non-opioid analgesics commonly used in the ICU are acetaminophen and NSAIDs (ketorolac, ibuprofen). These drugs can help decrease the amount of opioid use.

How Should the Patient's Oliguria Be Managed?

Oliguria in the presence of adequate fluid resuscitation indicates AKI. Patients in the ICU with AKI and septic shock may require renal replacement therapy, preferably CRRT.

What Is the Significance of a Low pH?

As tissue oxygenation decreases, anaerobic energy production increases and creates lactic acid as a byproduct. The acidosis activates potassium channel pumps and nitric oxide synthases to hyperpolarize and vasodilate vascular smooth muscle cells. The local effect of low pH coupled with the vasodilatory effects of inflammatory mediators perpetuates the hypotension in sepsis.

How Are Glucose Levels Managed in the Septic Patient?

Due to the high metabolic demand of a septic patient, insulin regimens are initiated when two consecutive blood glucose levels are >180 mg/dL. Intensive glycemic control is no longer favored as this has been shown to cause more morbidity than maintaining more moderate glycemic control (see NICE-SUGAR trial).

If the Patient Develops ARDS, What Are the Principles of Management?

Treatment of ARDS generally requires supportive care including lung-protective mechanical ventilation at low tidal volumes (6 mL/kg) to avoid barotrauma. For patients with moderate-to-severe ARDS, prone positioning for 12+ h per day may improve ventilation-perfusion matching and reduce mortality.

If the Patient Became Pulseless, How Should ACLS Be Executed?

For any emergency patient, assess the ABCs: airway, breathing, and circulation. Scan for breathing while firmly tapping and asking the patient to speak to check their airway. If there is no palpable carotid pulse, begin chest compressions immediately at a rate of 100 compressions/min.

Attach the monitor and defibrillator to the patient and continue chest compressions for 2 min. Then, check for a pulse and determine if the rhythm is shockable (pulseless ventricular tachycardia and ventricular fibrillation). If it is, shock the patient and immediately resume chest compressions. After 2 min, recheck the pulse and rhythm and shock again if warranted. If the patient does not respond after this second cycle of chest compressions, give 1.0 mg epinephrine. Continue to recheck pulse and rhythm, shock if warranted, and give epinephrine every 3–5 min.

If the rhythm is not shockable (pulseless electrical activity or asystole), resume chest compressions for 2 min, and administer 1.0 mg epinephrine. Continue CPR and epinephrine boluses every 3–5 min until the underlying cause is treated or the rhythm becomes shockable.

Watch Out
The only "shockable" rhythms are ventricular fibrillation and pulseless ventricular tachycardia.

What Is the Difference Between Synchronized and Desynchronized Shock?

Synchronized shock (cardioversion) is the delivery of a low-energy shock which synchronizes to the QRS complex. There is a delay after the shock button is pressed to allow synchronization to the heart's natural electrical beat to avoid shocking during the T wave, which can initiate ventricular fibrillation. It is used for unstable atrial fibrillation, atrial flutter, and supraventricular tachycardias unresponsive to medication.

Desynchronized shock (defibrillation) is the delivery of a random high-energy shock as soon as the shock button is pressed irrespective of the QRS complex. It is used when there is uncoordinated intrinsic electrical activity in the heart, such as pulseless ventricular tachycardia or ventricular fibrillation.

Areas of Controversy

Should Crystalloids or Colloids Be Used for Resuscitation in Septic Patients?

Intravenous fluids are necessary to improve cardiac output and tissue perfusion in patients with sepsis and septic shock, though the optimal type of fluid has been debated. There is belief that colloids (i.e., albumin) will maintain an osmotic pressure gradient, leading to greater intravascular volume resuscitation and decreased edema. However, colloids are much more expensive and have no proven clinical benefits compared to crystalloids. Therefore, crystalloids, like normal saline and lactated Ringer's, remain the preferred choice for resuscitation in the majority of patients. Among crystalloids, lactated Ringer's may be favored in many cases due to its more physiologic electrolyte composition and reduced risk of inducing hyperchloremic metabolic acidosis.

What Is the Role of Procalcitonin in Septic Patients?

Procalcitonin is a peptide precursor of calcitonin that is generally undetectable, but can rise in response to a bacterial infection. If the optimal duration of antibiotic therapy is unknown, procalcitonin may be used in combination with clinical evaluation to determine when antibiotics can be discontinued. While additional research is needed, there is evidence to suggest that monitoring procalcitonin may result in improved outcomes and shortened antibiotic duration. Most guidelines and clinical studies consider procalcitonin levels below 0.1 ng/mL as very unlikely to indicate a systemic bacterial infection. This threshold is commonly used to guide clinicians in reducing or withholding antibiotics in cases where bacterial infection is suspected but not confirmed.

Summary of Essentials

History and Physical

- Sepsis is defined as life-threatening organ dysfunction caused by a dysregulated host response to infection.
- Signs of infection: fever, warm and flushed skin, and leukocytosis.
  - Check for end-organ damage as evidenced by increased creatinine, decreased urine output, decreased platelet level, increased oxygen requirements, and mental status changes.
  - Shock: Vasopressors needed despite adequate fluids and a lactate >2.0 mmol/L.

Pathophysiology

- Septic shock is systemic inflammation characterized by poor utilization of oxygen
- Inflammatory mediators inhibit the body's ability to produce energy and cause vasodilation.
  - Cardiac output initially increases with the increased heart rate but is eventually compromised as venodilation pools venous return.

Workup

- CBC, CMP, coagulation studies, lactate, ABG, blood cultures, central venous catheter cultures, and urinalysis.
- Check for sources of infection based on patient's presentation and history.

Management

- IVF, broad-spectrum antibiotics, and vasopressors if needed.
  - Tailor the antibiotics based on cultures and sensitivities.
- ABCs: check airway, breathing, and circulation.
  - Intubate if GCS ≤8.
  - Achieve rapid sequence intubation with an induction agent (such as etomidate) and a paralytic (such as succinylcholine).
  - Use propofol or dexmedetomidine for sedation in a critically ill and intubated patient.
- Pulseless patient: start CPR.
  - Ventricular tachycardia or ventricular fibrillation: shock.
  - If patient remains unresponsive after two cycles of CPR, administer epinephrine.
  - Pulseless electrical activity or asystole: CPR with epinephrine and correct underlying cause (Hs and Ts).
- If renal replacement therapy is indicated for AKI, start CRRT in ICU patients who are hemodynamically unstable and requiring vasopressors despite adequate fluid resuscitation.
- Initiate insulin therapy at blood sugars above 180 mg/dL.

Acknowledgement The editors would like to acknowledge and thank the following authors for their contributions to the previous edition of the chapter: Monica Lee, Joanne M Bando

Suggested Reading

ARDS Definition Task Force, Ranieri VM, Rubenfeld GD, Thompson BT, et al. Acute respiratory distress syndrome: the Berlin definition. JAMA. 2012;30(23):2526–33.

Landry DW, Oliver JA. The pathogenesis of vasodilatory shock. N Engl J Med. 2001;345(8):588–95.

Nash DM, Przech S, Wald R, O'Reilly D. Systematic review and meta-analysis of renal replacement therapy modalities for acute kidney injury in the intensive care unit. J Crit Care. 2017;41:138–44.

Rhodes A, Evans LE, Alhazzani W, et al. Surviving sepsis campaign: international guidelines for management of sepsis and septic shock. Crit Care Med. 2017;45(3):486–552.

Russell JA, Rush B, Boyd J. Pathophysiology of septic shock. Crit Care Clin. 2018;34(1):43–61.

Nausea, Vomiting, and Left Groin Mass

Areg Grigorian, Amulya Vadlakonda, Christian de Virgilio, and David C. Chen

Contents

C. de Virgilio, A. Grigorian (eds.), *Surgery*, https://doi.org/10.1007/978-3-032-09799-6_2

Case Study

A 65-year-old obese woman presents to the emergency department with nausea and vomiting for the past day. The frequency of vomiting has increased despite the fact that she has not eaten for the past 12 h. Over the last few months, she has noticed a painful "lump" in her left groin that protrudes upon straining (i.e., coughing, bowel movements) but quickly disappears after lying down. She reports that the lump reappeared a few days ago but she can no longer push it back in. She has had no bowel movement and no flatus per rectum for the past 24 h. Her temperature is 37.9 °C, blood pressure 120/80 mmHg, and heart rate 120/min. She appears ill and uncomfortable with dry mucous membranes. Lung sounds are clear bilaterally. Her abdomen is mildly distended. Bowel sounds are high pitched with tinkles and rushes. Her abdomen is non-tender to palpation. There is a 2 × 2 cm mass in the left groin inferior to the inguinal ligament that is very painful to palpation. The overlying skin is slightly erythematous. The bulge is just medial to her femoral pulse, extending toward her thigh compartment. Laboratory studies are significant for white blood count of 14.7 × $10^3/\mu L$ (normal 4.1–10.9 × $10^3/\mu L$).

Diagnosis

What Is the Differential Diagnosis for a Groin Mass (Use *MINT* Mnemonic)? (Table 2.1)

Table 2.1 Differential diagnosis of groin mass

Type	Examples	Comments
*M*alformation	Undescended testicle, varicocele, hydrocele, hernias	Hernias will protrude with straining and may reduce with pressure
*I*nfectious/*i*nflammatory	Lymphadenopathy (reactive), mononucleosis (EBV), abscess, sarcoidosis, lymphogranuloma venereum	"Shotty," tender lymph nodes are typically reactive from local minor infections, scrapes, or cuts
*N*eoplastic	Lymphoma, lipoma, lymphadenopathy, metastatic cancer (anal, skin, genital)	Large non-tender lymph nodes limited to the inguinal region suggest metastatic cancer (melanoma, anal, or genital cancer)
*T*raumatic	Hematoma, femoral aneurysm, or pseudoaneurysm	Inquire about a history of recent trauma or intervention

EBV Epstein-Barr virus

What Is the Diagnosis for This Patient?

The presence of abdominal distention, a groin mass (below the inguinal ligament), and high-pitched bowel sounds in a patient with progressive nausea with vomiting is highly suggestive of a small intestinal obstruction from a strangulated hernia. The addition of systemic signs of inflammation or infection (fever, tachycardia, leukocytosis) and localized pain and redness of the skin overlying the hernia strongly suggests that the bowel within the hernia sac is ischemic or gangrenous. In this setting, emergent surgical intervention is necessary.

History and Physical

How Can Physical Exam Help Differentiate Between a Hernia and Other Causes of a Groin Mass?

A groin mass that enlarges with straining and reduces when supine is suggestive of a hernia, typically due to increased intra-abdominal pressure from factors such as chronic cough, constipation, or heavy lifting. In contrast, inguinal lymphadenopathy presents as firm or tender nodules that do not change with position or Valsalva. Small, tender, mobile nodes are often reactive, while large, non-tender nodes may indicate malignancy or systemic disease. Careful examination helps distinguish hernias from lymphadenopathy and directs appropriate workup.

What Are the Three Most Common Risk Factors for Developing a Hernia?

Obesity, chronic constipation, and occupations involving heavy lifting (such as delivery drivers) are among the most common risk factors for hernia development. Each contributes to repeated increases in intra-abdominal pressure, which can exploit or worsen areas of fascial weakness in the abdominal wall. Over time, this strain can lead to the formation or progression of hernias.

Pathophysiology

What Is a Hernia?

A hernia is a protrusion of tissue or organ(s) through a defect, most commonly in the abdominal wall. In abdominal hernias, peritoneal contents, such as the omentum and/or bowel, may protrude through a defect or weakness in the muscle or fascia. Hernias have three components: the abdominal wall defect, the hernia sac which protrudes through the defect, and the contents within the sac. The neck of a hernia is the part of the hernia sac adjacent to the abdominal wall defect. If the neck is narrow (as is the case for most femoral hernias), the bowel herniates less frequently. However, once it does enter, it has a higher chance of becoming constricted by the narrow neck and becoming incarcerated.

What Is the Difference Between a Reducible and an Incarcerated Hernia?

A hernia is considered reducible when its contents can be manually pushed back through the defect into the abdominal cavity. In contrast, an incarcerated hernia is irreducible, meaning the herniated contents are trapped outside the abdominal wall and cannot be returned. Incarcerated hernias may or may not be symptomatic and can sometimes remain stable for years, particularly if the hernia defect is large, as seen in some scrotal or incisional hernias.

What Is the Difference Between an Incarcerated and a Strangulated Hernia?

A strangulated hernia is a type of incarcerated hernia in which blood flow to the herniated contents is compromised, most commonly involving small bowel but potentially also omentum, large bowel, or ovary. This occurs more frequently when the hernia neck is narrow, leading to entrapment of bowel and possible closed-loop obstruction. As gas and secretions accumulate, the increasing intraluminal pressure further impairs perfusion. Strangulated hernias require urgent surgical intervention, as delay can result in bowel necrosis, sepsis, and death. Although the overall incidence of strangulation in inguinal hernias is less than 1%, the risk increases in symptomatic patients and those with risk factors such as advanced age, rapid onset, femoral hernia type, and significant comorbidities.

What Is the Pathophysiology of an Indirect Inguinal Hernia?

Indirect inguinal hernias are typically congenital and result from a patent processus vaginalis. During fetal development, the processus vaginalis, an outpouching of the peritoneum, follows the descent of the testicle into the scrotum and normally closes before birth. If it remains open, it can allow peritoneal contents such as bowel to herniate into the scrotum. In men, the hernia sac travels along the spermatic cord through the internal ring, whereas in women, it follows the round ligament toward the pubic tubercle. The neck of an indirect hernia is narrow as it passes through the internal ring, which increases the risk of incarceration or strangulation.

What Is the Pathophysiology of a Direct Inguinal Hernia?

Direct inguinal hernias are acquired and occur due to a weakness in the floor of the inguinal canal, specifically through the transversalis fascia in Hesselbach's triangle. These hernias protrude medial to the inferior epigastric vessels and are more common in older adults after years of chronic straining or increased intra-abdominal pressure. Unlike indirect hernias, direct hernias usually have a broad neck, which reduces the likelihood of strangulation. Because they result from wear and tear, direct hernias are rarely seen in younger individuals.

> **Watch Out**
> Indirect inguinal hernias traverse the deep ring and the superficial ring, while direct inguinal hernias *only* pass through the superficial ring.

What Are the Borders of Hesselbach's Triangle?

The lateral border is formed by the inferior epigastric vessels, the medial border by the rectus sheath, and the base by the posterior wall of the inguinal ligament.

What Are the Other Types of Hernias?

Femoral hernias occur in the femoral canal (◘ Fig. 2.1), inferior to the inguinal ligament traversing the empty space medial to the femoral vein. Although they appear infrequently in patients (10% of all hernias), they are much more common in women (particularly multiparous women) and have the *highest* rate of strangulation (◘ Table 2.2). *Umbilical hernias* (◘ Fig. 2.2) are prevalent in the pediatric population and common with congenital hypothyroidism. In children, most are asymptomatic and close spontaneously with no intervention (surgery if persists beyond age 4). In adults, umbilical hernias are associated with increased intra-abdominal pressure (pregnancy, ascites, weight gain). Surgery is recommended if symptomatic. *Ventral or incisional hernias* appear most commonly in the midline or at the site of a previous surgical incision and can occur weeks, months, or even years after the procedure.

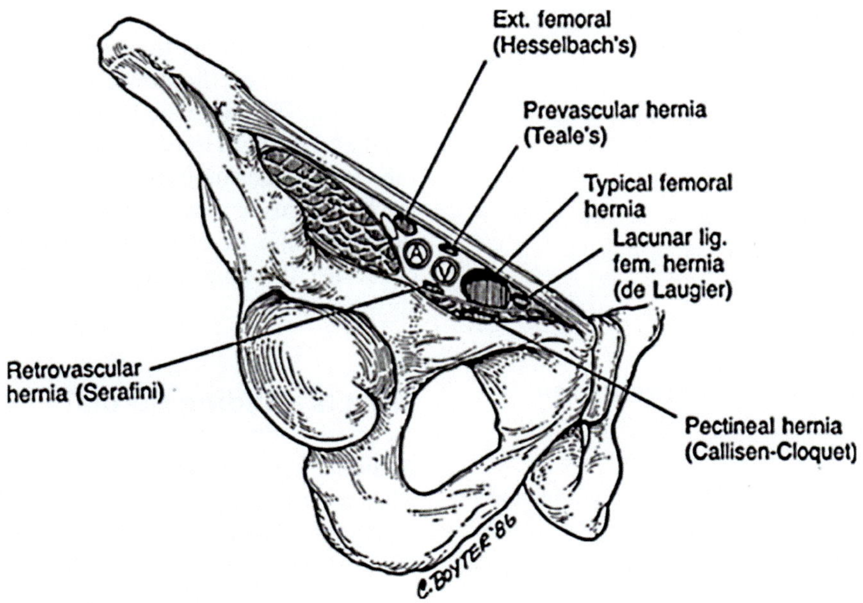

◘ **Fig. 2.1** Femoral hernia. (From: Ates M, et al. First laparoscopic totally extraperitoneal repair of Laugier's hernia: a case report. *Hernia*. 2013;17(1):121–3. Reprinted with permission from Springer Nature)

2

Table 2.2 Types of groin hernias

Type	Anatomy	Pathophysiology	Hernia sac lining	Other
Direct inguinal hernia	Protrudes through the abdominal wall (Hesselbach's triangle), *medial* to the inferior epigastric artery	Acquired weakness in the abdominal floor, chronic straining	Peritoneum	Least likely to incarcerate, more common in men
Indirect inguinal hernia	Protrudes through the internal inguinal ring *lateral* to the inferior epigastric artery	Congenital	Patent processus vaginalis, peritoneum	The most common hernia in men, women, and children
Femoral hernia	Passes through the femoral canal, into empty space medial to femoral vein	Multiple pregnancies increase risk for hernia though narrow femoral neck	Peritoneum	More common in women, most likely to incarcerate/strangulate

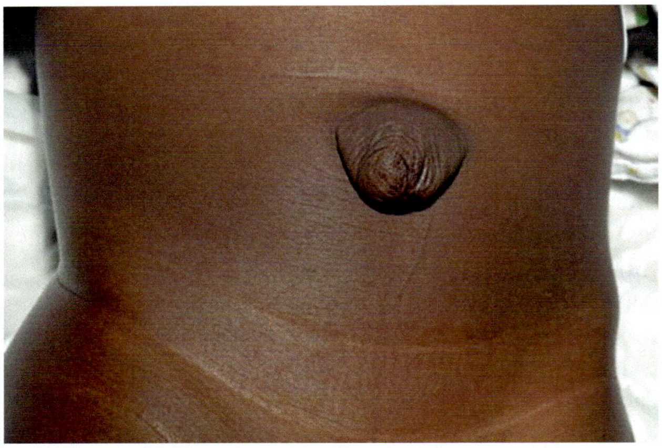

Fig. 2.2 Umbilical hernia. (From Miller R, et al. Umbilical hernia in babies and children. In: LeBlanc K, Kingsnorth A, Sanders D, editors. *Management of abdominal hernias*. Cham: Springer; 2018. Reprinted with permission from Springer Nature)

Watch Out

Recall the mnemonic "NAVEL" for a femoral hernia; from lateral to medial: femoral nerve, artery, vein, empty space (hernia protrudes), and lymphatic.

Why Are Femoral Hernias More Prone to Incarceration?

Bowel entering a femoral hernia passes down the narrow femoral canal. The femoral ring, which serves as the entrance to the femoral canal, is very rigid and unyielding. Thus, the fixed neck of a femoral hernia is prone to pinching off the bowel, putting the patient at risk for incarceration.

What Is the Significance of a Suspected Hernia Being Below as Opposed to Above the Inguinal Ligament?

A hernia below the inguinal ligament indicates that it is a femoral hernia, which passes under (posterior to) the inguinal ligament.

What Is a Richter's Hernia?

It is a type of hernia that occurs when only *part of the circumference* of the bowel wall is trapped within the hernia sac. The herniated segment can become strangulated and result in ischemia/gangrene. Since only part of the wall of the small intestine is herniated, patients do not have signs or symptoms suggestive of bowel obstruction. The absence of obstruction may mislead the clinician into thinking that the bowel is not at risk for strangulation.

What Is a Sliding Hernia?

A sliding hernia is a type of indirect hernia that occurs when a retroperitoneal organ (usually colon or bladder) typically herniates with the sac and essentially makes up the posterior wall of the sac. It usually occurs in males and more often on the left side. A sliding hernia should be suspected when the posterior wall of the hernia sac feels thickened. It is particularly dangerous because if it is not recognized, the bowel can easily be injured or transected when dividing the hernia sac. An indirect hernia sac should always be opened anteriorly as this will prevent making a hole in the bowel or bladder if a sliding hernia is present.

- **Watch Out**

A hernia containing the appendix is termed Amyand hernia, while one containing small bowel with a Meckel diverticulum is termed Littre hernia. Remember, *A*myand for *a*ppendix and *Litt*re for *litt*le kids (Meckel).

Workup

How Do You Diagnose a Hernia in an Adult?

Hernias are considered a clinical diagnosis. A good history (of a reducible mass that protrudes with straining) and a good physical exam are typically all that is needed. For both men and women, the patient is asked to stand. In men, the examiner's index finger is inserted in a cephalad direction through the scrotum, inverting it, and placed at the level of the external ring. The patient is asked to Valsalva or cough. If a hernia is present, a bulge will be palpated.

How Do You Diagnose a Hernia in an Infant?

Both indirect inguinal hernias and umbilical hernias are common in infants. The physical exam may be challenging as the infant cannot cough or strain on command. Thus, the history from the parent of a noticeable bulge with crying is important. Raising the infant's arms will make the infant struggle, increasing intra-abdominal pressure, often permitting visualization of the hernia bulge.

How Do You Distinguish Between a Direct and an Indirect Inguinal Hernia Intraoperatively?

Indirect inguinal hernias originate lateral to the inferior epigastric vessels, while direct inguinal hernias pass medial within Hesselbach's triangle. Indirect inguinal hernias travel through the internal ring along with the spermatic cord.

What Is the Role of Imaging Studies in the Diagnosis of Hernia?

Hernias are usually diagnosed based on history and physical exam, but imaging may be necessary when the exam is inconclusive, particularly in obese patients where palpation is limited. Ultrasound with Valsalva is cost-effective and often diagnostic but less reliable in obese individuals. CT scan or MRI may be needed, especially for occult hernias like Spigelian hernias that are not palpable. CT is more commonly used due to lower cost and wider availability. CT is also essential when evaluating for bowel obstruction, where a hernia may be the underlying cause (◘ Figs. 2.3 and 2.4).

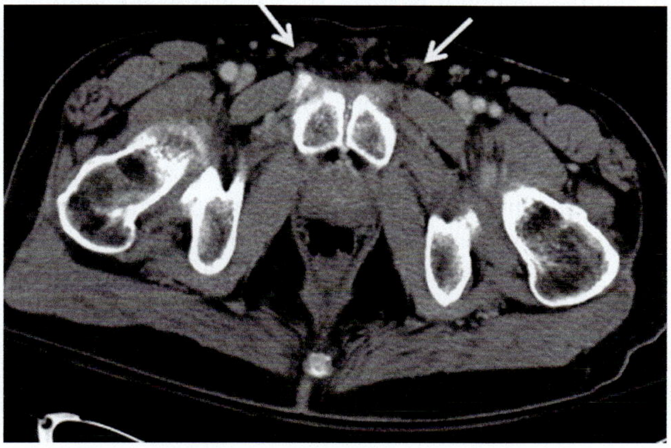

◘ **Fig. 2.3** Normal pelvic CT without hernia. *White arrows: normal inguinal canals*

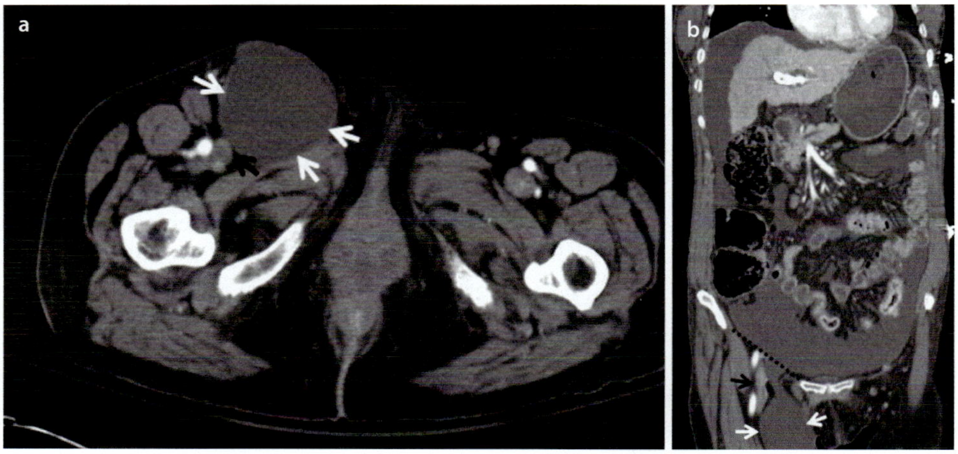

Fig. 2.4 Axial (**a**) and coronal (**b**) CT scans showing a right-sided femoral hernia. Note that it is medial to the femoral vein and inferior to the inguinal ligament. *White arrows: hernia sac. Black arrows: femoral vein. Black dotted line: location of inguinal ligament*

Management

What Is the Principle Component of the Operative Management of an Indirect Inguinal Hernia in an Adult? How About a Direct Inguinal Hernia?

In indirect inguinal hernias, the sac is opened, contents reduced, and a high ligation is performed at the internal ring to eliminate the patent processus vaginalis. In pediatric patients, high ligation alone is sufficient. In adults, however, the prolonged herniation weakens the inguinal floor, so a tension-free mesh repair (Lichtenstein) is added. In direct hernias, there is no patent processus vaginalis, so the sac is simply reduced, and the weakened floor is reinforced with mesh. Tissue-based repairs (Bassini, Shouldice, McVay) are reserved for cases where mesh is contraindicated. Laparoscopic mesh repair may be used for indirect, direct, and femoral hernias.

What Are the Principles of the Management of an Incarcerated Hernia?

Acutely incarcerated hernias are at risk of progressing to strangulation and require prompt attention. Provided there is no evidence of strangulation already (i.e., red skin, fever, leukocytosis), an attempt should be made to reduce the incarcerated hernia. This is typically done by placing the patient in slight Trendelenburg position, providing some sedation and analgesia, applying a cold compress, and then attempting gentle manual compression. The advantage of reduction is that it converts an emergent procedure into a semi-elective one and makes the operation easier as there will be less inflammation. If the hernia is not reducible, urgent surgical intervention is required.

What Is the Recommended Management for a Recurrent Inguinal Hernia?

For recurrent inguinal hernias, the recommended approach is to use the opposite technique from the initial repair to avoid operating through scarred or compromised tissue planes. If the first repair was open, a laparoscopic approach is preferred. Conversely, if the initial repair was laparoscopic, open repair is recommended. This strategy reduces operative difficulty and complication risk. Even in the setting of recurrence, mesh repair remains the standard unless there is a specific contraindication.

What Is the Recommended Management for an Umbilical Hernia in an Infant?

Umbilical hernias are very common in newborns. They rarely incarcerate and most close spontaneously by age 2. Indications for surgery are persistence beyond age 4, hernia defect larger than 2 cm in diameter (unlikely to close spontaneously), strangulation, or progressive enlargement after 1–2 years of age.

What Is a Cord Lipoma, and What Is the Recommended Management?

A cord lipoma is herniation of fat that may be incidentally found upon opening the hernia sac during an inguinal hernia repair. This fat typically originates from an extra-peritoneal source, and is found on the spermatic cord or round ligament. When found, it is recommended to carefully dissect the cord lipoma from the nearby cord structures and remove it, as it may cause recurrence if untreated.

Complications

What Nerves Can Be Injured During Hernia Repair? What Is the Mechanism of Injury? What Are the Consequences? (Table 2.3)

Watch Out

The most common nerve injured during open hernia repair is the *ilioinguinal nerve*. The most common nerve injured during laparoscopic repair is the *lateral femoral cutaneous nerve*.

Table 2.3 Nerve injuries during hernia repair

Injury	Deficit
Genital branch of the genitofemoral nerve	Loss of cremaster reflex and pain or loss of sensation in the anterior scrotum/labia majora (genital branch)
Ilioinguinal nerve	Pain or loss of sensation at the base of the penis, mons pubis, and inner thigh
Iliohypogastric nerve	Pain or loss of sensation in the suprapubic region
Lateral femoral cutaneous nerve (meralgia paresthetica)	Pain or loss of sensation in the lateral side of the thigh, commonly extending to the knee, more common during laparoscopic repair

Areas Where You Can Get in Trouble

Attempting to Reduce a Strangulated Hernia

Strangulated hernias imply that the bowel is compromised. Although the goal is to quickly restore blood flow to avoid bowel necrosis, this is not always possible, and the bowel may already be gangrenous upon presentation. If reduced, the gangrenous bowel will be pushed back into the peritoneal cavity, leading to sepsis and peritonitis. The only safe approach to reducing a strangulated hernia is in the operating room after confirming the bowel is not dead.

Open Hernia Repair in Women

Most surgeons recommend a laparoscopic approach for hernia repair in women, as the open approach appears to be associated with a higher recurrence rate. This may be due to the fact that women may have unrecognized femoral hernias, and the standard open hernia repair doesn't address a femoral hernia. Conversely, the laparoscopic approach allows visualization and repair of femoral hernias.

Reduced Hernia with Persistent Post-reduction Pain and SBO

Some patients may forcefully self-reduce their hernia repeatedly over many years. This can lead to scarring between the hernia sac and its contents, typically small bowel, eventually resulting in a rare condition known as "reduction en masse." In this condition, the hernia sac is reduced into the preperitoneal space, but the bowel remains incarcerated within the fibrosed, constrictive sac. This is particularly dangerous because there is no external evidence of an incarcerated or strangulated hernia on exam. Persistent pain following hernia reduction should prompt a CT scan to rule out this condition, which mandates emergency surgical exploration.

Areas of Controversy

Do You Repair or Observe Asymptomatic Inguinal Hernias?

There is ongoing debate as to whether asymptomatic inguinal (direct and indirect) hernias in male adults should be repaired or whether one should wait for symptoms to develop. A large prospective randomized controlled trial supports the premise of "watchful waiting," in men, provided no symptoms develop. More recent studies confirm the safety of watchful waiting but suggest that the majority of asymptomatic patients eventually do become symptomatic. Thus, most surgeons will offer elective repair of asymptomatic inguinal hernias. However, the "watchful waiting approach" does not apply to women as they are at greater risk of having a femoral hernia. Since femoral hernias are at higher risk of incarceration, routine laparoscopic repair of all groin hernias in women is recommended.

What Is the Recommended Management for an Inguinal Hernia in a Premature Infant?

Premature infants are at higher risk of incarceration, with bowel necrosis and gonadal ischemia. However, premature infants are also at much higher risk of complications from surgery (pulmonary from general anesthesia, injury to the vas deferens due to small size). A recent prospective randomized study demonstrated that delayed repair postdischarge from the ICU was associated with fewer complications than early surgery while still in the ICU.

Do You Repair Asymptomatic Ventral/Incisional Hernias? Is Mesh Needed for Repair?

Incisional hernias typically develop after prior abdominal surgery. De novo ventral hernias will typically arise in the midline linea alba. Most surgeons will offer watchful waiting for asymptomatic incisional/ventral hernias. Incisional hernia repairs, due to the fact that they are re-operative, have more risk, as adhesions may be encountered with potential bowel injury during surgery. Depending upon the size of the hernia defect, mesh is generally used for repair. Mesh decreases the chances of hernia recurrence compared to sutures alone. However, there are several potential mesh-related complications that arise including mesh infection, recurrence, adhesions, pain, and erosion into the bowel with fistula formation. Preferred techniques involve placing the mesh in an extraperitoneal position to avoid contact with the bowel.

Do You Repair Inguinal Hernias Laparoscopically or Open in Men?

Both laparoscopic and open inguinal hernia repair are acceptable options with comparable long-term outcomes. Laparoscopic repair is associated with faster return to work and less pain in bilateral or recurrent hernias, especially after prior open repair. Open repair may cause more postoperative discomfort but has similar efficacy. Laparoscopic repair is most commonly performed via the transabdominal preperitoneal (TAPP) approach, which involves entering the peritoneal cavity. An alternative is the total extraperitoneal (TEP) approach, which avoids peritoneal entry. TEP may reduce the risk of bowel injury, while TAPP allows inspection of both groins and detection of occult hernias. Evidence comparing the two approaches remains limited.

What Is the Role of Robotic-Assisted Surgery in the Repair of Inguinal Hernias?

Robotic-assisted inguinal hernia is one of the fastest-growing robotic operations. While initial studies appear to demonstrate equivalent risk of recurrence for both laparoscopic and robotic approaches, some studies suggest that the robotic approach takes longer and may be more costly.

Inguinal Hernia (◘ Fig. 2.5)

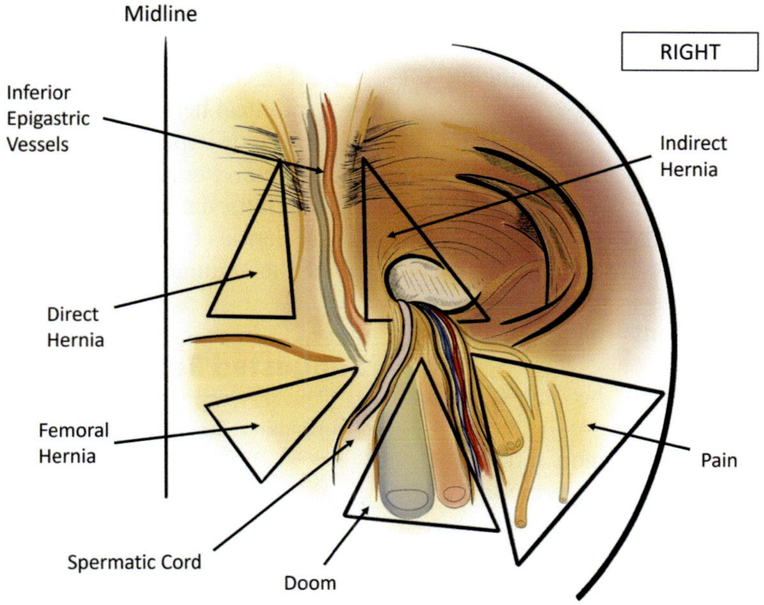

Fig. 2.5 Laparoscopic View of the Myopectineal Orifice. This view shows the landmarks for various hernias. An indirect hernia occurs lateral to the inferior epigastric vessels, a direct hernia occurs medial to the vessels, and a femoral hernia occurs inferior to the inguinal ligament. Also shown are the triangle of doom, which contains the external iliac vessels, and the triangle of pain, which contains sensory nerves

Summary of Essentials

History and Physical

- Must differentiate between inguinal and scrotal masses
- With hernias, look for factors that increase intra-abdominal pressure (straining with urination, cough, constipation, ascites, pregnancy)

Differential Diagnosis

- MINT: *M*alformation, *i*nfectious/*i*nflammatory, *n*eoplastic, *t*raumatic
  - The most common inguinal mass: enlarged lymph nodes
  - Autoimmune disease, malignancy, or as a response to a localized or systemic infection

Pathology/Pathophysiology

- Reducible hernia: contents can be pushed back through the defect into the peritoneal cavity
- Incarcerated hernia: contents are stuck in the hernia sac
- Strangulated hernia: a subset of incarcerated hernia with compromised blood flow to the bowel leading to ischemia
- Ventral or incisional hernia: at the site of a previous surgery
- Femoral hernias:
  - Rare, more common in multiparous women, and more prone to incarceration/strangulation
  - Posterior and inferior to the inguinal ligament and medial to the femoral vein
- Indirect inguinal hernia:
  - The most common hernia in men, women, and children
  - Congenital (patent processus vaginalis), lateral to inferior epigastric vessels, and through the deep and superficial ring
- Direct inguinal hernia:
  - More common in older men
  - Acquired weakness in Hesselbach's triangle, medial to inferior epigastric vessels, and only through the superficial ring

Workup

- Inquire about sources of increased straining/intra-abdominal pressure: urinary retention, constipation, heavy lifting, chronic cough, ascites, and weight gain

2

- A hernia is considered a clinical diagnosis; no imaging usually needed
- In morbidly obese, diagnosis can be difficult; CT scan when diagnosis unclear

Management

- Asymptomatic hernias can be observed:
  - Exception: inguinal hernias in women (performed laparoscopically) and infants (high ligation is all that is needed)
- Most inguinal hernias eventually become symptomatic
- Indirect hernia (most common in men and women)
  - Infants: Open the sac (anteriorly), reduce any contents, and perform a high ligation (at the internal ring) of the hernia sac
  - Adults: Same and add Lichtenstein repair
- Direct hernia (mostly in older men):
  - Do not open sac (no patent processus vaginalis), and reinforce floor with mesh (Lichtenstein) repair or laparoscopic repair
- Femoral hernia (mostly in women):
  - Medial to the femoral vein
  - Inferior to the inguinal ligament
  - Due to high incarceration risk, operative management is always indicated
- Incarcerated hernia:
  - Attempt reduction and then repair semi-electively
- Strangulated hernia:
  - Urgent surgery
- Umbilical hernia in children:
  - Repair if persists > age 4, defect >2 cm, and progressive enlargement after age 2
- In adults, definitive treatment of inguinal and femoral hernias typically includes strengthening the floor of the inguinal canal with mesh

Suggested Reading

Abi-Haidar Y, Sanchez V, Itani KM. Risk factors and outcomes of acute versus elective groin hernia surgery. J Am Coll Surg 2011;213:363.

Eklund A, Rudberg C, Leijonmarck CE, et al. Recurrent inguinal hernia: randomized multicenter trial comparing laparoscopic and Lichtenstein repair. Surg Endosc 2007;21:634.

HIP Trial Investigators. Effect of early vs late inguinal hernia repair on serious adverse event rates in preterm infants: a randomized clinical trial. JAMA 2024;331(12):1035–1044. doi:https://doi.org/10.1001/jama.2024.2302

Schmidt L, Öberg S, Andresen K, Rosenberg J. Recurrence rates after repair of inguinal hernia in women: a systematic review. JAMA Surg 2018;153(12):1135–1142. doi:https://doi.org/10.1001/jamasurg.2018.3102

Society for Surgery of the Alimentary Tract. SSAT patient care guidelines. Surgical repair of groin hernias. J Gastrointest Surg 2007;11:1228.

Wijsmuller AR, van Veen RN, Bosch JL, et al. Nerve management during open hernia repair. Br J Surg 2007;94:17.

Abdominal Pain, Nausea, and Vomiting

Jill Q. Dworsky and David C. Chen

Contents

C. de Virgilio, A. Grigorian (eds.), *Surgery*, https://doi.org/10.1007/978-3-032-09799-6_3

Case Study

A 38-year-old woman presents to the emergency department with colicky abdominal pain, nausea, and vomiting for the past day. She has had at least ten episodes of green, bilious emesis without blood. She has had no passage of stool or flatus per rectum since yesterday morning and has not eaten in 24 h due to the vomiting and abdominal pain. She denies a history of similar symptoms and has no other medical problems. Past surgical history is significant for a cesarean section 2 years ago. Her temperature is 37.8 °C, heart rate is 122/min, blood pressure is 124/78 mmHg, and respiratory rate is 14/min. Her mucous membranes are dry, and her abdomen is distended, with a well-healed low transverse abdominal incision. Auscultation reveals high-pitched tinkling bowel sounds. She has mild tenderness throughout the abdomen, but there is no rebound, guarding, or rigidity. No masses or hernias are identified. Rectal examination reveals normal tone, no gross blood, no masses, and no stool in the rectal vault. Laboratory examination reveals a white blood cell count of $8.2 \times 10^3/\mu L$ (normal $4.1–10.9 \times 10^3/\mu L$), hemoglobin 17 g/dL (12.3–15.7 g/dL), hematocrit 51% (37–46%), sodium 141 mEq/L (135–145 mEq/L), potassium 2.9 mEq/L (3.5–5.0 mEq/L), chloride 93 mEq/L (98–106 mEq/L), bicarbonate 34 mEq/L (24–30 mEq/L), BUN 36 mg/dL (7–22 mg/dL), and creatinine 1.2 mg/dL (0.56–1.0 mg/dL). Urinalysis demonstrates aciduria. Beta-HCG is negative. An abdominal X-ray is provided in ◘ Fig. 3.1.

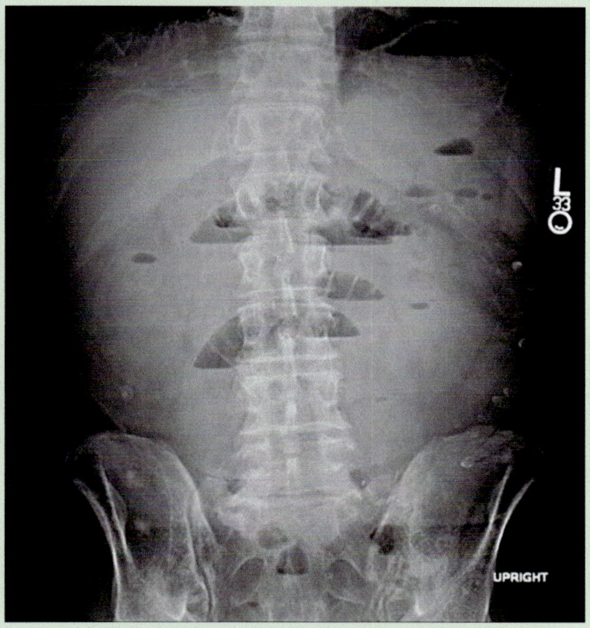

◘ **Fig. 3.1** Upright abdominal X-ray with air-fluid levels

Diagnosis

What Is the Differential Diagnosis? (◘ Table 3.1)

◘ **Table 3.1** Differential diagnosis of clinical presentation

Diagnosis	History and physical
Small bowel obstruction	Colicky abdominal pain, nausea, bilious vomiting, obstipation, abdominal distention, hyperactive bowel sounds (early) or hypoactive bowel sounds (late), prior abdominal surgery
Gastroenteritis	Cramping abdominal pain, fever, nausea, vomiting, diarrhea, hyperactive bowel sounds
Ileus	Diffuse abdominal discomfort but no sharp colicky pain, absent or hypoactive bowel sounds, stool in the rectum, may pass flatus and diarrhea, associated with recent surgery, narcotic use
Large bowel obstruction	Gradually increasing abdominal pain with longer intervals between episodes of pain, abdominal distention, obstipation, less vomiting (feculent), more common in the elderly
Colonic pseudo-obstruction (Ogilvie's syndrome)	Debilitated hospitalized medical or surgical patients; abdominal pain, nausea, vomiting, may continue to pass flatus, massive abdominal distention without mechanical obstruction; idiopathic
Acute mesenteric ischemia	Pain out of proportion to the physical exam; nausea, vomiting, anorexia, atrial fibrillation

What Is the Most Likely Diagnosis?

The history of acute onset of colicky abdominal pain, nausea, vomiting, and obstipation in a young patient with prior abdominal or pelvic surgery is highly suggestive of a mechanical *small bowel obstruction* (SBO) due to adhesions from prior surgery. This patient presents with uncomplicated or *simple* SBO. Treatment is necessary in order to avoid progression and potential complications such as strangulation, bowel necrosis, sepsis, and even death. This patient also presents with severe volume depletion as evidenced by dry mucous membranes, prerenal azotemia (BUN/creatinine ratio >20), hemoconcentration (elevated hemoglobin and hematocrit), and a *hypochloremic, hypokalemic metabolic alkalosis* as a result of volume losses from recurrent emesis and third spacing secondary to SBO.

> **Watch Out**
> A high bicarbonate level in the setting of vomiting is highly suggestive of metabolic alkalosis. Vomiting leads to the loss of gastric acid (hydrochloric acid), which decreases the hydrogen ion concentration in the body.

History and Physical Exam

3

What Is the Significance of SBO in a Patient Without a History of Abdominal Surgery?

In the case of a suspected SBO, it is important to ask the patient if they have a history of prior abdominal or pelvic surgery and to examine the abdomen for scars. The absence of prior abdominal or pelvic surgery lowers the likelihood of adhesions, which is the most common etiology of SBO in the United States. Adhesions typically result from prior surgeries but may also form due to prior abdominal infections, such as pelvic inflammatory disease or intestinal perforation. In 70–80% of cases, adhesive SBOs will resolve with conservative treatment.

> **Watch Out**
> While adhesions from prior abdominal surgery are the most common cause of SBO in the United States, hernias are the most common cause of SBO worldwide. Always make sure to examine the groins, the umbilicus, and the femoral region for masses in patients presenting with signs/symptoms suggestive of SBO.

What Is the Howship-Romberg Sign?

This is suggestive of an obturator hernia and consists of pain in the medial aspect of the thigh with abduction, extension, or internal rotation of the hip. The pain is due to compression of the obturator nerve by an obturator hernia, which is seen mostly in elderly multiparous females and in those with significant weight loss.

What Is the Significance of Severe Abdominal Pain and Localized Tenderness in Association with an SBO?

Severe abdominal pain and/or localized tenderness in association with SBO are suggestive of a complicated or *strangulated* SBO. In contrast to a simple SBO, where blood flow to the bowel remains intact, strangulated obstruction impairs vascular perfusion, leading to intestinal ischemia and ultimately necrosis and perforation. Although strangulation occurs in only a small percentage of SBOs, it increases the morbidity rate significantly. Early surgical intervention is essential to avoid morbidity and poor outcomes. Strangulated obstruction typically presents with continuous (as opposed to intermittent) abdominal pain, signs of a systemic response (fever, tachycardia, leukocytosis), peritoneal signs, acidosis, absence of bowel sounds, and localized abdominal tenderness. Occasionally, a painful mass or blood in the stool may be found. Unfortunately, these signs are neither particularly sensitive nor specific for early strangulation, but they should alert one to the possibility of strangulation and the need for early surgical intervention.

What Other Causes of Abdominal Pain Should Be Considered in a Young Woman?

Gynecologic etiologies should be considered, including pelvic inflammatory disease, often stemming from sexually transmitted infections; ectopic pregnancy, where the embryo implants outside the uterus; ovarian torsion, which may compromise blood supply; and a ruptured ovarian cyst.

Pathophysiology

What Is the Pathophysiology of SBO?

Gas and fluid accumulate proximal to the obstruction site, leading to bowel dilation and subsequent diffuse hypermotility as the bowel attempts to bypass the blockage. This heightened peristaltic activity in early SBO is responsible for the characteristic colicky (comes and goes in waves) pain. The non-localized increased motility can also occur distal to the obstruction, causing some patients to initially present with diarrhea. Distension of the small bowel stretches the visceral peritoneum, triggering autonomic responses that result in progressive nausea and vomiting. A complete mechanical obstruction of the small intestine typically presents with the absence of gas or stool in the rectum.

Are Bowel Sounds Helping in Diagnosing SBO?

Theoretically, bowel sounds are initially increased and should have a high-pitched, tinkling sound and rushes (air or fluid being forced through a narrowed area). As the bowel distends and intramural pressures rise, intestinal motility decreases, and bowel sounds diminish. Clinically, auscultation of the bowel is not particularly useful when differentiating normal versus pathologic bowel sounds.

What Are the Most Common Causes of an SBO? (◘ Table 3.2)

◘ **Table 3.2** Common causes of small bowel obstruction

Cause of SBO	Distinguishing features
Intra-abdominal adhesions	Most common cause *in the USA*; associated with prior abdominal or pelvic surgery
Hernia	Most common cause *worldwide*: bulge in the groin or abdominal wall
Crohn's	Terminal ileitis, strictures, perianal fistula, abscesses, fissures, and aphthous ulcers
Gallstone ileus	Elderly female; pneumobilia (air within the biliary tree) seen on CT, possible large calcification (gallstone) on plain film or CT in the right lower quadrant near the ileocecal valve
Intussusception	Target sign seen on CT; in adults, the lead point is more often a mass or tumor
Neoplasm	History of cancer; mass seen on CT
Volvulus	Whirl sign seen on CT
Radiation-induced stricture	History of pelvic radiation (e.g., prostate, gynecologic cancers)

RLQ right lower quadrant, *CT* computed tomography

What Is a Closed-Loop Obstruction?

A closed-loop obstruction is a severe form of bowel obstruction where a segment of the intestine is obstructed at both ends. In this scenario, neither vomiting nor nasogastric (NG) tube decompression resolves the obstruction due to the trapped gas and fluid within the affected segment. A volvulus is one example of a closed-loop obstruction. Rapid progression to strangulation increases the risk of ischemia and perforation. Closed-loop obstructions are more frequently associated with large bowel obstructions, largely because many individuals have competent ileocecal valves, which can act as natural points of obstruction.

What Is the Risk of Developing SBO After Different Operations?

In general, compared to upper abdominal operations, lower abdominal operations have a higher risk of postoperative adhesions that result in SBO. Adhesions after pelvic operations are responsible for more than 60% of SBOs in the USA. Appendectomy is the most common cause, followed by colorectal and gynecologic procedures. Adhesions may be caused by infection, foreign material (sutures), tissue ischemia, or handling of the bowel. Inflammatory processes such as appendicitis and diverticulitis may create adhesions as surrounding intestinal loops attempt to contain the source of inflammation and infection. Disruption of the visceral and parietal peritoneum with pelvic operations may lead to adhesions, especially in the dependent positions where the loops of the small intestine rest. Another possible explanation for the higher rate of SBOs after pelvic operations compared to upper abdominal operations is that the bowel is more mobile in the pelvis than in the upper abdomen and thus more likely to twist.

Does Laparoscopic Surgery Have a Lower Risk for SBO Compared to Open Surgery?

Yes. Open surgery may carry up to a fourfold increased risk in SBO.

What Are the Mechanisms of Fluid Loss in SBO?

Volume depletion is commonly observed in SBO, with fluid loss mechanisms varying by the obstruction's location and severity. In proximal obstructions, volume depletion primarily results from frequent vomiting and reduced oral intake due to anorexia, leading to significant electrolyte disturbances. Complete obstructions cause a transudative fluid shift into the peritoneal cavity. The intestine proximal to the obstruction site becomes distended from accumulated gastrointestinal secretions and gas, fostering bacterial overgrowth and further dilation from bacterial fermentation. This process increases hydrostatic pressure within the intestinal lumen, prompting fluid, electrolytes, and proteins to filter from the intravascular space into the bowel wall and lumen, a phenomenon known as *third spacing*. This third spacing contributes to volume depletion in both proximal and distal SBOs.

What Is the Mechanism of Metabolic Alkalosis and Aciduria in Patients with Ongoing Emesis?

The above patient presents with a hypochloremic, hypokalemic metabolic alkalosis as a result of volume losses from recurrent emesis. The volume loss activates the renin-angiotensin-aldosterone system to increase sodium and water absorption from the distal convoluted tubules in the kidneys. In order to maintain ion balance, potassium is excreted in exchange for sodium. As the patient becomes progressively more hypokalemic (which can lead to arrhythmias), the kidney will eventually excrete hydrogen ions instead of potassium ions, which perpetuates the systemic metabolic alkalosis and results in a *paradoxical aciduria*. This occurs in all processes that involve persistent emesis resulting in volume loss (e.g., pyloric stenosis).

Workup

What Laboratory Tests Should Be Obtained in the Initial Workup for SBO?

When working up SBO, it is important to obtain a complete blood count, chemistry panel, and serum lactate. While laboratory values do not play a significant role in the diagnosis of SBO, they are essential in assessing the degree of volume depletion and may raise the suspicion of bowel ischemia. Volume-depleted patients may exhibit hemoconcentration, as evidenced by elevated hemoglobin and hematocrit (as in this patient). A ratio of BUN/creatinine >20 is suggestive of prerenal azotemia, which can be caused by decreased blood flow to the kidneys (i.e., dehydration). A chemistry panel can reveal a hypochloremic, hypokalemic metabolic alkalosis, which often results from repeated bouts of emesis. Leukocytosis raises the possibility of an infectious etiology or bowel compromise.

What Imaging Is Recommended for an SBO?

When SBO is suspected, initial imaging should include an abdominal series. However, in clinical practice, a CT scan with IV contrast is usually obtained as well, even if the abdominal series confirms an SBO. The CT (oral contrast is usually not needed) provides additional information, such as identifying the location of the SBO, called a transition point (proximally dilated bowel and distally decompressed bowel), can assess for signs of bowel compromise, and potentially identify the cause of the SBO, such as intussusception, volvulus, and hernia.

What Findings on CT Scan Suggest That the Bowel Is Compromised (Ischemic/Gangrenous)?

Bowel wall thickening, pneumatosis intestinalis (gas within the bowel wall), portal venous gas, free intraperitoneal fluid, lack of bowel wall enhancement, and mesenteric stranding.

> **Watch Out**
> Remember the three films that comprise an abdominal series: upright chest x-ray (to look for free air under the diaphragm), upright abdominal x-ray (to look for air fluid levels), and supine abdominal X-ray (to look for dilated loops of bowel and absence of gas/stool in rectum). If the patient is critically ill and unable to sit upright, a lateral decubitus film is substituted.

How Do You Differentiate Large and Small Bowel on Radiographs?

The small bowel has lines (plicae circulares) going all the way around the circumference of the bowel (appearing like white lines going all the way across the bowel). The large bowel has lines (haustra) traversing only *halfway* through the bowel (appearing like lines partially indenting the bowel).

What Are the Different Radiologic Findings Associated with SBO? (◘ Table 3.3)

Table 3.3 Radiologic findings associated with small bowel obstruction

Radiologic finding	Radiologic appearance	Associated pathology in the context of SBO
SBO (abdominal series)	Dilated loops of small intestine (plicae circulares), air-fluid levels, bowel stacking	Classic radiographic findings of SBO
Target sign (CT)	Three concentric circles, with hyperdense inner and outer rings and a hypodense middle ring	Intussusception
Whirl or swirl sign (CT)	Twist of bowel wrapped around a single constrictive focus of mesentery or adhesion	Small bowel volvulus
Pneumatosis (CT)	Presence of gas within the wall of the intestine	Strangulated obstruction leading to intestinal ischemia and necrosis
Portal venous gas (CT)	Air in the periphery of the liver due to centrifugal portal flow	Late presentation of pneumatosis with air passing via portal venous circulation

How Is a Complete SBO Different from a Partial SBO?

The key difference between a complete SBO and a partial SBO lies in the extent of the blockage. In a complete SBO, there is a total blockage, preventing any passage of gas or fluids distal to the obstruction site. This condition typically requires surgical intervention if conservative management fails, as no material can get past. In contrast, a partial SBO allows some movement of gas and fluids past the obstruction, making it more amenable to conservative treatments such as fluid resuscitation and nasogastric decompression. Both types are initially managed conservatively in hemodynamically stable patients without signs of peritonitis, but the likelihood of requiring surgery is higher in complete SBOs.

How Do You Distinguish SBO from Large Bowel Obstruction (LBO)?

The clinical presentation of LBO is dependent upon the location and etiology of obstruction. If the proximal colon is involved, it is more likely to be mistaken for SBO (assuming the ileocecal valve is incompetent), as the small intestine will also become dilated, causing a similar clinical presentation. If a tumor is the cause of LBO, the course may be more insidious in onset, and a longer history of symptoms makes it less likely to be confused with SBO. In general, LBO causes gradually increasing abdominal pain, progressive distention, constipation, and occasionally feculent vomiting. Common causes of LBO include colon cancer, diverticular disease, and volvulus. On imaging, an "apple-core" lesion is characteristic of colon cancer, and a "coffee-bean" or "omega sign" tapering down toward the left lower quadrant is characteristic of sigmoid volvulus.

Watch Out

An obstructing sigmoid colon cancer can lead to a closed loop obstruction if the ileocecal valve is functional, as gas cannot exit into the small bowel or from rectum. A functional ileocecal valve is present in up to 80% of the population.

How Do You Distinguish Between Postoperative Ileus and Early SBO After Abdominal Surgery?

In the early postoperative period, it is important to distinguish between an obstruction, which occurs in less than 1% of those undergoing laparotomy, and an ileus, which is considered as the most common postoperative complication. Postoperative ileus results from reduced gastrointestinal motility due to stress-induced sympathetic responses, inflammatory mediators, and the effects of anesthetics and narcotics. Typically, normal motility resumes in the small intestine within 24 h post-surgery, 48 h for the stomach, and 3–5 days for the colon. Both conditions may present similarly with abdominal pain, nausea, vomiting, and distention. However, ileus is generally characterized by absent or hypoactive bowel sounds and a dull, constant pain. Radiographically, ileus is indicated by dilated bowel loops without air-fluid levels on plain films. If plain films are inconclusive, a CT scan is recommended to identify a transition point, a hallmark of SBO, differentiating it from ileus.

Watch Out

Gallstone ileus is a misnomer as this is a type of *mechanical* SBO where a large gallstone travels through a cholecystoduodenal (gallbladder to duodenum) fistula and becomes impacted in the terminal ileum near the ileocecal valve.

Management

What Are the Initial Steps in the Management of an SBO?

Patients with SBO are often significantly volume depleted. Aggressive fluid resuscitation (with an isotonic intravenous fluid such as normal saline) and electrolyte repletion are important initial steps in the management. Additionally, early placement of an NG tube to evacuate air and fluid is important because gastric decompression will decrease nausea, vomiting, distention, and the risk of aspiration. It may also resolve the SBO in combination with bowel rest.

What Is the Next Step?

After initial NG tube decompression, hemodynamically stable patients are admitted and observed. Most patients will then undergo an oral contrast challenge. This involves temporarily stopping the NG tube suction and administering a water-soluble contrast solution (such as Gastrograffin) either orally or via an NG tube, followed by a series of X-rays to track the contrast's progress.

Watch Out

A contrast challenge in a patient with SBO can be both diagnostic and therapeutic. Diagnostically, if contrast does not appear in the colon within 8 h of administration, it indicates that the patient is likely to fail conservative management, prompting consideration for early surgical intervention. Therapeutically, the contrast acts as an osmotic agent within the bowel lumen, potentially helping to alleviate the obstruction by drawing fluid into the bowel, which may assist in resolving the blockage.

Watch Out

Gastrografin (though via an enema) is also useful in resolving meconium obstruction in neonates.

Watch Out

Barium contrast is generally not be used in the setting of SBO. Barium can solidify in the small bowel, worsening the SBO or in the colon leading to constipation. If a perforation is present, leakage can lead to barium peritonitis.

When Should You Operate on a Patient with SBO?

While 70–80% of adhesive SBO cases resolve with conservative management, surgery becomes necessary if there is clear evidence of bowel compromise or ischemia, indicated by a rising lactate level, leukocytosis, significantly worsening abdominal pain, or the presence of shock. Although initial studies suggested an 8-h threshold for the failure of conservative management using contrast challenges, many surgeons opt to wait for 24 h before considering surgery. If there is no response to conservative measures after several days, evidenced by persistently high NG tube output or absence of contrast in the colon, surgical intervention may be warranted, even in the absence of overt signs or symptoms of bowel compromise.

What Should You Do If You Suspect Nonviable Bowel During Laparotomy for SBO?

Any obviously nonviable or necrotic bowel should be resected. For segments with questionable viability, they can be assessed using several methods such as checking the color (should be pink), presence of peristalsis, and arterial pulsations. A hand-held Doppler can also be used to detect arterial signals, and intravenous fluorescein dye may help identify viable tissue with commercial intraoperative cameras. Ischemic/necrotic bowel lacks peristalsis, has an absence of arterial Doppler signals, and fails to take up fluorescein dye. If a short segment appears to be of questionable viability, it should be resected. For larger segments, where resection risks short gut syndrome, the preferred approach is to leave the bowel intact, close the abdomen temporarily with a negative pressure wound covering, and perform a planned second-look operation the following day after further resuscitation to reassess viability.

Areas Where You Can Get in Trouble

Nausea and Vomiting Months to Years After Gastric Bypass

In patients who have undergone gastric bypass, internal hernias, particularly through defects in the mesentery, are the most common cause of SBO. Specifically, a Petersen's space hernia occurs when the bowel herniates through a mesenteric defect created to pass the Roux limb of small bowel connected to the stomach. While laparoscopic gastric bypass increases the risk for such herniation compared to open bypass, the presence of adhesions may actually reduce the risk by limiting bowel mobility and preventing herniation into Petersen's space. Stable patients suspected of having an internal hernia should be evaluated with a CT scan and undergo urgent surgical intervention. If there is evidence of peritonitis, immediate surgery is warranted.

Abdominal Complaints in Opioid Drug Users

Patients with substance use disorders that use opioids (e.g., IV heroin, oral narcotics, etc.) often have abdominal complaints ranging from bloating, distention, constipation, and diarrhea to generalized vague abdominal pain or discomfort. Chronic opioid users develop opioid-induced constipation, which is the most common adverse effect associated with prolonged use of opioids. Patients with chronic constipation should be evaluated for fecal impaction. In contrast, opioid users going through withdrawal may have increased GI motility and present with diarrhea. This may make it difficult to discern if serious abdominal pathology (e.g., small bowel obstruction, mesenteric ischemia) is present in a patient who uses opioids or is in withdrawal. Physical exam findings that will help differentiate opioid withdrawal from an acute abdominal process include the presence of *mydriasis, rhinorrhea, and diaphoresis* in those presenting with opioid withdrawal.

Areas of Controversy

Operating in Adults with Intussusception or SBO with No History of Abdominal Surgery

Historically, adult patients presenting with intussusception or those with SBO with no history of abdominal surgery underwent early surgical intervention. This practice stemmed from concerns that intussusception in adults (unlike infants) was almost always due to a pathologic "lead point" such as a tumor or Meckel's diverticulum, which requires resection. Similarly, SBO in the absence of prior abdominal surgery was thought to almost always be due to a pathologic process that would only resolve with surgery. However, recent reports indicate that some cases of intussusception and SBO without prior surgery can be transient and devoid of any pathology. Modern high-resolution CT scans are highly effective in identifying significant causes of obstruction, such as neoplasms. So in the setting of a CT that demonstrates no pathology, the likelihood of a serious underlying cause is very low, permitting non-operative management in cases where only minor or no clinical symptoms are present, and laboratory tests do not indicate severe abnormalities.

Clamp Trials with NG Tubes in SBO Patients

Removal of the NG tube is generally considered when the patient has symptomatic improvement (decreased bloating and nausea), signs of returning bowel function (flatus, stool), and a low volume of output from the NG tube. A low volume of output may be around 600–800 mL over a 24-h period but can vary based on the patient's size and clinician's preference. Prior to removing the NG tube, some clinicians may choose to do a "clamp trial." In this scenario, the NG tube remains in place but is not providing suction. If the patient develops nausea or vomiting, the tube can simply be unclamped to resume suction. At the end of the clamp trial, the NG tube is reconnected to suction; if a low volume of fluid returns and the patient remains asymptomatic, the NG tube can be removed. However, there is concern that an NG tube left in place and not connected to suction may increase the risk of aspiration, as it opens the lower esophageal sphincter. As such, other clinicians may choose to forgo a clamp trial and completely remove the NG tube when the patient is showing signs of resolution.

Closed-Loop Obstruction (◘ Fig. 3.2)

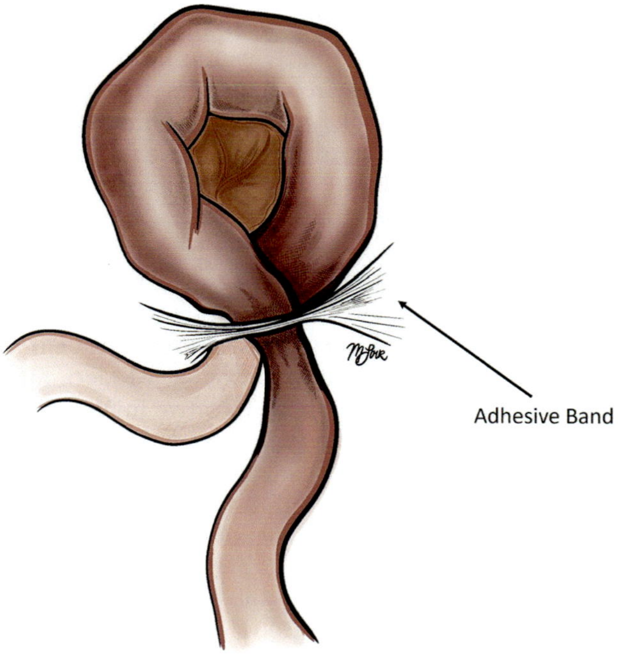

◘ **Fig. 3.2** Small Bowel Obstruction. A closed-loop obstruction of the small bowel is shown, caused by an adhesive band. This condition requires urgent surgery due to a high risk of strangulation and bowel ischemia

Summary of Essentials

History and Physical Exam

- Acute onset of colicky abdominal pain, nausea, vomiting, and obstipation
- History of previous pelvic or abdominal operations; examine for surgical scars
- Examine for hernias

Pathophysiology

- The most common cause of SBO in the USA is intra-abdominal adhesions from prior surgery
- Gas and fluid accumulate proximal to the site of obstruction
- Ongoing emesis and third spacing lead to volume depletion, prerenal azotemia, and hypochloremic, hypokalemic metabolic alkalosis

Diagnosis

- Classic radiographic findings of SBO: dilated loops of small intestine, air-fluid levels, bowel stacking
- CT can distinguish between postoperative ileus and SBO by demonstrating a transition point
- Contrast challenge can identify SBO patients likely to fail conservative management

Management

- Initial treatment includes NPO status, fluid resuscitation, electrolyte repletion, and placement of an NG tube
- 70–80% of patients with SBO will not need surgery
- Immediately proceed to operating room if any signs or symptoms of peritonitis or bowel ischemia
- Nonviable bowel must be resected
- Questionable bowel should be left alone with a planned second-look operation

Suggested Reading

Cheadle WG, Garr EE, Richardson JD. The importance of early diagnosis of small bowel obstruction. Am Surg 1988;54:565.

Duron JJ, Hay JM, Msika S, Gaschard D, Domergue J, et al. Prevalence and mechanisms of small intestinal obstruction following laparoscopic abdominal surgery: a retrospective multicenter study. Arch Surg 2000;135(2):208–12.

Felder S, Margel D, Murrell Z, Fleshner P. Usefulness of bowel sound auscultation: a prospective evaluation. J Surg Educ 2014;71(5):768–73.

Kozol R. Mechanical bowel obstruction: a tale of 2 eras. Arch Surg 2012;147:180.

Markogiannakis H, Messaris E, Dardamanis D, et al. Acute mechanical bowel obstruction: clinical presentation, etiology, management and outcome. World J Gastroenterol 2007;13:432.

Miller G, Boman J, Shrier I, Gordon PH. Natural history of patients with adhesive small bowel obstruction. Br J Surg 2000;87:1240.

Taylor MR, Lalani N. Adult small bowel obstruction. Acad Emerg Med 2013;20:528.

Right Leg Pain, Swelling, and Erythema for Two Days

Amulya Vadlakonda, David C. Chen, Areg Grigorian, and Christian de Virgilio

Contents

C. de Virgilio, A. Grigorian (eds.), *Surgery*, https://doi.org/10.1007/978-3-032-09799-6_4

Case Study

A 40-year-old male with diabetes mellitus and hepatitis C-related cirrhosis presents to the emergency department with a two-day history of right leg pain, redness, and swelling. He states that he thinks he may have been bitten in the leg by a bug while sleeping. On physical examination, his temperature is 37.8 °C, heart rate is 110/min, blood pressure is 90/60 mmHg, and respiratory rate is 18/min. His right leg is markedly swollen compared to the left. The skin overlying the calf region is erythematous, with one 3 cm bulla and an area of violaceous skin. There is no palpable crepitus. A plain X-ray of the leg demonstrates gas bubbles within the soft tissue in the calf. The foot itself is pink and warm, with normal pulses. Laboratory values are significant for a BUN of 40 mg/dL (normal 7–20 mg/dL), serum glucose of 200 mg/dL (70–100 mg/dL), creatinine of 1.6 mg/dL (0.8–1.4 mg/dL), white blood cell (WBC) count of 24×10^3/μL ($4.1–10.9 \times 10^3$/μL), hemoglobin of 9.5 g/dL (13.8–17.2 g/dL), and a serum sodium of 128 mEq/L (136–144 mEq/L).

Diagnosis

What Is the Differential Diagnosis? (▫ Table 4.1)

▫ **Table 4.1** Differential diagnosis of clinical presentation

Condition	Comments
NSTI	Acute infection of the deep fascia, often with crepitus, bullae, and necrosis of the subcutaneous tissue, mixed flora
Cellulitis	Infection of the deep dermis and subcutaneous fat, presenting with redness and erythema without the tissue destruction characteristics of NSTI
Cutaneous anthrax	Painless or pruritic eschar surrounded by edema
Hypersensitivity reaction	No fever or leukocytosis; history of exposure to plants or animals
DVT	Usually involves the leg, look for a history of hypercoagulability, immobility, and/or inflammatory state (e.g., postsurgical, malignancy)
Loxoscelism (brown recluse spider bite)	Necrotic ulcer often preceded by a small red papule, burning pain, and blister, look for a history of exposure to warm, dry places (e.g., cellars, attics)
Sweet's syndrome (acute febrile neutrophilic dermatosis)	Acute eruption of tender erythematous plaques with vesicles, fever, and neutrophilia; classically caused by treatment with G-CSF; may involve almost any other organ system, particularly the respiratory and GI tracts; also associated with pregnancy and malignancy
Pyoderma gangrenosum	Neutrophilic infiltration of the skin; exquisitely painful lesions; may involve almost any other organ system, associated with inflammatory bowel disease
Erythema multiforme	Erythematous or purpuric plaques and bullae with central clearing; involves the extremities, palms, and soles; associated with herpes simplex virus, mycoplasma, and malignancy
Stasis dermatitis	Dermal fibrosis and brawny edema secondary to venous incompetence; may become acutely inflamed with crusting and exudate; look for evidence or history of venous incompetence and DVT

G-CSF granulocyte colony-stimulating factor, *DVT* deep vein thrombosis, *GI* gastrointestinal, *NSTI* necrotizing soft tissue infection

4

What Is the Most Likely Diagnosis?

In a diabetic patient presenting with a painful, erythematous, swollen leg with bullae and violaceous skin, along with radiographic evidence of gas bubbles within the soft tissues of the leg, the most likely diagnosis is necrotizing soft tissue infection (NSTI). Additional key features supporting this critical diagnosis include high fever, leukocytosis, hypotension, and low serum sodium.

History and Physical

What Is the Implication of Crepitus?

Crepitus indicates the presence of gas within soft tissues, most often due to infection with gas-forming organisms such as *Clostridium* species.

What Are the Risk Factors for NSTI?

Factors that depress immunity and/or decrease tissue perfusion increase the risk for NSTI, including diabetes mellitus, malnutrition, intravenous (IV) drug abuse, obesity, chronic alcohol abuse, chronic lymphocytic leukemia, chronic steroid use, renal failure, peripheral arterial disease, and cirrhosis.

> **Watch Out**
> NSTI can also develop in postsurgical wounds, as well as following traumatic extremity injuries, particularly in association with gross wound contamination.

What Is the Implication of Bullae? Violaceous Skin?

The presence of bullae implies partial tissue death within the layers of the skin that allows for the collection of fluid between tissue layers. Violaceous skin (a violet or purple discoloration) implies ischemia.

What Are the "Hard Signs" of NSTI? What Percent of Patients with NSTI Have Such Hard Signs?

Hard signs are signs that, if present, are diagnostic of the disease. Crepitus, skin necrosis, bullae, or gas on X-ray are considered "hard signs" of NSTI when seen in association with a soft tissue infection. However, it has been shown that less than half of patients with NSTI will have hard signs.

> **Watch Out**
> NSTI may present with pain *out of proportion* to physical exam or cutaneous anesthesia (indicating necrosis of nerves/muscles).

Why Is It Important to Distinguish Between Cellulitis and NSTI? How do Laboratory Values Help?

Cellulitis and NSTI are surprisingly difficult to distinguish based on physical exam. Treatment of NSTI requires *emergent* surgical debridement of all infected tissue, whereas cellulitis simply requires antibiotics. As such, a high level of suspicion is required for a prompt diagnosis. A low serum Na or a very high WBC count is strongly suggestive of NSTI. The Laboratory Risk Indicator for Necrotizing Fasciitis (LRINEC) score has been developed in order to help distinguish NSTI from other soft tissue infections (▫ Table 4.2). A score ≥6 is concerning, and ≥8 is strongly predictive of NSTI.

▫ **Table 4.2** LRINEC score

Feature	Score
C-reactive protein >150 mg/L	4
WBC > 15 × 10^3/uL	1 (2 points if >25 × 10^3/uL)
Hemoglobin <13.5 g/dL	1 (2 points if <11 g/dL)
Na < 135 mEq/L	2
Creatinine >1.6 mg/dL	2
Glucose >180 mg/dL	1

Pathophysiology

What Is the Spectrum of NSTI?

NSTI can involve the skin and subcutaneous tissue (necrotizing cellulitis), the fascia (necrotizing fasciitis), and/or the muscle (necrotizing myositis). Another term used for necrotizing myositis is gas gangrene.

What Are the Typical Organisms Seen in NSTI?

NSTI may be monomicrobial or polymicrobial, and a classification scheme based on the infectious agent has been developed. Type-I NSTI is a *polymicrobial* infection and accounts for 70–80% of all NSTI cases. Of those caused by a single organism, the most common monomicrobial cause is *Staphylococcus aureus*, followed by *Klebsiella. Clostridium perfringens* is a rare cause of NSTI (and the classic organism associated with gas gangrene). Type II NSTI is an infection with group A *Streptococcus* with or without *Staphylococcus*. *Vibrio vulnificus* is a rare but aggressive cause of NSTI, particularly in patients with liver disease or iron overload who are exposed to seawater or raw seafood. It is associated with rapidly progressive soft tissue destruction and high mortality.

What Is the Implication of Culturing Clostridium Septicum from the Wound?

Clostridium septicum infection can lead to gas gangrene and is associated with occult malignancies, most often colon cancer and hematologic malignancies.

What Is the Term for NSTI That Involves the Scrotum and/or Perineum?

Fournier's gangrene. This is typically caused by infection with polymicrobial urogenital or colonic bacteria.

Management

What Are the Initial Steps in the Management of NSTI?

The initial treatment of a patient with suspected NSTI consists of intravenous fluids, broad-spectrum IV antibiotics, and aggressive emergent surgical debridement, which is the gold standard for both diagnosis and treatment for NSTI. When NSTI is suspected, clindamycin should be given empirically in addition to broad-spectrum IV antibiotics. Clindamycin inhibits bacterial protein synthesis and reduces toxin production in organisms such as Clostridium perfringens and Streptococcus pyogenes. Early use helps reduce tissue damage and systemic toxicity in toxin-mediated infections.

Watch Out

In patients with severe penicillin allergy, clindamycin is still essential due to its anti-toxin effects. Broad-spectrum coverage can be achieved with a combination of vancomycin and a carbapenem or aztreonam plus metronidazole.

How Do You Determine How Much Tissue to Debride?

All soft tissues, including the skin, subcutaneous fat, fascia, and muscle, that show any evidence of infection must be extensively debrided to the point of *seeing healthy bleeding tissue*. It is not acceptable to leave behind a tissue that is of borderline viability, as the infection will often continue to extend postoperatively. Current recommendations are that a second-look operation should be scheduled 24 h after the initial debridement to ensure that the infection has not reemerged. Patients may require multiple reoperations after the initial debridement.

Watch Out

Wet-to-dry dressings are used for infected or necrotic wounds. Once healthy granulation tissue appears, dressings should be switched to nonadherent, moisture-retaining types to promote re-epithelialization.

What If Extensive Muscle Necrosis Is Found?

If extensive muscle necrosis is discovered during surgery, amputation may be necessary.

What Are the Intraoperative Findings That Confirm NSTI?

Operative findings in NSTI include murky fluid (i.e., "dishwater" fluid), gray discoloration of the fascia , and lack of bleeding from the fascia. Additionally, the fascia may separate from the muscle easily, without the normal resistance on digital exploration.

What Do You Do If Your Suspicion for NSTI Is High But You Are Not Certain of the Diagnosis?

If the diagnosis of NSTI is uncertain, yet the suspicion is high, surgical exploration is undertaken, as this is the gold standard of both diagnosis and treatment. The incision must be taken down to the fascia and muscle so both can be inspected.

Is Imaging Beneficial in the Diagnosis of NSTI?

When the diagnosis is in question, plain X-rays are useful if they demonstrate gas in the soft tissue. However, most cases of NSTI do not demonstrate gas on plain films. A CT scan may also be beneficial. The primary finding to look for on CT imaging in patients with NSTI is *gas within deep tissues*.

What Is the Anticipated Mortality Risk Associated with NSTI?

The overall mortality rate for NSTI is very high, averaging 25%. The mortality has been largely unchanged for the past century. However, it is consistently lower in pediatric patients compared to adults.

Area Where You Can Get in Trouble

Postsurgical Wound with Dishwater Purulent Fluid

This is a rare but well-known complication after surgery, and the description of dishwater pus is classic for *post-operative clostridial wound infection*. The two most common organisms causing early postoperative necrotizing soft tissue infection are *Clostridium perfringens* and *Streptococcus pyogenes*. Like all cases of NSTI, the most important steps in management are IV fluids, broad-spectrum antibiotics, and emergent surgical debridement.

Assuming First Debridement Is Adequate

Even after adequate first debridement, NSTI can rapidly progress. As such, most surgeons recommend a mandatory second-look operative re-exploration within 24 h after initial surgery.

Area of Controversy

What Is the Role of Hyperbaric Oxygen?

The use of hyperbaric oxygen remains controversial but is a potential adjuvant therapy to aggressive surgical debridement and ICU care in the treatment of NSTI. A recent small study showed that hyperbaric oxygen reduced mortality in NSTI from 34% to 12%. However, hyperbaric oxygen should not replace or delay aggressive surgical debridement.

Summary of Essentials

History and Physical Examination

- Most present without a clear history of traumatic injury, even a small cut
- Acute onset of pain, swelling, and erythema
- Hard signs occur in less than half of patients
  - Air on plain X-ray

  - Crepitus
  - Bullae
  - Skin necrosis

Diagnosis

- NSTI is a clinical diagnosis
- Low serum sodium and very high WBC
- The LRINEC score can help distinguish NSTI from less life-threatening soft tissue infections

Management

- Immediate treatment includes IV fluids, broad-spectrum antibiotics, and emergent, aggressive surgical debridement
- Multiple reoperations for further debridement are often necessary
- Delay in recognition and treatment leads to an increase in mortality

Acknowledgements The editors would like to acknowledge and thank the following authors for their contributions to the previous edition of the chapter: Monica Lee, Paul N. Frank.

Suggested Reading

Chan T, Yaghoubian A, Rosing D, et al. Low sensitivity of physical examination findings in necrotizing soft tissue infection is improved with laboratory values: a prospective study. Am J Surg 2008;196(6):926–30.

Escobar SJ, Slade JB, Hunt TK, Cianci P. Adjuvant hyperbaric oxygen therapy (HBO2) for treatment of necrotizing fasciitis reduces mortality and amputation rate. Undersea Hyperb Med 2005;32(6):437–43.

McDermott J, Kao LS, Keeley JA, Grigorian A, Neville A, de Virgilio C. Necrotizing soft tissue infections: a review. JAMA Surg 2024;159(11):1308-1315. doi: https://doi.org/10.1001/jamasurg.2024.3365.

Wall DB, de Virgilio C, Black S, Klein SR. Objective criteria may assist in distinguishing necrotizing fasciitis from nonnecrotizing soft tissue infection. Am J Surg 2000;179(1):17–20.

Wong CH, Khin LW, Heng KS, Tan KC, Low CO. The LRINEC (Laboratory Risk Indicator for Necrotizing Fasciitis) score: a tool for distinguishing necrotizing fasciitis from other soft tissue infections. Crit Care Med 2004;32(7):1535–41.

Wysoki MG, Santora TA, Shah RM, Friedman AC. Necrotizing fasciitis: CT characteristics. Radiology 1997;203(3):859–63.

Acute Care Surgery

Question Set: Acute Care Surgery

Questions

1. A 64-year-old man is recovering in the intensive care unit (ICU) after colectomy for ischemic colitis. He has been intubated for 5 days and has a right internal jugular central line that was placed 10 days ago. He now has a fever of 38.7 °C, tachycardia, and leukocytosis. Blood cultures from both the central line and periphery grow Candida albicans. What is the most appropriate next step in management?
   (A) Start oral fluconazole and monitor for improvement
   (B) Remove the central venous catheter and start intravenous (IV) antifungals
   (C) Order serum beta-D-glucan and repeat cultures in 24 h
   (D) Continue observation as *Candida* often reflects colonization
   (E) Replace the central line over a guidewire and begin antibiotics

2. One week after open repair of a recurrent large right scrotal hernia, a 45-year-old male returns complaining of severe pain in his right testicle. The pain has gradually worsened since surgery. On physical exam, the testicle appears to be slightly swollen and very tender to palpation. Doppler study demonstrates no flow within the right testicle with normal flow in the left. Which of the following is true about this condition?
   (A) It is most commonly due to thrombosis of the pampiniform plexus
   (B) Urgent exploration of the right testicle is recommended
   (C) It is most likely due to transection of the testicular artery
   (D) It most likely represents testicular torsion
   (E) The testicle will likely remain permanently enlarged

3. A 65-year-old obese male with diabetes and a history of IV drug use presents with a painful swollen left leg. Exam reveals dark purple discoloration and several large bullae over the calf. On physical exam, his temperature is 38.3 °C, heart rate is 120/min, and blood pressure is 92/68 mmHg. The C-reactive protein (CRP) is 200 mg/L (normal <10 mg/L), and the white blood cell (WBC) count is 28.3 × 103/μL (normal 4.1–10.9 × 103/μL). Creatinine is 2.0 mg/dL (normal 0.5–1.5 mg/dL), and sodium is 127 mEq/L (normal 135–145 mEq/L). Distal pedal pulses are 1+. IV fluids and IV broad-spectrum antibiotics are administered. Which of the following is the next best step?
   (A) X-ray of the leg
   (B) CT scan of the leg with IV contrast
   (C) Venous duplex scan of the left leg
   (D) Measure compartment pressures
   (E) Emergent wide surgical debridement

4. A 66-year-old woman presents to her family doctor complaining of a pain in her left groin that has appeared intermittently over the past several months. On physical exam, a soft mass is palpated in her left groin, below the inguinal ligament, and near her femoral pulse. On palpation, the mass is soft and slightly tender and disappears with gentle compression. Which of the following is true regarding these types of hernias?
   (A) They are the most common hernia type in women
   (B) The risk of strangulation is relatively low
   (C) The hernia sac travels lateral to the femoral vein
   (D) If discovered incidentally and the patient is asymptomatic, repair is not indicated
   (E) It is associated with multigravida

5. Following open right inguinal hernia repair, a 50-year-old male complains of numbness and burning pain on the lateral right hemiscrotum. This most likely represents injury to:
   (A) The genital branch of the genitofemoral nerve
   (B) The femoral branch of the genitofemoral nerve
   (C) The ilioinguinal nerve
   (D) The lateral femoral cutaneous nerve
   (E) The iliohypogastric nerve

6. A 65-year-old male presents to the emergency department (ED) with nausea, vomiting, and severe abdominal pain. Past history is significant for prior sigmoid colectomy for diverticulitis 10 years ago. On physical exam, his temperature is 37.9 °C, blood pressure is 110/80 mmHg, and heart rate is 110/min. His abdomen has a well-healed midline scar and is distended. Bowel sounds are hyperactive with occasional rushes and tinkles. He has marked right upper quadrant (RUQ) tenderness to palpation with guarding. The rest of the abdominal exam is unremarkable. Abdominal series X-rays demonstrates one loop of markedly distended small bowel in the RUQ with an air-fluid level. No gas is seen in the colon or rectum. Laboratory values demonstrate a WBC of $18 \times 10^3/\mu L$ (normal $4.1–10.9 \times 10^3/\mu L$) with 15% bands and a serum lactate of 5 mmol/L (normal 0.5–1.6 mmol/L), blood urea nitrogen (BUN) 30 mg/dL (7–21 mg/dL), and creatinine 1.2 mg/dL (0.5–1.4 mg/dL). Amylase, lipase, and liver chemistries are normal. Nasogastric tube and IV fluids are given. What is the next step in the management?
   (A) Exploratory laparotomy
   (B) Admit for close observation
   (C) Upper gastrointestinal (GI) with small bowel follow through with barium
   (D) Upper GI with small bowel follow through with Gastrografin
   (E) Abdominal ultrasound

7. One day following extensive debridement of the right leg for a necrotizing soft tissue infection (NSTI), a 40-year-old male remains in the ICU, intubated, and requiring 70% fraction of inspired oxygen (FIO_2). WBC count has risen from a preoperative level of $16 \times 10^3/\mu L$ (normal $4.1–10.9 \times 10^3/\mu L$) to $34 \times 10^3/\mu L$. Serum lactate has also risen. Which of the following is the best next step in treatment?
   (A) Second-look operation
   (B) Amputation of the right leg
   (C) Broaden antibiotic coverage
   (D) CT scan of the leg
   (E) Start vasopressor

8. A 30-year-old woman is recovering from an open cholecystectomy in the hospital. On the second postoperative day, she begins to complain of cramping abdominal pain without vomiting. She has no past medical or surgical history, and her postoperative course has been unremarkable. She is receiving multiple doses of oral hydrocodone for pain and is tolerating a clear liquid diet. She has a temperature of 37.8 °C, blood pressure is 128/84 mmHg, and pulse is 82/min. Her physical exam is significant for absent bowel sounds, a mildly distended abdomen with mild diffuse tenderness without rebound or guarding. She is passing flatus. Which of the following is the best next step in management?
   (A) Obtain CT scan of the abdomen
   (B) Place a nasogastric tube
   (C) Neostigmine
   (D) Convert hydrocodone to a nonsteroidal anti-inflammatory drug (NSAID)
   (E) Return to the operating room for exploration

9. A Richter's hernia:
   (A) Describes a hernia in which a retroperitoneal organ protrudes into the hernia sac
   (B) Has a low risk of incarceration
   (C) Most commonly presents as a small bowel obstruction (SBO)
   (D) Can mislead the clinician as strangulated bowel can easily be missed
   (E) Should be manually reduced in the emergency department provided there is no evidence of bowel obstruction

10. A 55-year-old man with a history of schizophrenia arrives to the ED with abdominal pain and vomiting. He reports that the abdominal pain started yesterday and has been worsening. He is afebrile, blood pressure is 122/86 mmHg, and heart rate is 116/min. In the ED he vomits green emesis without blood. His last bowel movement was 48 h ago. Physical examination reveals a large scar in his right upper quadrant. On abdominal examination, the abdomen is distended, with hyperactive bowel sounds, and is tympanic to percussion, with mild diffuse tenderness, and no rebound or guarding. WBC is $9 \times 10^3/\mu L$ (normal $4.1–10.9 \times 10^3/\mu L$). Abdominal series shows dilated loops of bowel with multiple air–fluid levels. After fluid resuscitation, what is the most appropriate next step in management?
    (A) Nasogastric tube insertion
    (B) Laparoscopy
    (C) Exploratory midline laparotomy
    (D) Intravenous erythromycin
    (E) CT scan of the abdomen

11. A worried mother presents to you with concerns that her six-month-old boy has a protrusion at his belly button that is worse when he cries but reduces when he is sleeping. On exam you palpate a 1 cm fascial defect at his umbilicus. Which of the following is true about this condition?
    (A) Elective repair is recommended
    (B) The condition is associated with cardiac anomalies
    (C) The size of the defect predicts that it will not likely close on its own
    (D) The risk of incarceration is significant
    (E) Repair should be delayed until the child is 5 years old

Answers

1. Answer B
   This patient has candidemia, a bloodstream infection caused by *Candida* species, which is most often seen in ICU patients with central venous catheters. *Candida* normally colonizes the skin and mucosa but may enter the bloodstream in immunocompromised hosts or those with indwelling catheters. When *Candida* is isolated from blood cultures, it is never considered a contaminant and should be treated immediately with IV antifungals (e.g., echinocandins) and prompt catheter removal (C). Oral fluconazole is not the treatment of choice for unstable or critically ill patients (A). Beta-D-glucan may support diagnosis but cannot replace definitive blood culture results (C). Replacing the line over a guidewire is inappropriate in fungemia because the catheter is the likely source and must be removed (E).

2. Answer A
   This patient likely has ischemic orchitis secondary to damage or thrombosis of the pampiniform plexus. This is most likely to occur in patients with large or densely adhesed hernia sacs, such as in the case of prior surgery. The condition is usually self-limited, so urgent exploration is not indicated (B, E). Ischemic orchitis is more commonly caused by injury to the pampiniform plexus than to the testicular artery (C).

Testicular torsion is less likely than a vascular injury in this case, and although it will also have a decreased or absent Doppler signal, the pain occurs suddenly (D).

3. Answer E
Given leukocytosis, elevated CRP, elevated creatinine, hyponatremia, and the exam findings, there is a very high likelihood that this patient has a necrotizing soft tissue infection (NSTI). After IV fluids, blood cultures, and immediate broad-spectrum IV antibiotics, the next best step is to perform an emergent wide surgical debridement. If the diagnosis of NSTI is uncertain, yet the suspicion is high, surgical exploration is *still indicated*, as this is the gold standard of both diagnosis and treatment. The incision must be taken down to the fascia and muscle, so both can be inspected. When the diagnosis is in question, plain X-rays are useful as they may demonstrate gas in the soft tissue (A). CT scan may also be beneficial for the same reason (B). Duplex scan of leg veins is used to rule out deep venous thrombosis, which can present with leg swelling, but like compartment syndrome, it would not cause the laboratory abnormalities described (C, D).

4. Answer E
Multigravida causes stretching of the abdominal musculature and increases the risk of femoral hernia. Femoral hernias occur in the femoral canal, posterior to the inguinal ligament traversing the empty space medial to the femoral vein (recall the mnemonic "NAVEL" {from lateral to medial/femoral nerve, artery, vein, empty space, lymphatic}) (C). The most common type of hernia in women, and in men, is an indirect inguinal hernia (A). Although femoral hernias appear infrequently (10% of all hernias), they occur more commonly in females and have the highest risk of strangulation (B). Because of the high risk of strangulation, laparoscopic repair of a femoral hernia is indicated once diagnosed, regardless of whether the patient is having symptoms (D).

5. Answer A
The genital branch of the genitofemoral nerve provides sensation to the lateral aspect of the hemi-scrotum (and labia), as well as innervation of the cremaster muscle. The femoral branch of the genitofemoral nerve provides sensation to the proximal medial thigh (B). The ilioinguinal nerve provides sensation to root of the penis and upper/anterior medial scrotum, lower abdomen, as well as the adjacent medial upper thigh, and is the most commonly injured nerve in *open hernia repair* (C). The lateral femoral cutaneous nerve provides sensation to the lateral thigh as low as the knee and is the most common nerve injured during *laparoscopic hernia repair* (D). The iliohypogastric nerve supplies the skin overlying the pubis (E).

6. Answer A
Recognizing when to operate is critically important. This patient has small bowel obstruction (SBO) with evidence of ischemic or gangrenous bowel most likely secondary to adhesions from past surgery (e.g., sigmoidectomy). Necrotic bowel generally does not occur in association with SBO unless there is a closed-loop obstruction. A closed-loop obstruction is a particularly dangerous form of bowel obstruction in which a segment of intestine is obstructed both proximally and distally. This is more common in the large bowel as a competent ileocecal valve (present in 70–80% of the population) serves as one point of obstruction. Gas and fluid accumulate within this segment of bowel and cannot escape. This progresses rapidly to strangulation with risk of ischemia, gangrene, and subsequent perforation. Clues to ischemic bowel include the presence of acidosis, fever, leukocytosis, and severe localized pain (unusual for SBO). As such the patient will need exploratory laparotomy, and any bowel that is obviously nonviable needs to be resected. Most patients with SBO (without necrotic bowel) due to adhesions improve with conservative management and do not require surgery. Observation is not appropriate for this patient (B). Upper GI studies would not be indicated since this patient has strong evidence of necrotic bowel and requires urgent surgical intervention (C–D). Abdominal ultrasound is appropriate in the workup for cholelithiasis (E).

7. Answer A
A rising WBC and lactate after debridement are highly suggestive of progression of the NSTI. A second-look operation is often required but in this case would be essential in order to ensure that no additional tissues have become involved since the initial debridement. Amputation may be necessary, but only a second-look operation will indicate whether this is the case (B). CT scan in the postoperative setting would be difficult to interpret due to postsurgical changes (D). With severe sepsis, vasopressors may be necessary, but this would not be the definitive treatment (E). Furthermore, no hemodynamic parameters (blood pressure, central venous pressure) are provided that would indicate that vasopressors are needed. Patients with NSTI should always receive broad antibiotic coverage at initial presentation as it is often due to a polymicrobial infection. However, the cornerstone of management is surgical debridement (C).

8. Answer D
Always consider a nonmechanical postoperative ileus in patients that have had a recent surgery. This occurs in up to 50% of patients that have undergone abdominal surgery. Although the exact cause has not been elucidated, the etiology is likely multifactorial and involves dysfunction of the autonomic enteric nervous system. Inflammatory mediators (e.g., recent surgery) and opioid analgesics are thought to contribute to the development of postoperative ileus. Initial management should begin with changing pain medication to a non-opiate analgesic. Other options for analgesia include NSAIDs and acetaminophen. Encouraging ambulation is an important element of recovery in all postsurgical patients but is not as important as discontinuing opiates in the management of postoperative ileus. If the patient's symptoms worsen (e.g., emesis), bowel decompression with a nasogastric tube should be considered (B). In this case, an abdominal radiograph should be obtained to look for a large gastric bubble and dilated loops of bowel, consistent with ileus. If the ileus persists or there is any indication of sepsis (leukocytosis, fever, tachycardia), a CT scan of the abdomen should be obtained (A). Neostigmine is used in patients with pseudo-obstruction (Ogilvie's syndrome) (C). Returning to the OR for exploration is inappropriate for postoperative ileus (E).

9. Answer D
A retroperitoneal organ (such as colon) protruding into a hernia sac describes a sliding hernia (A). With a Richter's hernia, only part of the circumference of the bowel wall is trapped within the hernia sac. That segment of bowel is prone to incarceration and strangulation but does so without associated symptoms, signs, or radiologic evidence of SBO (C). Therefore, it may easily mislead clinicians into thinking that the hernia is not incarcerated (B). Manual reduction in hernias (including Richter's) should not be attempted if strangulation is suspected as dead bowel will be reduced into the peritoneum. Strangulation should be suspected in the presence of fever, leukocytosis, acidosis, severe pain, or marked erythema overlying the skin of the hernia. It is often difficult to palpate a Richter's hernia, and it should be reduced in the operating room (E).

10. Answer A
This patient has evidence (on history, physical, and radiologic imaging) of an SBO that is most likely secondary to adhesions from prior surgery (abdominal scar). SBO from adhesions can present many years after surgery. The initial management of SBO includes placing the patient nothing by mouth (NPO), aggressive intravenous fluid resuscitation (the patient is tachycardic and likely very dehydrated), and nasogastric tube placement. Aside from the salutatory effect of gastric decompression on the distended bowel, patients with SBO are at risk of aspiration. Once the patient has been adequately resuscitated, CT scan with oral contrast is recommended as it is useful in confirming the diagnosis of SBO, determining if the SBO is partial or complete, and ruling out other diagnosis (E). Oral contrast may also have a therapeutic effect in resolving the SBO. Most patients with SBO due to adhesions improve with these maneuvers and do not require surgery. Operative management with laparotomy and lysis of adhesions should be considered in the following conditions: if the patient demonstrates evidence

of clinical deterioration as manifest by increasing pain, tenderness, fever, leukocytosis, or acidosis (C). Operative management can be achieved either via open laparotomy or laparoscopy (B). Evidence of a *complete SBO* is a relative indication for surgery, but recent studies suggest that some of these patients resolve with nonoperative management as well. Intravenous erythromycin acts as a prokinetic agent and has some utility for gastroparesis, but not for SBO (D). In cases where a mechanical obstruction is suspected, prokinetic agents should be avoided.

11. Answer E
This patient has an umbilical hernia, which is a common finding in newborns. It is recommended that repair be delayed until after the child is 5 years old, unless the defect is larger than 2 cm, the defect is growing, or there is evidence of strangulation (A). Umbilical hernias are not associated with the VACTERL (vertebral, anal, cardiac, tracheoesophageal fistula, renal, limb) complex of anomalies (B). Defects smaller than 2 cm will likely close spontaneously (C). It is very rare for umbilical hernias in children to incarcerate (D).

Breast and Skin

Danielle M. Hari

Contents

Abnormal Screening Mammogram

Areg Grigorian, Christian de Virgilio, and Danielle M. Hari

Contents

C. de Virgilio, A. Grigorian (eds.), *Surgery*, https://doi.org/10.1007/978-3-032-09799-6_5

Case Study

A 40-year-old woman sees her doctor for an annual physical exam. She is healthy and does not take any medications. She has a family history of breast cancer. Her physical examination is normal with no palpable breast masses. Her doctor recommends that she get a screening mammography as part of her routine health maintenance screening, which she agrees to do. A week later, she gets a call from her doctor to inform her that the mammogram is abnormal (BI-RADS 4). Her left breast was found to have multiple clusters of fine linear microcalcifications, with the largest cluster measuring 2 mm in diameter.

Diagnosis

What Is the Differential Diagnosis for an Abnormal Mammogram in the Absence of a Palpable Breast Mass? (Table 5.1)

Table 5.1 Differential diagnosis of clinical presentation

Select benign calcifications	
Skin calcifications	May be secondary to dermatitis or topical hygiene products (e.g., deodorants, ointments) which can appear as skin calcifications but are not true skin calcifications
Vascular calcifications	Linear or parallel tracks; may be associated with underlying vascular disease
Coarse or "popcorn"-like calcifications	Dystrophic in origin and usually associated with underlying fibroadenoma
Round and punctate calcifications	Associated with fibrocystic changes of the breast, adenosis, and skin calcifications
Eggshell or rim calcifications	Appear to be deposited on the surface of a sphere; can be seen in fat necrosis or fibrocystic changes of the breast
Dystrophic calcifications	Coarse, irregular shaped; seen in irradiated breast or following trauma
Suspicious calcifications	
Amorphous calcifications	Without a clearly defined shape or form; small and hazy appearance
Coarse heterogeneous calcifications	Irregular, conspicuous calcifications typically larger than 0.5 mm; associated with benign (e.g., fibroadenoma, fibrosis) and malignant conditions (e.g., DCIS)
High probability of malignancy	
Fine pleomorphic calcifications	Classified as BI-RADS 5; typically associated with DCIS
Fine linear/linear branching calcifications	Represent casts of the ducts ("casting" type) in which they lie; often associated with comedo subtype of intraductal carcinoma, typically high grade or poorly differentiated

DCIS ductal carcinoma in situ

What Is the Most Likely Diagnosis?

Fine, linear calcifications on mammogram are highly suggestive of malignancy. Such calcifications form in areas of necrosis and in a linear pattern. This is likely from dead cancer cells lining the ducts that outgrow their blood supply. Thus, the most likely diagnosis is malignancy. Since the lesion is small and there is no palpable mass, it most likely represents ductal carcinoma in situ (DCIS) as opposed to invasive ductal carcinoma. In addition, she has a family history of breast cancer which increases her risk.

Screening

Should Women Perform Self Breast Examinations?

The age and frequency of screening are controversial (see below Areas of Controversy section). While women are encouraged to monitor their breasts for any changes, self-breast examinations are no longer recommended at any age, as there is minimal evidence that they help detect early breast cancer. Breast awareness is still recommended so that patients can alert their providers of changes such as nipple discharge, skin changes, and masses. Clinical breast exams are still recommended by medical providers during clinical encounters to evaluate symptoms and to perform physical examinations of patients.

> **Watch Out**
> If the surgery shelf exam asks about screening for breast cancer, the likely answer is starting at age 40 and continuing annually.

What Are the Risks of Mammography?

Mammograms utilize small doses of radiation, which, over time, can place patients at an increased risk for cancer. However, for most women over 40, the benefits of regular mammograms far outweigh any potential radiation risks. Additionally, mammograms can miss up to 20% of cancers, particularly small ones, and those that are in areas that are difficult to view. On the other end of the spectrum, it may detect cancers that would have otherwise never led to symptoms, subjecting the patient to the adverse effects of intervention or additional testing (e.g., biopsy). Lastly, mammograms are not always accurate. Mammographic findings are heavily dependent on the technique used in attaining the images, the experience of the radiologist evaluating the images, and the breast density of the patient.

Why Is Mammography Not Useful in Young Women (<30 Years Old)?

Younger women tend to have denser breast tissue due to an increased ratio of dense breast tissue to fatty tissue. Dense breasts make it difficult to detect abnormal calcifications or masses. Ultrasound is the typical first imaging modality used for young patients (<30 years) with breast symptoms.

History and Physical

What Is the Gail Risk Model?

The most commonly implemented risk assessment model is the Breast Cancer Risk Assessment Tool (BCRAT), also known as the Gail model. The BCRAT is a mathematical model used to calculate the risk of developing breast cancer. The model considers factors such as age, age at menarche, reproductive history, family history in first-degree relatives, and prior biopsies. One disadvantage of the model is that it can underestimate breast cancer risk in women with a strong family history of breast or ovarian cancer that does not involve first-degree relatives; if this is the case, alternative risk models should be implemented such as the Tyrer-Cuzick Risk Model. The Gail model should not be used for women under the age of 35.

> **Watch Out**
> Age of menopause is *not* a factor in the Gail model. This is important as it allows this tool to be used in all women, including those that are postmenopausal.

Pathophysiology

What Is One Characteristic of Mammographic Calcifications that Helps Differentiate Between Benign and Malignant Conditions?

Larger calcifications (macrocalcifications) are almost always benign, while smaller calcifications (microcalcifications) are more frequently seen in patients with breast cancer.

What Are the Primary Features of Ductal Carcinoma In Situ (DCIS)?

DCIS is characterized by malignant epithelial cells within the mammary ductal system, without invasion into the surrounding stroma. DCIS has several histological patterns, including comedo with prominent central necrosis, cribriform with back-to-back glands, and papillary. Comedo-type DCIS is typically high grade and associated with a worse prognosis. DCIS is often multifocal and can be associated with a concurrent invasive carcinoma. In addition, DCIS lesions have a 20–50% risk of progression to invasive carcinoma if left untreated.

What Are the Primary Features of Lobular Carcinoma In Situ (LCIS)?

LCIS is characterized by atypical epithelial cells that arise from the lobules and terminal ducts of the breast. Unlike DCIS, it is *not* a premalignant lesion but rather is a marker for the development of future ipsilateral as well as contralateral invasive breast cancer (ductal or lobular) (◘ Table 5.2). It is almost always incidentally found on a breast biopsy that is performed for some other reason. LCIS itself is not thought to progress to invasive lobular carcinoma, so there is no role for resecting it to attain clear margins. However, *excisional biopsy* is still recommended to rule out concurrent invasive cancer. Two forms of LCIS have been associated with microcalcifications on mammography: the classic form with small uniform cells and the pleomorphic form with larger cells. The pleomorphic form is clinically more aggressive and must be treated with a wide excision in contrast to classic LCIS. The relative risk of developing an invasive cancer in women with LCIS is approximately 7× higher compared to women without LCIS.

◘ **Table 5.2** Ductal carcinoma in situ (DCIS) versus lobular carcinoma in situ (LCIS)

	DCIS	LCIS
Typical presentation	Incidental microcalcifications on mammography	Incidental finding on histopathology
Location	Ducts, multifocal	Lobules
Pattern	Comedo (prominent necrosis in the center of the involved spaces), micropapillary, cribriform (back-to-back glands)	Solid
Axillary metastasis	Present in up to 10% of patients	Usually absent
Incidence of concurrent invasive carcinoma	High	Low
Risk of progression to invasive carcinoma if untreated	High	Low

How Does Breast Cancer Metastasize to the Spine?

Batson plexus is a network of valveless veins that are thought to be the route for metastasis of breast cancer to the spine.

Workup

How Are Mammograms Used in Staging Breast Lesions?

Mammogram abnormalities include masses, microcalcifications, and asymmetry. The radiologist summarizes the mammographic findings using the American College of Radiology's Breast Imaging Reporting and Data System (BI-RADS) final assessment (◘ Table 5.3), which standardizes the reporting of mammographic findings and indicates the relative likelihood of a normal, benign, or malignant diagnosis. It is important to note that the BI-RADS category only refers to the imag-

5

Table 5.3 BI-RADS

BI-RADS category	Interpretation
0	Incomplete assessment; needs additional imaging and/or old imaging comparison
1	Negative; continue screening based on current screening guidelines
2	Benign findings; continue screening based on current screening guidelines
3	Probably benign; recommend shorter interval follow-up (e.g., diagnostic mammography and/or ultrasound at 6-month intervals for 1 year)
4	Suspicious abnormalities; biopsy should be considered. Further categorized as: 4a. Low likelihood of cancer (2–10%); biopsy recommended 4b. Moderate likelihood of cancer (10–50%); biopsy recommended 4c. High likelihood of cancer (50–95%); biopsy recommended
5	Highly suggestive of malignancy; biopsy recommended
6	Known biopsy-proven malignancy

ing findings and does not take clinical information into account with the exception of BI-RADS 6 which indicates biopsy-proven cancer (Figs. 5.1 and 5.2).

Watch Out

Beware of discordant findings. Clinically suspicious masses in a patient with a low BI-RADS score *still* require biopsy. Similarly, BI-RADS-5 lesions found to be benign on core needle biopsy are considered "benign-discordant" and should undergo a second core biopsy before performing an excisional biopsy as a last resort to diagnose the lesion.

What Is the Next Step in Management for the Above Patient?

An abnormal mammogram, in particular a BI-RADS 4 or BI-RADS 5, requires further workup. The appropriate next step is a stereotactic core needle biopsy.

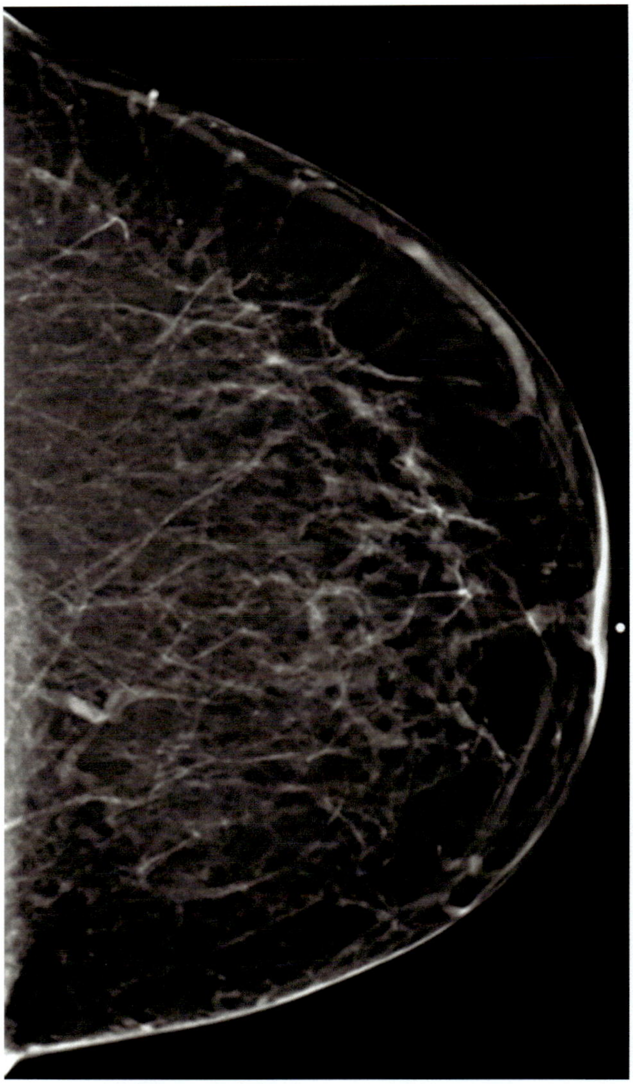

Fig. 5.1 Normal screening mammogram, craniocaudal (CC) view

What Is a Stereotactic Core Needle Biopsy?

A stereotactic core needle biopsy is performed on lesions that are *not palpable* and only visible on mammography. The lesion is biopsied with a hollow needle using image guidance by a radiologist with a special stereotactic mammography machine that pinpoints the location of the abnormal area.

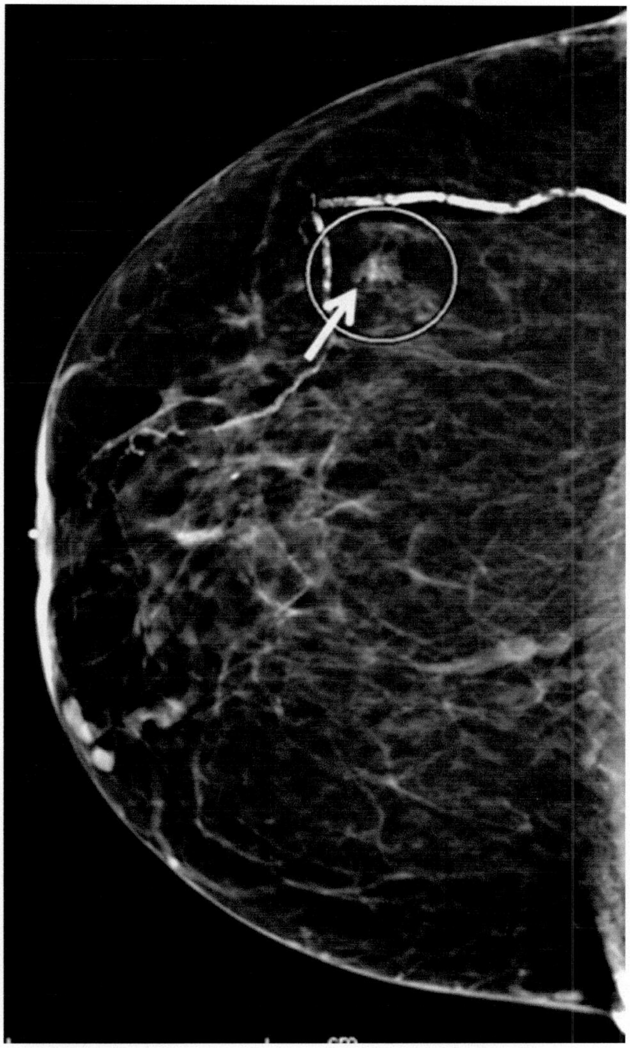

Fig. 5.2 Abnormal screening mammogram (CC view) showing 1 cm foci of microcalcifications in the upper outer quadrant BI-RADS (category 0)

How Does One Interpret the Results of a Stereotactic Core Needle Biopsy?

The biopsy may be benign or malignant. If the result is benign, the radiologist assesses whether the pathology is concordant with the mammographic findings. If the biopsy is benign and concordant, no further intervention is needed. If the findings are discordant, meaning the biopsy is benign but the imaging remains suspicious, a repeat core needle biopsy is preferred if feasible. If not, a surgical excisional biopsy may be performed to obtain a definitive diagnosis.

What Is the Next Step If the Repeated Stereotactic Biopsy Is Still Discordant?

The lesion needs to be removed via an excisional biopsy. However, since the lesion is not palpable, the surgeon needs a guide. This has classically been done with wire localization. This involves coordination between the radiologist and the surgeon. The radiologist marks the lesion by inserting a wire through the skin, directly into the area of suspicious calcification under radiologic guidance. The tip of the wire has a hook to keep it in place. The patient is then taken to the operating room, where the surgeon makes an incision over the protruding wire and excises a core of tissue around the tip of the wire. An X-ray image of the specimen is obtained to confirm that all of the suspicious calcifications have been removed. There are now various other options to localize the lesion including radioactive seed localization or nonradioactive infrared or magnetic technologies. A tiny radioactive seed or infrared reflectors/magnetic marker is placed under imaging guidance. During surgery, a handheld probe is used to locate the seed, reflector, or marker, and the surgeon then excises the surrounding tissue.

What Other Findings on Core Needle Biopsy Require Surgical Excisional Biopsy?

Certain findings on core needle biopsy have higher risk for concurrent malignancy, so a localized surgical excisional biopsy is recommended to evaluate for malignancy in the vicinity of these lesions. These include LCIS, atypical ductal/lobular hyperplasia, flat epithelial atypia, and radial scar. However, since these lesions themselves do not lead to progression to cancer, the excisional biopsy does not require negative margins.

What Constitutes Positive Margins on a Malignant Specimen?

After excision, the margins of the specimen are inked, and the pathologist must confirm that there is *no invasive tumor on the ink*. If there is tumor on the ink, it is considered a positive margin. If the lesion is DCIS, a 2-mm margin is required.

Management

What Is the Next Step If the Stereotactic Needle Biopsy Demonstrates DCIS?

DCIS, if left unresected, will often progress to invasive ductal cancer. Thus, the mainstay of DCIS treatment is typically breast-conserving therapy (lumpectomy with negative margins followed by adjuvant radiation) or a mastectomy. If the margins are <2 mm after lumpectomy, a re-excision or mastectomy is indicated.

What Is the Next Step If the Stereotactic Biopsy Demonstrates LCIS?

If LCIS is found on core needle biopsy, one would perform a surgical excisional biopsy. This is done to rule out the presence of adjacent cancers that are sometimes found. Unlike DCIS which leads to an invasive cancer directly in the lesion, LCIS does not directly lead to invasive cancer. Therefore, a negative margin is not necessary. If the excisional biopsy only shows LCIS, then no further surgery is recommended. LCIS is a risk factor for developing invasive cancer in either breast (any type, not just lobular).

What Is the Difference Between an Excisional Biopsy and a Lumpectomy?

A lumpectomy is a treatment procedure aimed at removing a known cancerous tumor from the breast. During a lumpectomy, the surgeon excises the tumor along with a margin of healthy surrounding tissue to ensure complete removal of the cancer, often followed by radiation therapy to eliminate any remaining cancer cells and reduce the risk of recurrence. In contrast, an excisional biopsy is primarily a diagnostic procedure used to remove a suspicious lump or area of abnormal tissue for pathological examination. The goal of an excisional biopsy is to determine whether the lesion is benign or malignant by removing the entire suspicious area with minimal surrounding tissue. If cancer is found in the excisional biopsy, further treatment, such as a lumpectomy or mastectomy, may be required. Essentially, a lumpectomy aims to treat cancer by ensuring clear margins around the tumor, while an excisional biopsy focuses on obtaining a pathologic diagnosis of a suspicious lesion with minimal tissue removal.

> **Watch Out**
> Pleomorphic subtype of LCIS is considered an aggressive subtype. As such, pleomorphic LCIS needs an excisional biopsy *with negative margins* but does not require additional treatment (such as radiation) unless an invasive component is found.

What Are the Treatment Options for LCIS?

There are two main options for management: monitoring and chemoprevention. Monitoring involves increased surveillance with regular clinical breast exams every 6–12 months and annual mammography or MRI to detect any new changes in the breast tissue. Chemoprevention includes the use of medications like tamoxifen (premenopausal) or aromatase inhibitors (postmenopausal) to significantly reduce the risk of developing invasive breast cancer. Lifestyle modifications, such as maintaining a healthy diet, regular exercise, and limiting alcohol intake, are also recommended to help lower cancer risk. Surgical options, such as bilateral prophylactic mastectomy, may be considered for high-risk patients, especially those with a strong family history or genetic predisposition (i.e., BRCA), but are no longer routinely offered since the benefits from chemoprevention are similar to prophylactic surgery.

> **Watch Out**
> Tamoxifen should not be used in pregnant women due to its teratogenicity, or in lactating women as it may suppress milk production.

What If the Stereotactic Biopsy Demonstrates Invasive Ductal Carcinoma?

The two primary surgical options are breast-conserving therapy, which includes lumpectomy followed by radiation therapy to reduce the risk of local recurrence, or total (simple) mastectomy. In both cases, a sentinel lymph node biopsy should also be performed to assess for nodal involvement.

Can You Get Lymph Node Metastasis with DCIS?

DCIS is, by definition, confined within the mammary duct and has not breached the basement membrane. Therefore, it cannot enter the surrounding tissue or the lymph system. However, when DCIS is multifocal, comedo subtype, or high grade, it may have an invasive component that is missed and subsequently result in lymph node metastasis. This occurs in a small number of DCIS cases. As such, SLNB is generally not recommended for DCIS. However, for certain high-risk lesions such as extensive microcalcifications on mammogram >3 cm, or DCIS associated with a palpable mass, SLNB should be performed. It is also recommended if the patient opts for a mastectomy, as it is not possible to perform a SLNB after the breast has been removed.

What Should You Consider for a Patient with Mastitis that Does Not Resolve with Antibiotics?

Mastitis most often occurs in lactating patients and presents with a warm, erythematous, and tender breast. The most common organism is *Staphylococcus aureus*. The treatment includes antibiotics covering *S. aureus*, continued breast-feeding (this does not pose a risk to the infant), and lactation consultation. Women that are not lactating can also develop mastitis when there is an obstruction or pseudo-obstruction of the lactiferous duct. Risk factors include trauma to the nipple (e.g., scarring from nipple piercing), granulomatous disease of the breast, smoking (leads to keratinizing squamous metaplasia), and hidradenitis. Alcohol has not been demonstrated to be associated with mastitis and breast abscesses. If mastitis does not resolve or recurs, a mammography and skin biopsy should be performed to rule out inflammatory breast cancer.

Areas of Controversy

Prophylactic Bilateral Mastectomy

Women with strong family histories of breast cancer, genetic mutations (BRCA-1 or BRCA-2), radiation therapy to the chest before age 30, or conditions that place them at increased risk for developing invasive cancer may consider prophylactic surgery to remove both breasts. LCIS is a marker for increased risk of developing cancer in either breast. Patients with LCIS and a family history of breast cancer could be considered suitable candidates for prophylactic bilateral mastectomy. Patients without a family history may not benefit from such aggressive intervention because of such a low risk of progression to cancer and as such bilateral prophylactic mastectomy is no longer routinely offered to patients with LCIS.

Controversy in Breast Cancer Screening Guidelines

One of the most contentious debates in breast cancer screening revolves around the appropriate age and frequency of mammography. Different organizations provide varying recommendations, with some advocating for annual screening starting at age 40 while others suggest beginning at age 45. The US Preventive Services Task Force (USPSTF) now recommends biennial screening for women aged 40–74, while the American Cancer Society advises starting at age 45 with the option to begin at 40 and to "continue for as long as a woman is in good health and is expected to live at least 10 more years." This discrepancy highlights the challenges in balancing the benefits of early cancer detection against the risks of overdiagnosis, false positives, and the associated anxiety and unnecessary interventions. The lack of consensus also emphasizes the need for personalized screening strategies that consider individual risk factors and patient preferences.

Summary of Essentials

Diagnosis

- DCIS and LCIS do not typically present as palpable masses
- Benign calcifications: skin, vascular, popcorn-like, plasma cell mastitis, lucent-centered, eggshell or rim, milk of calcium, suture, or dystrophic
- Suspicious calcifications: fine, linear, branching, and pleomorphic microcalcifications

Screening

- Age and frequency of screening are controversial
- Some cancer societies recommend screening in normal-risk women starting at age 40, while others recommend starting at age 45
- USPSTF recommends that women ages 40–74 years undergo screening mammography every other year

5

History and Physical

- Gail risk model to help calculate risk of developing breast cancer

Etiology/Pathophysiology

- Macrocalcifications are almost always benign, while microcalcifications are more concerning for cancer
- DCIS can progress to invasive cancer if left unresected
  - Can be multifocal
  - Can be associated with a concurrent invasive carcinoma
- LCIS is not premalignant, but is associated with an increased risk of future ipsilateral as well as contralateral invasive breast cancer (either lobular or ductal)

Workup

- BI-RADS (0–6) is a standardized summary of mammographic findings
- BI-RADS 3 is probably benign (2% chance of cancer); BI-RADS 4 is suspicious
- Stereotactic biopsy is indicated for BI-RADS 4a/b/c or BI-RADS 5
- Repeat core biopsy or localized excisional biopsy for discordant findings

Management

- DCIS: lumpectomy to 2 mm margin or mastectomy
- LCIS (found on excisional biopsy): observation, chemoprevention, or surgery depending on patient's risk factors
- LCIS found on core biopsy requires excisional biopsy to rule out adjacent or associated ductal or lobular cancer
- ILC or IDC: lumpectomy to negative margins "no ink on tumor"

Suggested Reading

Chala LF, de Barros N, de Camargo MP, et al. Fat necrosis of the breast: mammographic, sonographic, computed tomography, and magnetic resonance imaging findings. Curr Probl Diagn Radiol 2004;33:106–12.

Demetri-Lewis A, et al. Breast calcifications: the focal group. Am J Roentgenol 2012;198:W325.

Fisher B, Costantino JP, Wickerham DL, Redmond CK, Kavanah M, Cronin WM, Vogel V, Robidoux A, Dimitrov N, Atkins J, Daly M, Wieand S, Tan-Chiu E, Ford L, Wolmark N, other NSABP investigators. Tamoxifen for prevention of breast cancer: Report of the National Surgical Adjuvant Breast and Bowel Project P-1 Study. J Natl Cancer Inst 1998;90(18):1371–88.

Kuerer HM, Albarracin CT, Yang WT, et al. Ductal carcinoma in situ: state of the science and roadmap to advance the field. J Clin Oncol 2009;27:279.

Miller AB, et al. Twenty five year follow-up for breast cancer incidence and mortality of the Canadian National Breast Screening Study: randomised screening trial. BMJ 2014;348:g366.

Muttarak M, et al. Breast calcifications: which are malignant? Singapore Med J 2009;50:907.

New Palpable Mass in the Right Breast

Junko Ozao-Choy, Areg Grigorian, Christian de Virgilio, and Danielle M. Hari

Contents

C. de Virgilio, A. Grigorian (eds.), *Surgery*, https://doi.org/10.1007/978-3-032-09799-6_6

Case Study

A 55-year-old postmenopausal female presents with a new mass in her right breast. She states that the mass has been there for about 3 months and has slowly grown in size. She first noticed it when she was taking a shower. The mass is not painful. She reports no nipple discharge, no nipple inversion, and no skin changes. She had her first menstrual period at age 11. Her only pregnancy was at age 35. Her mother and sister both had breast cancer. On physical examination, she has a 2 cm palpable, hard, ill-defined, immobile, non-tender mass in the upper outer quadrant of her right breast. There is no palpable axillary or supraclavicular adenopathy.

Diagnosis

What Benign Conditions Are in the Differential Diagnosis of a Palpable Breast Mass? (Table 6.1)

Table 6.1 Differential diagnosis of a palpable breast mass

Condition	History and physical	Features
Fibrocystic change	Vague irregularity of breast tissue (lumpy breast), often in upper quadrants, cysts have a blue-dome appearance on exam	Most common *overall breast mass* in women; found in 60–90% of breasts during routine autopsy; normal variant of premenopausal breast
Fibroadenoma	Well-circumscribed, mobile, rubbery, encapsulated mass	Most common *benign tumor*; typically affects women <30 years; estrogen sensitive causing it to grow during pregnancy (most commonly identified benign breast mass during pregnancy)
Intraductal papilloma	Classically presents as unilateral bloody nipple discharge in premenopausal women	Most common cause of bloody nipple discharge in women aged 20–40 years; usually do not show up on mammogram; papilloma is lined by epithelial (luminal) and myoepithelial cells in contrast to cancer cells which are only lined by luminal cells
Fat necrosis	Following trauma or recent breast surgery; feels hard like cancer, can cause skin dimpling, may be accompanied by pain	Abnormal calcification on mammogram secondary to saponification
Abscess	Painful mass typically in lactating breast, erythematous and warm, fevers, purulent drainage from mass or nipple discharge	Could be caused by postpartum mastitis (localized cellulitis caused by bacterial invasion through an irritated or fissured nipple), blockage of ducts, nipple piercings, rarely underlying breast mass
Galactocele	Painful or painless aseptic mass in lactating breast that is not warm or erythematous	Typically occurs on cessation of lactation; can be managed by massaging the breast or aspiration
Mondor's disease	Tender lump, sudden onset	Thrombosis of a superficial chest wall vein, warm compress, NSAIDs

What Malignant Lesions Are in the Differential Diagnosis of a Palpable Breast Mass? (Table 6.2)

Table 6.2 Malignant lesions of the breast

Type	History and physical	Features	Prognosis
Ductal carcinoma in situ (*DCIS*)	Does *not* usually present as a palpable mass	Malignant cells in ducts with no invasion of the basement membrane; incidental microcalcifications on mammogram; if present as a mass, higher chance of concurrent invasive carcinoma; considered premalignant	Majority do well
Lobular carcinoma in situ (*LCIS*)	Does *not* usually present as a palpable mass	Abnormal growth of benign cells that arise from the lobules and terminal ducts of the breast; *not* premalignant	Majority do well
Invasive ductal carcinoma	Firm, immobile, discrete mass, nipple retraction, painless	Malignant cells in ducts with stromal invasion and microcalcifications, the most common form of invasive breast cancer	Dependent on stage
Invasive lobular carcinoma	Firm, immobile, discrete mass, nipple retraction, painless, frequently bilateral	Malignant cells in breast lobules with insidious infiltration; higher risk of multicentric and bilateral disease	Dependent on stage
Mucinous carcinoma	Gelatinous well-circumscribed mass	Well-circumscribed mass, slow growth, more common in elderly, pure mucinous type (not mixed) less likely to metastasize to lymph nodes	More favorable but stage dependent
Inflammatory carcinoma	Inflamed, tender, warm, erythematous breast, peau d'orange	Carcinoma that has infiltrated the subdermal lymphatics, rapid progression, angioinvasive behavior	Poor
Phyllodes tumor	Can be fast growing, firm, and rubbery or hard; typically mobile until malignant, at which point fixation may occur	Benign, borderline, or malignant, hard to diagnose with needle biopsy, wide local excision, locally recurrent, does not metastasize to lymph nodes, can behave like sarcoma	Dependent on whether malignant

What Is the Most Likely Diagnosis for This Patient?

Invasive breast cancer is the most likely diagnosis in a postmenopausal woman with a new palpable breast mass that is non-tender, hard, ill-defined, immobile, and in the upper outer quadrant. In addition, she has other risk factors for breast cancer, including family history in a first-degree relative and early menarche. Most women who detect breast masses do so in the shower or after trauma to the chest, which brings attention to a palpable mass.

History and Physical

What Features on Physical Examination Are Suggestive of Breast Cancer?

Physical exam findings of benign breast masses can be hard to differentiate from cancer, since normal variants of breast tissue may feel nodular. A careful inspection for asymmetry, skin changes, and nipple discharge (or crusting) should be done for each patient reporting a newly found breast mass. A bimanual examination of the breasts should then be performed with the patient in a supine position, with the ipsilateral arm raised above her head, palpating for any obvious masses. A single dominant lesion that is hard and immobile, with irregular borders, is suspicious for breast cancer. The cervical, supraclavicular, infraclavicular, and axillary nodes should also be examined. Enlarged, firm, immobile, and/or matted lymph nodes suggest disseminated cancer.

What Are the Risk Factors for Breast Cancer?

The most important risk factors for breast cancer are female gender, increasing age, and a family history of premenopausal breast cancer. In particular, a family history of breast cancer in males or premenopausal women, bilateral breast cancer, a history of ovarian cancer, and multiple relatives with cancer should prompt investigation for the presence of a gene mutation. The majority of inherited breast cancers are associated with BRCA1 or BRCA2 gene mutations. Other important risk factors associated with a higher risk of developing breast cancer include increased lifetime estrogen exposure. This prolonged exposure may be due to factors such as early menarche, nulliparity or childbirth after age 30, and/or late menopause. ◘ Table 6.3 shows the relative risk of developing breast cancer for common clinical risk factors.

◘ **Table 6.3** Relative risk (RR) for breast cancer

Low (<2 RR)	Moderate (2–4 RR)	High risk (>4 RR)
Age at menarche <12	Age at first birth >30	BRCA1/BRCA2 mutation
Age at menopause >55	Mother or sister with breast cancer	Age >70
Nulliparity	Previous breast cancer	
Obesity	Radiation exposure	
Hormone replacement therapy		

What Are the Different Types of Nipple Discharge and What Is the Differential Diagnosis for Each?

Nipple discharge is categorized as normal milk production (lactation), physiologic nipple discharge, or pathologic nipple discharge. Benign nipple discharge tends to be nonspontaneous, clear, bilateral, and multiductal. Physiologic discharge can be related to post-lactation (up to 2 years following birth), fluctuating hormone levels (puberty and menopause), or nipple stimulation. Pathologic nipple discharge can be due to medical conditions such as prolactinoma, hypothyroidism (thyroid-releasing hormone stimulates prolactin), Cushing's disease, or medications (e.g., antipsychotics, cimetidine, spironolactone). The most common cause of pathologic nipple discharge (spontaneous, unilateral, clear, or bloody) is a papilloma, which is a benign tumor growing from the lining of the breast duct. Nevertheless, malignancy can be found in up to 15% of patients that present with nipple discharge. The likelihood of cancer is higher if the discharge is bloody (versus non-bloody), spontaneous, unilateral, uniductal, and associated with a breast mass or if it occurs in women older than 40 years.

What Should You Suspect If a Patient Has a Diagnosis of Breast Infection That Does Not Respond to Antibiotics?

If a breast infection does not improve with antibiotics, consider the possibility of inflammatory breast carcinoma. Key clinical clues include persistent erythema, warmth, edema, and peau d'orange involving a large area of the breast, typically without fever or systemic symptoms. In cases where these signs persist or worsen despite antibiotic treatment, further evaluation with imaging and biopsy is warranted to rule out malignancy.

Pathology/Pathophysiology

What Histologic Features of Fibrocystic Changes Are Associated with Increased Risk for Cancer?

Most cases of fibrocystic-related changes are benign, but certain features place patients at an increased risk for invasive carcinoma in both breasts. Whereas apocrine metaplasia has no increased risk for cancer, ductal hyperplasia or sclerosing adenosis doubles the risk of cancer development. Atypical ductal hyperplasia has the highest risk for cancer.

What Is the Pathophysiology of "Peau d' Orange"?

Peau d'orange is a French term meaning "skin like an orange peel." It is caused by tumor cells invading local lymphatics, leading to lymphedema of the skin, expansion of the interfollicular dermis, and characteristic dimpling resembling the texture of an orange peel. When deeper subcutaneous layers are involved, it can also cause pitting.

What Is the Pathophysiology of Nipple Retraction?

The suspensory ligaments of the breasts are called *Cooper's ligaments*. When a breast tumor infiltrates these ligaments, it can retract the skin, often at or around the nipples.

Workup

How Does the Age of the Patient Affect the Workup of a New, Palpable Breast Mass?

In women under 30, ultrasound is the first-line imaging due to dense breast tissue and a low likelihood of malignancy. Ultrasound can distinguish cystic from solid masses and guide aspiration if needed. Simple cysts may be observed unless painful or enlarging; bloody aspirates should be sent for cytology. Solid masses require image-guided core needle biopsy, which is preferred over surgical biopsy. In women over 30, mammography is typically the first imaging modality. Breast MRI is not routinely used for initial evaluation and is reserved for diagnostic uncertainty, high-risk patients, or lesions suspected to be mammogram-occult. It has a high false-positive rate.

What Imaging Is Recommended for Working up a New Breast Mass in Women over 30?

A bilateral diagnostic mammogram and focused ultrasound should be ordered in a woman over the age of 30 with a new breast mass to better characterize the mass, and identify other non-palpable lesions in the affected breast, as well as examine the contralateral breast. Certain mammographic features such as asymmetry, clustered pleomorphic calcification, increasing density, or a new mass with irregular borders or spiculation are suggestive of malignancy. Once a mass is identified, a core needle biopsy should be performed to exclude cancer (◘ Fig. 6.1).

Watch Out
Some breast cancers may not be seen on mammogram or ultrasound but only on breast MRI. In these cases, an MRI-guided core needle biopsy should be performed.

What Metastatic Workup Is Recommended Following a Diagnosis of Breast Cancer?

For clinically early-stage breast cancer, an extensive metastatic workup is generally unnecessary. Additional work-up should be ordered only if the patient has signs and symptoms of metastatic disease or is clinically at high risk for metastatic disease.

How Is Breast Cancer Staged Clinically?

The most commonly used staging system is the one described by the American Joint Committee on Cancer (AJCC). *T* (tumor) describes the size of the tumor and/or its depth of invasion. *N* (node) describes spread to regional lymph nodes. *M* (metastasis) indicates if the

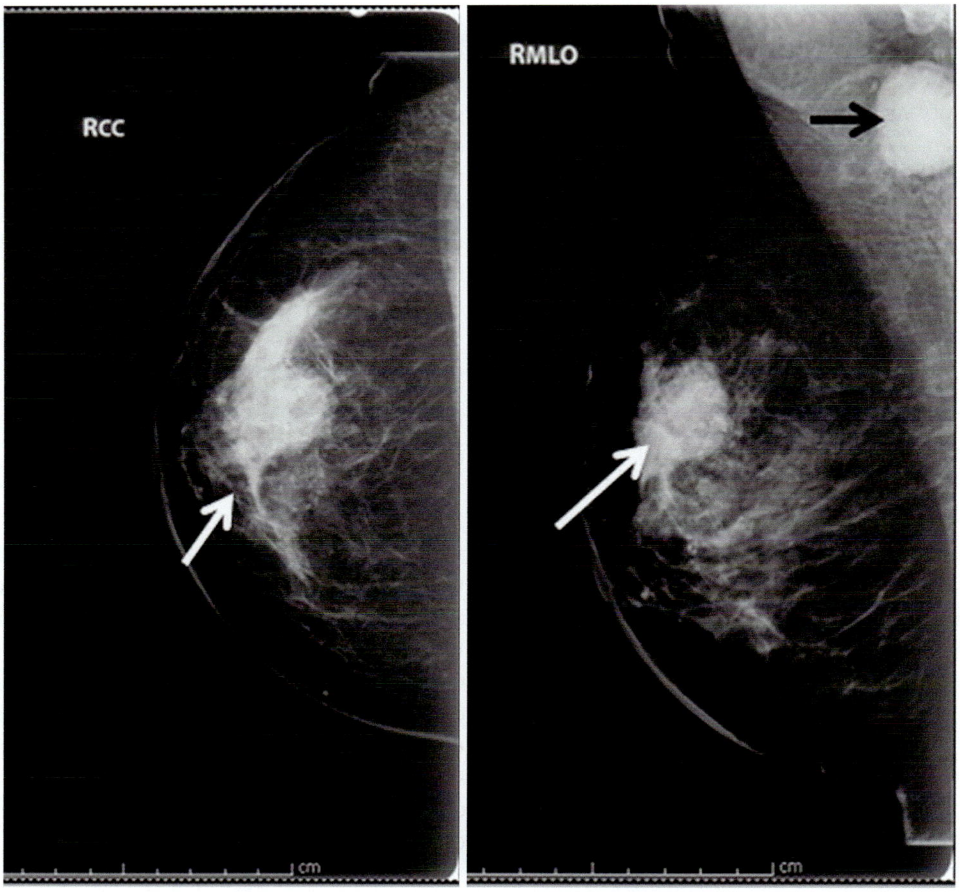

Fig. 6.1 Diagnostic mammogram with craniocaudal (CC) view (*left*) and mediolateral oblique (MLO) view (*right*). *White arrows: mass suspicious for malignancy. Black arrow: enlarged axillary lymph node suspicious for malignant involvement*

tumor has metastasized remotely. Differentiating between the different stages based on TNM classification is beyond the scope of this book.

Are Tumor Markers for Breast Cancer Utilized?

Although tumor markers for breast cancer exist (CA-15-3, CA 27.29, and CEA), they are not used routinely as not all patients with breast cancer have elevated levels. Additionally, these tumor markers have poor sensitivity and specificity, making them poor choices for screening tools.

What Is a Triple-Negative Breast Cancer?

This refers to breast cancer that is negative for estrogen (ER), progesterone (PR), and human epidermal growth factor-2 (HER-2) receptors. The fact that these breast cancers do not express these receptors makes them more difficult to treat with conventional therapy. Tumors that express ER/PR receptors are favorable because it allows for the option to employ hormonal drugs as adjuvant therapy to treat breast cancer. HER-2 is a protein that is found in approximately 20% of breast cancer, and anti-HER-2 therapy can help stop proliferation of cancer cells. However, HER-2-positive cancers tend to be more aggressive, and, in the past, breast cancer that is HER-2 positive was considered to have worse prognosis. With new therapies targeting HER-2, the prognosis for HER-2-positive breast cancer patients has improved considerably such that in the most recent AJCC prognostic staging, many HER-2-positive patients are now down-staged. The prognosis for triple-negative breast cancer has continued to be typically worse, requiring more aggressive therapy, although new combination systemic therapy has improved outcomes as well.

Watch Out

The majority of HER2-positive and triple-negative breast cancers are treated with neoadjuvant chemotherapy before surgery except in the earliest stages of breast cancer.

What Breast Cancer Subtype Do Patients with BRCA Develop?

Triple-negative tumors typically are the most common subtype in BRCA-1 carriers, demonstrate high histological grade, occur at a younger age (<40 years), and are found more commonly in Black women.

What Are the Unique Features of Invasive Lobular Carcinoma?

Invasive lobular carcinoma is typically hormone receptor positive and occurs more commonly in *premenopausal* women. The growth pattern is linear, making it difficult to visualize on mammogram and ultrasound.

How Is a Diagnosis of Inflammatory Breast Carcinoma Confirmed?

A core needle biopsy of the breast parenchyma showing malignancy is required to diagnose inflammatory breast carcinoma. Although not mandatory, a full-thickness punch biopsy of the dermis showing cancer cells invading dermal lymphatics can further support the diagnosis. The diagnosis is confirmed in a patient who has tissue-confirmed breast cancer along with physical findings of inflammation—such as erythema, swelling, and peau d'orange—that involve at least one-third of the breast.

How Should Fat Necrosis Be Worked Up?

Fat necrosis of the breast is a benign condition but can mimic breast cancer on physical exam and imaging, often presenting with skin or nipple retraction, calcifications on mammography, and a fixed, irregular mass. A core-needle biopsy can be performed if the diagnosis is unclear on imaging, which will demonstrate findings consistent with fat necrosis, such as fat globules and foamy histiocytes. Surgical excision is not recommended unless the diagnosis continues to be inconclusive.

Management

What Surgical Options Are Available for Patients with Early Breast Cancers Without Metastatic Spread?

The two basic options are breast-conserving therapy (BCT) and simple/total mastectomy. BCT consists of a lumpectomy (partial mastectomy) *and* radiation therapy (to decrease the risk of local recurrence). For patients with invasive breast cancers or for some patients with DCIS without palpable lymphadenopathy, a sentinel lymph node biopsy (SLNB) is also performed during breast surgery. BCT is typically reserved for early-stage breast cancers. The survival rate after BCT is equivalent to simple mastectomy while providing a more cosmetically appealing option for women.

> **Watch Out**
> High-risk features of DCIS include comedo-type, high-grade, >5 cm, palpable, and multifocal lesions.

What Is the Premise Behind SLNB?

A sentinel lymph node is the first node or group of nodes to which the lymphatics of the breast drain. The premise behind SLNB is that if the sentinel node is free of metastasis, then other lymph nodes in the axilla will also be disease-free, and, therefore, there is no need to remove the remaining lymph nodes in the axilla. SLNB is used for staging breast cancers and is performed intraoperatively by identifying, removing, and histologically examining the lymph node to determine if the cancer has spread to the lymph system. A radioactive technetium tracer and/or a blue dye (taken up by lymphatics) is first injected subareolarly. The lymph nodes that are radioactive and/or blue are then identified and considered the sentinel nodes and are removed.

> **Watch Out**
> Radioactive technetium tracer used in SLNB in patients undergoing BCT or simple mastectomy has been demonstrated to be safe for use in pregnancy, as the tracer remains localized in the breast tissue that is then removed. The blue dye should be avoided as it can potentially harm the fetus.

Why Does SLNB Need to Be Performed at the Same Time as a Mastectomy and Not Later?

If a mastectomy is planned, the SLNB needs to be performed at the same time. Once the breast is removed, SLNB is difficult to perform, as the breast tissue with accompanying lymphatics has been removed.

Can There Be More Than One Sentinel Node?

Yes, in most cases, there are 2–4 sentinel nodes.

What Do You Do If During SLNB No Sentinel Lymph Node Is Identified?

In most cases, the surgeon would proceed to axillary lymph node dissection (ALND). Whether to proceed with ALND depends on several factors, including the tumor status and patient comorbidities (a very elderly patient may forgo ALND).

What Are Contraindications to BCT?

Absolute contraindications are multiple primary tumors in two or more quadrants, diffuse malignant-appearing microcalcifications throughout the breast, previous history of chest wall radiation, positive surgical margins despite repeat excision, and first trimester pregnancy (as radiation cannot be given during pregnancy). However, it is possible to perform BCT in the second and third trimesters of pregnancy and then receive radiation therapy after childbirth. Relative contraindications are a history of collagen vascular disease and large tumors in a small breast in which adequate margins would result in a cosmetically undesired appearance.

Watch Out

In a woman with a history of non-Hodgkin lymphoma (mantle cell lymphoma) who now presents with invasive breast cancer, prior chest wall radiation therapy constitutes a contraindication to breast-conserving therapy. In such cases, the appropriate treatment is a simple or total mastectomy.

Can the Nipple and Breast Skin Be Spared During a Simple Mastectomy?

Yes, two other options for tumor resection are skin-sparing and nipple-sparing mastectomy. These approaches provide a skin envelope in order to accommodate a breast reconstruction with a better cosmetic outcome. Contraindications to nipple-sparing mastectomy include a breast cancer in close proximity to the nipple (<2 cm), nipple skin involvement, nipple discharge, previous breast surgery or radiation therapy that compromises blood flow to the nipple areolar complex, active smoking, significant comorbidities such as uncontrolled diabetes, and morbid obesity.

What Are the Management Options for Clinically Advanced Breast Cancers?

Clinically advanced breast cancer includes tumors >5 cm, skin involvement (e.g., inflammatory breast cancer), or large, matted axillary nodes. These patients typically receive neoadjuvant chemotherapy followed by surgery. Large tumors generally preclude breast conservation, requiring simple mastectomy. If axillary nodes are clinically positive and matted, sentinel lymph node biopsy is not appropriate, and axillary lymph node dissection (ALND) is required. When both a large tumor and clinically positive nodes are present, a modified radical mastectomy is performed. Inflammatory breast cancer also requires neoadjuvant chemotherapy, followed by modified radical mastectomy to ensure clear margins.

When Do You Perform ALND?

ALND involves removing Level I (lateral to the pectoralis minor muscle) and II (under the pectoralis minor muscle) axillary nodes. If the sentinel lymph node(s) is (are) positive for metastatic cancer, complete ALND is not necessarily needed. Recent studies have shown the safety of excluding ALND in patients with only 1–2 positive nodes who had undergone breast conservation therapy. Such patients should receive radiation to the remaining breast and low axilla.

What Are the Boundaries in the Axilla for Breast Dissection?

There are four boundaries: axillary vein (superior), floor of the axilla/subscapularis (posterior), latissimus dorsi muscle (lateral), and medial border of the pectoral minor muscle (medial).

To What Structure Are Axillary Lymph Node Levels Referenced?

Axillary lymph node levels are based on their location relative to the *pectoralis minor muscle*. Level I nodes are lateral to the muscle border, Level II nodes are located behind, and Level III nodes are medial. Rotter nodes are interpectoral (between pectoralis major and minor) and are technically Level II nodes.

Watch Out

In breast cancer, ALND requires removal of Level I and II nodes, while in melanoma, ALND requires removal of Level I, II, and III nodes.

What Is the Purpose of Axillary Lymph Node Dissection? Does It Affect Survival?

Axillary lymph node dissection is used for staging of breast cancer; removing the lymph nodes per se has not been shown to improve survival.

What Is the Treatment for Inflammatory Breast Carcinoma?

Treatment involves three phases: neoadjuvant chemotherapy to reduce tumor burden, followed by a modified radical mastectomy, and concluding with adjuvant radiation therapy to address any residual disease.

What Are the Options for Hormonal Therapy, and What Is the Premise Behind It?

Cancers that are ER + or PR + are candidates for (◘ Table 6.4). These drugs work by either decreasing the level of steroid hormones in the body or antagonizing the receptors that promote growth of cancer cells. They are most often used as adjuvant therapy to prevent recurrence.

What Study Must Be Done Prior to Starting Trastuzumab?

Since there is a high risk of cardiomyopathy in patients receiving trastuzumab, it is recommended that all patients receive an echocardiogram or a MUGA scan (more sensitive) to determine their ejection fraction.

Why Is an Aromatase Inhibitor (AI) Only Effective in Postmenopausal Women?

AI work by inhibiting the aromatase enzyme, located in fat tissue, which is responsible for making small amounts of estrogen in postmenopausal women. AIs are only effective in women with ovaries that have stopped producing estrogen, which occurs after menopause. The primary source of estrogen for these women is that which is produced in fat cells.

◘ Table 6.4 Hormonal therapy in breast cancer

Drug	Mechanism	Features
Tamoxifen	Blocks estrogen receptors	Acts like estrogen in some tissues (endometrial) but antiestrogen in others (*selective estrogen receptor modulator or SERM*); can be used to decrease incidence in high-risk women; increases risk for *endometrial cancer and blood clots*; taken for 5–10 years following surgery; can cause fatigue, hot flashes, and vaginal dryness
Raloxifene	Blocks estrogen receptors	Decreased risk of endometrial cancer when compared to tamoxifen, as effective as tamoxifen in reducing incidence of invasive breast cancer in high-risk postmenopausal women but does not reduce incidence of DCIS or LCIS
Fulvestrant	Blocks estrogen receptors	Works systemically (not a SERM), severe osteoporosis risk, only approved for *postmenopausal* women that have failed therapy with tamoxifen
Anastrozole	Aromatase inhibitor	Decreases estrogen levels, only effective in *postmenopausal* women, no risk of endometrial cancer, less risk of blood clots when compared to SERMs
Trastuzumab	Monoclonal antibody blocking HER-2 receptors	Reduces recurrence, improves overall survival, expensive, risk of cardiomyopathy

Does Everyone with Breast Cancer Require Chemotherapy?

No. Patients with noninvasive breast cancers (carcinoma in situ) do not benefit from systemic chemotherapy because the cancer cells have little risk for dissemination. In addition, certain very small invasive cancers (<0.5 cm) with favorable tumor receptors and a negative SLNB may not benefit from chemotherapy. In hormone receptor-positive, HER2-negative patients larger than 0.5 cm, the a 21-gene RT-PCR assay is strongly recommended. This test examines the individual patient's tumor characteristics at the molecular level, enabling the clinician to predict the likelihood of chemotherapy benefit as well as recurrence in early-stage breast cancer. Most patients that are ER-/PR-, HER2-positive or triple-negative should receive chemotherapy.

What Are the Most Common Chemotherapy Regimens?

Many options are available and should be tailored to the patient's type of breast cancer and personal medical history. The most commonly used drugs fall into four categories (■ Table 6.5).

Watch Out

Chemotherapy timed preoperatively (neoadjuvant) versus postoperatively (adjuvant) has the same survival outcome for all breast cancer subtypes.

What Are the Options for Breast Reconstruction? What Is the Timing?

Women undergoing a mastectomy may choose to have additional breast reconstruction surgery to retain their breast shape. The options are to perform an immediate or delayed reconstruction. Immediate reconstruction can be done with an autologous tissue flap (transverse rectus abdominal muscle or latissimus dorsi) or with a temporary tissue expander. The tissue expander is later replaced by a permanent implant once the skin is sufficiently stretched. If the patient desires an autogenous reconstruction but requires postoperative radiation therapy, then the reconstruction is often delayed (as the radiation may compromise the flap). On the other hand, tissue expanders can be placed immediately, regardless of whether radiation therapy is needed. The decision to perform a delayed reconstruction is based on several factors, including patient preference, surgeon availability, and patient risk factors.

■ **Table 6.5** Chemotherapeutic regimens for breast cancer

Class	Representatives	Mechanism	Risks
Anthracyclines	Doxorubicin, epirubicin, and idarubicin	Inhibits DNA/RNA synthesis, inhibits topoisomerase II, halting cell growth and division	Hair loss, vomiting, cardiomyopathy
Alkylating agent	Cyclophosphamide	Promotes DNA damage by alkylating guanine bases	Risk of leukemia, cystitis, and bladder cancer
Antimetabolites	Methotrexate and 5-FU	Interferes with DNA synthesis, halting cell growth and division	Hair loss, vomiting, bone marrow suppression
Taxanes	Paclitaxel and docetaxel	Inhibits mitotic phase in cell cycle	Neuropathy

Complications

What Nerves Are at Risk for Damage During ALND? (Table 6.6)

Table 6.6 Nerves at risk during axillary lymph node dissection

Nerve	Location	Muscle innervated	Deficit if damaged
Long thoracic	Travels along midaxillary line	Serratus anterior	Upward rotation, abduction, and weak elevation of the scapula (winged scapula)
Thoracodorsal	Travels lateral to long thoracic nerve	Latissimus dorsi	Weak extension, adduction, and internal rotation of shoulder joint
Medial pectoral	Travels lateral to or through the pectoral minor muscle and lateral to the lateral pectoral nerve	Pectoral minor *and* major	Weak internal rotation of humerus
Lateral pectoral	Travels medial to the medial pectoral nerve	Pectoral major	Weak flexion, adduction, and internal rotation of humerus

What Is the Most Morbid Complication of Lymph Node Dissection?

Lymphedema is the most morbid complication, resulting from the disruption of the normal flow within the lymph system. ALND is associated with a greater risk of lymphedema than SLNB. Lymphedema can lead to significant pain and disability in the affected arm. Patients with lymphedema also have an increased risk of cellulitis owing to the inability to properly mobilize the immune system.

What Does Long-Standing Lymphedema Increase Risk For?

In chronic cases, patients may develop lymphangiosarcoma (*Stewart-Treves syndrome*). Patients with lymphangiosarcoma will present with rapidly progressive, purpuric papulonodular lesions or red, bruise-like plaques with indistinct borders on the breast, axilla, or upper arm. These lesions arise due to tumor spread within the vasculature. Although primary angiosarcoma of the breast can also develop, secondary angiosarcoma is more likely to result in patients with chronic lymphedema. Diagnosis is confirmed via biopsy, and the prognosis remains poor even after limb amputation.

Watch Out

The use of sentinel lymph node biopsy (SLNB) in breast cancer can reduce the need for axillary lymph node dissection (ALND), thereby minimizing the risk of chronic lymphedema and its complications.

Areas You Can Get in Trouble

Ignoring a Breast Mass During Pregnancy

Traditionally, breast cancer in pregnancy has been rare. Stage for stage, prognosis appears to be the same as for nonpregnant women. However, pregnant women with breast cancer are often diagnosed at later stages. This is a result of denser breast tissue, which can make breast masses harder to visualize on mammogram. In addition, the hormonal changes that take place during pregnancy can obscure any signs or symptoms that may have otherwise prompted a patient to seek a doctor's advice. A pregnant patient's breast is larger, more tender, and lumpier. Delayed diagnosis remains to be the biggest challenge in dealing with breast cancer in pregnancy. Radiation and hormonal therapy are *never* recommended during pregnancy. Neoadjuvant chemotherapy is an option in the second trimester. BCT is an appropriate option during the second and third trimester with the radiation postponed until after delivery.

Ignoring a Breast Mass in an Elderly Male

Men have breast tissue and as such can also develop breast cancer. Breast cancer in males is rare (1% of all breast cancers), with most cases identified as invasive ductal carcinoma. DCIS is less common, as most men present late, with a palpable mass. Since lobules are not fully formed in men, LCIS and lobular breast cancer are extremely rare. The biggest risk factor is age, with most men diagnosed between 65 and 70 years. High estrogen levels promote breast cell growth, which can lead to cancer. Hormonal medications, obesity, alcohol abuse, cirrhosis, and Klinefelter syndrome can all lead to high serum estrogen levels. Additional risk factors include family history of breast cancer, genetic defects (BRCA-2 is a stronger risk factor in men), and radiation therapy to the chest wall (e.g., Hodgkin's disease). The impression that breast cancer in males has a worse prognosis when compared to women may be a result of diagnosing men at later stages of the disease. However, the overall survival, stage for stage, is similar to that of women with the same stage of breast cancer.

Watch Out

Gynecomastia is *not* a risk factor for male breast cancer.

Area of Controversy

How Aggressive Should Therapy Be for Early-Stage Breast Cancer?

Several randomized controlled trials have recently been published on the subject of de-escalation of therapy for patients with early-stage breast cancer. There is now evidence that in many patients, especially in the postmenopausal patient population, traditional surgical procedures and adjuvant therapies such as SNLB, radiation therapy, and chemotherapy can be omitted to avoid unnecessary interventions or treatments.

Summary of Essentials

History and Physical

- A new breast mass in postmenopausal women is cancer until proven otherwise
- Breast cancer: firm with irregular borders
- Nipple discharge that is bloody, spontaneous, unilateral, uniductal, and associated with a breast mass or occurs in women over 40 years is more suspicious for cancer
- Risk factors: family history, genetic mutations (BRCA-1 or BRCA-2), obesity, early menarche, late menopause, nulliparity or childbirth after age 30, alcohol, and radiation to the chest

Etiology/Pathophysiology

- Fibrocystic disease: most common cause of a palpable breast mass
- One in eight women in the United States will develop breast cancer
- Invasive ductal carcinoma: most common malignant breast neoplasm
- Fibroadenoma: most common benign breast tumor
- Triple-negative breast cancer: negative for estrogen, progesterone, and HER-2 receptors

Diagnosis

- Apply triple test (physical exam, imaging, tissue sample) to all new breast masses.
- Imaging:
  - ≤30 years old—ultrasound
  - >30 years old—mammogram plus ultrasound
- Tissue diagnosis is indicated for any clinically suspicious mass regardless of imaging findings; core-needle biopsy is preferred

Management

- For early stage (no nodal-disease or distant metastasis)
  - Lumpectomy, SLNB, and radiation (BCT)
  - Total/simple mastectomy and SLNB
- Equal in terms of survival
- SLNB:
  - Average 2–4 sentinel nodes
  - Less lymphedema than ALND
  - If positive for metastasis may need ALND
- ALND:
  - Level I and II nodes
  - Part of a modified radical mastectomy procedure
- For advanced or high-risk cancers, treatment must be individualized:
  - For inflammatory breast cancer, neoadjuvant chemotherapy followed by modified radical mastectomy and then radiation therapy
  - For large tumors, BCT not an option
  - For clinically positive axillary lymph nodes, SLNB not an option; proceed to ALND
- Drugs:
  - Trastuzumab for HER-2 positive
  - Tamoxifen for premenopausal estrogen receptor positive
  - Anastrozole (aromatase inhibitor) for postmenopausal estrogen receptor positive
  - Most patients receive hormonal therapy

Complications

- ALND can lead to significant morbidity
  - Lymphedema
  - Lymphangiosarcoma
  - Nerve injury (long thoracic, thoracodorsal, medial, and lateral pectoral nerves)

Watch Out

- Men can get breast cancer (usually invasive ductal carcinoma)
- Do not confuse inflammatory breast cancer with cellulitis
- Do not ignore breast masses during pregnancy or in younger women

Suggested Reading

Anderson WF, Althuis MD, Brinton LA, Devesa SS. Is male breast cancer similar or different than female breast cancer? Breast Cancer Res Treat 2004;83:77.

Bauer K, Brown M, Cress RD, Parise CA, Caggiano V. Descriptive analysis of estrogen receptor (ER)-negative, progesterone receptor (PR)-negative, and HER2-negative invasive breast cancer, the so-called triple-negative phenotype: a population-based study from the California cancer Registry. Cancer 2007;109(9):1721–8.

Edge SB, Byrd DR, Compton CC, et al., editors. AJCC (American Joint Committee on Cancer). Cancer staging manual. 7th. New York: Springer; 2010. p. 347.

Nelson HD, Tyne K, Naik A, et al. Screening for breast cancer: an update for the U.S. Preventive Services Task Force. Ann Intern Med 2009;151:727.

Sullivan T, Raad RA, Goldberg S, et al. Tubular carcinoma of the breast: a retrospective analysis and review of the literature. Breast Cancer Res Treat 2005;93:199.

Vaidya JS, Wenz F, Bulsara M, et al. Risk-adapted targeted intraoperative radiotherapy versus whole-breast radiotherapy for breast cancer: 5-year results for local control and overall survival from the TARGIT-A randomised trial. Lancet 2014;383(9917):603–13.

Recently Changed Skin Lesion

James McDermott, Arezou Yaghoubian, and Junko Ozao-Choy

Contents

C. de Virgilio, A. Grigorian (eds.), *Surgery*, https://doi.org/10.1007/978-3-032-09799-6_7

Case Study

A 44-year-old fair-skinned Caucasian male who works as a lifeguard presents with a 1 cm pigmented skin lesion on the right forearm that has recently changed colors and become larger in diameter. The patient denies itching, oozing, or bleeding associated with the lesion. He has a history of severe blistering sunburns during childhood. The lesion is slightly elevated and asymmetric with ill-defined borders. There is no evidence of bleeding, ulceration, or excoriation. There are no satellite lesions seen. Examination of the patient's right axilla and neck reveals no obvious lymphadenopathy. No other skin lesions are identified on physical examination.

Diagnosis

What Is the Differential Diagnosis? (Table 7.1)

Table 7.1 Differential diagnosis of clinical presentation

Diagnosis	Malignant?	Comments
Junctional nevi	No	Dark, flat, smooth lesions; they are occasionally hairy and develop from the basal layer of epidermis; nevi on palms and soles are usually junctional; benign lesions with very low risk of malignant degeneration; the *most common mole in children*
Compound nevi	No	Brown to black, well-circumscribed, <1 cm in diameter; may be elevated, frequently hairy, arise from epidermal-dermal interface and from within dermis; malignant transformation is rare
Intradermal nevi	No	Light-colored, well-circumscribed, <1 cm in diameter; hairs are usually present, cell distribution occurs in the dermis; the *most common mole in adults*
Giant congenital nevi	No	Brown to black, hairy, >20 cm in diameter, irregular nodular surface; frequently described as a bathing trunk or coat sleeve type of lesion; *excision is recommended*
Spitz nevi	No	Smooth, round, pink-black, 1–2 cm in diameter, found mainly in children; increased cellularity occurs in nests within the upper dermis; atypical nevi have a small risk of malignant degeneration
Pigmented actinic keratosis	No	Premalignant, caused by sun exposure, sandpaper texture, small, rough, erythematous, or brownish papules, often on the face, back, or neck, also called "cutaneous horn"
Keratoacanthoma	No	Well-differentiated, originating from the pilosebaceous glands, develo+ps rapidly and regresses spontaneously (outgrows blood supply and necroses) and presents as a cup-shaped tumor filled with keratin debris
Seborrheic keratosis	No	Common in the elderly, presents as raised, discolored plaques, coin-like, waxy, "stuck-on" appearance
Dysplastic nevus	No	Large, pigmented, irregular border, frequently occurs on the back, chest, buttocks, breast, and scalp, and can be found in sun-exposed and sun-protected areas; typically excised
Melanoma	Yes	Proliferation of melanocytes, the most common cause of death from skin cancer, presents as a mole-like growth with "ABCDE" (see below)
Squamous cell carcinoma (SCC)	Yes	Proliferation of squamous cells characterized by formation of keratin pearls presents as an ulcerated, nodular mass with no telangiectasias, usually on the face (classically involving the lower lip)
Basal cell carcinoma (BCC)	Yes	Most common cutaneous malignancy presents as an elevated, pearl-like nodule with a central, ulcerated crater surrounded by telangiectasias (classically involving the upper lip)
Metastatic tumors to the skin	Yes	In males, the most common sources are malignant melanoma (30%), lung, colon, carcinoma of the oral cavity, larynx, and kidney; in females, the most common sources are breast (70%), followed by melanoma, and ovary

What Is the Most Likely Diagnosis?

In a patient presenting with a recently changed skin lesion that has become variegated and larger in diameter with an asymmetric, irregular border, the most likely diagnosis is melanoma. Additionally, the patient's fair skin, occupation as a lifeguard, and history of blistering childhood sunburns further increase his risk of developing skin cancer.

History and Physical

What Risk Factors for Skin Cancer Are Common to SCC, BCC, and Melanoma?

A common pathway for increased risk for skin cancer (SCC, BCC, and melanoma) is excessive exposure to ultraviolet (UV) light, particularly UV-B (remember, B for Bad). Occupations that involve long-term sun exposure place patients at higher risk, such as a lifeguard, farmer, construction worker, gardener, and field worker. Immunosuppression is another recognized risk factor. For SCC and BCC, the risk is greatest with cumulative long-term UV exposure. With melanoma, both blistering sunburns and overall sun exposure are risk factors. Skin cancer is also more common in patients who have fair skin and hair, as well as in those with blue eyes.

What Factors During Childhood/Teen Years Are Associated with an Increased Risk of Skin Cancer?

A blistering sunburn in childhood or adolescence more than doubles the chance of developing skin cancer, as does the use of a tanning salon.

What Genetic Conditions Are Associated with an Increased Risk of Skin Cancer?

Xeroderma pigmentosum is a rare autosomal recessive condition that leads to photosensitivity due to deficient repair of DNA damaged by UV radiation. It leads to a very high rate of melanoma, BCC, and SCC at an early age.

What Are Findings on Physical Examination That Differentiate a Benign Nevus from Melanoma?

The "ABCDEs" of melanoma (◘ Table 7.2) can serve as a memory tool to help remember the common differentiating characteristics. However, not all melanomas follow the ABCDE rule (i.e., nodular melanomas).

◘ **Table 7.2** "ABCDEs" of melanoma

A	Asymmetry of lesion	Is the lesion round and symmetric (mole) or does it look asymmetric (melanoma)?
B	Border irregularity	Do the borders of the lesion seem smooth and circumscribed (mole) or are they jagged and indistinct (melanoma)?
C	Color variegation (different colors)	Does the lesion have one even pigmented color (mole) or does it have several shades of pigment (melanoma)?
D	Diameter >6 mm	Is the lesion bigger than about the size of a pencil eraser (melanoma)?
E	Evolution (changing lesion)	Are there any big changes, such as rapid growth, bleeding, or ulceration in the lesion (melanoma)?

> **Watch Out**
> Hair growth on a skin lesion suggests that it is a benign nevus. Melanomas destroy hair follicles.

What Is the Ugly Duckling Sign?

The ugly duckling sign is a concept that emerged after recognizing the limitations in the ABCDE mnemonic. Any skin lesion that looks different or out of place (and thus, an "ugly duckling") in a nest of other similar appearing lesions is suspicious and recommended for biopsy.

Why Is It Important to Inquire About and Examine Areas of Chronic Skin Inflammation?

Chronic skin inflammation is a known risk factor for SCC. It can develop in chronic open burn wounds (Marjolin's ulcer), chronic venous ulcers, and hidradenitis suppurativa.

> **Watch Out**
> Chronically non-healing wounds should be biopsied to rule out malignancy, particularly SCC.

On What Areas of the Skin Are Melanomas Most Likely to Occur in Non-White Patients?

In Black, Asian, and Hawaiian populations, melanomas most commonly occur on nonexposed areas of skin with less pigmentation, such as the palms, soles, mucous membranes, and nail beds.

What Is the Most Common Site of Melanoma in Men Versus Women?

For men, the back is the most common site, while the legs are the most common site for women.

What Is the Most Common Site of Digital Melanoma?

Great toe. Toe amputation and sentinel lymph node biopsy are the preferred treatment.

Does the Regular Use of SPF Protection Reduce the Risk of Skin Cancer?

Yes, regular daily use of an SPF-15 or higher sunscreen reduces the risk of developing SCC and melanoma by about half.

What Is Suggested by a Bright, Red, Raised Plaque in an Infant?

An infantile hemangioma is a benign vascular tumor that appears as a bright red, raised plaque within days to weeks after birth. It proliferates rapidly during infancy and typically begins to regress spontaneously in early childhood. Most hemangiomas are managed with observation. However, certain features, such as a segmental distribution, scarring, or a periorbital location, warrant further evaluation or treatment. Oral propranolol is the preferred treatment for high-risk hemangiomas, as it promotes regression through vasoconstriction.

Pathophysiology

What Is a Nevus? What Are Dysplastic Nevi? Are Nevi at Risk for Malignant Transformation?

A nevus is a mole. It is very rare for common moles to become malignant. Dysplastic nevi are irregular moles, often with a central elevation and a peripheral pigmented rim, giving a "fried egg" appearance. Though they are benign, there is a low risk that they can become malignant. Patients with 50 or more common moles or those with 10 or more dysplastic nevi are at increased risk of developing melanoma. However, melanoma most often develops in areas of skin without nevi. As such, there is no reason to remove common nevi, but dysplastic nevi should be excised. If the nevus is severely dysplastic with positive or close margins, the patient may require re-excision.

What Is Dysplastic Nevus Syndrome?

Dysplastic nevus syndrome (also called familial atypical multiple mole-melanoma syndrome) is an autosomal dominant disorder characterized by multiple dysplastic nevi with an increased risk of progression to melanoma (10% risk). These patients have a family history of melanoma, 100 or more moles, and at least 2 large dysplastic nevi.

From Where Does Melanoma Arise?

Melanoma originates from melanocytes, which are derived from neural crest cells. It can arise from a preexisting nevus or de novo as a new pigmented lesion (although a small percentage can be *amelanotic*).

What Is the Most Common Skin Cancer? Second Most Common? Which Skin Cancer Is Associated with the Greatest Number of Deaths?

7

BCC is the most common skin cancer (and the most common overall cancer), followed by SCC, whereas melanoma accounts for the most deaths. An elderly patient with significant sun exposure, presenting with an ulcerated nodule on a sun-exposed area featuring prominent telangiectasias, would raise concern for BCC, often described as a “pink, pearly papule.”

What Is the Most Common Precancerous Skin Lesion?

Actinic keratosis is the most common precancerous skin lesion. It is a rough, scaly epidermal lesion that occurs in an area of the body subjected to chronic sun exposure. The risk of actinic keratosis undergoing malignant transformation to SCC is about 1% per year. Some actinic keratoses can be pigmented.

Watch Out
A keratoacanthoma presents as a rapidly growing nodule with ulceration and a central keratin plug. Although it frequently regresses and may resolve spontaneously over several months, some keratoacanthomas can progress to invasive squamous cell carcinoma.

What Is Bowen’s Disease?

Bowen’s disease is a squamous cell carcinoma (SCC) in situ, confined to the epidermis without dermal invasion. It typically presents as a well-demarcated, erythematous plaque with a scaly or crusted surface. Although it does not metastasize in its in situ form, untreated lesions may gradually evolve into invasive squamous cell carcinoma, at which point there is a risk of regional or distant spread.

What Is the Metastatic Risk of BCC, SCC, and Melanoma?

BCC can be locally destructive; however, metastases are rare. SCC does metastasize, but much less commonly than melanoma. The most common site for melanoma to metastasize is to *other areas of the skin including subcutaneous tissues*, followed by the lung, liver, brain, and bone.

Watch Out
The most common metastasis to the small bowel is melanoma.

What Are the Four Subtypes of Melanoma? (Table 7.3)

Table 7.3 Four subtypes of melanoma

Type	Prevalence	Features
Superficial spreading	50–60%	Most common type; typically has a long horizontal growth phase before the vertical growth phase
Lentigo maligna	4–10%	Lentiginous proliferation indicates the tumor remains at the junction (in situ); best prognosis; aka “Hutchinson freckle”
Acral lentiginous	2–3%	Typically found in the subungual, sole, or palm location; common in ethnic groups of color; *not* related to UV light exposure
Nodular	10–30%	Worst prognosis due to rapid vertical growth; increased metastatic potential; 5% amelanotic (very difficult to detect)

> **Watch Out**
> Lentigo maligna has the best prognosis of the four melanoma subtypes; remember, *Lentigo is Least aggressive*.

What Is the Breslow Depth?

Breslow depth is based on the actual depth of invasion, which is the vertical height of the melanoma from the granular layer to the deepest area of penetration and is measured in millimeters (Table 7.4). Breslow thickness correlates directly with the risk of local recurrence, metastasis, and survival rate.

Table 7.4 Breslow thickness 5-year survival

Depth	5-year survival
<0.75 mm	95–100%
0.75–1.5 mm	80–96%
1.5–4.0 mm	60–75%
>4.0 mm	50%

Workup

What Are the Different Types of Skin Biopsy?

Suspicious skin lesions should undergo biopsy to establish a diagnosis, with options including excisional and incisional biopsies. An excisional biopsy removes the entire lesion, making it ideal for small lesions, as it provides a complete sample for thorough examination. In contrast, an incisional biopsy removes only part of the lesion, which is useful when the lesion is large or located in a cosmetically sensitive area, as it avoids unnecessary removal of the entire lesion if it is benign.

Shave biopsies, performed with a razor blade or scalpel, remove a slice or disk of skin and are suitable for lesions that appear confined to the epidermis, such as skin tags, warts, suspected actinic keratosis, or basal cell cancer. However, shave biopsies are not recommended for suspected melanoma because they can lead to inaccurate measurement of Breslow thickness.

Punch biopsies, which extend into the dermis and subcutaneous tissue, are used for larger lesions, when a sample of deeper tissue is needed, or when the lesion is in a cosmetically sensitive location like the face. This method is advantageous for large suspicious moles, as it avoids complete excision unless the lesion is confirmed to be malignant, in which case the entire lesion will need to be excised with appropriate margins.

For the patient in the vignette with a small forearm lesion suspected to be melanoma, a shave biopsy would be inappropriate due to the risk of miscalculating Breslow depth. Instead, a punch biopsy or an excisional biopsy would be more suitable options.

Once the Diagnosis of Melanoma Is Established, What Additional Studies Should Be Obtained?

If the patient has no symptoms or signs of advanced disease, no additional workup is recommended. Additional workup is recommended if the patient has enlarged lymph nodes, unexplained weight loss, or jaundice. If clinically palpable lymph nodes are present, the patient should have lactate dehydrogenase (LDH) drawn and undergo a CT scan of the chest, abdomen, and pelvis, and a PET scan to rule out metastatic disease. An ultrasound of the enlarged node and a core biopsy of the nodes prior to surgery may also be recommended. An MRI of the brain may also be indicated if the patient has symptoms of CNS metastasis (e.g., motor deficits, seizures, headaches). LDH is a prognostic indicator in melanoma and has been found to be indicative of liver metastases.

What Are Poor Prognostic Indicators with Melanoma?

Thicker lesions, *ulceration*, high mitotic rate, lymph node involvement, distant metastasis, elevated LDH level, location on trunk, and male gender.

Management

What Treatment Options Exist for Skin Cancers? (Table 7.5)

Table 7.5 Treatment options for skin cancer

Treatment	Comments
Electrodissection/curettage	Can result in a 95% cure rate in BCC; however, the disadvantage is a lack of specimens for determining the adequacy of resection
Topical therapies	Includes imiquimod and 5-FU (for BCC when surgical treatment is not feasible)
Surgical excision	Removes entire skin cancer with a border of normal appearing skin; this is the preferred treatment for skin cancers
Radiation	Recommended choice when excision is not possible or used as adjuvant therapy when there are high-risk lesions
Cryotherapy	Liquid nitrogen is used to freeze and destroy cancerous tissue; it is best for precancerous or very superficial lesions

7

What Is the Primary Therapy for BCC/SCC Skin Cancers?

Complete surgical excision of the lesion with negative margins. Patients with lesions in cosmetically sensitive areas, aggressive tumor features, ill-defined lesions, or recurrent BCC/SCC are candidates for Mohs surgery (discussed below).

What Type of Surgical Margins Do You Need for BCC Versus SCC?

BCC needs 3–5 mm, while SCC needs 5–10 mm.

Watch Out
If margins are positive, it is essential to re-excise the incision to clear margins.

How Is Melanoma Surgically Managed?

If the patient underwent an excisional biopsy, since the intent is to establish a diagnosis and not perform a curative resection, the area needs to be surgically re-excised with appropriate margins once the diagnosis of melanoma is established (Table 7.6). In select cases, a sentinel lymph node biopsy (SLNB) is also performed. The extent of margins and need for SLNB are determined by tumor thickness.

Table 7.6 Melanoma excision

Tumor thickness	Excision margin	Lymph node management
Melanoma in situ	0.5–1 cm	None
≤1 mm	1 cm	Consider SLNB for high-risk features[a]
1–2 mm	1–2 cm	SLNB
>2 mm	2 cm	SLNB

[a]Lymphovascular invasion, positive deep margin on biopsy (0.8 mm), ulceration, high mitotic rate, younger patients (<40 years)

What Is the Purpose of the SLNB, and How Is It Performed?

SLNB is used to detect clinically occult regional lymph node metastases in patients with melanoma. After lymphoscintigraphy is performed to identify the primary draining lymph node (sentinel node), this node is excised and examined histologically. SLNB is primarily a prognostic tool in selected high-risk patients. If the sentinel node is negative for malignancy, no further nodal surgery is needed, thereby avoiding the morbidity of complete lymph node dissection (CLND), which carries a significant risk of lymphedema. If the sentinel node is positive, the benefit of proceeding with CLND remains an area of ongoing debate (see below).

How Is Melanoma of the Fingernail Managed?

Acral-lentiginous melanoma is found beneath the nail, on the palm of the hand, or on the sole of the foot. These lesions represent approximately 3% of all cutaneous melanomas. The prognosis for subungual melanomas is worse than that of other cutaneous melanomas, probably because of the delay in diagnosis. Management requires amputation of the digit at the joint just proximal to the lesion, as well as an SLNB if indicated by Breslow depth.

What Is the Prognosis for Melanoma?

When disease is confined to the primary site, 5-year survival is >99%. If lymph nodes are involved, this decreases to 75%. For those with distant metastases, the 5-year survival is 35%.

What Is the Follow-Up Protocol for Melanoma?

Melanoma surveillance protocols depend on the stage of disease. Most patients with advanced melanoma require a physical examination at 3–6-month intervals over the course of the first 3–5 years. Regional lymph node disease is the most common type of recurrence.

What Is Mohs Surgery? What Are the Main Indications for Its Use? Is It Appropriate for the Treatment of Melanoma?

Mohs micrographic surgery is a technique that combines surgical excision with immediate microscopic examination of margins, allowing for precise, layer-by-layer removal of cancerous tissue. This approach enables maximal tissue preservation while achieving clear margins, reducing the need for wide excisions. Mohs surgery is considered first-line treatment for high-risk nonmelanoma skin cancers such as basal cell carcinoma and squamous cell carcinoma, particularly when lesions are located in cosmetically or functionally sensitive areas like the face. It is generally not used for invasive melanoma due to the difficulty of assessing melanocytes on frozen sections and the need for wider margins; however, it may be considered for select cases of melanoma in situ when appropriate immunostaining techniques are available.

Areas Where You Can Get in Trouble

Assuming That a Discolored Nail Bed Is a Benign Condition

Blackened or darkened toenails may represent benign conditions and may be difficult to distinguish from a subungual melanoma on physical examination. Benign conditions include subungual hematoma (bleeding under the nail bed from trauma), benign streaks in the nail plate, benign subungual nevus, and onychomycosis. Subungual hematomas grow out with the nail. Dermoscopy can be helpful in distinguishing melanoma from a subungual hematoma. If the area is suspicious, a full-thickness biopsy through the nail bed should be performed. The presence of atypia or melanoma in situ requires complete excision with clear margins.

Pink Nodule Progressing to a Blue Color in an Immunocompromised Patient

Elderly patients that are immunocompromised (e.g., HIV, lymphoma, leukemia) may develop Merkel cell carcinoma (MCC) which is now thought to arise from epidermal or dermal stem cells, as opposed to Merkel cells (specialized touch receptor cells in the epidermis of the skin). Though the exact cause of MCC is unclear, MCC has been linked to exposure to UV light and infection by the Merkel cell polyomavirus. The nodule first appears pink and progresses to a blue-violaceous color and rapidly expands. Treatment involves wide local excision with 1–2 cm margins, SLNB, radiation, chemotherapy, and/or immunotherapy depending on the stage and extent of the disease.

Pyoderma Gangrenosum

Pyoderma gangrenosum is a rare, non-infectious, and non-cancerous ulcerative condition characterized by rapidly progressive, painful ulcers with a purulent base and violaceous border, often following minor trauma (pathergy). This condition is frequently associated with systemic inflammatory diseases, such as rheumatoid arthritis and inflammatory bowel disease. Diagnosis is clinical, typically following a biopsy to exclude other etiologies. Treatment generally involves corticosteroids.

Melanoma Recurring Many Years After Initial Presentation

Recurrence of melanoma may present years or even decades later (dormant melanoma). These patients will often have a clue on H&P that indicates a resected melanoma from early in life (i.e., missing toe). A patient with a history of melanoma who presents with a small bowel obstruction should be suspected of having metastatic melanoma to the small bowel.

Areas of Controversy

Is There Any Benefit for Surgical Resection for Stage IV (Distant Metastasis) Melanoma?

The MSLT-I trial demonstrated the benefit of metastasectomy (resection of metastatic lesions) in patients with stage IV resectable disease. The National

Comprehensive Cancer Network (NCCN) guidelines support considering surgical resection of metastatic melanoma lesions in select patients, particularly when the metastases are limited and can be completely resected. This approach should be considered as part of a multimodal treatment strategy that may include systemic therapies such as immunotherapy or targeted therapy.

Role for Completion Lymph Node Dissection (CLND)

One area of controversy is the role of CLND in patients with a positive sentinel lymph node biopsy. While CLND can improve staging and regional control, it has not demonstrated a survival benefit compared to observation with ultrasound surveillance, as indicated by the MSLT-II and DeCOG-SLT trials. The NCCN guidelines now suggest that the decision to perform CLND should be individualized. Patients with a positive SLNB may be managed with ultrasound surveillance rather than routine CLND, particularly in the absence of clinically palpable lymph nodes. The choice between CLND and ultrasound surveillance should consider the patient's morbidity risks (lymphedema, nerve damage), tumor burden, high-risk features, and patient preference.

Summary of Essentials

History and Physical

- New skin lesions require a thorough skin assessment and clinical evaluation of relevant nodal basins
- ABCDEs of melanoma can help differentiate it from a benign nevus

Differential Diagnosis

- Benign nevi
  - Spitz tumor, junctional nevi, compound nevi, intradermal nevi, and giant/congenital pigmented nevi
- Other benign and precancerous
  - Actinic keratosis, dermatofibroma, keratoacanthoma, seborrheic keratosis, and dysplastic nevus
- Cancer
  - BCC, SCC, and melanoma

Pathology/Pathophysiology

- Skin cancer incidence: BCC > SCC > melanoma
- Metastatic risk: melanoma > SCC > BCC (can be locally destructive; metastasis is rare)
  - Melanoma is a proliferation of melanocytes, derived from neural crest cells
  - Staged by Breslow thickness based on depth of invasion

Workup

- Biopsy all suspicious lesions
  - Excisional biopsy if small
  - Punch biopsy if large
- Melanoma
  - CXR, LFTs, LDH, and CBC if clinical evidence of advanced disease
  - PET and CT if clinically palpable nodes

Management

- Melanoma
  - Re-excise with margins based on Breslow depth
  - Selective SLNB based on Breslow depth
  - Adjuvant immunotherapy for high-risk patients
- BCC/SCC
  - 3–5 mm margins (BCC)
  - 5–10 mm margins (SCC)
  - Mohs
    - Tissue sparing
    - For cosmetically sensitive areas

Watch Out

- Shave biopsies should not be performed for suspected melanoma
- Nodular and amelanotic melanomas do not follow the ABCDE rule

Suggested Reading

American Cancer Society. Survival rates for melanoma skin cancer. Last Revised: January 17, 2024

Balch CM, Gershenwald JE, Soong SJ, et al. Final version of 2009 AJCC melanoma staging and classification. J Clin Oncol 2009;27:6199.

Bello DM, Faries MB. The landmark series: MSLT-1, MSLT-2 and DeCOG (management of lymph nodes). Ann Surg Oncol 2020;27(1):15-21. doi:https://doi.org/10.1245/s10434-019-07830-w

Markovic SN, Erickson LA, Rao RD, et al. Melanoma Study Group of the Mayo Clinic Cancer Center, Malignant melanoma in the 21st Century, part 1: epidemiology, risk factors, screening, prevention, and diagnosis. Mayo Clin Proc 2007;82(3):364–80.

Rigel DS, Russak J, Friedman R. The evolution of melanoma diagnosis: 25 years beyond the ABCDs. CA Cancer J Clin 2010;60:301.

Swetter SM, Tsao H, Bichakjian CK, Curiel-Lewandrowski C, Elder DE, Gershenwald JE, Guild V, Grant-Kels JM, Halpern AC, Johnson TM, Sober AJ, Thompson JA, Wisco OJ, Wyatt S, Hu S, Lamina T. Guidelines of care for the management of primary cutaneous melanoma. J Am Acad Dermatol 2019;80(1):208-250. doi: https://doi.org/10.1016/j.jaad.2018.08.055. Epub 2018 Nov 1.

Breast and Skin

Question Set: Breast and Skin

Questions

1. A 34-year-old woman presents to the clinic with recurrent painful bumps in her groin and axillae. She reports that these areas frequently swell, and drain foul-smelling fluid. She has been treated in the past with incision and drainage of abscesses, but the lesions keep returning. On physical exam, there are several tender subcutaneous nodules in the bilateral axillae without sinus tracts or scarring. Which of the following is the most appropriate next step in management?
   (A) Incision and drainage
   (B) Oral corticosteroids
   (C) Wide local excision
   (D) Oral tetracycline
   (E) Radiation therapy

2. A 25-year-old female lifeguard presents to her doctor to discuss a new 10 mm skin lesion that she found on her right forearm that has been growing over the last month. The lesion is a dark blue color, is symmetric, and has been growing vertically. What is the most likely diagnosis?
   (A) Impetigo
   (B) Melanoma
   (C) Nevus
   (D) Molluscum contagiosum
   (E) Squamous cell carcinoma (SCC)

3. A 36-year-old woman is evaluated for a lump in her right breast that she noticed 5 months ago. She denies any nipple discharge, retraction, or skin changes. She has no family history of breast cancer. On physical exam, the breasts appear normal. Palpation reveals a 1 cm dominant lump in the upper outer quadrant of the right breast that does not appear to be fixed to the surrounding structures. The patient has no other dominant masses in either breast. There is no axillary lymphadenopathy. Mammogram and ultrasound do not demonstrate any suspicious lesions. What is the next step in the management?
   (A) Ultrasound-guided core needle biopsy
   (B) Fine-needle aspiration (FNA)
   (C) MRI
   (D) Follow-up clinical breast exam in 3 months
   (E) Genetic testing

4. A 31-year-old breastfeeding female comes to the doctor for localized swelling, redness, and pain of the left breast. She also reports muscle aches and fatigue. On physical exam her temperature is 38.0 °C, pulse is 82/min, blood pressure is 126/68 mmHg, and respirations are 16/min. Physical exam reveals a localized area of erythema and warmth in the left breast with no palpable masses. There is no axillary lymphadenopathy. What is the most likely next course of action?
(A) Biopsy
(B) Antibiotic treatment and continue breastfeeding
(C) Antibiotic treatment and encourage bottle-feeding only
(D) Diagnostic mammography
(E) Incision and drainage

5. A 33-year-old female of Scottish descent presents with a nodule on her face near the corner of her eye. The lesion measures 13 mm in diameter. The borders are irregular, and the center of the lesion is dark. Which of the following is the best recommendation?
(A) Shave biopsy
(B) Punch biopsy
(C) Excisional biopsy with 1 mm margin
(D) Excisional biopsy with 5 mm margin
(E) Reexamination in 2 months

6. A 71-year-old woman is evaluated for a lump in her right breast that she noticed 3 weeks ago. She denies any nipple discharge, retraction, or skin changes. She has a sister diagnosed with breast cancer at the age of 57. The patient had menarche at the age of 9 and menopause at the age of 56. She had two children, one at the age of 39 and the other at the age of 41. On physical exam, the breasts are normal on inspection. Palpation reveals a 1.5 cm dominant lump that does not appear to be fixed to the surrounding structures. The patient has no other dominant masses in either breast. There is no axillary lymphadenopathy. What is the strongest risk factor in this patient predisposing her to breast cancer?
(A) Early menarche
(B) Family history of breast cancer
(C) Older age
(D) Age at first pregnancy
(E) Late menopause

7. A 50-year-old woman comes to the clinic to discuss treatment for a new diagnosis of breast cancer. Her annual screening mammogram revealed a 2.3 cm mass in the right breast. The patient does not have any other breast masses, skin changes, nipple discharge, or axillary adenopathy. Mammography revealed no other suspicious calcifications within the breast. Biopsy of the mass was performed and revealed infiltrating ductal carcinoma. Estrogen receptor (ER), progesterone receptor (PR), and HER2/neu receptor testing were negative. Which of the following is the best option for the management of this patient's breast cancer?
(A) Lumpectomy and breast irradiation
(B) Lumpectomy and hormone therapy
(C) Lumpectomy and chemotherapy
(D) Lumpectomy, sentinel node biopsy, and breast irradiation
(E) Lumpectomy, sentinel node biopsy, breast irradiation, and chemotherapy

8. A 65-year-old woman presents to her family physician with a pruritic, erythematous, ulcerated rash surrounding the areola of her right breast. She recently started a new medication, hydrochlorothiazide, for hypertension. She is prescribed hydrocortisone 1% ointment, but the lesion persists 3 months later. She has no history of skin diseases in the family. She takes warfarin for atrial fibrillation. Otherwise, she is healthy. What is the best next step in the management of this patient?
   (A) Punch biopsy of the skin lesion
   (B) Change hydrocortisone 1% to triamcinolone to treat eczema
   (C) Treatment with antibiotics
   (D) Oral steroid course to treat psoriasis
   (E) Increase the dose of hydrocortisone

9. A 64-year-old man who emigrated from Japan arrives to his doctor to discuss new skin lesions. His wife first noticed two discolored plaques on his back 2 weeks ago, but he now has multiple lesions all over his back, chest, and face. They are the size of a coin and appear to have a "stuck-on" appearance. He is afebrile, blood pressure is 136/86 mmHg, and he has a pulse of 90/min. The skin lesions do not itch, and they are not tender. He has no other complaints, and a review of systems is only remarkable for recent weight loss. He is more concerned about his cosmetic appearance. What is the best next step in management?
   (A) Reexamine in 2 weeks
   (B) Skin biopsy
   (C) Abdominal CT scan
   (D) Mohs procedure
   (E) Corticosteroids

10. A 45-year-old female undergoes screening mammography which demonstrates an area of suspicious microscopic calcification in her right upper outer breast. Stereotactic-guided biopsy confirms ductal carcinoma in situ (DCIS). Which of the following is true about this condition?
   (A) It should be excised to a negative margin
   (B) It is considered a marker for malignancy in either breast
   (C) The cribriform type has a worse prognosis than the comedo type
   (D) It does not occur in men
   (E) Radiation therapy is an acceptable alternative to surgical excision

11. A 30-year-old female presents with bloody discharge from her left breast that she has noticed intermittently for the past month. She denies any palpable breast mass, weight loss, fevers, or night sweats. She has no medical history or family history of breast cancer. The skin around the breast and areola are normal with no rashes or lesions. No breast mass is palpable, and there is no axillary lymphadenopathy. Ultrasound did not reveal any masses. What is the most likely diagnosis?
   (A) Fibrocystic changes
   (B) Intraductal papilloma
   (C) Ductal carcinoma in situ (DCIS)
   (D) Paget's disease of the breast
   (E) Infiltrating ductal carcinoma

12. A 61-year-old female presents with swelling and redness of her entire left breast that has persisted for 4 weeks. On physical exam her temperature is 37.6 °C, pulse is 82/min, blood pressure is 136/78 mmHg, and respirations are 16/min. Her left breast appears larger than her right one. The entire breast is warm, and the skin is edematous. No breast masses are palpable. There is no nipple discharge or rashes. There are several palpable enlarged lymph nodes in her left axilla. Ultrasound and mammography show thickening of the skin but otherwise no masses. Which of the following is the best option for further management?
(A) Punch biopsy of skin
(B) Oral antibiotics
(C) Intravenous antibiotics
(D) Nonsteroidal anti-inflammatory drug (NSAID)
(E) Incision and drainage

13. A 17-year-old female presents with breast pain that she noticed for several months. She states that she feels multiple breast masses in both breasts. She denies any weight loss, fevers, or night sweats. She has no medical history or family history of breast cancer. The skin around the breast and areola is normal with no rashes or lesions. No solitary breast masses are palpable, but both breasts are lumpy and painful to palpation, most notably in the upper outer quadrants. There is no axillary lymphadenopathy. What is the most appropriate next step in management?
(A) Diagnostic mammography
(B) Excisional biopsy
(C) Ultrasound-guided core needle biopsy
(D) Reassurance and reexamine in 1 month
(E) Fine-needle aspiration (FNA)

14. A 15-year-old girl develops short gut syndrome following resection of bowel secondary to leiomyosarcoma in the small intestinal wall. She is subsequently placed on long-term total parenteral nutrition (TPN) and is recovering well. A month later, she develops red and inflamed patches of dry and scaly skin around her mouth and eyes. Her hair also begins to thin, and she notices a bad taste when she gets her daily cherry-flavored Chloraseptic spray to prevent dry throat. What is the most likely underlying etiology of her skin lesions and thinning hair?
(A) Zinc deficiency
(B) Copper deficiency
(C) Pemphigus vulgaris
(D) Chromium deficiency
(E) Psoriasis

15. Which of the following would be best suited for Mohs surgery?
(A) Superficial spreading melanoma in the arm
(B) Nodular melanoma on the back
(C) Basal cell carcinoma on the face
(D) Subungual melanoma
(E) Squamous cell carcinoma of the neck

16. Where are melanomas in patients with dark skin most likely to occur?
(A) Back
(B) Arms
(C) Legs
(D) Palms, soles, and mucous membrane
(E) Face

17. A 50-year-old field worker arrives to a free clinic to discuss a "sore" on his lower lip. He has had no trauma to the face. He reports that he first noticed the "sore" 6 months ago, and it has slowly gotten bigger. On physical exam, he has an ulcerated 1 cm nodule on his lower lip. There are no telangiectasias present. What is the most likely diagnosis?
    (A) Basal cell carcinoma
    (B) Squamous cell carcinoma
    (C) Lichen planus
    (D) Dermatitis herpetiformis
    (E) Melanoma

18. Which of the following melanomas have the best prognosis?
    (A) Superficial spreading
    (B) Nodular
    (C) Lentigo maligna
    (D) Acral lentiginous
    (E) Subungual

19. Which of the following melanomas do not follow the ABCDE mnemonic?
    (A) Superficial spreading
    (B) Nodular
    (C) Amelanotic
    (D) Acral lentiginous
    (E) Amelanotic and nodular

20. Which of the following is the most common precancerous skin lesion?
    (A) Actinic keratosis
    (B) Seborrheic dermatitis
    (C) Seborrheic keratosis
    (D) Compound nevi
    (E) Keratoacanthoma

21. A 45-year-old female presents with a recent change in a preexisting mole on her anterior thigh. She states that the mole keeps bleeding, is darker, and has grown. The mole is 8 mm in diameter on physical exam. There are no palpable nodes in the groin. An excisional biopsy is performed with a 1 mm margin and to a depth of the subcutaneous fat. Pathology reveals a melanoma that is 0.8 mm in thickness with ulceration. The margins are negative. What is the next step in the management?
    (A) No further treatment
    (B) Re-excision with 1 cm margins
    (C) Re-excision with 1 cm margins and sentinel lymph node biopsy (SLNB)
    (D) Granulocyte-macrophage colony-stimulating factor (GM-CSF)
    (E) Interferon alpha

22. A 57-year-old woman comes to the clinic to discuss surgical treatment for a new diagnosis of breast cancer. Her annual screening mammogram revealed a 1.7 cm mass in the right breast. Biopsy of the mass was performed and revealed infiltrating ductal carcinoma. Estrogen receptor and progesterone receptor testing were negative, while HER2 receptor testing was positive. In addition to lumpectomy and breast irradiation, the treating doctor decides to add targeted therapy with trastuzumab to the treating regimen. What study must be done prior to starting trastuzumab?
(A) Thyroid-stimulating hormone (TSH)
(B) Liver function tests
(C) Echocardiogram
(D) Creatinine clearance
(E) Chest X-ray

Answers

1. Answer D
This patient has classic findings of hidradenitis suppurativa, a chronic inflammatory condition of apocrine gland-bearing areas such as the axillae, groin, and perianal region. It presents with recurrent inflamed nodules, subcutaneous abscesses, scarring, and sinus tract formation. The first-line treatment is a prolonged course of oral antibiotics such as tetracyclines, which have both antibacterial and anti-inflammatory effects. Incision and drainage may temporarily relieve symptoms but does not reduce recurrence and is not definitive treatment (A). Oral corticosteroids are not standard treatment and have limited evidence for long-term control (B). Wide local excision is reserved for severe, refractory disease after medical therapies fail (C). Radiation therapy is not a first-line treatment and is rarely used due to the risk of local tissue damage (E).

2. Answer B
Nodular-variant melanomas grow vertically, not horizontally. They are usually a uniformly dark blue or black "berry-like" lesion that is mostly symmetric, elevated, and one color. Impetigo is a superficial bacterial infection oftentimes due to *Staphylococcus aureus*. It presents first as a flat macule and then a raised pustule that erodes and oozes a dry, honey-crusted serum (A). A nevus, or a mole, is described as a *small* (<6 mm) macule with sharp, symmetric borders, and an evenly distributed color (C). Molluscum contagiosum is caused by the *poxvirus* and occurs most commonly in children and immunocompromised adults (D). It is characterized by small, firm, pink, and umbilicated papules. Squamous cell carcinoma is a malignant proliferation of epithelial cells that presents as an ulcerated, nodular mass in sun-exposed areas (E).

3. Answer A
A diagnostic mammogram and ultrasound should be ordered in a woman over the age of 30 years who presents with a new breast mass. Mammography helps to look for suspicious calcifications in other areas of the affected breast, characterize the mass, as well as evaluate the contralateral breast. It is important to note that the mammogram may be normal despite the presence of a palpable breast cancer. For this reason, a tissue biopsy is recommended for palpable breast masses regardless of the mammogram results. In a palpable nodule, tissue sampling is best performed via ultrasound-guided core needle biopsy. Ultrasound also provides more information about the mass (cystic vs. solid). FNA is rarely used as it provides only cytology rather than histology (B). MRI would be a useful adjunct in patients with high risk of breast cancer (e.g., BRCA-1) (C). Follow-up examination in 3 months without a biopsy to rule out a malignant lesion would be inappropriate (D). Genetic testing would be indicated if this patient had a strong family history of breast or ovarian cancer but would not be done until tissue diagnosis of breast cancer is confirmed (E).

4. Answer B

The patient most likely has mastitis. This is a localized, painful inflammation of the breast accompanied by fever and malaise usually occurring in breastfeeding women but can affect non-lactating women as well. The diagnosis of mastitis is made clinically based on an erythematous, tender, swollen area of one breast associated with fever. Although this occurs most commonly in nursing mothers, it can also occur in non-nursing women. Other symptoms may include muscle pain (myalgias) and malaise. Transmission occurs via introduction of bacteria in small breaks in the skin caused by the trauma of breast-feeding. Most cases of lactation mastitis are a result of an infection by *Staphylococcus aureus*. Treatment consists of antibiotics to cover skin flora, symptomatic relief with analgesics including anti-inflammatory agents such as ibuprofen, and cold compresses to reduce local pain and swelling. Patients should be encouraged to continue breastfeeding as this helps relieve any ductal obstruction that might be contributing to the infection (C). The breast milk in a woman with mastitis is not dangerous to the baby. Biopsy would be appropriate if the patient has suspected inflammatory breast carcinoma (A). Although very rare, inflammatory breast carcinoma can occur during pregnancy. If mastitis fails to resolve after antibiotics, then consideration should be given to performing a biopsy of the skin. At that time, diagnostic mammography should also be ordered (D). Incision and drainage are rarely used for localized abscess with fluctuance. Instead, needle aspiration is preferred, as it is associated with reduced healing time, decreased risk of fistulas, and greater patient satisfaction (E). Ultrasound can help differentiate mastitis from a breast abscess.

5. Answer B

The lesion is concerning for melanoma and as such will require tissue confirmation to rule out cancer. Excisional biopsy (removing the entire lesion), down to the subcutaneous fat, would be the preferred approach for a lesion on an extremity or torso (C). However, depending on the size of the lesion and its location (not desirable to make a cosmetically unappealing large incision if the lesion ends up being benign), an initial incisional biopsy (taking only a small sample) is preferred. Punch biopsy down through the dermis (to calculate Breslow thickness) is the preferred method in this setting. Shave biopsies are not recommended if melanoma is suspected as the true Breslow thickness may not be measurable (A). During the initial biopsy, no attempts are made to achieve a wide margin. If the pathology comes back benign, no further treatment may be necessary. Excisional biopsy should aim to remove the entire lesion with narrow margins (typically 1–2 mm) to allow for accurate Breslow depth assessment while preserving tissue for staging (D). Reexamination is not appropriate for a patient suspected of having melanoma (E).

6. Answer C

The most important risk factors for breast cancer are female gender, increasing age, and a family history of premenopausal breast cancer. A new breast mass in a woman over the age of 50 should be considered cancer until proven otherwise, as it carries the highest relative risk of being cancer. A family history of breast cancer can also significantly increase the risk of breast cancer, particularly if diagnosed in a premenopausal woman (B). The majority of inherited breast cancers are associated with BRCA-1 or BRCA-2 gene mutations. Other important risk factors associated with a slightly higher risk of developing breast cancer include early menarche, nulliparity or older age at first full-term pregnancy, and/or late menopause (A, D–E). Increased lifelong exposure to estrogen is common among these risk factors.

7. Answer E

Understanding when to offer surgery, radiation, chemotherapy, hormone therapy, trastuzumab, or SLNB to a breast cancer patient is important, and variations in this question will undoubtedly show up on the surgical shelf exam. There is a formula to answering these questions. First, this patient is diagnosed with infiltrating ductal carcinoma and so should be offered total mastectomy or breast conserving therapy, which consists of lumpectomy *and* radiation. Most elect the latter because it provides better cosmesis. Since this patient has an invasive carcinoma >2 cm, a SLNB is also indicated. If she had DCIS, a SLNB would only be indicated if the lesion was high risk (>5 cm, comedo type, or high grade). Additionally, if she was undergoing total mastectomy (for any size invasive carcinoma or DCIS), a SLNB should be performed as it would *not be possible* to do so at a later time. Hormone receptor (ER/PR)-negative breast cancers are thought to have a worse prognosis as adjuvant hormone therapy is not available. As such, there patients should receive chemotherapy (which is given preoperatively in some cases). Similarly, triple-negative breast cancers have an even worse prognosis, and so chemotherapy should be given to these patients as well. Trastuzumab (HER2 receptor blocker) is indicated in patients with HER2-positive breast cancer. In the case of ER/PR-negative but HER2-positive breast cancers, chemotherapy and trastuzumab should be given.

8. Answer A

The presentation is concerning for Paget's disease of the breast. This presents as an eczematous, scaling, and ulcerating lesion around the areola. Paget's disease of the breast is a type of DCIS that extends into the ducts to involve the skin of the nipple. Patients are initially misdiagnosed with a skin condition, including eczema and psoriasis, and receive a variety of ointments that do not resolve the lesion. Paget's disease of the breast is almost always associated with an underlying carcinoma and must be diagnosed via biopsy of the lesion. Trying different regimens of steroids and antibiotics is inappropriate given the high likelihood that she has cancer (B–E).

9. Answer C

The skin lesions described are most likely to be seborrheic keratosis (SK). Isolated SKs occur commonly in the elderly. Sudden onset of multiple SKs (*Leser-Trelat sign*) suggests an underlying carcinoma of the gastrointestinal (GI) tract, most often gastric cancer. It is considered to be a result of a paraneoplastic syndrome associated with the cancer. The best next step in working up a suspected GI malignancy is an abdominal CT scan. Given the high likelihood of malignancy, it would be inappropriate to only reexamine the patient in 2 weeks (A). SKs have a characteristic appearance and typically do not need to be confirmed with a skin biopsy (B). Mohs is a specialized tissue-sparing procedure for treating skin cancer (D). It involves tangential excisions of the lesion until margins are negative. Mohs has the advantage in that definitive excision and closure can be achieved on the same day. Corticosteroids are not used in the management of SKs (E).

10. Answer A

DCIS is characterized by malignant epithelial cells within the mammary ductal system, without invasion into the surrounding stroma. Comedo-type DCIS is high grade and associated with a worse prognosis (C). DCIS lesions have a high risk of subsequent invasive carcinoma at the site of the DCIS. As such if left unresected, it will often progress to invasive ductal cancer. Thus, the mainstay of DCIS treatment is breast-conserving therapy (excision of entire lesion with negative margins and radiation). Radiation therapy is used in combination with surgical excision but cannot replace it (E). Lobular carcinoma in situ (not DCIS) is considered a marker for malignancy in either breast (B). Breast cancer in males is rare (1% of all breast cancers) with most cases identified as invasive ductal carcinoma. DCIS can occur in men but is even more rare, as DCIS most often presents as abnormal calcifications on mammogram (D).

11. Answer B
Although bloody nipple discharge should raise concern for cancer, intraductal papilloma is the most common cause of bloody nipple discharge. This is a benign breast tumor arising from the proliferation of mammary duct epithelium that classically occurs in females 20–40 years of age. Treatment includes excision, which is diagnostic as well as curative. Fibrocystic changes are a common cause of breast pain in young females but do not present with bloody discharge (A). Patients report painful breast tissue before menses with improvement during menstruation. Physical exam reveals fibrotic tissue and cystic, lumpy tissue. DCIS and infiltrating ductal carcinoma are more common in older women (C, E). Although breast cancer can present with bloody nipple discharge, it is less common than intraductal papilloma, especially in a young woman. Paget's disease of the breast causes an eczematous lesion on the breast that is associated with an underlying breast carcinoma (D).

12. Answer A
The patient most likely has inflammatory breast carcinoma, an especially aggressive type of breast cancer. Inflammatory breast cancer can be easily confused with mastitis, as there is usually no palpable breast mass and ultrasound and mammography similarly are *often negative*. The lack of systemic signs of infection and persistence despite antibiotics points toward inflammatory breast cancer, not mastitis. As such, it is imperative to perform a biopsy of the skin, which may show cancer cells invading the subdermal lymphatics. Additional workup should include a breast MRI (which is more likely to show the breast cancer in this setting than ultrasound and mammogram), as well as consideration for needle biopsy of the lymph nodes. Antibiotics or NSAIDs would be inappropriate in a patient with high suspicion for cancer (B–D). Incision and drainage would be appropriate if there was an indication on physical examination or evidence of a breast abscess on ultrasound (E). Inflammatory breast carcinoma typically presents as swelling of the breast and with edematous skin due to obstruction of subdermal lymphatics by tumor (termed *peau d'orange*, meaning orange peel in French). At presentation, positive lymph node involvement is frequent, and approximately one-third of patients have distant metastases.

13. Answer D
The history and physical exam are most consistent with a diagnosis of fibrocystic changes of the breast, which is considered a *normal variant* of the breast in adolescents and young adults. Patients will present with painful breast tissue before menses that improves during menstruation. On examination, fibrotic tissue may be palpated and is generally found in the upper outer quadrants of the breast. This patient should be counseled and instructed to look for these changes with a follow-up appointment in a month. Persistent cystic breast lesions can be evaluated and treated with FNA, although this is not needed in children and adolescents (E). Cystic lesions that resolve with aspiration should be reevaluated with ultrasonography 3 months after aspiration, but a core needle biopsy would not be indicated (C). Excisional biopsy is warranted for cystic lesions that do not resolve with aspiration or for suspicious solid lesions (B). Diagnostic mammography is not indicated for adolescents and should be reserved for females >30 years old who present with a breast mass (A).

14. Answer A

Zinc deficiency can occur in surgical patients on long-term TPN or in patients diagnosed with a malabsorption syndrome. This can present with alopecia, red, and inflamed patches of dry and scaly skin around the mouth and eyes, abnormal taste, and impaired wound healing. Zinc supplementation will remedy this condition. Copper and chromium deficiency are rare but can also affect this patient population. The most common manifestations of copper deficiency include hematologic abnormalities (anemia, leukopenia) and myeloneuropathy (B). Chromium deficiency presents with impaired glucose tolerance and peripheral neuropathy (D). Pemphigus vulgaris occurs as a result of autoimmune destruction of desmosomes between keratinocytes and is characterized by multiple skin and oral mucosa bullae (C). Psoriasis is believed to have an autoimmune etiology and presents as salmon-colored plaques with a silvery scale that occur on extensor surfaces (e.g., patella) (E).

15. Answer C

Mohs is a specialized tissue-sparing technique of treating skin cancer in which the tumor is removed in a series of thin layers as opposed to one wide excision. The advantage is that it prevents excising excessive normal tissue and allows for immediate confirmation of negative surgical margins intraoperatively. It is best suited for basal cell and squamous cell carcinoma in cosmetically sensitive areas such as the face. Mohs is not generally recommended for melanoma. This is because it is difficult to distinguish the normal skin from melanoma on frozen section (immunohistochemical stains are sometimes needed). Because of this, Mohs is considered by most surgeons to be an unreliable method of resection for melanoma (A, B, D). The treatment of choice for subungual melanoma is digital amputation.

16. Answer D

Melanocytes are found in equal numbers in most people (black or white). However, individuals with darker skin have melanocytes that produce more melanin, a protein which makes skin darker and helps protect from skin cancer by absorbing UV-B (B for bad) radiation. As such, in dark-skinned patients, melanomas are more likely to occur in areas that have less pigmentation such as the palms, soles, and mucous membranes (A–C, E). In general, men more commonly have melanoma on the back, while women more commonly have melanoma on the legs.

17. Answer B

The most common type of lip cancer is squamous cell carcinoma (SCC). Lip cancer occurs much more commonly on the lower lip, as it gets more sun exposure than the upper lip. Occupations that involve long-term sun exposure (e.g., lifeguard, farmer, construction worker, gardener, and field worker) place patients at higher risk for developing skin cancer. SCC is described as an ulcerated, nodular mass without any telangiectasias. Basal cell carcinoma presents as a pearly white nodule with a central ulcerated crater surrounded by dilated vessels (telangiectasias) (A). Lichen planus can be remembered as the "5 Ps:" pruritic, planar, polygonal, purple papules (C). It commonly involves the wrists and elbows and is associated with chronic hepatitis C infection. One of the manifestations of celiac disease includes dermatitis herpetiformis (D). It presents as pruritic vesicles and bullae that are grouped together (herpetiform). It only occurs in a minority of celiac patients and typically resolves with a gluten-free diet. Melanoma presents as a mole-like growth and follows the ABCDE rule (E).

18. Answer C
Lentigo maligna has the best prognosis of the melanoma subtypes (remember, lentigo is least aggressive). Nodular-variant melanomas are characterized by the absence of a radial growth phase. They are usually a uniformly dark blue or black "berry-like" lesion that is mostly symmetric, elevated, and one color. They are considered to be the most rapidly growing and aggressive variant of malignant melanoma (B). Typically, it arises on apparently normal skin (the head, trunk, and neck are the most common locations) versus preexisting lesion. Ulceration is common, giving a poorer prognosis. Superficial spreading is the most common type of melanoma (A). It typically has a long horizontal growth phase before the vertical growth phase which confers a better prognosis. Acral lentiginous melanomas are typically found in the subungual, sole or palm location, and common in ethnic groups of color (D–E). Subungual melanomas tend to present late as they are often confused with a subungual hematoma.

19. Answer E
Amelanotic and nodular melanomas do not follow the ABCDE rule (A–D). As previously mentioned, nodular-variant melanomas are characterized by the absence of a radial growth phase. Amelanotic melanomas are notoriously difficult to identify because this variant is deficient in pigment or is unable to produce any pigment at all. For this reason, they typically go unrecognized until the disease advances enough to locally invade the surrounding tissue. Superficial spreading is the most common type of melanoma. It typically has a long horizontal growth phase before the vertical growth phase which confers a better prognosis. Acral lentiginous melanomas are typically found in the subungual, sole or palm location, and common in ethnic groups of color.

20. Answer A
Actinic keratosis presents as a rough, scaly patch of the skin that can vary in color (pink, red, brown). It is the *most common precancerous skin lesion* and thus can progress to squamous cell carcinoma. Seborrheic dermatitis (cradle cap) is a self-limited condition that commonly affects infants and presents as a yellow, greasy plaque on the scalp (B). Seborrheic keratosis is a common tumor in the elderly and presents as raised, discolored plaques that appear coin-like, waxy, and with a "stuck-on" appearance (C). Both of these conditions are benign and *not considered to be precancer*ous. Compound nevi are brown-black, well-circumscribed lesions that are <1 cm in diameter (D). They may be elevated and are frequently hairy, arising from the epidermal-dermal interface and from within the dermis. Malignant transformation is rare. Keratoacanthoma is a low-grade subtype of squamous cell carcinoma that can grow rapidly and become large in size (E). Most will spontaneously get better within a year, but removal with surgery is still recommended.

21. Answer C
Once the diagnosis of melanoma is established by punch or excisional biopsy, the area needs to be re-excised to obtain wider margins, and in select cases, SLNB is obtained (A). The extent of margins and need for SLNB are determined by tumor thickness. Patients with tumor thickness <1 mm (considered a thin melanoma) require an excision margin of only 1 cm. Additionally, for tumors <1 mm with ulceration, a SLNB is also performed (B). For melanomas that are thin with no ulceration, SLNB is not performed. For thick melanomas >2 mm, a 2 cm margin is recommended. Interferon alpha, GM-CSF, and dacarbazine are all adjuvant therapy options for patients with melanoma (D–E). There has been no concrete evidence that adjuvant therapy prolongs survival in melanoma. However, there is some evidence to suggest that there is an improved relapse-free survival and overall survival with high-dose interferon alpha.

✓ 22. Answer C

Trastuzumab is a monoclonal antibody that blocks the HER2 receptors. The medication is used in the treatment of HER2-positive breast cancers to help reduce recurrence and improve survival. Since there is a high risk of cardiomyopathy in patients receiving trastuzumab, it is recommended that all patients receive an echocardiogram prior to initiating therapy with trastuzumab. An alternative is to obtain a MUGA scan (multi-gated acquisition scan), which is a nuclear study that evaluates ventricular function with better fidelity. MUGA scan is considered superior to an echocardiogram but is not widely available. Trastuzumab-related cardiotoxicity is most often manifested by an asymptomatic decrease in ejection fraction. The optimal surveillance for trastuzumab-related cardiotoxicity is not well defined. The remaining answer choices are not needed prior to starting trastuzumab (A–B, D–E).

Cardiothoracic

Peyman Benharash

Contents

Chest Pain, Diaphoresis, and Nausea

Joanna Curry, Areg Grigorian, and Peyman Benharash

Contents

C. de Virgilio, A. Grigorian (eds.), *Surgery*, https://doi.org/10.1007/978-3-032-09799-6_8

Case Study

A 68-year-old male presents to the emergency roon with four hours of severe chest discomfort, cold sweats and nausea. He describes the pain as heavy pressur over the entire chest that is 9/10 in intensity and radiate to his neck. He is mildly short of breath. He denies bacl pain. He has noted reduced exercise tolerance over th past few months, only being able to walk for ½ blocl before having to stop to catch his breath. He is able to li flat without any shortness of breath. He smokes abou one pack of cigarettes per day and was recently diag nosed with diabetes mellitus and hypertension. He denies a history of cardiac events or stroke. Physical examination reveals a blood pressure of 144/78 mmHg, a heart rate of 97/min, and a respiration rate of 28/min. Breath sounds are equal without crackles. Cardiac examination reveals a regular rate without murmurs and an S4. An ECG was obtained, which shows sinus rhythm with ST-segment elevations in V2, V3, and V4. A stat troponin is ordered and returns above the normal range. Chest X-ray is normal.

Diagnosis

What Is the Differential Diagnosis? (Table 8.1)

Table 8.1 Differential diagnosis of clinical presentation

Diagnosis	Comments
Aortic dissection	Acute, tearing chest pain radiating to the back, associated with hypertension and Marfan's syndrome, can present with stroke, MI, tamponade, and acute aortic insufficiency; CXR: widened mediastinum
Acute coronary syndrome	Includes STEMI, NSTEMI, and UA; chest pain described as an "elephant on chest," with shortness of breath, diaphoresis, nausea, vomiting, tachycardia, and hypotension
Coronary vasospasm	Common in younger patients, cocaine users, and women; coronary narrowing caused by autonomic dysfunction and mimics typical angina associated with a true MI
Pericarditis	Pleuritic chest pain (i.e., worse with inspiration) that improves with leaning forward, dyspnea, cough, friction rub, and pulsus paradoxus (drop in blood pressure on inspiration) if tamponade is present
Pulmonary embolism	Pleuritic chest pain, dyspnea, hypoxia, and hypotension if embolus is massive; right heart strain and abnormal ECG findings may be present
Diffuse esophageal spasm	Esophageal motility disorder presenting with chest pain, dysphagia, and food regurgitation; may be triggered by reflux, caffeine, and spicy foods
Esophageal perforation	Most commonly after invasive procedures such as endoscopy, also in heavy alcohol consumption with forceful vomiting (i.e., Boerhaave syndrome)
Spontaneous Pneumothorax	Collapsed lung in tall, thin patients may present as acute pain and shortness of breath

MI myocardial infarction, *CXR* chest x-ray, *STEMI* ST-elevated myocardial infarction, *NSTEMI* non-ST-elevated myocardial infarction, *UA* unstable angina

What Is the Most Likely Diagnosis?

Given the patient's history of severe chest pain with radiation to the neck, reduced exercise tolerance, and ST elevations in V2, V3, and V4, the patient is likely suffering from an acute coronary syndrome (ACS), specifically a STEMI secondary to an occluded left anterior descending coronary artery.

> **Watch Out**
> A Stanford type A aortic dissection (i.e., involving the ascending aorta) can cause acute coronary artery occlusion and can present in a similar fashion. However, there may be a diastolic murmur from aortic regurgitation and a widened mediastinum on CXR.

History and Physical

What Are the Risk Factors for MI?

Diabetes, smoking, and hypertension are the three most significant risk factors for MI. Additional risk factors include increased age, male sex, hypercholesterolemia, and family history of coronary artery disease.

What Elements of the History and Physical Exam Make MI Less Likely in a Patient Presenting with Chest Pain?

It is highly unlikely that patients under the age of 40 and older healthy patients (e.g., 60-year-old swimmers) with no cardiovascular risk factors experience an MI. Pain that is reproducible by palpation, localized pain that is described as being sharp, and chest pain associated with eating are less likely to be related to heart disease.

What Is Suggested by Episodic Chest Pain Unrelated to Exertion in a Young Person?

Prinzmetal (vasospastic) angina is characterized by episodic chest pain unrelated to exertion. It is caused by coronary artery vasospasms, which result in transient decreased myocardial perfusion and reversible myocyte injury. The ECG may show ST-segment elevation during episodes, reflecting transmural ischemia. However, Prinzmetal angina is not caused by coronary artery disease. Calcium channel blockers are typically used to treat the underlying cause.

What Are the Classic History and Physical Exam Findings Seen in MI?

Chest pain, diaphoresis, anxiety, tachycardia, tachypnea, and nausea/vomiting are classic findings. If there is a large area of ischemic damage to the heart, the patient may have heart failure presenting with bilateral rales (pulmonary edema), jugular venous distention, new S3 or S4 heart sounds, new murmurs, and hemodynamic instability (i.e., cardiogenic shock).

What Group of Women Is at Highest Risk for MI? Why?

Postmenopausal women are at higher risk for MI. In fact, heart disease is the leading cause of death in women over the age of 40. The decline in estrogen levels is believed to contribute to the increased risk. Estrogen promotes growth and maintenance of the intimal layer of the arterial wall, maintaining its ability to expand and accommodate blood flow. However, exogenous estrogen supplementation has not been shown to reduce cardiovascular risk in women.

> **Watch Out**
> Up to 25% of MIs are silent or atypical and do not present with the classic symptoms including chest pain. This most often occurs in women, elderly, patients with diabetes, and in post-operative MIs (due to receiving pain medication).

What Are the Differentiating Features of Various Cardiac Murmurs? (Table 8.2)

Table 8.2 Differentiating features of cardiac murmurs

Murmur	Description	Location
Aortic stenosis	Mid-systolic crescendo-decrescendo	Upper right sternal border
Aortic regurgitation	Decrescendo diastolic murmur	Lower left sternal border (valvular); right sternal border (root dilation)
Mitral stenosis	Diastolic opening snap, low-pitched diastolic murmur. As stenosis worsens, the opening snap occurs earlier in diastole	Apex
Mitral regurgitation	Holosystolic murmur, decreased or absent S1	Apex, radiating to the axilla
Mitral valve prolapse	Mid/late systolic click, possibly followed by a late systolic crescendo-decrescendo murmur	Apex
Hypertrophic obstructive cardiomyopathy	Systolic crescendo-decrescendo murmur	Upper left sternal border
Tricuspid regurgitation	Holosystolic	Lower left sternal border
Atrial septal defect	Mid-systolic murmur; wide fixed split S2	Second left intercostal space
Ventricular septal defect	Harsh holosystolic murmur; louder in smaller defects	Lower left sternal border

Changes Seen in Systolic Murmurs with Various Maneuvers (Table 8.3)

Table 8.3 Effects of maneuvers on systolic murmurs

	Valsalva (decreases preload)	Handgrip (increases afterload)	Leg raise (increases preload)
Aortic stenosis	↓	↓	↑
Hypertrophic cardiomyopathy	↑	↓	↓
Mitral regurgitation	↓	↑	↑
Ventricular septal defect	↓	↑	↑

Watch Out

Valve repair should be considered in patients with severe valve defects (based on echocardiography), progressively worsening symptoms, evidence of heart remodeling, or if planning pregnancy.

What Are the Three Classic Symptoms of Aortic Stenosis?

The three classic symptoms of aortic stenosis are dyspnea, angina, and syncope. High myocardial wall tension coupled with left ventricular hypertrophy increases myocardial oxygen demand, which is further compromised by decreased diastolic coronary blood flow.

What Is the Dreaded Consequence of Aortic Stenosis?

Patients with aortic stenosis are at increased risk of sudden death. It has been hypothesized to be caused by ventricular arrhythmias or an abnormal baroreceptor reflex. This risk is about 2% in asymptomatic individuals and up to 30% in symptomatic individuals. Sudden death can occur during anesthetic induction, so it is essential that the aortic stenosis murmur be recognized prior to any surgical procedure.

> **Watch Out**
> Dyspnea is the most concerning symptom in aortic stenosis, as it indicates the onset of congestive heart failure (CHF). Without surgical valve replacement, approximately 50% of patients with CHF due to aortic stenosis will die within 2 years.

Pathophysiology

What Is Meant by ACS?

ACS entails varying degrees of acute myocardial ischemia, the end result of coronary artery disease. There are three types of ACS: unstable angina (UA), NSTEMI, and STEMI (Table 8.4).

Table 8.4 Acute coronary syndrome

Condition	Comments
UA	Nonocclusive thrombosis causes reduced myocardial perfusion, but no myonecrosis (death of cardiac myocytes), hence no elevation in cardiac enzymes
NSTEMI	Occlusive thrombosis eliminates perfusion to only the partial thickness of the myocardial wall (affects the subendocardial side) and causes myonecrosis, leading to elevation in cardiac enzymes and possibly ECG findings suggestive of ischemia (but not ST-segment elevation)
STEMI	Occlusive thrombosis eliminates perfusion to full thickness of the myocardial wall and causes myonecrosis, leading to elevation in cardiac enzymes and characteristic elevation of the ST-segment on ECG

What Are the Series of Events That Take Place During an Acute MI?

Thrombus formation following plaque rupture is the primary mechanism involved in coronary vessel obstruction leading to ischemia and, eventually, myocyte necrosis and tissue death.

What Coronary Vessel Is Most Often Affected?

The left anterior descending (LAD) artery is the most commonly affected coronary vessel.

Are There Different Mechanisms of MI?

Yes. MIs are categorized based on their underlying mechanism. Type 1 MIs are due to a primary coronary event, such as plaque rupture with subsequent thrombosis. Type 2 MIs occur in the setting of an imbalance between myocardial oxygen supply and demand and are often seen with conditions like hypoxia, hypotension, anemia, sepsis, or tachyarrhythmias. Postoperative MIs are typically type 2 and result from a combination of factors rather than acute plaque rupture. Type 1 MIs require urgent revascularization, while Type 2 MIs are managed by treating the underlying cause.

Workup

What Are the Initial Diagnostic Steps for Suspected MI?

In addition to a relevant history (i.e., prior MI, chest pain) and physical exam, the patient should have a 12-lead ECG and blood test for cardiac enzymes. A chest radiograph will help rule out other diagnoses like pneumothorax and aortic dissection.

What Is the Role of Measurement of Cardiac Enzyme Levels in the Blood?

Cardiac enzymes, including troponin-I and creatine phosphokinase myocardial fraction (CKMB), are measured every 8 hours in the first 24 hours of a suspected

MI. CKMB is the first to rise, but it has a low specificity. Troponin-I has the highest sensitivity for MI and increases in 3 hours, peaks in 6 hours, and gradually decreases over 7 days.

Watch Out
Ischemia causing death of cardiac myocytes can cause elevation in cardiac enzymes in both NSTEMI and STEMI, but not in UA.

What Is the Best Cardiac Enzyme to Diagnose a Second MI on Top of a Recent MI?

CKMB is the best marker to look for a secondary MI following a recent MI. Its levels peak within 12–40 hours following MI and decrease after 2–3 days. Therefore, in a subsequent MI, there will be a new increase in CKMB.

Watch Out
Both CKMB and troponin are cleared through the kidneys and may have a much longer half-life in the presence of kidney disease.

What Is the Role of ECG?

ECG will help determine the location of the ischemia or infarction (Table 8.5). ECG may potentially identify non-ischemic causes of the patient's symptoms, such as pericarditis, pulmonary embolism, and arrhythmia.

Table 8.5 Coronary anatomy and ECG changes

Coronary artery	Branch of	Supplies	ECG leads changes
LAD	Left coronary artery	Anterior wall of left ventricle, anterior 2/3 of intraventricular septum	V2, V3, V4
Circumflex branch	Left coronary artery	Lateral and posterior wall of left ventricle, left atrium	aVL, V5, V6
Posterior descending artery	Right coronary artery (80% of patients)	Inferior wall of left ventricle, posterior 1/3 of intraventricular septum	II, III, aVF

What Is the Role of Imaging?

Unless other diagnoses are suspected, imaging has a limited role in the setting of ACS, as time is of the essence in establishing coronary reperfusion. If the chest pain is atypical for MI (e.g., ripping, tearing), a CXR should be obtained to rule out other causes of chest pain, such as aortic dissection. Echocardiography can also be obtained to examine wall motion abnormalities when the diagnosis is uncertain. However, this should not delay reperfusion therapy, as that is key to improving outcomes of STEMI.

Management

What Is the Initial Management of STEMI?

Initial management of STEMI follows the B-MONA mnemonic: Beta-blocker, Morphine, Oxygen, Nitrates, and Aspirin. Aspirin should be given immediately, along with clopidogrel and anticoagulation (e.g., IV heparin). Urgent percutaneous coronary intervention (PCI) is the definitive treatment and should be performed within 90 minutes of first medical contact. If PCI is not available within that time frame, systemic thrombolysis with tissue plasminogen activator (tPA) is indicated. In the catheterization lab, the occluded vessel is opened, and a stent (either bare-metal or drug-eluting) is placed. Additional therapies depend on hemodynamic status and complications (Table 8.6).

Table 8.6 Management of STEMI

Intervention	Rationale
Aspirin	Inhibits platelet aggregation; given before PCI or fibrinolysis
Clopidogrel	P2Y12 inhibitor; used with aspirin to prevent further thrombosis before PCI or fibrinolysis
Platelet glycoprotein IIb/IIIa antagonist	Potent platelet aggregation inhibitor; often used during PCI for high thrombus burden
Heparin	Prevents clot propagation; used before PCI or fibrinolysis
β-blocker	Reduces myocardial oxygen demand by lowering heart rate and contractility; avoids reinfarction/arrhythmias; contraindicated in cardiogenic shock

(continued)

Table 8.6 (continued)

Intervention	Rationale
Nitroglycerin	Alleviates chest pain by causing vasodilation, thereby reducing preload and afterload (reduces oxygen demand) and improving myocardial perfusion (increases oxygen supply); avoid in right ventricular infarct or severe aortic stenosis
Morphine	Analgesic used only if chest pain persists despite nitrates; may cause hypotension or heart block
Angiotensin-converting enzyme (ACE) inhibitor	Reduces mortality in anterior MI or EF <40%; prevents remodeling
Angiotensin receptor blocker (ARB)	For patients who cannot tolerate an ACE inhibitor (e.g., cough)
High-intensity statin (e.g., atorvastatin)	Lowers LDL; reduces ischemic complications; improves outcomes post-PCI
Supplemental oxygen	Only indicated if oxygen saturation < 90%

Watch Out

An arteriovenous fistula (AVF) is a potential complication of vascular access during cardiac catheterization. A large coronary AVF can present with angina, A femoral AVF can present with leg swelling and a continuous bruit with a palpable thrill over the catheterization site. Large fistulas can lead to high-output heart failure.

What If PCI Is Unsuccessful?

If adequate flow cannot be established using percutaneous techniques in the catheterization laboratory, the patient may be referred for emergency coronary artery bypass grafting (CABG). Emergency operations for STEMI continue to have a high mortality despite many technological advances in myocardial protection.

Should Oxygen Always Be Administered for a Patient with ACS?

No, oxygen should only be administered if a patient's oxygen saturation is below 90%. Supplemental oxygen in a patient that is well oxygenated can further reduce blood flow to the myocardium through coronary artery vasoconstriction.

What Is the Initial Management of NSTEMI?

Initial management is similar to STEMI and includes B-MONA (β-blocker, Morphine, Oxygen if $SpO_2 < 90\%$, Nitrates, and Aspirin), dual antiplatelet therapy (aspirin + clopidogrel), IV heparin, and possibly a glycoprotein IIb/IIIa inhibitor. The main difference is that NSTEMI does not require immediate reperfusion. Instead, patients undergo risk stratification (e.g., Thrombolysis in Myocardial Infarction {TIMI} score) to determine timing of cardiac catheterization—typically within 24–72 hours for moderate-to-high risk patients.

What Is the Most Important Determinant of Long-Term Outcome After STEMI? Is There a Role of Emergency CABG After a STEMI?

The most important determinant is the speed at which blood flow is restored to the ischemic myocardium. In most cases, fibrinolysis or PCI would be able to accomplish this much faster than CABG, largely attributable to delays in getting the patient to the operating room. Indications for emergent CABG after STEMI include failed PCI, cardiogenic shock, and free rupture.

What Are the Indications for CABG in the Elective Setting?

CABG is rarely performed in the emergent setting (<5% of cases). In the elective setting, this procedure is reserved for stable patients with the following conditions:

- >50% stenosis of the left main coronary artery
- >70% stenosis in three major coronary arteries (two major arteries if the patient has diabetes)
- Significant stenosis in the proximal LAD plus one other major vessel
- Refractory angina despite optimal medical therapy
- Lesions not amenable to PCI, such as complex bifurcation lesions or diffuse disease

What Does the Traditional CABG Entail?

Traditional CABG involves performing a median sternotomy and placing the patient on a heart-lung machine (pump) while the heart is temporarily arrested. The ascending aorta is clamped, and then a cold solution high in potassium is administered into the aortic root to induce cardiac arrest and help protect the heart while vascular grafts are placed. The coronary artery blockages are bypassed using various grafts, including the internal mammary artery (IMA), greater saphenous vein, radial artery, and even the gastroepiploic artery

What Is the Best Conduit for CABG?

The IMA, a branch of the subclavian artery, is the best conduit for CABG. Greater than 95% of these bypasses to the LAD are patent at 10 years. This bypass is referred to as a LIMA to LAD.

Should More Than One Coronary Artery Be Bypassed During CABG?

Several studies have suggested that long-term survival is superior in patients receiving two or more coronary bypass grafts compared to patients receiving only one. In addition, the rates of postoperative cardiac events (e.g., angina, MI, graft occlusion, or PCI) and death are lower in patients receiving multiple grafts.

How Does CABG Compare to Coronary Artery Stenting in Patients with Multivessel Coronary Artery Disease?

Despite the improvement in stent technology (drug-eluting stents), CABG continues to be superior to stenting in terms of lower rates of mortality, MI, and revascularization, and thus remains the standard for multivessel disease.

What Are the Predictors of Mortality Following CABG?

Preoperative cardiogenic shock, emergent surgery, age > 65, and depressed left ventricular ejection fraction.

Complications

What Are the Complications of MI? (Table 8.7)

Table 8.7 Complications of MI

Complication	Characteristics	Post-MI timing
Cardiogenic shock	Large infarcts impair contractility and reduce cardiac output; the most common cause of in-hospital mortality	Immediate
Congestive heart failure	Reduced ejection fraction post-MI may lead to pulmonary edema or cardiogenic shock	Immediate
Arrhythmia	Occur in ~90% of patients; ventricular fibrillation is the most fatal and is the leading cause of out-of-hospital death	First 2 days
Peri-infarction pericarditis	Pleuritic chest pain that decreases with leaning forward, dyspnea, cough, fever, and a friction rub	2–4 days
Papillary muscle rupture	Sudden acute mitral regurgitation: dyspnea, pulmonary edema, hypotension	3–5 days
Interventricular septum rupture	Can cause left-to-right shunt, acute-onset right heart failure; may present with a new holosystolic murmur over the left sternal border	3–7 days
Ventricular free wall rupture	Most cases occur following anterior MI; sudden cardiac tamponade and death; may present with Beck's triad: hypotension, JVD, muffled heart sounds	5–14 days
Ventricular aneurysm	Occur as a result of a weakened ventricular wall; persistent ST elevations with deep Q waves; risk of embolic stroke, arrhythmias, or heart failure	5–90 days
Dressler's syndrome	Autoimmune condition where antibodies form against the pericardium (post-CABG too) with pleuritic chest pain, fever, and friction rub; responds to NSAIDs	1 month

How Does Cardiac Tamponade Lead to Obstructive Shock?

Cardiac tamponade increases pericardial pressure, which restricts ventricular diastolic filling. This impairs preload, reduces stroke volume, and results in obstructive shock due to severely decreased cardiac output.

What Is Suggested by Fever, Chills, and Leukocytes in a Patient with Pericardial Effusion?

Fever, chills, and leucocytosis in a patient with a pericardial effusion are concerning for purulent pericarditis. This is an acute infection most often caused by hematogenous spread of *Staphylococcus aureus*. Echocardiography-guided pericardiocentesis is necessary for diagnosis and source control.

How Does Papillary Muscle Rupture Lead to Acute Mitral Regurgitation?

Papillary muscle rupture causes loss of mitral valve support, resulting in acute mitral regurgitation. Blood flows abruptly from the left ventricle into the left atrium during systole, which the noncompliant atrium cannot accommodate, leading to elevated left atrial and ventricular filling pressures and acute pulmonary edema.

Areas You Can Get in Trouble

Valvular Heart Disease

Patients with prosthetic heart valves, prosthetic cardiac grafts, or congenital heart abnormalities should receive antibiotic prophylaxis (e.g., amoxicillin) prior to invasive procedures to prevent infective endocarditis (IE). IE can cause embolic stroke due to vegetations dislodging from the affected valve. Nonbacterial thrombotic endocarditis presents similarly, with stroke-like symptoms and repeated negative blood cultures, and is often associated with hypercoagulable states. A regurgitant murmur over a prosthetic valve is concerning for prosthetic valve dysfunction. Prosthetic valve endocarditis should be suspected if this murmur is accompanied by fever, leukocytosis, and bacteremia and requires transesophageal echocardiography to identify valvular vegetations.

Summary of Essentials

History and Physical

- Most significant risk factors: Diabetes, smoking, and HTN
- Other risk factors: Age, male sex, hyperlipidemia, and family history
- Classic symptoms: Chest pain, diaphoresis, nausea/vomiting, tachycardia, and anxiety
- Postmenopausal women are at higher risk due to decreased estrogen
- Up to 25% of MIs are silent or atypical, especially in the elderly, diabetics, and post-op patients
- Murmurs and physical exam findings may suggest valvular disease, papillary muscle rupture, or septal rupture
- Aortic stenosis: classic triad = dyspnea, angina, and syncope; dyspnea indicates CHF and poor prognosis

Pathophysiology

- Acute coronary syndrome includes unstable angina, NSTEMI, and STEMI
- Most MIs result from plaque rupture with thrombus formation (type 1 MI)
- Type 2 MIs result from supply-demand mismatch (e.g., sepsis, anemia)
- LAD is most commonly involved; it supplies the anterior LV and septum
- STEMI shows ST elevations in V2–V4

Workup

- ECG and troponin are first-line; ECG helps localize ischemia
- Cardiac enzymes: Troponin-I (most sensitive), CKMB (best for reinfarction)
- Enzymes measured every 8 hours × 3

- CXR may rule out aortic dissection, pneumothorax
- Echocardiogram helps identify wall motion abnormalities or complications but should not delay PCI
- Risk stratify NSTEMIs (e.g., TIMI score)

Management

- Initial treatment = B-MONA: Beta-blocker, Morphine, Oxygen (if SpO_2 <90%), Nitrates, Aspirin; also give: Clopidogrel, heparin, statin, ± GPIIb/IIIa inhibitor
- STEMI: PCI within 90 min of first medical contact; if PCI unavailable, give IV tPA
- NSTEMI: No immediate PCI unless high risk; most undergo delayed angiography within 24–72 hours
- CABG: Emergent if failed PCI or mechanical complications (e.g., rupture, shock); elective for left main disease, multivessel disease, or refractory angina; IMA is preferred conduit for LAD; multiple grafts improve long-term outcomes

Acknowledgement The editors would like to acknowledge and thank the following authors for their contributions to the previous edition of the chapter: Ryan Ou, Paul N. Frank.

Suggested Reading

Anderson JL, Adams CD, Antman EM. 2012 ACCF/AHA focused update incorporated into the ACCF/AHA 2007 guidelines for the management of patients with unstable angina/non-ST-elevation myocardial infarction. Circulation. 2013;127:e000.

Gaudino M, Benedetto U, Fremes S, Biondi-Zoccai G, et al. Radial-artery or Saphenous-vein grafts in coronary-artery bypass surgery. N Engl J Med. 2018;378(22):2069–77.

Goldman S, Zadina K, Moritz T, et al. Long-term patency of saphenous vein and left internal mammary artery grafts after coronary artery bypass surgery: results from a Department of Veterans Affairs Cooperative Study. J Am Coll Cardiol. 2004;44(11):2149–56.

Hannan EL, Wu C, Walford G, et al. Drug-eluting stents vs coronary-artery bypass grafting in multivessel coronary disease. N Engl J Med. 2008;358:331–41.

Hillis LD, Smith PK, Anderson JL, et al. 2011 ACCF/AHA guideline for coronary artery bypass graft surgery. Circulation. 2011;124:e652–735.

Medvedofsky D, Goldenberg I, Fefer P, et al. Statins loading before PCI on STEMI. J Am Coll Cardiol. 2013;61(10):E65.

Muneretto C, Negri A, Manfredi J, et al. Safety and usefulness of composite grafts for total arterial myocardial revascularization: a prospective randomized evaluation. J Thorac Cardiovasc Surg. 2003;125:826.

O'Gara PT, Kushner FG, Ascheim DD, et al. 2013 ACCF/AHA guideline for the management of ST-elevation myocardial infarction. Circulation. 2013;127:e362–425.

Ruttmann E, Fischler N, Sakic A, et al. Second internal thoracic artery versus radial artery in coronary artery bypass grafting: a long-term, propensity score-matched follow-up study. Circulation. 2011;124:1321.

Chest and Back Pain

James McDermott and Peyman Benharash

Contents

C. de Virgilio, A. Grigorian (eds.), *Surgery*, https://doi.org/10.1007/978-3-032-09799-6_9

Case Study

A 26-year-old male presents to the emergency department complaining of sudden-onset severe chest pain radiating to the upper back for the past 3 hours. He describes it as a tearing sensation in his back. He denies any fevers or chills but reports an episode of syncope prior to arriving at the hospital. He is in significant pain and is unable to remain still. His past medical history is negative. His blood pressure is 140/50 mmHg in the right arm and 110/50 in the left, with a heart rate of 102 beats per minute. He appears to be tall and thin, with long arms, long thin fingers, and hypermobile joints. His sternum has a concave deformity. Cardiac examination reveals a regular rhythm, an early diastolic murmur at the left upper sternal border, and muffled heart sounds. Breath sounds are equal bilaterally without crackles. His radial pulse on the left is diminished compared to the right. ECG demonstrates nonspecific ST-segment changes. Troponin and CK-MB are within normal ranges. A chest X-ray demonstrates a widened mediastinum (◘ Fig. 9.1).

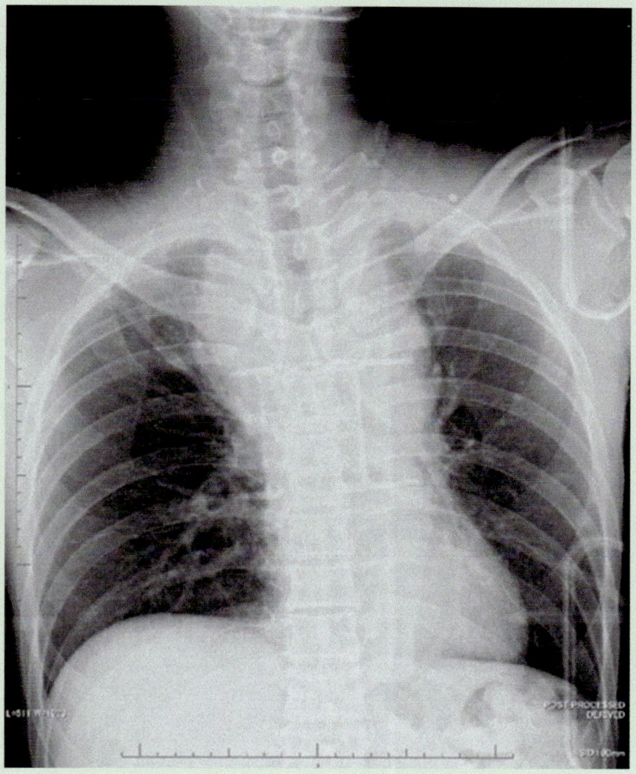

◘ **Fig. 9.1** Chest radiograph on admission showing widening of the upper mediastinum

Diagnosis

What Is the Differential Diagnosis? (Table 9.1)

Table 9.1 Differential diagnosis of clinical presentation

Condition	History and physical
Aortic dissection	Sudden onset of tearing chest pain radiating to the back or scapula, syncope, hypertension, connective tissue disorders (e.g., Marfan's syndrome)
Aortic regurgitation	Diastolic murmur loudest at the upper right sternal border with increased pulse pressure; may occur acutely with aortic dissection or endocarditis
Endocarditis	History of rheumatic heart disease, congenital anomalies (e.g., bicuspid aortic valve), or IV drug use; fever, new murmur, positive blood cultures, Janeway lesions (nontender lesions on palms and soles), and Osler nodes (tender lesions on digits)
Cardiac arrhythmia	Unprovoked syncope, dizziness, and hypotension
Acute pericarditis	Substernal, pleuritic chest pain, worse supine, better leaning forward, fever, tachycardia, friction rub, pulsus paradoxus
Unstable angina	Episodic chest pain of cardiac origin that occurs at rest; may be relieved with nitroglycerin
Non-cardiac causes of chest pain	Pulmonary (e.g., pulmonary embolus, pneumonia, pneumothorax), GI (e.g., esophageal spasm, GERD, Boerhaave syndrome), pancreatitis
Musculoskeletal	Muscle strain, rib fractures, costochondritis (tenderness with point palpation)

GERD gastroesophageal reflux disease, *GI* gastrointestinal

What Is the Most Likely Diagnosis?

The history is classic for an aortic dissection secondary to Marfan's syndrome. Additionally, the history and physical exam suggest the patient has suffered complications secondary to the aortic dissection, including acute aortic insufficiency (early diastolic murmur and increased pulse pressure) and pericardial effusion (muffled heart sounds). The clinical features also point toward Marfan's syndrome, which typically presents with a tall and thin body habitus and associated cardiac, skeletal (pectus excavatum, arachnodactyly, hyperflexible joints), and/or ocular (ectopic lentis: displacement of the crystalline lens) abnormalities. It is important to rapidly establish the diagnosis of aortic dissection and classify it by type (Stanford A or B), as the management strategies differ significantly between aortic dissection and other conditions, as well as between types A and B (discussed further below).

History and Physical

What Are the Risk Factors for Aortic Dissection?

The risk factors for aortic dissection are hypertension (most prevalent), connective tissue disease (e.g., Marfan and Ehlers-Danlos), advanced age, atherosclerosis, pregnancy, drug use (cocaine, methamphetamines, anabolic steroids), and aortic injury (e.g., trauma, cardiac catheterization, bicuspid aortic valve). Structural abnormalities like a bicuspid aortic valve and aortic coarctation also elevate risk. In patients with Turner syndrome, particularly those with cardiovascular manifestations such as a bicuspid aortic valve, aortic coarctation, aortic root dilation, or hypertension, the risk is notably heightened. Acute, severe chest pain in a patient with Turner syndrome features (e.g., short stature, primary amenorrhea) should prompt consideration of aortic dissection.

Watch Out

Systemic hypertension is the most common risk factor for aortic dissection.

What Is the Significance of Unequal Pulses in the Upper and Lower Extremities in Patients with Aortic Dissection?

Unequal pulses suggest that the blood supply to one of those extremities is adversely affected and therefore provide a clue as to the location of the dissection. An upper extremity pulse discrepancy (or blood pressure difference > 20 mm Hg, as in this patient) is consistent with a dissection involving the aortic arch, whereas a lower extremity pulse discrepancy suggests involvement of the descending aorta all the way down to one of the iliac arteries.

What Is the Significance of an Increased Pulse Pressure?

Patients with aortic insufficiency will present with a widened pulse pressure (as in this patient). Diastolic pressure decreases due to regurgitation, while systolic pressure increases secondary to the increased stroke volume as a result of the backflow of the blood from the aorta (increased preload).

What Is the Significance of New Diastolic Murmur?

A new diastolic murmur may indicate aortic insufficiency, a common finding in 50–75% of cases of ascending (Stanford type A) aortic dissection. In these cases, the aortic valve becomes incompetent due to either annular dilation or cusp prolapse. This occurs when the aortic dissection extends into the aortic root, causing the aortic valve leaflets to detach from the wall. Annular dilation prevents the valve leaflets from meeting properly (coaptation), allowing blood to regurgitate back into the heart during diastole.

What Is the Significance of a History of Intravenous Drug Use Disorder?

Patients with a history of IV drug use are at risk for endocarditis due to the introduction of bacteria into the bloodstream. Endocarditis often presents with fever and valvular regurgitation. Classic physical findings for endocarditis are listed in ◘ Table 9.2.

◘ **Table 9.2** Physical findings for endocarditis

Finding	Pathophysiology
Petechiae	Septic emboli or vasculitic processes
Splinter hemorrhages	Microscopic blood clots underneath the nail
Osler nodes	Septic emboli to small vessels in the skin, causing *tender* microabscesses
Janeway lesions	Small erythematous or hemorrhagic *nontender* lesions on the palms, soles, or distal finger pads
Roth spots (retinitis septica)	Retinal hemorrhages, a white spot close to the optic disk surrounded by hemorrhage

Pathophysiology

What Is the Initial Event Leading to an Aortic Dissection?

An aortic dissection begins with a tear in the intima, allowing blood to enter and dissect through the media, splitting the aortic wall into an inner layer (intima and inner media) and an outer layer (outer media and adventitia). This process creates a true lumen, which is the normal channel for blood flow, and a false lumen, formed between the intimal flap and the outer media. As blood enters the false lumen, the tear propagates, potentially enlarging the false lumen. The initial intimal tear typically results from shear stress, most often occurring in regions of high mechanical force, such as the aortic arch and proximal descending aorta just distal to the left subclavian artery.

Why Are Patients with Marfan's Syndrome at Increased Risk for Aortic Dissection?

Marfan syndrome is an autosomal dominant connective tissue disorder characterized by misfolded fibrillin proteins, leading to cystic medial necrosis in large vessels like the aorta. This structural weakness in the medial layer predisposes the aorta to dissection. Patients with Marfan syndrome should avoid activities that significantly elevate blood pressure, such as weight lifting and contact sports, to reduce their risk of dissection.

Why Are Patients with Vascular Ehlers-Danlos Syndrome (EDS) at Increased Risk for Aortic Dissection?

Patients with vascular EDS are at increased risk for aortic dissection due to defects in the synthesis or processing of connective tissue components, such as collagen and the extracellular matrix. This connective tissue disorder manifests with multiple joint dislocations, easy bruising, poor wound healing, and wide, atrophic scars—all signs of tissue fragility. In vascular EDS, the weakened structure of the aortic wall, especially in the media layer, makes it prone to dissection under normal circulatory pressures.

Are Dissections and Aneurysms the Same Disease?

No, aortic dissections and aneurysms are different conditions, although they may occur together and share some risk factors. An aortic aneurysm involves the dilation and weakening of all three layers of the aortic wall, leading to an increased vessel diameter. In contrast, an aortic dissection occurs when a tear in the aortic intima allows blood to enter and separate the layers of the vessel wall.

How Are Aortic Dissections Classified?

Two traditional classification schemes exist (DeBakey and Stanford), both of which describe dissections based on the segments of the aorta involved (◘ Fig. 9.2). A Stanford type A dissection involves the ascending aorta/aortic arch, whereas a type B dissection begins in the descending aorta, distal to the takeoff of the left subclavian artery. The main disadvantage of the Stanford classification is that it does not distinguish between patients with isolated ascending aorta/aortic arch dissection and patients with dissection involving the entire aorta.

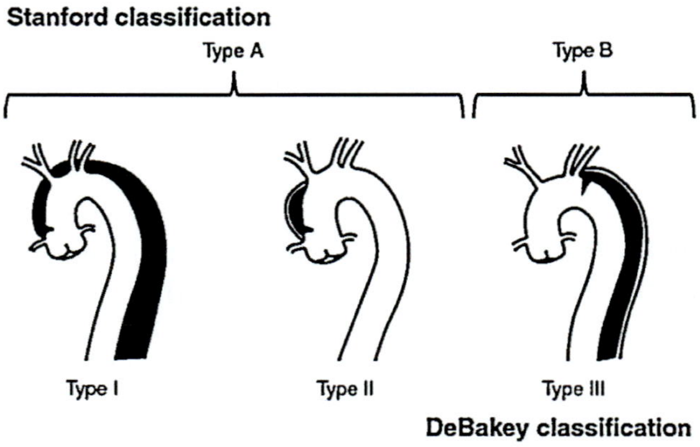

◘ **Fig. 9.2** Aortic dissection classification scheme diagram. (Illustration by Anne-Sophie Sillesen; From: Pandey and Hamady (2012). Reprinted with permission)

However, since the most important determinant of therapy is whether the ascending aorta/aortic arch is (Stanford A) or is not (Stanford B) involved, the Stanford classification is more commonly used. Remember, Type **A** is **A**nything involving **A**scending.

> **Watch Out**
> Stanford type B aortic dissections are the most common type overall. However, Marfan's patients more often present with type A aortic dissections.

How Do Aortic Dissections Cause Complications?

An aortic dissection may occlude major arteries, leading to ischemia. As blood enters the false lumen, it may partially or completely compress the true lumen. The complications and subsequent clinical presentation are highly dependent on the anatomic location of the dissection and whether the dissection affects major arterial branches. Additionally, aortic dissections can lead to aortic rupture, which is often fatal. A rupture may result in a hemothorax, commonly on the left side due to the aorta's left-sided course in the chest. Thus, aortic dissection should be suspected in patients presenting with hypotension and fluid in the left pleural space.

What Life-Threatening Complications Are Specific to Dissections That Involve the Ascending Aorta/Aortic Arch (Stanford Type A)?

Type A dissections may dissect into and obstruct blood flow in the coronary arteries, causing myocardial infarction (MI). They may disrupt blood flow in the carotid arteries, which can cause ischemic stroke. They may also dissect into the pericardial sac, causing acute tamponade, or dissect the aortic valve, leading to acute aortic insufficiency.

What Major Complications Are Specific to Dissections That Involve the Descending and Infrarenal Aorta (Stanford Type B)?

Type B dissections are much less likely to cause acute complications since the ascending aorta/aortic arch is not involved. Since they begin distal to the left subclavian artery and the descending thoracic aorta does not have any major arterial branches (other than to the spinal cord), the dissection can extend for a long distance without causing ischemic symptoms. Depending on which artery becomes occluded, the dissection can lead to ischemia of the liver (celiac artery), bowel (superior mesenteric artery), kidneys (renal arteries), limbs (iliac arteries), or spinal cord (spinal arteries, artery of Adamkiewicz). Collectively, ischemia to any of these areas is termed malperfusion syndrome. Note that type A dissections can extend into the descending aorta and have similar manifestations.

Workup

What Tests Should Be Ordered Immediately?

Blood typing with crossmatching, cardiac biomarkers (e.g., troponin, CK-MB), and ECG should be ordered.

What Is the First Imaging Modality Recommended in a Patient Who Presents with Acute Chest Pain?

Chest X-ray should be obtained as it may demonstrate a widened mediastinum in most patients with dissection. However, 15–20% of patients will have a normal chest X-ray. If the chest X-ray shows a widened mediastinum, particularly in a patient with non-traumatic chest pain, then a chest CT angiogram with intravenous contrast should be obtained to look for aortic dissection (◘ Figs. 9.3 and 9.4). Even if the CXR is negative, a CT angiogram should still be obtained if clinical suspicion for aortic dissection is high based on the history.

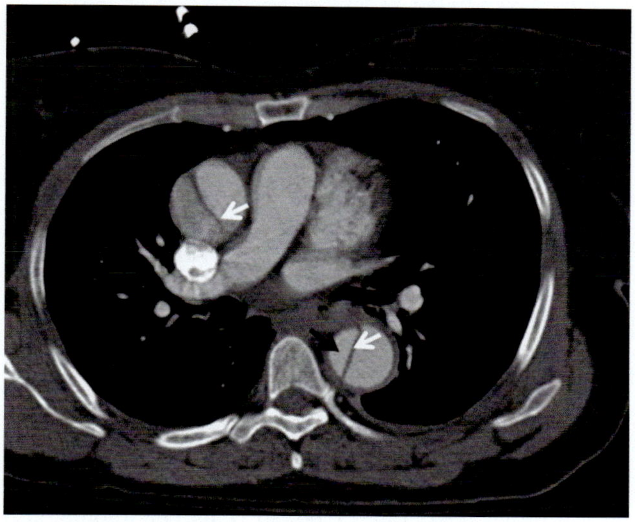

◘ **Fig. 9.3** Axial CT showing a Stanford type A aortic dissection involving the ascending and descending aorta. *White arrows: intimal flap. Black arrow: true lumen*

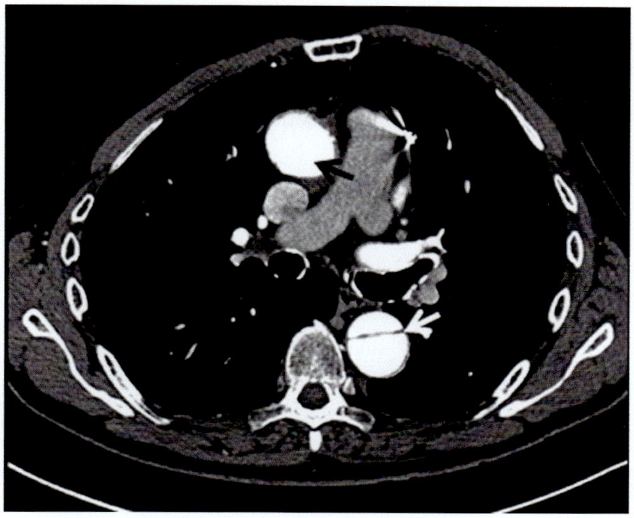

◘ **Fig. 9.4** Axial CT showing a Stanford type B aortic dissection involving the descending aorta. *White arrow: intimal flap. Black arrow: normal ascending aorta*

What Imaging Is Recommended If the Patient Is Hemodynamically Unstable and an Aortic Dissection Is Highly Suspected?

Hemodynamically unstable patients suspected of having a type A aortic dissection should be taken to the OR immediately, without a chest CT scan, for surgical intervention. Transesophageal echocardiography (TEE) can be performed in the operating room, while the patient is under general anesthesia, and if confirmatory, surgery can begin immediately.

Management

What Is the First Step in the Management of an Aortic Dissection?

Impulse control measures are the first step to reduce the risk of dissection extension or rupture by decreasing the force of blood ejection against the aortic wall. This is achieved through strict control of heart rate and blood pressure. Beta-blockers are used to slow the heart rate, with a target heart rate of 60–80 beats per minute, and reduce blood pressure, thereby reducing the force of each heartbeat and decreasing shear stress on the aorta. Esmolol is particularly effective due to its being an ultra-short acting, selective beta-1 antagonist. Additional blood pressure agents, such as intravenous nitroprusside or nicardipine, can be given to lower systolic blood pressure to a target range of 100–120 mm Hg in acute cases. Together, these interventions help stabilize the patient, minimizing the risk of further aortic dissection (◘ Table 9.3).

Watch Out

Cocaine use increases the risk of aortic dissection. In this case, a combined alpha- and beta-blocking drug such as labetalol should be used to prevent unopposed vasoconstriction.

What Is the Next Step (After Starting Antihypertensives) Once the Diagnosis of Type A Dissection Is Established?

The patient should be taken urgently to the operating room for repair via median sternotomy, as time is of the essence. Mortality has been quoted as 1–2% for every hour of delay. Thus, these patients should not first be admitted to the ICU; instead, impulse control measures can be initiated en route to the operating room. Depending on the exact location of the dissection, in addition to replacing part of the ascending aorta with a synthetic graft, a new aortic valve may need to be placed, and the coronary arteries may need to be reimplanted into the new graft.

What Is the Next Step (After Starting Antihypertensives) Once a Diagnosis of Type B Dissection Is Established?

The patient should be admitted to the ICU for impulse control.

◘ Table 9.3 Characteristics of Stanford type A versus type B aortic dissection

	Type A dissection	Type B dissection
Prognosis	50% of patients die within 48 hours without surgical intervention, <10% will live beyond 1 month, MI and stroke portend an even worse prognosis	80% of patients survive with appropriate medical therapy
Management	Begin with medical therapy (e.g., β-blocker) and urgent surgical intervention	Begin with medical therapy only (in the absence of malperfusion syndrome): β-blocker (first line), nitroprusside, calcium channel blockers, and morphine for analgesia (surgical repair is indicated if there is malperfusion)

When Should Patients with Type B Dissection Undergo Surgical Repair?

Urgent surgical intervention is reserved for patients who demonstrate or develop evidence of malperfusion as described above.

What Are the Surgical Options for a Type B Dissection?

The preferred approach in most cases is thoracic endovascular aortic repair (TEVAR) with placement of a stent graft. Open repair via a thoracotomy is rarely performed today due to higher morbidity and mortality. Spinal cord ischemia is a complication specific to the repair of dissections involving the thoracic aorta, as the blood supply to the spinal cord (via the artery of Adamkiewicz) may be interrupted. It is much less common with TEVAR than with open repair.

What Are the Differences in Prognosis and Definitive Management Between Type A and Type B Aortic Dissections?

What Are Some of the Post-Operative Complications After Sternotomy?

Sternotomy involves separating the sternum to access the heart and thoracic aorta and is associated with several major complications, including sternal dehiscence and mediastinal infection (mediastinitis). Sternal dehiscence is the separation of the sternum and may present with post-operative chest wall pain and instability in the absence of systemic signs of infection. Patients may describe a "clicking" with chest movement. Once confirmed radiographically (i.e., displaced sternal wire) or clinically (palpable rocking or clicking of sternum), dehiscence should be repaired urgently in the operating room. Post-sternotomy mediastinitis may result from intraoperative wound contamination and is associated with a high mortality rate. It often presents with signs of a systemic inflammatory response (fevers, chills, tachycardia, hypotension), chest pain, chest wall edema/crepitus, purulent drainage from the incision site, and leukocytosis. Mediastinitis requires urgent surgical exploration, debridement, and antibiotic therapy.

Areas Where You Can Get in Trouble

Giving Beta-Blockers to a Patient with Aortic Dissection Complicated by Cardiac Tamponade or Severe Aortic Regurgitation

Beta-blockade in these patients will worsen hypotension and may precipitate cardiac arrest.

Confusing Type-A Aortic Dissection with Acute MI

Patients with type A aortic dissection can present with coronary artery malperfusion and thus have a similar presentation as an acute MI. In patients with acute MI without aortic dissection, the MI is generally due to acute occlusion of a coronary artery due to rupture of an atherosclerotic coronary plaque. Treatment consists of antiplatelet agents, therapeutic anticoagulation with a heparin infusion, possibly fibrinolytic drugs, and emergent coronary catheterization to relieve the obstruction and possibly place a stent. If the diagnosis of a type A aortic dissection is missed, the patient may be incorrectly given heparin and taken to the coronary catheterization lab instead of the operating room for a sternotomy.

Area of Controversy

Endovascular Repair of a Stable Asymptomatic Type B Aortic Dissection

In patients with type B dissection, the descending aorta can progressively dilate with time, eventually requiring surgery if the diameter of the aneurysm exceeds 6 cm. Since endovascular repair of type B dissections is less invasive and is associated with fewer complications, some centers advocate early repair of stable type B dissections in order to prevent a chronic enlargement of the aorta. At present, the role of prophylactic TEVAR for uncomplicated, stable type B dissections remains controversial. Early TEVAR (within 2 weeks) is associated with a higher risk of procedural complications.

Aortic Dissection (◘ Fig. 9.5)

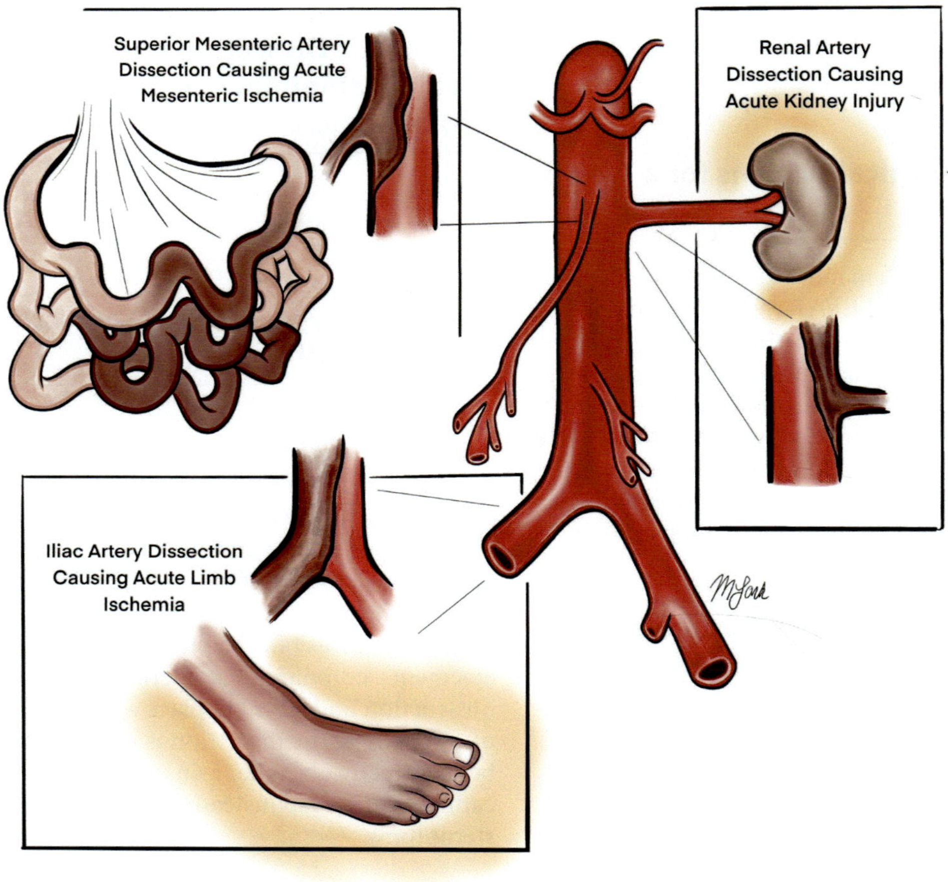

◘ **Fig. 9.5** **Complications of Aortic Dissection.** An aortic dissection can occlude major arteries, leading to severe complications. These include superior mesenteric artery occlusion causing bowel ischemia, renal artery occlusion causing impaired renal perfusion, and iliac artery occlusion causing acute limb ischemia

Summary of Essentials

History and Physical Exam

- Sudden onset of severe tearing chest pain radiating to the upper back
- Risk factors: severe hypertension, atherosclerosis, advanced age, connective tissue disorders (Marfan, Ehlers-Danlos), pregnancy, and cocaine use
- Look for evidence of acute aortic insufficiency, cardiac tamponade
- Check for diminished pulses in an extremity or a difference in blood pressure in each arm
- Look for evidence of malperfusion
  - Stroke
  - Elevated liver enzymes
  - Paraparesis
  - Limb ischemia
  - Severe abdominal pain
  - Renal insufficiency
- Aortic dissection can easily be missed
  - Acute MI can be caused by a type A dissection

Pathophysiology

- High shear stress and pulsatile blood flow can cause a tear that begins in the intima and splits the media, creating a true and a false lumen
- Expansion of the false lumen may occlude branch vessels and cause ischemia to the brain, spinal cord, viscera, or extremities

Classification

- Stanford A: involves ascending aorta/aortic arch
  - Can also involve the descending aorta
- Stanford B: descending aorta (distal to left subclavian) only

Diagnosis

- Chest X-ray: widened mediastinum (not present in 15–20%)
- CT chest with IV contrast: if the mediastinum is wide or suspicion for dissection is high
- Unstable patient: directly to OR, intraop TEE

Management

- Immediate control of blood pressure: Beta-blocker (esmolol) preferred unless there is suspected tamponade or severe aortic regurgitation
- Type A dissection: immediate operative repair
  - Median sternotomy (replace ascending aorta with graft)
  - Possible aortic valve replacement
  - Possible reimplantation of coronary arteries
- Type B dissection: admit to ICU for blood pressure control
  - Surgery only if evidence of malperfusion, ongoing pain, or refractory hypertension
  - TEVAR preferred

Acknowledgement The editors would like to acknowledge and thank the following authors for their contributions to the previous edition of the chapter: Ryan Ou, Paul N. Frank.

Suggested Reading

Braverman AC. Acute aortic dissection clinician update. Circulation. 2010;122:184–8.

Hiratzka LF, Bakris GL, Beckman JA, et al. ACCF/AHA/AATS/ACR/ASA/SCA/SCAI/SIR/STS/SVM Guidelines for the diagnosis and management of patients with thoracic aortic disease. A report of the American College of Cardiology Foundation/American Heart Association Task Force on Practice Guidelines, American Association for Thoracic Surgery, American College of Radiology, American Stroke Association, Society of Cardiovascular Anesthesiologists, Society for Cardiovascular Angiography and Interventions, Society of Interventional Radiology, Society of Thoracic Surgeons, and Society for Vascular Medicine. J Am Coll Cardiol. 2010;55(14):e27–e129.

Isselbacher EM, Preventza O, Hamilton Black J 3rd, et al. 2022 ACC/AHA Guideline for the Diagnosis and Management of Aortic Disease: A Report of the American Heart Association/American College of Cardiology Joint Committee on Clinical Practice Guidelines. *Circulation*. 2022;146(24):e334–e482. https://doi.org/10.1161/CIR.0000000000001106

Pandey VA, Hamady M (2012) Aortic dissection. In: Hoballah J, Lumsden A (eds) *Vascular surgery*. New Techniques in Surgery Series, vol 6. Springer, London

Hemoptysis, Cough, and Weight Loss

Joanna Curry and Peyman Benharash

Contents

C. de Virgilio, A. Grigorian (eds.), *Surgery*, https://doi.org/10.1007/978-3-032-09799-6_10

Case Study

A 71-year-old female presents to her primary care physician with an 8-week history of cough with intermittent blood-tinged sputum. She reports a 20-pound weight loss and increasing fatigue over the last three months. She denies fevers or sick contacts. She is a current smoker with a 40-pack-year smoking history. She previously worked as a welder in a shipyard for 30 years before retiring five years ago. Her past medical history includes hypertension. Breath sounds are equal without crackles. Cardiac exam reveals a regular rate and rhythm. Her blood pressure is 120/80 mmHg, and her heart rate is 88/min. An initial chest x-ray reveals blunting of the right costophrenic angle, an enlarged cardiac silhouette, and a mass in the right hilar region measuring 3.1 cm × 3.5 cm.

Diagnosis

What Is the Differential Diagnosis? (Table 10.1)

Table 10.1 Differential diagnosis of clinical presentation

Diagnosis	Comments
Primary Lung Cancer	Malignancy arising from lung epithelial or parenchymal cells
Metastatic Disease	Pulmonary metastasis is the most common form of lung tumors, most commonly from colon, breast, prostate, and bladder primaries
COPD	Chronic inflammatory lung disease causing obstructed airflow from the lungs
CHF	CHF can cause increased congestion, leading to backup into the pulmonary vasculature and parenchyma
Pneumonia	Infection and irritation of the lung parenchyma can present with cough and hemoptysis
Tuberculosis	Infection by *Mycobacterium tuberculosis* often affects the lungs. Symptoms include fevers, hemoptysis, and weight loss
HIV	Respiratory manifestations of *HIV* include cough, dyspnea, and pleuritic chest pain; cough can be productive of clear, purulent, or blood-streaked sputum
Other causes	Rheumatic (e.g., amyloidosis, sarcoidosis); infection (e.g., Abscess, fungal infection, viral)

COPD chronic obstructive pulmonary disease, *CHF* congestive heart failure, *HIV* human immunodeficiency virus

What Is the Most Likely Diagnosis?

The chronicity of the patient's symptoms, history of cigarette smoking, and occupational exposure, along with the chest x-ray (CXR) findings of a blunted costophrenic angle, an enlarged cardiac silhouette, and a pulmonary lesion, are highly suggestive of lung malignancy.

History and Physical

What Are the Risk Factors for Lung Cancer?

Cigarette smoking is the primary risk factor, accounting for the vast majority of cases, although nonsmokers may also develop lung cancer, particularly adenocarcinoma. Risk increases with cumulative tobacco exposure. Other risk factors include secondhand smoke exposure, environmental toxins such as radon and asbestos, and underlying lung disease such as COPD or pulmonary fibrosis.

What Is the Importance of Occupational Exposure?

Historically, shipyard workers have been frequently exposed to asbestos. Asbestos is a fibrous silicate mineral that is classically associated with the development of mesothelioma. While up to 90% of mesothelioma is associated with asbestos exposure, only about 1% of patients with a history of asbestos exposure develop mesothelioma. Mesothelioma presents with similar symptoms to primary lung malignancies but will demonstrate pleural thickening on imaging. Smoking has not been shown to increase the risk of mesothelioma. Other exposures are listed in ◘ Table 10.2.

What Is the Significance of a Pleural Effusion?

Primary lung malignancy can cause an exudative pleural effusion due to pleural invasion or lymphatic obstruction. These effusions typically appear as unilateral blunting of the costophrenic angle on CXR. Cytologic analysis of pleural fluid may confirm malignancy in many cases. The light criteria are used to distinguish exudative from transudative effusions (◘ Table 10.3).

What Is the Significance of an Enlarged Cardiac Silhouette?

Primary lung malignancy can cause a pericardial effusion, which may be identified as an enlarged cardiac silhouette on CXR. These malignant pericardial effusions are often large and prone to recurrence. Acute management consists of pericardiocentesis, and recurrence is prevented with a pericardial window or prolonged catheter drainage.

◘ Table 10.2 Occupational exposure

Occupational exposures	Source	Comments
Asbestos	Mining, construction, and ship repair	Chronic inflammatory response leads to fibrosis, pleural disease, and mesothelioma
Silica	Mining, stone cutting, quarry	Chronic inflammation leading to PMF, COPD, and cancer
Beryllium	Alloy processing	Pneumonitis, chronic granulomatous disease, and possibly lung cancer
Coal	Mining	PMF, COPD
Other metals (aluminum, chromium, nickel, cobalt, titanium, etc.)	Various sources	Ranges from pneumonitis to lung cancer

PMF progressive massive fibrosis, *COPD* chronic obstructive pulmonary disease

Table 10.3 Light's Criteria for Pleural Effusion Classification

	Laboratory Parameters			
Classification	**Pleural fluid protein/serum protein ratio**	**Pleural fluid LDH/serum LDH ratio**	**Pleural fluid LDH**	**Causes**
Transudative	≤0.5	≤0.6	<2/3 ULN serum	CHF, cirrhosis, nephrotic syndrome, CKD
Exudative	>0.5	>0.6	>2/3 ULN serum	Infection, malignancy, autoimmune disease, hemothorax/chylothroax

LDH lactate dehydrogenase, *ULN* upper limit of normal, *CHF* congestive heart failure, *CKD* chronic kidney disease

Pathophysiology

Does This Patient Have a Solitary Pulmonary Nodule (SPN)?

No. A SPN is defined as a single, well-circumscribed lesion within the lung parenchyma that is 3 cm or less in diameter, completely surrounded by normal lung tissue, and not associated with lymphadenopathy, pleural effusion, or other pulmonary abnormalities. Lesions larger than 3 cm are considered pulmonary masses and have a higher risk of malignancy. This patient's lesion exceeds 3 cm and is associated with symptoms, classifying it as a pulmonary mass rather than an SPN. In patients with a history of malignancy, any new lung lesion is presumed to represent metastatic disease unless proven otherwise.

Watch Out

Pulmonary nodules must be at least 1-cm in size to be seen on CXR, whereas CT scan can detect subcentimeter nodules.

How Is Lung Cancer Classified? Why Is It Important?

Lung cancer is divided into non-small cell lung cancer (NSCLC, 80–85%) and small cell lung cancer (SCLC, 10–15%). NSCLC is further categorized into three major histologic subtypes: adenocarcinoma, squamous cell carcinoma, and large cell carcinoma (Table 10.4).

What Is the Epidemiology of Lung Cancer?

Lung cancer is the second most commonly diagnosed cancer in both men and women, following prostate and breast cancer, respectively. However, it remains the leading cause of cancer-related death in the United States. This is due in part to its typically late presentation and aggressive clinical course. The majority of cases are diagnosed at an advanced stage, often after metastasis has occurred.

Table 10.4 Lung cancer subtypes

Tumor type	Incidence	Comments
Adenocarcinoma	40%	Often located peripherally; the most common primary lung cancer; most likely to arise in nonsmokers
Squamous cell carcinoma	20%	Often hilar mass arising from the bronchus; can have cavitations; associated with smoking
Large cell carcinoma	20%	Often located peripherally; highly anaplastic; strong association with smoking
Small cell carcinoma	15%	Often centrally located; neoplasm of neuroendocrine Kulchitsky cells; undifferentiated and very aggressive
Other	5%	Can be peripheral or central; carcinoid tumors, nests of neuroendocrine cells; symptoms often due to mass effect

What Syndromes Are Often Associated with Lung Cancers? (Table 10.5)

Table 10.5 Syndromes associated with lung cancer

Tumor type	Common syndromes
Adenocarcinoma	Hypertrophic pulmonary osteoarthropathy (clubbing, periostitis of hand joints); Trousseau syndrome (migratory superficial thrombophlebitis)
Squamous cell carcinoma	Ectopic production of PTH-related protein, resulting in hypercalcemia and hypophosphatemia (endogenous PTH will be low); Pancoast tumor (syndrome), due to location of the lesion (superior sulcus) this results in compression of the thoracic inlet with involvement of brachial plexus and cervical sympathetic nerves, causing severe pain in shoulder, atrophy of upper extremities, and Horner's syndrome (ptosis, miosis, anhidrosis)
Large cell carcinoma	Gynecomastia from secretion of *beta*-HCG; SVC syndrome (presents with increased dyspnea, increased jugular venous pressure, and facial swelling)
Small cell carcinoma	Ectopic production of ACTH or ADH; Lambert-Eaton syndrome (proximal muscle weakness, improves with activity)
Carcinoid	Carcinoid syndrome (flushing, diarrhea, wheezing, and salivation); the most common lung mass in adolescents and young adults

PTH parathyroid hormone, *HCG* human chorionic gonadotropin, *SVC* superior vena cava, *ACTH* adrenocorticotropic hormone, *ADH* antidiuretic hormone, *Ach* acetylcholine

Watch Out

Trousseau's syndrome (superficial migratory thrombophlebitis) is also associated with pancreatic cancer. Trousseau's sign (carpopedal spasm with blood pressure cuff inflated) is a sign of hypocalcemia.

What Are Common Sites of Metastasis for Primary Lung Cancer?

Primary lung cancer commonly metastasizes to the brain, bone, adrenal glands, liver, and kidneys. These sites are often involved at the time of diagnosis, particularly in advanced-stage disease. Neurologic symptoms such as headache or focal deficits may suggest brain metastases, while bone pain or pathologic fractures may indicate skeletal involvement. Hypercalcemia may occur due to bony metastases or, less commonly, from ectopic production of parathyroid hormone–related protein by squamous cell carcinoma. Adrenal involvement is frequently asymptomatic and detected incidentally on imaging, whereas hepatic metastases may present with elevated liver enzymes or hepatomegaly.

Is Universal Screening for Lung Cancer Appropriate?

Although universal screening for lung cancer could theoretically improve early detection and survival, it is not currently recommended due to concerns over false positives, overdiagnosis, and the potential harms of unnecessary invasive procedures. Additionally, repeated imaging exposes patients to ionizing radiation, which may carry its own long-term risks. As a result, emphasis remains on primary prevention through smoking cessation rather than widespread screening of asymptomatic individuals.

Is Screening of Benefit to Any Group?

The US Preventive Services Task Force recommends an annual low-dose CT for lung cancer screening in adults aged 50–80 with a 20-pack-year smoking history who currently smoke or quit within the last 15 years. However, despite guideline support, actual screening rates remain low, often due to limited access, lack of patient awareness, and variability in clinician implementation.

Workup

What Are the Initial Diagnostic Steps for Suspected Lung Cancer?

A CXR is often obtained initially and may reveal a suspicious lesion; however, CXR has limited sensitivity, and findings must be followed up with a chest CT, which provides detailed information about lesion size, morphology, location, and potential involvement of lymph nodes or other thoracic structures. When available, comparison with prior imaging is helpful to assess for lesion stability or growth. A new or enlarging lesion on CT warrants further evaluation, often with PET imaging, tissue diagnosis, and staging workup.

Should a Biopsy Be Performed?

The decision to biopsy a lung nodule or mass depends on radiographic features and patient-specific risk factors. Concerning imaging findings include size greater than 8 mm, spiculated or irregular borders, upper lobe location, and absence of benign patterns such as dense central calcification. High-risk patient factors include older age, current or former smoking history, a personal or family history of malignancy, and female sex. If malignancy is suspected, tissue diagnosis is typically necessary to confirm the histologic subtype and guide management. The method of biopsy is determined by lesion location. Peripheral nodules are best sampled with CT-guided transthoracic needle aspiration, whereas central or endobronchial lesions are often biopsied using bronchoscopy. Endobronchial ultrasound may be used to assess and sample mediastinal lymph nodes when nodal involvement is suspected. In patients with high pretest probability of malignancy and good operative candidacy, it may be appropriate to proceed directly to surgical resection without prior biopsy.

Management

How Are SPNs Managed?

Management depends on nodule size, radiographic features, and patient risk factors such as age and smoking history. Nodules smaller than 6 mm in low-risk patients typically do not require follow-up. Nodules measuring 6–8 mm often warrant serial CT imaging to assess for growth. Nodules larger than 8 mm may require further evaluation with PET/CT or tissue sampling, depending on the clinical context. Features concerning malignancy include spiculated borders, upper lobe location, absence of calcification, and documented growth over time.

How Does the Lung Cancer Type Influence Management?

Treatment is determined based on cancer type and stage. SCLC is a disseminated disease in most patients at the time of presentation, and initial treatment primarily involves a combination of chemotherapy and radiation therapy. For NSCLC, surgical resection is the treatment of choice. Unfortunately, by the time the patient presents with symptoms of lung cancer, many are already beyond curative resection.

What Is the Importance of Preoperative Evaluation?

A preoperative evaluation with forced expiratory volume in 1 second (FEV1) and diffusing capacity for carbon monoxide (DLCO) is recommended in all patients in whom a lung resection is considered. Patients with predicted postoperative FEV1 and DLCO greater than 60% are generally considered low risk for lobectomy, while values greater than

80% are typically required to proceed safely with pneumonectomy. If values are borderline or low, further testing, such as quantitative perfusion scanning or exercise testing, may be used to refine risk assessment.

Areas You Can Get in Trouble

What If the Patient Has a History of Lung Transplant?

In a lung transplant recipient, hemoptysis is concerning and warrants prompt evaluation. The differential includes infection, rejection, and malignancy. The first step is bronchoalveolar lavage to assess for infectious pathogens, as immunosuppressed patients are at high risk for opportunistic infections. If infection is ruled out, transbronchial biopsy should be performed to evaluate for acute cellular rejection. Rejection is typically treated with high-dose (pulse) corticosteroids. Additionally, transplant recipients have an increased risk of malignancy due to chronic immunosuppression, including both recurrent and de novo primary lung cancers, which should be considered in the diagnostic workup.

What Are Potential Infectious Complications in Patients with Suspected or Confirmed Lung Cancer?

Patients with suspected or confirmed lung cancer, particularly those who are hospitalized, immunosuppressed, or have central venous catheters, are at increased risk for bloodstream infections. Central venous catheters are the most common source of hospital-acquired bloodstream infections, and catheter-associated bacteremia should be considered in any patient presenting with fever or signs of systemic infection. Gram-positive organisms such as *Staphylococcus aureus* are frequently involved, although fungal pathogens including *Candida* may occur in immunocompromised individuals. Diagnostic evaluation includes blood cultures and, when applicable, removal and culture of the catheter tip. Management includes intravenous antimicrobial therapy and prompt source control.

Summary of Essentials

History and Physical Exam

- Chronic cough with hemoptysis and unintentional weight loss
- Risk factors include tobacco use, advanced age, pulmonary fibrosis, HIV, and occupational exposures (e.g., asbestos, silica)
- Physical exam may reveal no pertinent findings; imaging is critical in diagnosis

Pathophysiology

- Lung cancer is the second most common malignancy and the leading cause of cancer-related death in both men and women
- Risk of disease is proportional to the magnitude of cigarette consumption
- Tumors may produce paraneoplastic syndromes (e.g., SIADH, hypercalcemia, hypertrophic osteoarthropathy)

Classification

- Divided into adenocarcinoma, squamous cell carcinoma, large cell carcinoma (NSCLC), SCLC, and other (carcinoid tumor)

Diagnosis

- Initial workup includes CXR and chest CT, with CT being the preferred modality for lesion characterization
- PET/CT and biopsy (via bronchoscopy or CT-guided) are used to confirm diagnosis and stage disease
- Malignant pleural and pericardial effusions may be present

Management

- SPN management is based on size, features, and risk profile; lesions >8 mm or with high-risk features often require biopsy or resection
- Annual screening with low-dose CT for patients aged 50–80 with a 20-pack-year smoking history, who are actively smoking, or who quit within 15 years
- NSCLC
  - Stage I/II: surgery ± adjuvant therapy
  - Stage III: chemoradiation ± surgery in select cases
  - Stage IV: systemic therapy or palliative care
- SCLC
  - Limited stage: chemoradiation
  - Extensive stage: chemotherapy followed by prophylactic cranial irradiation

Acknowledgement The editors would like to acknowledge and thank the following authors for their contributions to the previous edition of the chapter: Ryan Ou.

Suggested Reading

Aberle DR, Adams AM, Berg CD, et al. Reduced lung-cancer mortality with low-dose computed tomographic screening. N Engl J Med. 2011;365(5):395–409.

Dela Cruz CS, Tanoue LT, Matthay RA. Lung cancer: epidemiology, etiology, and prevention. Clin Chest Med. 2011;32(4) https://doi.org/10.1016/j.ccm.2011.09.001.

Herbst RS, Heymach JV, Lippman SM. Lung cancer. N Engl J Med. 2008;359(13):1367–80.

Jemal A, Ward E, Hao Y, Thun M. Trends in the leading causes of death in the United States, 1970–2002. JAMA. 2005;294(10):1255–9.

Cardiothoracic

Question Set: Cardiothoracic

Questions

1. An otherwise healthy 17-year-old boy presents to the emergency department with sudden-onset chest pain and shortness of breath that began shortly after a prolonged coughing episode during an upper respiratory illness. He reports feeling a "crunching sensation" in his chest when breathing. He is tall and thin and has no history of trauma. Vital signs are stable, and oxygen saturation is 98% on room air. On physical examination, his lungs are clear to auscultation, but there is mild palpable crepitus in the suprasternal region. Chest X-ray shows linear lucencies tracking along the mediastinum but no lung collapse or pleural effusion. What is the most appropriate next step in management?
   (A) Emergent needle thoracostomy
   (B) Chest tube placement
   (C) Supportive care and observation
   (D) Intravenous (IV) corticosteroids and bronchodilators
   (E) Surgical consultation for mediastinal exploration

2. A 75-year-old male with severe aortic stenosis has a routine checkup at his primary care doctor. Which of the following symptoms portends the worst prognosis?
   (A) Exertional chest pain
   (B) Dyspnea
   (C) Fainting spells
   (D) Mid-systolic murmur heard loudest at the upper right sternal border
   (E) Small head nodding movements at each heartbeat

3. Which of the following is the most important risk factor for aortic dissection?
   (A) History of coronary artery bypass grafting (CABG)
   (B) Giant cell arteritis
   (C) Pregnancy
   (D) Hypertension
   (E) Bicuspid aortic valve

4. A patient is diagnosed with type A aortic dissection, and there is concern for cardiac tamponade. Which of the following findings would be the *most* consistent with cardiac tamponade?
   (A) Pulsus bisferiens
   (B) Watson's water hammer pulse
   (C) Peaked T-waves
   (D) Equalization of central pressures
   (E) Pulsus alternans

5. A 17-year-old male presents for a pre-participation physical before track season. A harsh systolic murmur is heard at the second right intercostal space. He denies ever experiencing chest pain, dizziness, or difficulty breathing. Which of the following would be expected on further workup?
(A) T-wave inversion on electrocardiogram
(B) Laterally displaced point of maximum impulse (PMI) on palpation
(C) Weak femoral pulses compared to brachial pulses
(D) Increased intensity of the murmur with Valsalva maneuver
(E) Increased intensity of the murmur with squatting

6. A 65-year-old woman arrives to the emergency department complaining of chest pain. Her past medical history includes hypertension, atherosclerosis, and coronary artery disease. She underwent a coronary artery bypass graft (CABG) 3 weeks ago for three-vessel disease. She reports that her chest pain worsens with inspiration and lessens when leaning forward. A friction rub is heard on auscultation. Electrocardiogram shows global ST elevation. What is the most likely diagnosis?
(A) Myocarditis
(B) Myocardial infarction (MI)
(C) Cardiac tamponade
(D) Acute pericarditis
(E) Pulmonary embolism

7. A 65-year-old female has breast cancer and a remote history of congestive heart failure (CHF). Her physician is planning to administer a chemotherapeutic agent that has potential for cardiac toxicity. Which of the following is considered the gold standard for accurately assessing her ejection fraction (EF)?
(A) Multigated acquisition (MUGA) scan
(B) Echocardiography
(C) Electrocardiogram
(D) Coronary angiography
(E) Cardiac MRI

8. A 76-year-old man is driven to the emergency department by his wife and is complaining of severe chest pain that started 30 min prior. He denies abdominal or extremity pain. Pulses in the arms and legs are 2+. His kidney function is normal. CT scan shows an aortic dissection. Which of the following findings on CT scan would most strongly indicate the need for urgent surgery?
(A) Dissection of the entire descending thoracic aorta
(B) Involvement of common iliac arteries
(C) Involvement of renal arteries
(D) Extension into mesenteric vessels
(E) Involvement of origin of innominate artery

9. A 65-year-old female is diagnosed with aortic dissection beginning 2 cm distal to the left subclavian artery and extending distally. Her blood pressure is 180/70 mmHg, and her heart rate is 88/min. Peripheral pulses are all 2+, and her abdomen is soft and nontender. What is the next best step in treatment?
(A) Surgical repair
(B) Aggressive IV fluids
(C) Labetalol drip
(D) Endovascular repair
(E) Nicardipine drip

10. A 65-year-old man is rushed to the emergency department by ambulance after he suddenly lost strength and sensation in his left leg and arm. He was hospitalized 2 months ago with a non-ST elevated myocardial infarction (NSTEMI). He is compliant with all of his medications and had been recovering well until the present episode. Electrocardiogram shows normal sinus rhythm without evidence of ischemia. Chest X-ray is unremarkable. Carotid ultrasound demonstrates <30% stenosis bilaterally. What is the most likely etiology of the patient's present symptoms?
    (A) Ventricular thromboembolism
    (B) Septic embolism to the brain
    (C) Type A dissection involving the right carotid artery
    (D) Thromboembolism from the left atrial appendage
    (E) Paradoxical venous thromboembolism

11. A 66-year-old man is recovering in the intensive care unit (ICU) after receiving a coronary artery bypass graft (CABG). On the fourth postoperative day, he complains of chest pain. He is sweating, anxious, short of breath, and nauseated. Electrocardiogram shows evidence of right-sided myocardial infarction (MI). His blood pressure is 98/65 mmHg. What is the next best step in management?
    (A) Administer 1 L of normal saline
    (B) Nitroglycerin
    (C) Nitroprusside
    (D) Nifedipine
    (E) Lisinopril

12. A 65-year-old male presents with a painful nodule in his wrist that is determined to be a ganglion cyst. Despite attempts at aspiration, it recurs. He is unable to work as a computer programmer, is on disability, and is feeling depressed. He is scheduled for wrist surgery. He reports having been discharged 1 week ago for an episode of chest pain. Troponins were elevated at that time, but there was no elevation of his ST segment. Which of the following is the best recommendation?
    (A) Proceed with surgery with intraoperative transesophageal echocardiography
    (B) Proceed with surgery but perform under local anesthesia with sedation
    (C) Proceed with surgery only if echocardiogram shows normal ejection fraction
    (D) Proceed with surgery after aggressive beta blockade to get heart rate into low 60s
    (E) Postpone surgery for at least 4 weeks

13. A 65-year-old male is about to undergo an elective inguinal hernia repair. Which of the following findings on history or physical would portend the highest operative risk?
    (A) Systolic, crescendo–decrescendo murmur at the sternal border of the right second intercostal space radiating into the neck
    (B) A history of myocardial infarction 10 years ago
    (C) Insulin-dependent diabetes mellitus with an elevated hemoglobin A1C (Hb-A1C)
    (D) Renal insufficiency not yet on dialysis
    (E) Smoking

14. A 65-year-old male undergoes a videoscopic right upper lobectomy for squamous cell lung cancer. On postoperative day 1, he suddenly develops chest pain and diaphoresis. Blood pressure is 120/60 mmHg, and heart rate is 80/min. Serial highly sensitive troponin-I assays demonstrate levels of 0.4, 0.3, and 0.01 ng/mL. Electrocardiogram demonstrates nonspecific T-wave changes with no ST-segment elevation. Following the administration of oxygen, morphine, aspirin, and a beta-blocker, his symptoms resolve. What is the next step in the management?
(A) Intravenous thrombolytic therapy
(B) Percutaneous coronary intervention (PCI) with stenting
(C) PCI without stenting
(D) Coronary artery bypass graft (CABG)
(E) Continue medical management and reevaluate as outpatient in 4–6 weeks

15. A 67-year-old male is diagnosed with a type B aortic dissection. At the time of initial presentation on the previous day, his blood pressure was 178/110 mmHg. He was treated with intravenous beta-blocker, and his blood pressure was reduced to 112/60 mmHg and has remained in that range. However, 1 day later, he suddenly develops severe abdominal pain. His blood pressure is measured to be 110/56 mmHg. Which of the following is the most likely explanation?
(A) *Clostridium* difficile infection
(B) Occlusion of the superior mesenteric artery
(C) Pancreatitis
(D) Aortoenteric fistula
(E) Diverticulitis

16. An obese 52-year-old man with a 50-pack-year smoking history and hypertension controlled with chlorthalidone presents to a remote hospital without interventional capabilities with 30 min of crushing chest pain radiating to his left arm and jaw. Troponin and Creatine Kinase-MB levels are elevated, and electrocardiogram shows ST-segment elevations in leads V1 through V4. He is treated with thrombolytic therapy, and his symptoms resolve. The next morning, the patient is found dead in his bed. Which of the following is the most likely cause of death?
(A) Ventricular free wall rupture
(B) Embolic stroke
(C) Ventricular arrhythmia
(D) Post-MI pericarditis
(E) Overwhelming infection

17. A 40-year-old male presents with acute chest pain and nausea. Serum troponin levels are elevated, and the electrocardiogram demonstrates ST-segment elevation. Which of the following would be the strongest contraindication to intravenous thrombolytic therapy?
(A) Right knee arthroscopic surgery 1 month ago
(B) Recently completed antibiotic course for Helicobacter pylori infection
(C) Wide mediastinum on chest X-ray
(D) History of alcohol use disorder
(E) Endovascular aortic aneurysm repair 1 month ago

18. A 63-year-old woman with diabetes is recovering in the ICU after receiving a coronary artery bypass graft (CABG). On the sixth postoperative day, she starts complaining of chest pain. Her temperature is 38.7 °C, blood pressure is 108/72 mmHg, and pulse is 125/min. On physical exam, there is drainage from her sternal wound, and there is a crunching sound heard with a stethoscope over the precordium during systole. The sternum feels somewhat unstable to palpation. Her laboratory examination is significant for an elevated white blood count ($16.7 \times 10^3/\mu L$). Chest X-ray is pending. What is the most likely diagnosis?
    (A) Acute pericarditis
    (B) Postoperative myocardial infarction (MI)
    (C) Empyema
    (D) Acute mediastinitis
    (E) Pneumonia

Answers

1. Answer C
This patient has a classic presentation of spontaneous pneumomediastinum, most commonly seen in tall, thin adolescent males following intense coughing or an asthma exacerbation. The elevated intra-alveolar pressure leads to alveolar rupture and air dissection along bronchovascular sheaths into the mediastinum and subcutaneous tissues. Symptoms include pleuritic chest pain, dyspnea, and subcutaneous emphysema (palpable crepitus). Chest X-ray typically shows air tracking along the mediastinum without evidence of lung collapse. In uncomplicated cases, the condition is self-limited and managed with supportive care including rest, analgesia, and close monitoring. Emergent needle thoracostomy is indicated for tension pneumothorax, a life-threatening condition characterized by hypotension, tracheal deviation, and unilateral breath sound absence. This patient is hemodynamically stable and lacks these findings (A). Chest tube placement is used for pneumothorax, especially if large or symptomatic. This patient has no evidence of lung collapse or air in the pleural space, making this option inappropriate (B). Intravenous corticosteroids and bronchodilators are appropriate in asthma exacerbations with bronchospasm. While coughing may be the inciting event, there is no evidence of active bronchospasm or asthma decompensation in this case (D). Surgical consultation for mediastinal exploration is unnecessary for spontaneous pneumomediastinum without signs of esophageal rupture (E).

2. Answer B
The classic symptoms of aortic stenosis are angina, syncope, and dyspnea. Of these, dyspnea due to congestive heart failure portends the worst prognosis, with approximately 50% mortality within 2 years without valve replacement (A, C). A loud midsystolic murmur indicates hemodynamically significant obstruction but is a better prognostic sign than an absent murmur, which indicates low blood flow across the valve (D). Small head nodding movements with each heartbeat are known as de Musset's sign and is found in aortic regurgitation (E).

3. Answer D
All of the above are risk factors for aortic dissection. However, the most significant risk factor for aortic dissection is systemic hypertension (A–C, E).

4. Answer D

In cardiac tamponade, fluid (blood or effusion) in the pericardial space externally compresses the heart, which limits diastolic filling and reduces stroke volume. Since pericardial fluid is free flowing, the pressure is distributed equally along the pericardium. As this continues the rising pressure in the pericardium is transmitted to all four cardiac chambers resulting in equalization of central pressures. Pulsus bisferiens, also known as a biphasic pulse, refers to two strong systolic pulses with a mid-systolic dip, in other words, two pulses during systole (A). It can be seen in aortic regurgitation with or without aortic stenosis and hypertrophic cardiomyopathy. Watson's water hammer pulse is a pulse with a rapid upstroke and descent seen in patients with aortic regurgitation (B). Peaked T-waves are most often associated with hyperkalemia (C). It is unlikely to be seen in patients with cardiac tamponade since their electrocardiogram findings are characteristically low voltage. Pulsus alternans is a physical exam finding wherein the amplitude of a peripheral pulse changes from beat to beat associated with changing systolic blood pressure (E). It is most commonly caused by left ventricular failure.

5. Answer D

The patient likely has hypertrophic obstructive cardiomyopathy, an asymmetric thickening of the ventricular septum that creates a narrowing of the left ventricular outflow tract. Vigorous exercise places him at increased risk of sudden cardiac death. Murmur intensity increases with Valsalva because decreased preload further narrows the left ventricular outflow tract, intensifying the obstruction. In contrast, squatting increases preload and reduces murmur intensity. T-wave inversion would be found in ischemic heart disease and would be very unlikely in an otherwise healthy 17-year-old (A). Laterally displaced PMI would be found in patients with congestive heart failure, also very unlikely in this patient (B). Weak femoral pulses compared to brachial pulses are a finding in coarctation of the aorta and would not create a harsh systolic murmur (C). Murmurs due to aortic regurgitation, mitral regurgitation, and ventricular septal defect increase in intensity with squatting (E).

6. Answer D

Acute pericarditis is inflammation in the pericardial sac accompanied by pericardial effusion. It can occur following post-MI (termed Dressler's syndrome), chest radiation, or recent heart surgery. Patients present with pleuritic chest pain that lessens when leaning forward, friction rub heard on auscultation, global ST elevation, and PR depression. Patients with myocarditis (A) usually present with signs and symptoms of acute decompensating heart failure (e.g., tachycardia, gallop, mitral regurgitation, and edema) (A). Chest pain accompanied with MI would not be expected to lessen with leaning forward (B). Furthermore, global ST elevation would not be expected. Cardiac tamponade can occur once the effusion reaches a critical mass in which cardiac output is compromised (C). Pulmonary embolism can present with pleuritic chest pain, but it will not be influenced by positioning and is more likely to have electrocardiogram findings suggestive of right heart failure (E).

7. Answer E

Cardiac MRI is considered the gold standard for measuring ejection fraction due to its superior spatial resolution and reproducibility. It allows precise quantification of ventricular volumes and function, without relying on geometric assumptions. In addition to assessing systolic function, cardiac MRI provides detailed information on myocardial fibrosis, viability, and infiltration, which is particularly useful in patients at risk of cardiotoxicity from chemotherapy. While MUGA scans were previously favored for EF assessment due to reproducibility, they involve radiation exposure and have limited additional diagnostic capabilities (A). Echocardiography is widely available and typically used for initial evaluation, but it is operator-dependent and less accurate than MRI (B). Electrocardiogram and exercise stress test are unable to measure a patient's ejection fraction (C). Coronary angiography is considered the gold standard in identifying coronary artery disease and can estimate ejection fraction but is not as accurate (D).

8. Answer E
It is important to rapidly identify Stanford type A dissections, as they require urgent surgical intervention due to the fact that they can lead to cardiac tamponade, acute aortic valve insufficiency, acute myocardial infarction, and stroke. A Stanford type A dissection involves the ascending aorta and/or the aortic arch. Thus, an aortic dissection involving the innominate artery is a Stanford type A (A–D). Stanford type B aortic dissection is more common. It begins in the descending aorta, distal to the takeoff of the left subclavian artery. Stanford type B dissections are much less likely to cause acute complications since the ascending aorta/aortic arch is not involved. A type B dissection may involve the mesenteric, renal, or iliac arteries, but not occlude them, as blood may continue to flow normally (either though the true or the false lumen). Most can be managed medically with blood pressure control (beta-blockers). Surgical intervention is needed if the involvement of these vessels leads to malperfusion (such as leg ischemia, bowel ischemia, or renal failure).

9. Answer C
Based on the description of the site of the dissection, this is a type B aortic dissection. These are usually managed medically unless the patient has evidence of malperfusion (A). Since her peripheral pulses are all 2+ and her abdomen is soft and non-tender, there is no evidence of malperfusion. The goal is to maintain a relatively low blood pressure in order to minimize stress on the aorta. Aggressive IV fluids will not reduce blood pressure and may actually raise it (B). Nicardipine will lower blood pressure, but intravenous beta-blocker is the treatment of choice because it also reduces the rate of pressure increase with each beat of the heart, which lowers the stress on the aortic wall (E). Endovascular therapy is not routinely needed for most type B dissections (D).

10. Answer A
Patients with a recent myocardial infarction are at risk of developing a left ventricular thrombus, particularly when the infarct involved the anterior wall or apex. These thrombi can embolize, leading to ischemic stroke. The most likely etiology in this patient with a recent NSTEMI and no evidence of carotid disease is embolization from a ventricular thrombus. While warfarin was historically used to prevent thromboembolism, direct oral anticoagulants (DOACs) are increasingly preferred due to their fixed dosing and reduced bleeding risk. Thromboembolism from the left atrial appendage is a concern in patients with atrial fibrillation (D). Paradoxical venous thromboembolism is a concern in patients with an atrial septal defect or patent foramen ovale, wherein a deep venous thrombus can travel through the defect into the left heart and ultimately to the brain (E). Septic embolism is a concern in patients with a history of IV drug use and can lead to cerebral abscess (B). Type A dissection would usually present with severe chest pain radiating to the back (C).

11. Answer A
This patient has a postoperative right-sided MI, resulting in compromised cardiac output secondary to decreased preload. One of the steps in the management of *right-sided* MI is to administer fluids to help increase filling of the heart. Avoid nitrates in these patients as it may further reduce preload (B–C). Acutely, patients with MI need oxygen, aspirin, analgesics, and beta-blockers. Oxygen should be used selectively as it is considered a systemic vasoconstrictor and can further reduce coronary blood flow. Dihydropyridine calcium channel blockers, such as nifedipine, are contraindicated in MI

because of the associated peripheral vasodilation that may lead to reactive tachycardia and subsequently result in even more stress on the heart (D). Angiotensin-converting enzyme (ACE) inhibitors (e.g., lisinopril) should be considered for long-term treatment after the acute episode has resolved (E).

12. Answer E

This patient has a NSTEMI. Proceeding with elective surgery 1 week after an acute MI is inappropriate (A–D). Patients with a recent MI are at significantly increased cardiac risk during non-cardiac surgery, particularly within the first month after MI. Although performing the operation under local anesthesia with sedation seems appealing, there is still considerable stress and cardiac risk with such an approach (B). The best recommendation for this patient is to postpone surgery for at least 4 weeks. At that point, consideration should still be given to cardiac stress testing prior to surgery or even further surgical delay, as the cardiac risk persists for at least 6 months after an MI.

13. Answer A

Major predictors of adverse postoperative cardiac events must be identified prior to elective non-cardiac surgery. These include recent (within 1 month) myocardial infarction, unstable or severe angina, decompensated congestive heart failure, and significant arrhythmias. Such cardiac conditions require postponing surgery and performing further cardiac workup. A systolic, crescendo–decrescendo murmur at the sternal border of the right second intercostal space radiating into the neck is highly suggestive of aortic stenosis and would require an echocardiogram to rule out severe aortic stenosis. Aortic stenosis impairs coronary perfusion, which can become further exacerbated during induction of anesthesia. From all the choices listed, it portends the highest operative risk. Even in asymptomatic patients, severe aortic stenosis significantly increases the risk of perioperative hypotension, myocardial ischemia, and sudden cardiac death, particularly during anesthesia induction. Lee's revised cardiac risk index identifies intermediate risk factors; these include known coronary artery disease, history of CHF, history of stroke or transient ischemic attack, insulin-dependent diabetes, creatinine >2.0 mg/dL, and high-risk surgery (i.e., aortic) (B–D). Adding a point for each factor and assigning a score (from 0–6) are highly effective in stratifying cardiac risk. Interestingly, smoking has not been shown to be an independent risk factor for adverse perioperative cardiac events in most studies (E).

14. Answer E

The patient has suffered a postoperative NSTEMI. Most NSTEMI (as opposed to a STEMI) in the postoperative setting are managed without PCI with a combination of oxygen, morphine for pain relief, aspirin, and a beta-blocker. Optimally, an additional antiplatelet agent (such as clopidogrel) and intravenous heparin are also given, but this depends on how recent the operation was and the potential for postoperative bleeding. Consideration should be given to stress testing at 4–6 weeks after surgery, and depending on the results, PCI is then considered. Urgent PCI is indicated in the setting of a STEMI, and in certain high-risk NSTEMIs (continued rise in troponins, ongoing chest pain), but will require clopidogrel (again may not be desirable so soon after surgery) if a stent is placed (B–C). The patient described has a down trend of troponins and relief of symptoms, further supporting medical management. Emergent CABG would be considered if PCI fails or is not technically feasible with severe three-vessel disease (D). Emergent operations for acute MI continue to have a high mortality despite many technological advances in myocardial protection. Thrombolytic therapy is an alternative when PCI is not available but would be contraindicated within 2–3 weeks of major surgery (A).

15. Answer B
Sudden onset of severe abdominal pain in association with an aortic dissection should always raise suspicion for malperfusion of the bowel which can lead to bowel ischemia, gangrene, and death. This most likely would occur if the dissection extends into, and suddenly occludes, the superior mesenteric artery, which supplies blood to the bowel from the ligament of Treitz to the mid-transverse colon. It is also important to recognize that bowel ischemia early on causes excruciating pain in the absence of peritonitis ("pain out of proportion to physical exam"). He has not been on broad-spectrum antibiotics and has no reason to have *C. difficile* infection, which most often presents with vague abdominal pain and diarrhea (A). Pancreatitis presents with epigastric pain radiating to the back, nausea, vomiting, anorexia, fever, and tachycardia and is most commonly associated with cholelithiasis and alcohol abuse (C). Aortoenteric fistula is a possible long-term sequela in patients who have had an intra-aortic synthetic graft placed (D). Diverticulitis is a common cause of left lower quadrant abdominal pain in elderly patients and does not typically cause such sudden severe pain (E).

16. Answer C
This patient is presenting with ST-elevation myocardial infarction (MI). It is important to know the timing of causes of death after MI. In the first 48 h after MI, death is likely due to ventricular arrhythmia. If arrhythmia occurs after 48 h, an implantable defibrillator should be placed. Ruptures of the myocardium, either as a ventricular septal rupture or free wall rupture, usually do not occur until 4–5 days after MI, at which point the dead myocardium has been weakened by the body's inflammatory response (A). Post-MI pericarditis, also known as *Dressler's syndrome*, usually occurs weeks or months after MI or cardiac surgery (D). An embolic stroke would present with sudden onset of numbness on one side of the body, cranial nerve deficits, and/or aphasia (B). It is unlikely to cause death so quickly. There is no reason to believe the patient has sustained an overwhelming infection (E).

17. Answer C
Wide mediastinum on chest X-ray is concerning for aortic dissection. Patients with type A aortic dissection can present with coronary artery malperfusion and thus have a similar presentation as an acute myocardial infarction. Suspected aortic dissection is considered an absolute contraindication to thrombolysis in patients with myocardial infarction. The remaining choices are all relative contraindications for intravenous thrombolytics (A–B, D–E).

18. Answer D
This patient's presentation is most concerning for acute mediastinitis. This is a life-threatening infection of the mediastinum with a very high mortality rate that is most commonly associated with cardiac surgery. The incidence rate is 1–2% following CABG. The source of infection may be a sternal wound infection, combined with instability of the sternum that permits bacteria to enter the mediastinum. *Hamman's sign* is

a crunching sound heard with a stethoscope over the precordium during systole and is suggestive of acute mediastinitis. Patients will frequently present with chest pain, increased drainage from the sternal wound, fevers, and leukocytosis. Chest radiograph findings include a widened mediastinum with or without pneumomediastinum or air–fluid levels within the mediastinum. A CT scan can also support the diagnosis by demonstrating dehiscence of the sternum and stranding, fluid and air pockets within the anterior mediastinum. Management includes surgical debridement, drainage, antibiotics, and rewiring the sternum. Acute pericarditis will present with pleuritic chest pain that lessens when leaning forward, friction rub heard on auscultation, and characteristic electrocardiogram findings (global ST elevation) (A). Pneumonia would present with shortness of breath, productive cough, and abnormal lung sounds (E). Postoperative MI would not be expected to present with evidence of systemic inflammation (B). Empyema is defined as pus in the pleural space and would not explain the physical exam findings of sternal instability and Hamman's sign (C). CT scan would demonstrate a loculated fluid collection within the right or left pleural cavity.

Endocrine

Michael W. Yeh

Contents

Incidentally Discovered Adrenal Mass on CT Scan

Eugene J. Park, Masha J. Livhits, and Michael W. Yeh

Contents

C. de Virgilio, A. Grigorian (eds.), *Surgery*, https://doi.org/10.1007/978-3-032-09799-6_11

Case Study

A 55-year-old female was involved in a motor vehicle accident, at which time she underwent an abdominal CT scan that was negative for any injury. However, a 1.7-cm right adrenal nodule was incidentally noted. The patient complains of difficulty losing weight but denies any recent weight gain, abnormal hair growth, or muscle weakness. She has a long-standing history of diabetes and hypertension. She denies headache, palpitations, and flushing. A physical exam is significant for central obesity, but she does not have supraclavicular fat accumulation or purple striae. Workup for the adrenal mass revealed an elevated 24-hour urine cortisol level (170 mcg/dL; normal <45 mcg/dL). This was followed by a low-dose dexamethasone suppression test, which resulted in a lack of cortisol suppression (AM cortisol 14.2 mcg/dL, normal <2 mcg/dL). Further biochemical workup, including catecholamines and metanephrines as well as plasma aldosterone and renin levels, was normal.

Diagnosis

What Is the Differential Diagnosis?

The differential for an adrenal mass is broad, given the variety of cell types present in the adrenal gland. The two key defining characteristics are whether the nodule is functional (associated with hormone hypersecretion) and whether it is malignant (either metastatic or primary adrenocortical). The majority of incidentally discovered adrenal nodules are both benign and nonfunctional. These include nonfunctional adenomas, myelolipomas, and cysts. Functional tumors typically secrete one of three hormone types: cortisol, aldosterone, or catecholamines (epinephrine and norepinephrine). Primary malignancies, typically adrenocortical carcinoma, are defined by the presence of local invasion into adjacent organs, blood vessels, or lymph nodes, or distant metastasis. Of note, adrenocortical carcinomas are often associated with hormone hypersecretion. Finally, the adrenal glands are a frequent site for metastasis, most commonly from lung and breast cancer. The following chart (▪ Table 11.1) provides an overview of common adrenal incidentalomas:

▪ **Table 11.1** Common adrenal incidentalomas

Diagnosis	Percentage	Clinical presentation
Benign, nonfunctional mass (myelolipoma, adenoma, cyst, hematoma, granulomalinfection)	80%	Often asymptomatic; may have a specific history related to trauma or infection (e.g., tuberculosis)
Hypercortisolism (Cushing's syndrome)	7%	Weight gain, central obesity, muscle weakness, poor wound healing, hirsutism, amenorrhea, depression, hypertension, diabetes mellitus
Catecholamine hypersecretion (pheochromocytoma)	5%	Episodic tachycardia, sustained or episodic hypertension, headache, flushing, palpitations
Adrenocortical carcinoma	5%	Abdominal pain (mass effect); symptoms related to functional tumor, large >6 cm
Metastasis	2%	History of extra-adrenal tumor (most commonly lung or breast tumor; also melanoma, lymphoma, and kidney and ovary tumors)
Hyperaldosteronism (Conn's syndrome)	1%	Muscle cramps, weakness, hypertension
Androgen hypersecretion	<1%	Virilization, hirsutism, menstrual abnormalities

What Is the Most Likely Diagnosis?

Given the small size of the mass and the evidence of cortisol hypersecretion, it is most likely a benign cortisol-secreting adrenal adenoma. An adrenal incidentaloma is an incidentally discovered mass seen on imaging performed for an unrelated reason (▪ Fig. 11.1). Approximately 5% of patients who undergo an abdominal CT scan will have an incidentally discovered adrenal mass.

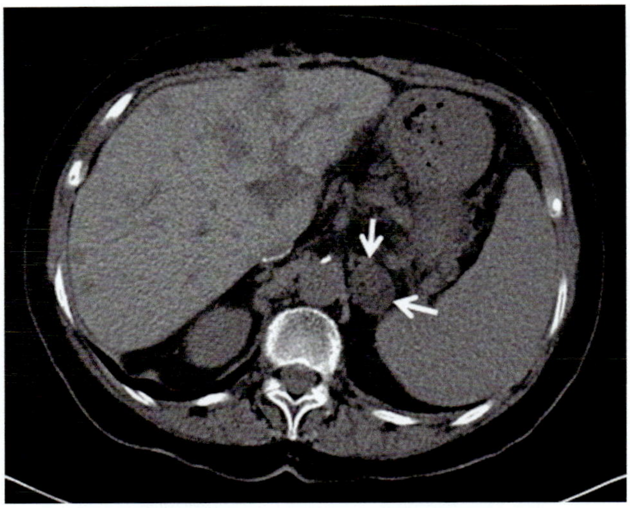

Fig. 11.1 Axial CT showing a small incidentaloma—an asymptomatic adrenal nodule discovered incidentally

History and Physical

What Are the Findings on History and Physical Examination in a Patient That Hypersecretes Cortisol?

11

Physical exam findings include truncal obesity and fat accumulation around the head (moon facies) and neck (buffalo hump). Proximal muscle wasting can make it difficult for patients to stand from a seated position or climb stairs. The skin thins out, resulting in purple striae on the abdomen and extremities, easy bruising, and a reddish coloration of the face (plethora). Women may present with amenorrhea and hirsutism. Patients often have associated metabolic conditions (i.e., obesity, diabetes, elevated cholesterol or lipid levels, and hypertension). Hypercortisolism is also associated with osteoporosis, poor wound healing, and psychiatric symptoms.

What Is the Difference Between Cushing's Syndrome and Cushing's Disease?

Cushing's Syndrome (Fig. 11.2) refers to the collection of signs and symptoms resulting from glucocorticoid excess, regardless of the source. It is often caused by exogenous glucocorticoids, commonly prescribed for immunosuppression in autoimmune diseases or following organ transplants. Endogenous Cushing's syndrome can be ACTH-dependent or ACTH-independent. The majority of endogenous cases are ACTH-dependent, stemming from excess ACTH secretion (secondary hypercortisolism). *Cushing's Disease* is a specific form of ACTH-dependent Cushing's syndrome, where hypercortisolism arises from an ACTH-secreting pituitary adenoma. This distinguishes it from other causes of ACTH-dependent Cushing's syndrome, such as ectopic ACTH production from non-small cell lung cancer or bronchial carcinoid tumors. In contrast, ACTH-independent Cushing's syndrome (primary hypercortisolism) usually results from a single adrenal adenoma, though some patients may have bilateral adrenal hyperplasia or multiple adrenal nodules.

What Is the Clinical Presentation of an Adrenal Nodule That Hypersecretes Aldosterone?

The classic hallmark of hyperaldosteronism is hypertension with hypokalemia; however, hypokalemia is seen in less than 40% of cases. Hyperaldosteronism should be considered in patients with refractory hypertension requiring three or more antihypertensive agents. Hypokalemia, if present, may present with muscle cramping, muscle weakness, or rarely paralysis. Patients with hyperaldosteronism often show an excellent response to spironolactone, an aldosterone antagonist.

What Is the Clinical Presentation of a Pheochromocytoma?

Patients with pheochromocytoma most often present with sustained or episodic hypertension. Though only a minority present with the classic triad of headache, flushing, and palpitations, more than 90% complain of at least one of these symptoms.

What Signs and Symptoms Should Raise Suspicion for an Adrenocortical Carcinoma?

Adrenocortical carcinomas are highly lethal malignancies (5-year survival <25%) which often present at an advanced stage after having grown in a quiescent fashion. Approximately 60% are functional. The most common hormone hypersecretion associated with adrenocortical carcinoma is cortisol, followed by androgens, and very rarely, aldosterone. Patients with non-functional tumors may present with an abdominal mass, abdominal pain, nausea, anorexia, early satiety, or weight loss. Approximately 75% of adrenocortical carcinomas are >6 cm at the time of presentation (Figs. 11.3 and 11.4).

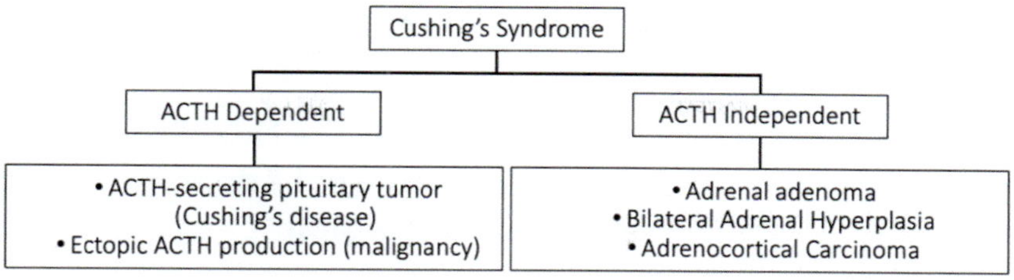

Fig. 11.2 Cushing's syndrome

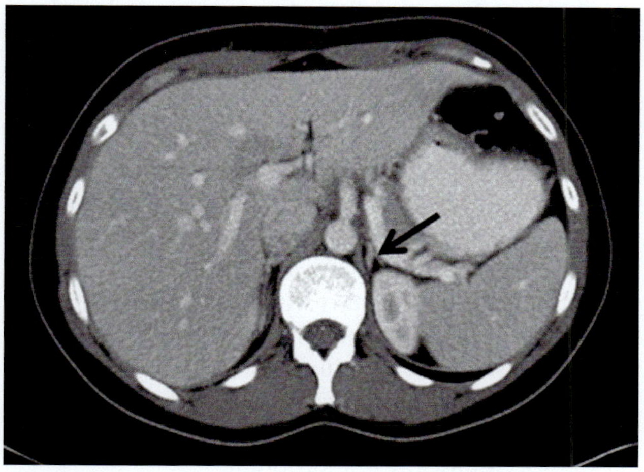

Fig. 11.3 Axial CT of the normal left adrenal gland

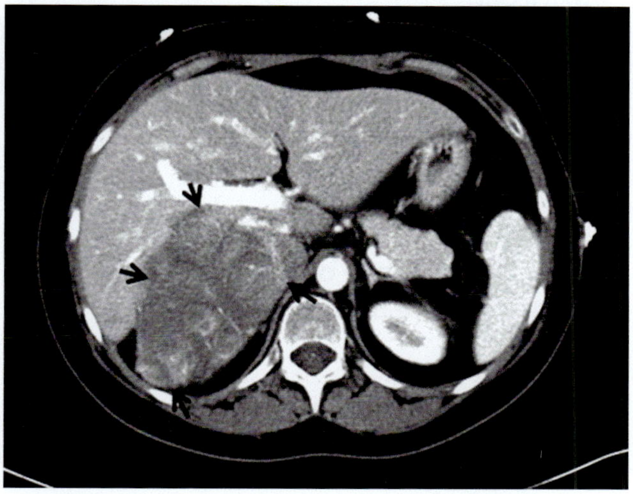

Fig. 11.4 Axial CT showing a large adrenal mass consistent with malignant adrenal cortical carcinoma

Pathophysiology

What Is the Most Common Adrenal Mass?

The most common adrenal mass is a nonfunctional benign adrenocortical adenoma. Only 20% of adrenal adenomas are associated with hormone hypersecretion. The most common functional lesion discovered incidentally is a cortisol-secreting adenoma.

What Are the Zones of the Adrenal Gland and What Hormones Do They Produce?

Each adrenal gland has an outer cortex and an inner medulla. The cortex is composed of three zones (from outer to inner): glomerulosa, fasciculata, and reticularis. The outer zona glomerulosa is the site of mineralocorticoid (aldosterone) production. The middle zona fasciculata is the site of glucocorticoid (cortisol) production. The inner zona reticularis is the site of sex hormone (dehydroxyepiandrosterone, dehydroxyepiandrosterone-sulfate, and androstenedione) synthesis. The adrenal medulla is the location for catecholamine synthesis.

Watch Out

Remember the names of each layer of the adrenal gland by knowing that the adrenals are close to the kidneys and that you monitor kidney function with "GFR" (glomerulosa, fasciculata, reticularis) and their corresponding hormones as "Salt, Sugar, Sex."

What Are the Physiologic Effects of Normal and Excessive Cortisol Secretion?

Cortisol binds to intracellular cytoplasmic receptors and influences transcriptional activation of genes, specifically affecting glucose metabolism, intravascular volume, and immune modulation. The primary action of cortisol is to increase blood glucose levels via inhibition of insulin-mediated cellular glucose uptake, stimulation of glycogenolysis, stimulation of hepatic gluconeogenesis, and stimulation of peripheral proteolysis and lipolysis. Excessive cortisol secretion therefore causes hyperglycemia, muscle wasting, and fat redistribution, which presents as central obesity. Cortisol also regulates intravascular volume and blood pressure by increasing renal reabsorption of sodium, raising peripheral vascular resistance, and having direct chronotropic and inotropic effects on the heart. Excessive secretion results in hypertension. Cortisol impairs cellular immunity by inhibiting cytokine production, inhibiting T-cell activation, and impairing monocyte and neutrophil chemotaxis. Hypercortisolism impairs wound healing and increases the risk of infection.

What Is the Cause of Hypertension and Hypokalemia in Hyperaldosteronism?

Aldosterone acts on the distal convoluted tubule of the kidney to increase sodium reabsorption (active process). This causes passive reabsorption of water and increases extracellular volume and blood pressure. To balance the positively charged sodium ions, potassium is excreted in the urine.

Watch Out

In cases of excess volume loss (e.g., emesis), the renin-angiotensin-aldosterone system is initiated to replete intravascular volume. Persistent potassium excretion can lead to severe hypokalemia and subsequent arrhythmia. Eventually, the kidneys secrete hydrogen instead of potassium, resulting in acidic urine (paradoxical aciduria) in the context of metabolic alkalosis.

Workup

What Is the Next Step in Workup When an Adrenal Adenoma Is Suspected or Seen on Imaging?

An evaluation (Fig. 11.5) must be performed to determine if the adrenal mass is associated with hormone hypersecretion. A thorough history and physical should be performed, followed by biochemical analysis. Suspected *Cushing's syndrome* can be evaluated with a 24-hour urine cortisol *or* low-dose dexamethasone suppression test *or* midnight salivary cortisol. If any of these are abnormal, the next step is to order a plasma ACTH level *and* high-dose dexamethasone suppression test. Due to the wide circadian variability of plasma cortisol levels (highest at 8:00 a.m., lowest at midnight), a single random cortisol level is not helpful. If hyperaldosteronism is suspected, start with a plasma aldosterone/renin ratio and serum potassium. Suspected pheochromocytoma should be evaluated with a 24-hour urine/plasma metanephrines or catecholamines. If no clinical symptoms are present, sending all the above biochemical studies empirically is appropriate.

Watch Out

A careful medication history should be performed to examine for exogenous sources of glucocorticoids, including those contained in herbal or "alternative" supplements.

What Is the Purpose of the Low-Dose Dexamethasone Suppression Test?

The low-dose dexamethasone suppression test is a screening tool for hypercortisolism. It involves administering 1 mg of dexamethasone orally at night, followed by a morning plasma cortisol measurement. Dexamethasone is a synthetic glucocorticoid that suppresses ACTH secretion from the anterior pituitary through negative feedback, thereby lowering cortisol

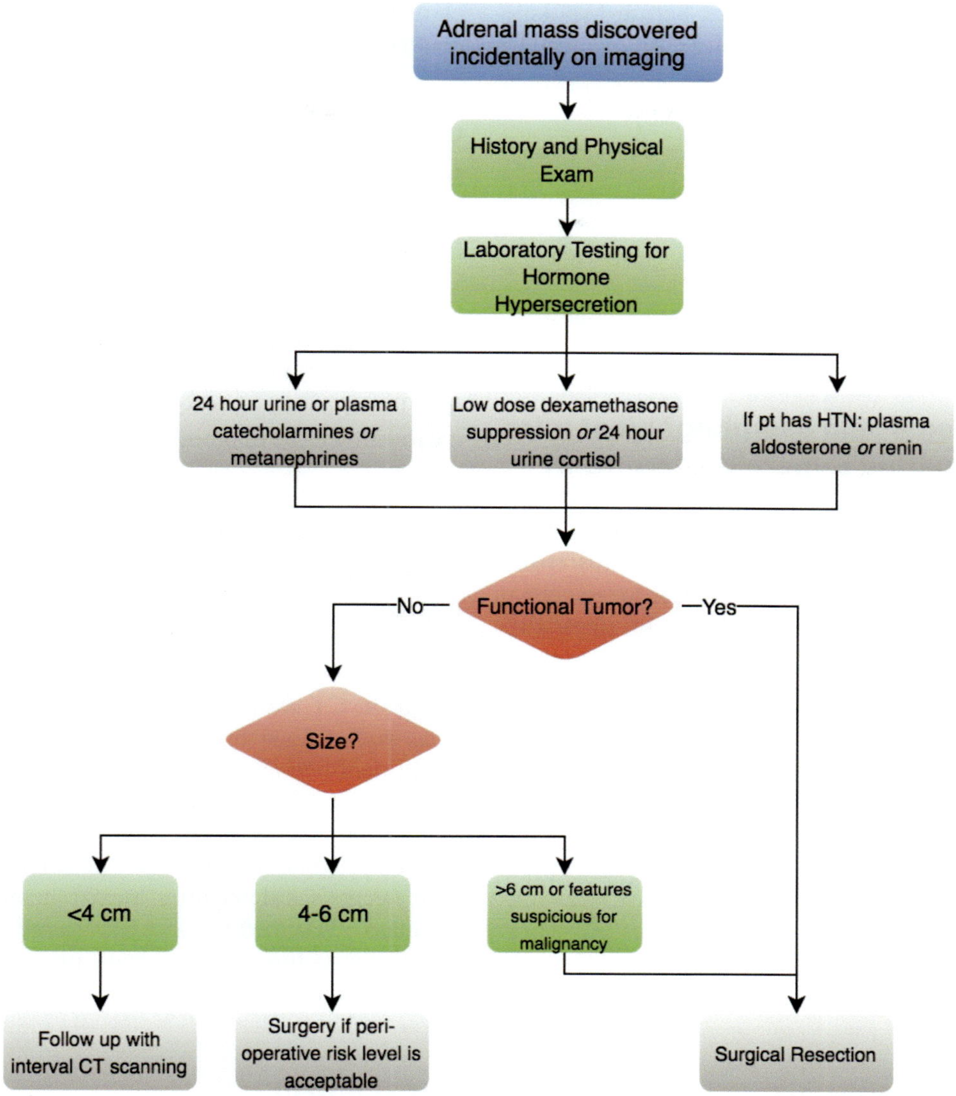

Fig. 11.5 Algorithm for workup and management of incidental adrenal mass

production by the adrenal glands. In normal individuals, this suppression results in a morning cortisol level below 5 μg/dL. A persistently elevated cortisol level suggests endogenous cortisol production, provided exogenous steroid use has been excluded.

How Do ACTH Levels and the High-Dose Dexamethasone Test Help Identify the Source of Hypercortisolism?

If cortisol remains elevated after low-dose dexamethasone, the next step is to measure plasma ACTH. A low ACTH level (<5 pg/mL) suggests an adrenal tumor producing cortisol independently. A normal or elevated ACTH level indicates ACTH-dependent Cushing syndrome, due to either a pituitary adenoma or an ectopic ACTH-secreting tumor. The high-dose dexamethasone test helps differentiate these: pituitary adenomas typically show cortisol suppression with high-dose dexamethasone, while ectopic ACTH sources do not respond to suppression.

What Laboratory Testing Can Identify Hyperaldosteronism?

Patients with hyperaldosteronism generally have increased aldosterone levels (>20 ng/dL), but the most sensitive screening test is to calculate the ratio between the serum aldosterone level and the plasma renin activity (measured in ng/mL/h). Normal ratios are in the 4–10 range, while patients with hyperaldosteronism have ratios >20. An elevated ratio in a hypertensive patient indicates autonomous aldosterone secretion and normal feedback inhibition of renin release. Serum hypokalemia and increased urinary potassium excretion may also be observed.

> **Watch Out**
> A patient with hypertension who requires potassium supplements (clue for hypokalemia) is suggestive of hyperaldosteronism.

What Is Adrenal Vein Sampling? What Is Its Role in Evaluating Hyperaldosteronism?

Primary hyperaldosteronism can be caused by bilateral adrenal hyperplasia or a unilateral aldosterone-secreting adenoma. Because aldosterone-secreting adenomas are usually small (1–2 cm in size), they may not be visualized on cross-sectional imaging such as CT or MRI. As the prevalence of nonfunctional adrenal nodules increases with patient age, adrenal vein sampling by central vein catheterization can be useful to confirm the functional status of an adrenal nodule. Adrenal vein sampling is recommended when the patient is being considered for adrenalectomy, and CT is equivocal or shows bilateral adrenal masses.

> **Watch Out**
> Another source of hypertension is renal artery stenosis due to atherosclerosis (in the elderly) or fibromuscular dysplasia (in young women). Narrowing of the renal arteries leads to decreased blood flow to the kidney, activation of the renin-angiotensin-aldosterone system, and increased aldosterone. If this is suspected, ultrasound can be used to evaluate stenosis of the renal arteries.

What Laboratory Testing Can Identify a Pheochromocytoma?

Plasma metanephrines are highly sensitive and serve as an effective screening test when pheochromocytoma is strongly suspected. If plasma results suggest pheochromocytoma, a 24-hour urine collection measuring catecholamines and metanephrines can then be used to confirm the diagnosis, given its high specificity.

What Is the Best Imaging Modality to Evaluate an Adrenal Nodule? What Is Another Option?

Contrast-enhanced CT scan with fine cuts is generally the preferred imaging modality. It is fast, widely available, and has excellent spatial resolution to evaluate the adrenal gland. MRI is an alternative that is comparable to CT and based on specific characteristics can help to narrow down the diagnosis.

What Imaging Characteristics Help to Differentiate a Benign from Malignant Lesion?

The following characteristics are suggestive of a benign lesion on CT scan: size <4 cm, homogeneous appearance, well-defined borders, high levels of intracellular lipid (identified as ≤10 Hounsfield units (HU) on non-contrast CT scan), rapid washout of contrast, and low amount of vascularity. Features that are more concerning for malignancy include size >6 cm, irregular borders with necrosis, calcification and/or hemorrhage within the mass, ill-defined borders with possible invasion into adjacent structures, low levels of intracellular lipid, and high vascularity.

Management

What Is the Treatment for a Nonfunctional Adrenal Mass? How Does the Size Impact Management?

The management of a nonfunctional adrenal adenoma is based on the likelihood of malignancy. Lesions smaller than 4 cm with benign imaging features have a very low risk of malignancy (<5%); these should be observed with interval CT scanning. Lesions greater than 6 cm or those with concerning imaging features should be resected (adrenalectomy). For lesions between 4 cm and 6 cm, either observation or resection is acceptable and should be decided based on other imaging characteristics and/or patient-specific factors such as the level of perioperative risk.

What Is the Surveillance Protocol for an Adrenal Nodule That Will Not Be Resected?

There is no universally agreed upon surveillance protocol, but a reasonable follow-up strategy consists of repeat imaging at 6, 12, and 24 months, as well as repeat biochemical evaluation for hormone levels yearly for 4 years.

What Is the Treatment for a Functional Adrenal Mass?

Any functional adrenal mass should undergo adrenalectomy regardless of size, as long as the patient is medically fit to undergo an operation.

What Are Important Perioperative Management Principles?

Patients with *Cushing's syndrome* require perioperative and postoperative glucocorticoid replacement, as ACTH secretion from the pituitary can remain suppressed for months and sometimes years after surgery. These patients are therefore at risk for postoperative adrenal insufficiency. Patients with an aldosterone-secreting mass are treated with spironolactone and potassium preoperatively. Pheochromocytoma patients require preoperative alpha-blockade for 10–14 days prior to surgery and close intraoperative hemodynamic monitoring.

> **Watch Out**
> Beta-blockers should only be used after adequate alpha-blockade in patients with pheochromocytoma because unopposed alpha-receptor stimulation may result in severe vasoconstriction and malignant hypertension.

What Are the Key Surgical Principles During an Adrenalectomy?

Laparoscopic adrenalectomy is now the standard surgical treatment for most adrenal tumors, unless the tumor is large (> 6 cm) or there is suspicion for invasive carcinoma. In these latter cases, open adrenalectomy is preferred. The operation can be performed either transabdominally or retroperitoneally. The arterial supply of the adrenal gland is derived from branches of the inferior phrenic artery (superiorly), aorta (medially), and renal artery (inferiorly). Venous drainage from the left adrenal vein empties into the left renal vein, while the right adrenal vein empties directly into the inferior vena cava (IVC). Control of the right adrenal vein is the critical step during right adrenalectomy.

Prognosis

What Is the Prognosis of an Adrenal Adenoma?

For patients with benign lesions, the prognosis is excellent. Surgery usually results in biochemical cure in patients with functional adenomas. Adrenalectomy for an aldosterone-secreting adenoma results in durable improvement of hypertension in 70–90% of patients.

Key Areas Where You Can Get in Trouble

What Is the Role of Percutaneous Needle Biopsy in the Workup of an Adrenal Mass?

Percutaneous biopsy is generally not part of the standard workup for an adrenal mass. If a functional tumor is identified by biochemical testing, a biopsy is unnecessary because these tumors require surgical removal. Importantly, performing a biopsy on a pheochromocytoma is contraindicated, as it can trigger a dangerous surge in catecholamines. Similarly, biopsy of a suspected adrenocortical carcinoma is not recommended because histopathology is often unreliable for distinguishing benign from malignant disease, and there is a risk of bleeding or tumor seeding along the biopsy tract. The only appropriate indication for adrenal biopsy is in patients with a known extra-adrenal primary malignancy, when imaging findings are indeterminate and the biopsy result would confirm metastatic disease and alter management.

Medical or Surgical Therapy for Hyperaldosteronism?

Surgery is the preferred treatment for patients with a unilateral aldosterone-secreting adrenal adenoma. For patients with bilateral adrenal hyperplasia, medical therapy is preferred, as the removal of both adrenal glands will lead to primary adrenal insufficiency

(Addison's disease). Medical therapy often includes anti-hypertensives in addition to potassium-sparing diuretics (i.e., spironolactone) and potassium supplementation.

Summary of Essentials

History and Physical

- Look for evidence of hormonal hypersecretion

Etiology/Pathophysiology

- Most common incidentaloma is a nonfunctional benign adrenocortical adenoma
- Most common functional incidentaloma is associated with hypercortisolism
- Other functional adrenal masses include pheochromocytoma and aldosteronoma
- Rarely, adrenal masses can be due to adrenocortical carcinoma
- Consider metastasis if positive history of extra-adrenal malignancy

11

Diagnosis

- Hypercortisolism
  - 24-hour urine free cortisol level
  - Low-dose dexamethasone suppression test
  - High-dose dexamethasone suppression test if both cortisol/ACTH remain elevated
  - Salivary cortisol level
- Hyperaldosteronism
  - Serum aldosterone/plasma renin ratio >20
- Pheochromocytoma
- Urine or plasma metanephrine levels
- CT scan
  - Benign- <4 cm, homogenous, lipid rich
  - Malignant >6 cm, heterogenous, lipid poor

Management

- Functional adenoma—adrenalectomy
- Nonfunctional adenoma
  - <4 cm: observation
  - 4–6 cm: adrenalectomy if features concerning for malignancy
  - >6 cm: adrenalectomy.

Watch Out

- Do not biopsy adrenal masses
  - Beware of short posterior adrenal vein entering IVC with right adrenalectomy

Suggested Reading

Fassnacht M, Arlt W, Bancos I, et al. Management of adrenal incidentalomas: European Society of Endocrinology Clinical Practice Guideline in collaboration with the European Network for the Study of Adrenal Tumors. Eur J Endocrinol. 2016;175(2):G1–G34.

Iacobone M, Citton M, Scarpa M, Viel G, Boscaro M, Nitti D. Systematic review of surgical treatment of subclinical Cushing's syndrome. Br J Surg. 2015;102(4):318–30.

Lockhart ME, Smith JK, Kenney PJ. Imaging of adrenal masses. Eur J Radiol. 2002;41(2):95–112.

Mansmann G, Lau J, Balk E, Rothberg M, Miyachi Y, Bornstein SR. The clinically inapparent adrenal mass: update in diagnosis and management. Endocr Rev. 2004;25(2):309–40.

Newell-Price J, Bertagna X, Grossman AB, Nieman LK. Cushing's syndrome. Lancet. 2006;367(9522):1605–17.

Nieman LK. Approach to the patient with an adrenal incidentaloma. J Clin Endocrinol Metab. 2010;95(9):4106–13.

Ogilvie JB, Duh QY. New approaches to the minimally invasive treatment of adrenal lesions. Cancer J. 2005;11(1):64–72.

Rossi GP, Auchus RJ, Brown M, et al. An expert consensus statement on use of adrenal vein sampling for the subtyping of primary aldosteronism. Hypertension. 2014;63(1):151–60.

Terzolo M, Bovio S, Pia A, Reimondo G, Angeli A. Management of adrenal incidentaloma. Best Pract Res Clin Endocrinol Metab. 2009;23(2):233–43.

Young WF. Clinical practice. The incidentally discovered adrenal mass. N Engl J Med. 2007;356(6):601–10.

Zeiger MA, Siegelman SS, Hamrahian AH. Medical and surgical evaluation and treatment of adrenal incidentalomas. J Clin Endocrinol Metab. 2011;96(7):2004–15.

Zeiger MA, Thompson GB, Duh QY, Hamrahian AH, Angelos P, Elaraj D, et al. The American Association of Clinical Endocrinologists and American Association of Endocrine Surgeons medical guidelines for the management of adrenal incidentalomas. Endocr Pract. 2009;15(Suppl 1):1–20.

Fatigue, Constipation, and Depressed Mood

Joanna Curry, James X. Wu, and Michael W. Yeh

Contents

C. de Virgilio, A. Grigorian (eds.), *Surgery*, https://doi.org/10.1007/978-3-032-09799-6_12

Case Study

A 62-year-old woman presents to your office after being diagnosed with osteoporosis by her primary care physician. Her T-score is −4.2 at the lumbar spine. Further testing reveals a serum calcium level of 11 mg/dL (normal 8.5–10.5 mg/dL), a phosphate level of 1.7 mg/dL (normal 2.5–4.8 mg/dL), an intact parathyroid hormone level of 83 pg/mL (normal 15–75 pg/mL), and elevated urinary calcium levels. She denies any previous fractures. She reports fatigue and difficulty concentrating. She denies any history of neck irradiation or family history of thyroid or parathyroid disease. She has no significant past medical or surgical history. She has no known allergies. She occasionally takes ibuprofen for joint pain in her hands. She is a retired schoolteacher who is physically active and enjoys traveling. On review of systems, the patient reports constipation and occasional depressed mood. Physical examination is unremarkable; her neck is supple without masses or adenopathy.

Diagnosis

What Is the Differential Diagnosis of Hypercalcemia?

See Table 12.1 for the differential diagnosis of hypercalcemia. A commonly used mnemonic is "CHIMPANZEES."

What Is This Patient's Diagnosis?

An elevated serum calcium combined with an elevated parathyroid hormone (PTH) level and high urinary calcium confirms the diagnosis of primary hyperparathyroidism (HPT). In addition, this patient endorsed fatigue, constipation, and depressed mood, which are all symptoms associated with hypercalcemia.

Table 12.1 Differential diagnosis of hypercalcemia

Etiology	Differentiating lab finding	Comment
*C*alcium supplementation	None	Calcium carbonate, calcium citrate
*H*yperparathyroidism	↑ or high-normal PTH	Primary hyperparathyroidism is the most common *outpatient* cause of hypercalcemia
*H*yperthyroidism	↓ TSH	Leads to increased bone resorption
*I*mmobility	None	Causes rapid bone turnover due to increased osteoclastic activity, usually young patients following trauma
*I*atrogenic	None	Thiazide diuretics: Increase calcium absorption at distal tubule;
*M*ilk-alkali syndrome	↑ HCO3	Excess ingestion of calcium from antacids
*P*aget's disease	↑ alkaline phosphatase, ↑ serum and urine hydroxyproline	Excessive, disorganized bone remodelling
*A*ddison's disease	↑ ACTH	Unclear, glucocorticoid deficiency may increase bone resorption
*A*cromegaly	↑ IGF1	
*N*eoplasm	↑ PTHrP	Most common cause of *inpatient* hypercalcemia; can be due to cytokines or PTHrP
*Z*ollinger-Ellison syndrome	↑ Gastrin	Associated with multiple-endocrine neoplasia (hyperparathyroidism)
*E*xcessive vitamin D	↑ Increased vitamin D	Excess GI calcium absorption, increased bone resorption
*E*xcessive vitamin A	↑ increased vitamin A	Unclear etiology
*S*arcoidosis/granulomatous disease	↑ Vitamin D	Granuloma macrophages activate 25-OH vitamin D

PTH parathyroid hormone, *TSH* thyroid stimulating hormone, *ACTH* Adrenocorticotropic hormone, *IGF1* Insulin-like growth factor 1, *PTHrP* parathyroid hormone-related protein

What Condition Can Mimic Primary HPT?

Familial hypocalciuric hypercalcemia (FHH) is a benign, autosomal dominant disorder that causes mild hypercalcemia with normal or mildly elevated PTH levels. It is often mistaken for primary HPT but can be distinguished by low urinary calcium excretion (calcium-to-creatinine clearance ratio <0.01). FHH results from inactivating mutations in the calcium-sensing receptor (CASR) gene, leading to altered calcium sensing in the parathyroid glands and kidneys. As a result, PTH secretion is inappropriately maintained despite hypercalcemia, and renal calcium reabsorption is increased. This condition does not require surgical treatment, so accurate diagnosis is important to avoid unnecessary parathyroidectomy.

Watch Out

Humoral hypercalcemia of malignancy is caused by parathyroid hormone-related peptide (PTHrP) in 80% of cases (squamous cell cancers), while 20% of cases are caused by cytokines/chemokines (breast cancer).

History and Physical

What Is the Typical Presentation for Patients with Hypercalcemia?

12

Prior to the widespread use of routine laboratory testing, hypercalcemia typically presented with nephrolithiasis, bone pain, or pathologic fractures. These manifestations are encapsulated by the classic mnemonic “stones, bones, groans, and moans,” referring to renal calculi, skeletal discomfort, gastrointestinal symptoms, and neuropsychiatric disturbances. However, due to increased routine serum calcium screening, most patients are now diagnosed at an earlier stage often before the onset of overt clinical symptoms.

What Are the Renal Manifestations of Hypercalcemia?

Nephrolithiasis (most common in men under age 60), as well as nephrocalcinosis, polyuria, polydipsia, and renal hypertension. Over time, some patients will experience a decline in renal function.

What Are the Gastrointestinal Manifestations of Hypercalcemia?

Constipation, nausea, vomiting, heartburn, and vague abdominal pain. Rarely, peptic ulcer disease and pancreatitis.

What Are the Neurological Manifestations of Hypercalcemia?

Fatigue, depressed mood, difficulty concentrating, impaired memory, anxiety, sleep disturbance, proximal muscle weakness, and psychomotor symptoms. Stupor and coma can occur in severe hypercalcemia (serum calcium >14 mg/dl) or the elderly.

What Is Chvostek's Sign?

Facial twitch in response to tapping on the facial nerve anterior to the external auditory canal. This reflects early tetany and is a sign of *hypocalcemia* that may arise after parathyroidectomy.

What Is Trousseau's Sign?

This refers to the involuntary muscle spasms of the arm and hand occurring when blood flow to the arm is temporarily restricted, typically by inflating a blood pressure cuff above systolic pressure. Similar to Chvostek's sign, this marks early tetany due to hypocalcemia.

> **Watch Out**
> Massive blood transfusion is an often overlooked cause of *hypocalcemia*. Citrate in transfused blood binds ionized calcium, leading to symptomatic hypocalcemia, which may present with paresthesias, Trousseau sign, or Chvostek sign. Patients with liver dysfunction are at higher risk due to impaired citrate metabolism.

What Is a Hypercalcemic Crisis?

Patients with severe hypercalcemia (>14 mg/dl) may present with nausea, vomiting, confusion, and mental status changes. This is a medical emergency, as severe hypercalcemia can lead to cardiac arrhythmias and coma.

What Are the Risk Factors for Primary HPT?

Increased age, female sex, exposure to low-dose therapeutic ionizing radiation, family history of HPT, and lithium therapy for mood stabilization.

Why Is Family History Important?

HPT occurs in a number of inherited diseases, such as multiple endocrine neoplasia (MEN) 1, MEN-2A, familial isolated HPT, and HPT-jaw tumor syndrome.

> **Watch Out**
> MEN-1 (3 Ps) consists of hyper**p**arathyroidism, **p**ituitary adenomas, and **p**ancreatic neuroendocrine tumors. MEN-2A (2 Ps) is characterized by hyper**p**arathyroidism, **p**heochromocytoma, and medullary thyroid cancer. MEN-2B (1 P) is characterized by marfanoid habitus, mucosal neuromas, medullary thyroid cancer, and **p**heochromocytoma.

What Are the Physical Exam Findings of HPT? What Is the Significance of an Anterior Neck Mass Palpated in a Patient with HPT?

Physical exam findings are typically not useful in HPT, as the great majority of enlarged parathyroid glands are soft, <2 cm in diameter, and non-palpable. An anterior neck mass in a patient with HPT is most commonly a thyroid nodule but can rarely represent a parathyroid carcinoma.

What Is T-Score?

The T-score is a test of bone density. The T-score refers to the number of standard deviations away from the average for a young adult at peak bone density. Normal bone has a T-score greater than −1. Patients with osteopenia have scores between −1 and − 2.5, whereas those with osteoporosis have a score less than −2.5.

Anatomy

Describe the Location of the Parathyroid Glands. What Is Their Embryological Development?

There are typically four parathyroid glands: two superior (laterally) and two inferior (medially) (◘ Fig. 12.1). The superior parathyroids develop from the fourth pharyngeal pouch, migrate with the thyroid gland, and are usually located near the tubercle of Zuckerkandl, posterior to the point where the recurrent laryngeal nerve enters the larynx. These glands have a consistent anatomical position, found in this location in approximately 95% of individuals. The inferior parathyroid glands develop from the third pharyngeal pouch and migrate inferiorly in conjunction with the thymus. About 65% are located on the inferior surface of the thyroid gland, with most of the remainder being found within the thyrothymic ligament or the thymus. Supernumerary glands are present in up to 15% of individuals.

> **Watch Out**
> The parathyroid glands can sometimes be hidden in the mediastinum (within the thymus), within the carotid sheath and thyroid gland or behind the esophagus.

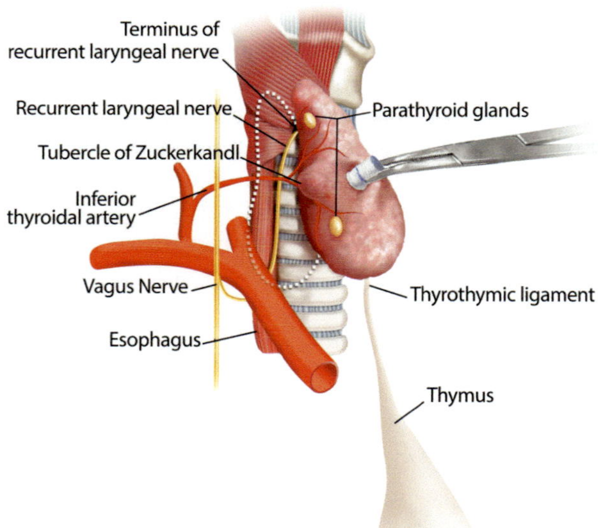

◘ **Fig. 12.1** Parathyroid glands

Pathology/Pathophysiology

What Pathology Causes Primary HPT?

Primary hyperparathyroidism is most commonly caused by a parathyroid adenoma, accounting for approximately 80% of cases. Parathyroid adenomas are typically solitary. The next most common cause is hyperplasia, which affects all four glands. Rarely the cause can be parathyroid carcinoma.

What Is the Typical Pathology in Primary HPT Associated with the MEN Disorders?

In MEN disorders, the gene is expressed in all glands and is thus characterized by four-gland hyperplasia.

What Is the Pathophysiology of Secondary HPT?

It is an adaptive response to prolonged hypocalcemia and hyperphosphatemia from chronic kidney disease, or from vitamin D deficiency due to malabsorption. This leads to parathyroid hyperplasia with excessive PTH secretion. Serum calcium levels can be low or normal. Secondary HPT requiring surgery is uncommon (about 1%).

What Causes Tertiary HPT?

Persistent excess secretion of PTH following renal transplantation in patients with long-standing secondary HPT. Renal transplantation restores normal vitamin D homeostasis and reverses secondary HPT in >95% of cases within 1 year. Patients with tertiary HPT generally manifest with hypercalcemia, inappropriate PTH level excess, and parathyroid hyperplasia. ◘ Table 12.2 summarizes the key differences in the three types of HPT.

What Are the End Organs Affected by PTH?

PTH primarily targets the skeleton and kidneys. In bone, PTH stimulates osteoblasts to express RANKL, which binds to RANK receptors on osteoclast precursors, promoting their maturation and activity. In the kidneys, PTH increases calcium reabsorption and pro-

Table 12.2 Different types of hyperparathyroidism

Condition	Ca^{2+}	PO4	PTH	Comments
Primary HPT	↑	↓	↑	Most often found incidentally on routine lab studies in *otherwise healthy* patients who are *asymptomatic* Cl: PO4 > 33:1
Secondary HPT	↓or normal	↑	↑	Hypocalcemic stimulus due to poor calcium reabsorption, lack of vitamin D activation
				Renal transplant usually curative
Tertiary HPT	↑	↓	↑	History of corrected renal failure with transplant
				Adenoma formed in setting of chronic hypocalcemia with persistent PTH stimulation
				Hypercalcemia can harm graft function

HPT hyperparathyroidism, *PTH* parathyroid hormone

motes phosphate excretion. PTH also drives hydroxylation of 25-OH vitamin D to the active 1,25-OH vitamin D via the upregulation of renal 1-alpha-hydroxylase. The active form of vitamin D then increases intestinal calcium absorption, further contributing to serum calcium homeostasis.

What Is the Basic Physiology of Calcium Metabolism?

Calcium homeostasis in humans is principally regulated by PTH. Calcitonin, a counter-regulatory hormone that lowers the serum calcium, is very weak and has a negligible effect in humans (Table 12.3).

What Is the Most Common Cause of PTH Deficiency? How Does It Manifest?

The most common cause of PTH deficiency is iatrogenic destruction or removal of parathyroid glands at the time of parathyroid or thyroid surgery. Autoimmune destruction of the parathyroid glands is very rare. Patients with PTH deficiency will present with *hypo*calcemia and hyperphosphatemia in the presence of normal renal function.

Table 12.3 Calcium metabolism

Hormone	Stimulus	Effect on the kidney	Effect on the bone	Effect on the intestine
PTH	↓ca, ↑PO4, ↓1,25-OH vitamin D, mildly ↓Mg	↑1,25-OH vitamin D production, ↓tubular reabsorption of PO4 and HCO3	↑bone resorption	–
1,25-OH vitamin D	PTH	↓Tubular reabsorption of Ca	↑Ca uptake	↑Absorption of Ca and PO4
Calcitonin	↑Ca, gastrin	–	↓bone resorption	–

PTH parathyroid hormone

Work-Up

What Laboratory Tests Are Used for the Diagnosis of Primary HPT?

Serum calcium and PTH level. Other useful tests include phosphate, chloride, bicarbonate, magnesium, serum creatinine, 24-h urinary calcium (to rule out FHH which is characterized by low urinary calcium), and 25-OH vitamin D level.

What Is the Difference Between Total Serum Calcium Level and Ionized Calcium Level?

Total serum calcium is the sum of protein-bound calcium and free calcium. Ionized calcium reflects free (nonprotein bound) calcium and functions as the main regulator of PTH secretion.

If the Serum Calcium Is High, But the PTH Level Is Normal, Does That Rule Out Primary HPT?

12

No. In the setting of high serum calcium, the PTH level should be low. An *inappropriately normal* (nonsuppressed) PTH level in the setting of hypercalcemia would strongly suggest primary HPT. Impaired negative feedback is often diagnostic of endocrine disease.

How Can the Serum Chloride to Phosphate Ratio Suggest Primary HPT?

A serum chloride to phosphate ratio >33 is highly suggestive of HPT. PTH acts on the kidney and increases calcium reabsorption as well as excretion of bicarbonate and phosphate, assuming normal kidney function. Excretion of bicarbonate results in a rise in serum chloride to balance ion charges, resulting in hyperchloremic metabolic acidosis.

> **Watch Out**
> Remember PTH's effect on phosphate by "PTH is the **P**hosphate **T**rashing **H**ormone."

What Other Tests Should Be Ordered in a New Diagnosis of HPT?

Bone mineral density testing via dual-energy X-ray absorptiometry (DEXA) is indicated in asymptomatic patients, all postmenopausal women, and patients with a history of fragility fractures. A T-score is calculated. Patients with HPT often have osteopenia or osteoporosis. Cortical bone sites, such as the distal radius, are more commonly affected in primary HPT, while trabecular-rich areas like the spine may be relatively spared. This distribution helps distinguish it from postmenopausal osteoporosis. Renal ultrasound or abdominal plain films may be used in patients with symptoms suggestive of nephrolithiasis.

> **Watch Out**
> Gastrointestinal disorders, such as celiac and inflammatory bowel disease, can cause osteoporosis due to malabsorption of fat-soluble vitamins and secondary HPT.

What Radiologic Findings Are Suggestive of Bony Involvement in HPT?

Plain films of the hands can reveal subperiosteal cortical bone resorption, most commonly in the distal phalanges. In rare cases of advanced disease, osteitis fibrosa cystica may be found on plain films, as manifested by brown tumors—lucent areas left by overactive bone breakdown and subsequent fibrosis.

What Tests Help Localize the Involved Gland in HPT?

99-m technetium sestamibi scanning (◘ Fig. 12.2) and ultrasound are the most frequently used imaging tests to localize the involved gland(s) in primary HPT. Dynamic parathyroid CT, sometimes termed 4D-CT, is also used by some centers. Localizing studies are generally not indicated in secondary or tertiary HPT, since multiple-gland hyperplasia is the expected underlying pathology.

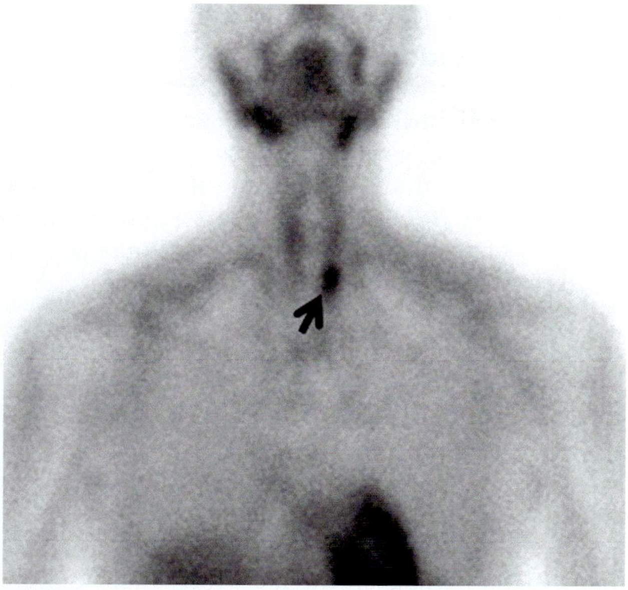

Fig. 12.2 Sestamibi scan showing a hyperactive parathyroid adenoma

Watch Out

Sestamibi is also taken up by the thyroid tissue. Hence, a thyroid nodule can mimic the appearance of a parathyroid adenoma.

What If All Localizing Scans Fail to Localize the Abnormal Parathyroid Gland(s)?

In about 85% of patients, imaging will localize the abnormal parathyroid gland, and a great majority will have a single parathyroid adenoma. If localizing scans are negative, yet the diagnosis of primary HPT is clearly established, surgery should still be considered but will be more challenging. Hence, patients with negative imaging should be referred to an experienced surgeon for treatment.

Management

What Are the Indications for Parathyroidectomy in Primary HPT?

Parathyroidectomy is indicated in all patients with symptomatic hypercalcemia. For patients with asymptomatic HPT diagnosed through a laboratory screening, a 2020 consensus statement recommended surgery by an experienced parathyroid surgeon in those with any of the following indications:

1. Serum calcium level of 1.0 mg/dL greater than the upper limit of normal
2. Creatinine clearance reduced to <60 mL/min
3. Elevated 24-h urine calcium (>250 mg/day in women; > 300 mg/day in men)
4. Presence of asymptomatic nephrolithiasis or nephrocalcinosis seen on imaging
5. Bone mineral density with T-score less than −2.5 at any site
6. Evidence of vertebral fracture
7. Age <50

What Are the Indications for Parathyroidectomy in Secondary HPT?

Patients with very high PTH levels (>800 pg/ml) despite best medical management, bone pain, pruritus, progressive renal disease, fragility fractures, or calciphylaxis, a rare but serious condition involving vascular calcification and skin necrosis, often associated with ESRD.

What Is the Nonoperative Management of Patients with HPT?

Patients not selected for surgical therapy require biochemical monitoring of serum calcium and serum creatinine annually. Bone mineral density should be measured every 1–2 years. Bisphosphonates may stabilize or improve bone mineral density. Cinacalcet, a calcimimetic, may be used to reduce the serum calcium, though it has no benefit with regard to bone density.

Watch Out

In patients who are not candidates for parathyroidectomy, bisphosphonates may be used to improve bone mineral density. However, prolonged or high-dose bisphosphonate therapy, particularly in those receiving treatment for malignancy or severe osteoporosis, carries a risk of osteonecrosis of the jaw.

What Is the Role of Intraoperative PTH Monitoring?

Because of the short half-life of PTH (about 4 min), intraoperative rapid PTH testing may aid in determining the completeness of parathyroid resection. The most commonly used protocol involves drawing PTH levels at the time of gland excision and again 10 min post-excision. A fall of >50% in the PTH level is associated with a 98% long-term cure rate.

What Are the Surgical Options for HPT?

If the patient has a single enlarged parathyroid adenoma, the affected gland is removed. This is typically done with a unilateral neck exploration with excision of a solitary parathyroid adenoma. If the patient has hyperplasia of all four glands, most surgeons recommend either removing 3½ of the glands or all four glands and reimplanting ½ (about 40 g) of one of the glands into the forearm muscle or into the sternocleidomastoid. The latter is most appropriate for patients with a high likelihood of recurrent disease, such as MEN-1.

Why Is It Not Advised to Remove All Four Parathyroid Glands?

Removal of all four glands usually results in permanent hypocalcemia that is very difficult to control. The reimplantation preserves some parathyroid tissue. Typically, the non-dominant forearm is favored over the sternocleidomastoid, that way if the patient develops recurrent HPT, it avoids reoperation in the neck.

What Is the Postoperative Management Following Parathyroidectomy?

Monitor for neck hematoma, voice changes (injury to recurrent laryngeal nerve), perioral numbness, or tingling in fingers (hypocalcemia). Postoperative oral calcium supplementation may alleviate minor symptoms of relative hypocalcemia and is routinely used. Intravenous calcium supplementation is not commonly needed.

What Is the Treatment for a Neck Hematoma with Stridor?

Immediately open neck wound at the bedside to decompress the hematoma followed by evacuation of hematoma and hemostasis in the operating room.

What Are the Benefits of Parathyroidectomy?

Successful parathyroidectomy results in sustained increases in bone mineral density at multiple sites and decreases the risk of kidney stone formation. Approximately 70% of patients report improvements in quality of life attributed to relief of constitutional, musculoskeletal, and neuropsychiatric symptoms.

What Syndrome Causing Postoperative Hypocalcemia Can Occur Following Parathyroidectomy?

Hungry bone syndrome is a well-recognized cause of postoperative hypocalcemia following parathyroidectomy. In the setting of chronic hyperparathyroidism, sustained elevations in PTH lead to increased bone resorption and a state in which the skeleton is deprived of calcium. After surgical correction, this suppression is lifted, and the bone rapidly takes up calcium, phosphate, and magnesium in a process of remineralization. The condition is most commonly seen in patients with secondary hyperparathyroidism, particularly those on long-term dialysis. Affected individuals may also exhibit hypophosphatemia and hypomagnesemia. Management often requires inpatient calcium repletion and close monitoring for up to a week following surgery.

Areas Where You Can Get in Trouble

Assuming Normal Calcium Rules Out HPT

A low serum albumin can lead to a falsely low total calcium level. The formula for correction is corrected Ca = serum Ca + [(0.8) (4.0—serum albumin)]. This correction is typically applied when serum albumin is below 4.0 g/dL. Alternatively, ionized calcium can be measured, which is unaffected by albumin but is pH-dependent.

Hypocalcemia That Does Not Respond to Calcium Replacement

If a patient with hypocalcemia does not respond to calcium repletion, check the magnesium level. Hypomagnesemia can cause refractory hypocalcemia by inhibiting the bioactivity of PTH.

Special Situations

How Do You Treat Hypercalcemic Crisis?

The initial treatment of hypercalcemic crisis begins with aggressive intravenous hydration using normal saline, as most patients are volume depleted due to impaired renal concentrating ability caused by hypercalcemia. Volume repletion enhances urinary calcium excretion and dilutes serum calcium. Once euvolemia is achieved, loop diuretics may be considered to promote calciuresis, though their routine use is limited to patients with volume overload. Calcitonin may be administered early for rapid but short-term calcium lowering; it is particularly useful in patients with normal renal and cardiac function. Bisphosphonates, such as pamidronate or zoledronic acid, are effective for sustained calcium reduction, especially in cases of hypercalcemia of malignancy, by inhibiting osteoclast-mediated bone resorption. Medications that worsen hypercalcemia, including thiazide diuretics and digoxin, should be discontinued. If the underlying cause is primary hyperparathyroidism, urgent parathyroidectomy may be required. In cases of severe renal dysfunction or life-threatening hypercalcemia unresponsive to medical therapy, hemodialysis may be necessary to rapidly lower calcium levels.

Algorithm for the Work-Up and Management of HPT (◘ Figs. 12.3 and 12.4)

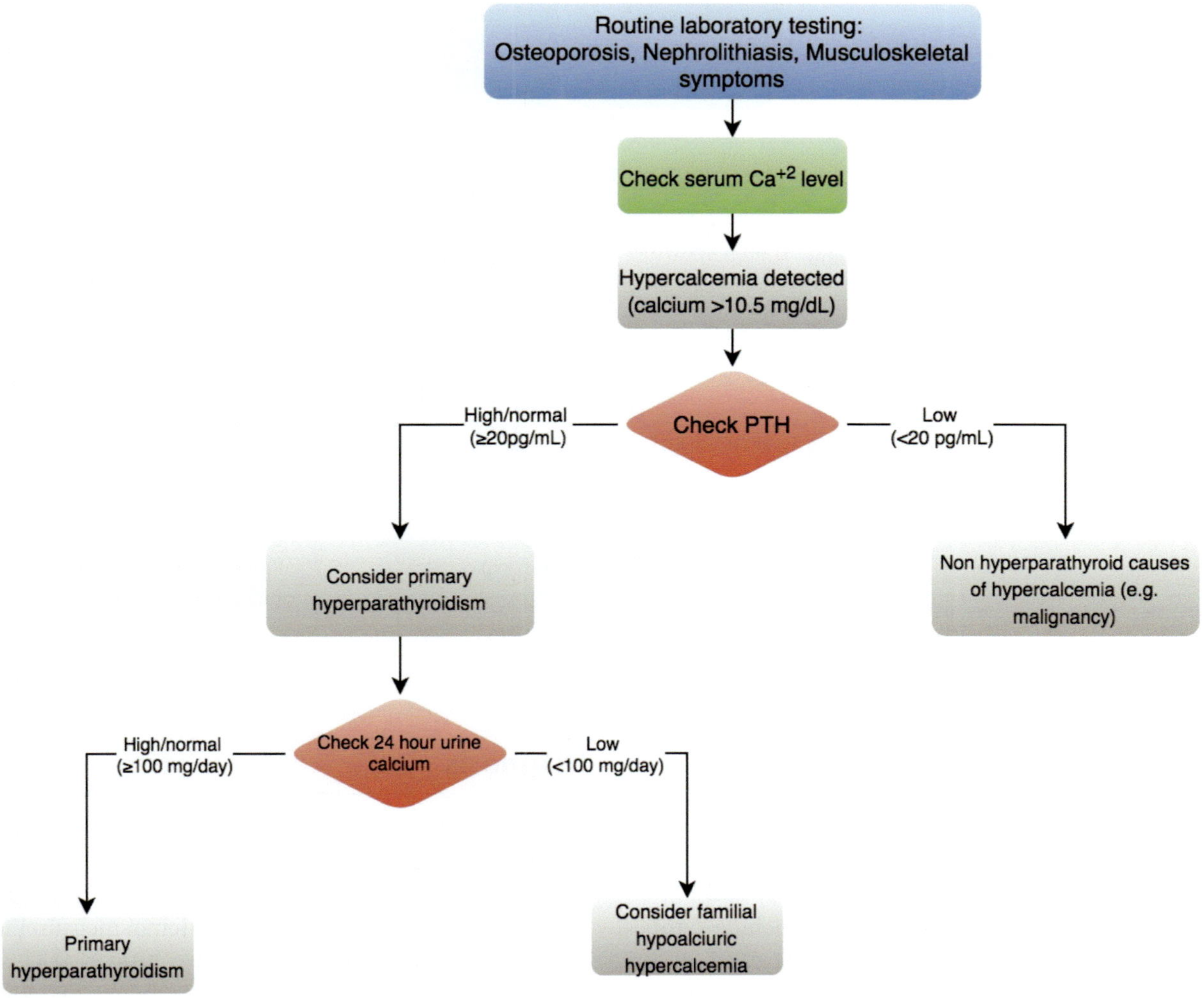

◘ **Fig. 12.3** Diagnostic algorithm for primary hyperparathyroidism

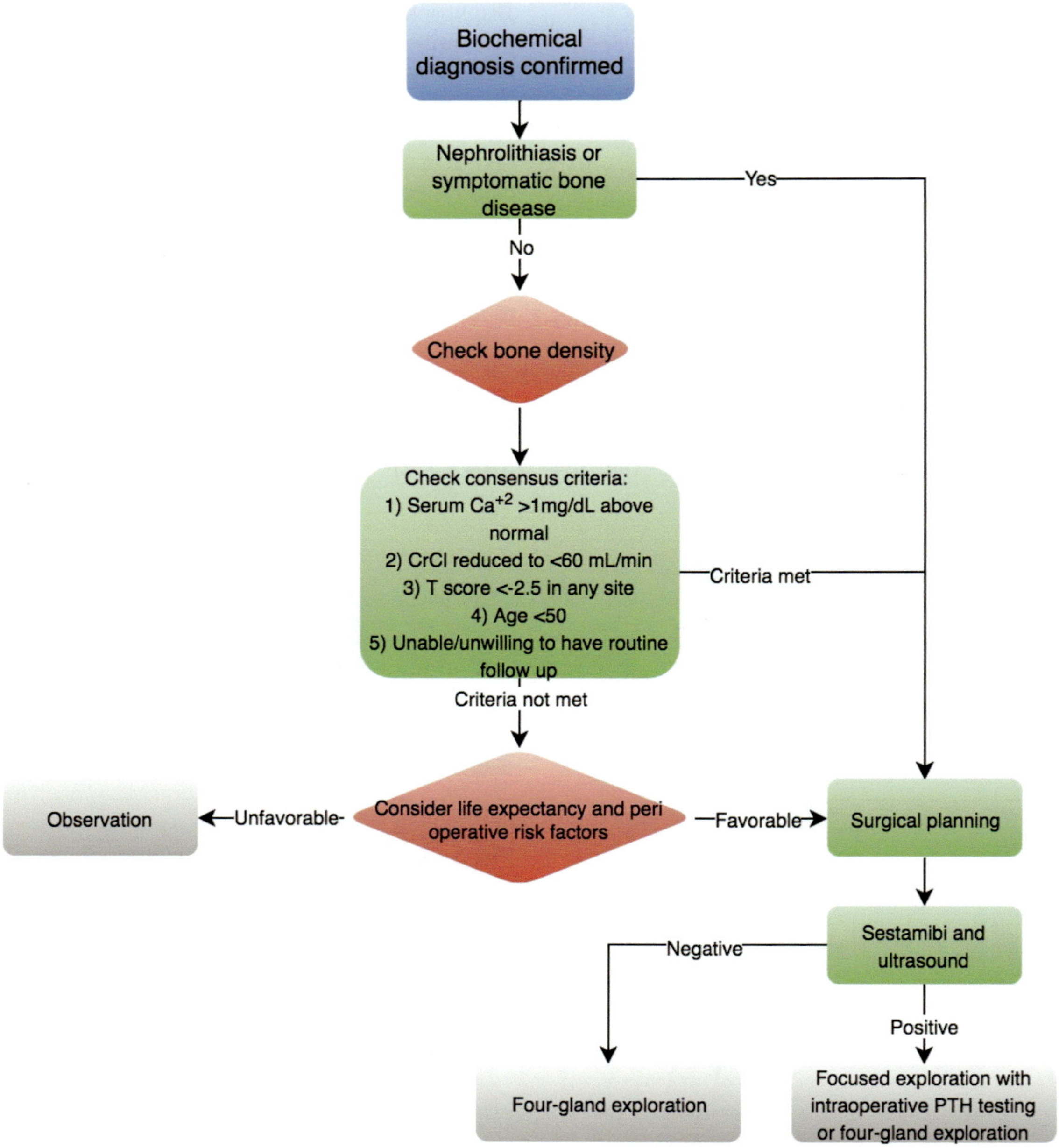

Fig. 12.4 Management algorithm for primary hyperparathyroidism

12

Summary of Essentials

History and Physical

- Classic symptoms of hypercalcemia include "stones, bones, groans, and moans," but most cases of primary HPT are now discovered incidentally via routine laboratory testing
- Hypercalcemia of malignancy is the most common cause of inpatient hypercalcemia; primary HPT is the most common outpatient cause

Diagnosis

- Primary HPT: elevated calcium with high or inappropriately normal PTH level
- Differentiate from familial hypocalciuric hypercalcemia (FHH) using a 24-h urine calcium measurement; a calcium-to-creatinine clearance ratio < 0.01 supports FHH
- Obtain bone densitometry in asymptomatic patients

Pathophysiology

- PTH affects the bones and kidneys directly, increasing bone breakdown and calcium absorption and vitamin D activation in the kidneys
- Primary HPT is most often caused by a solitary adenoma, while MEN syndromes cause four-gland hyperplasia
- Secondary HPT results from chronic hypocalcemia (e.g., chronic kidney disease, vitamin D deficiency); tertiary HPT arises after renal transplantation due to autonomous PTH secretion

Management

- Indications for parathyroidectomy in asymptomatic patients include: serum calcium >1 mg/dL above normal, CrCl <60 mL/min, osteoporosis (T-score < −2.5), vertebral fracture, nephrolithiasis or nephrocalcinosis, elevated 24-h urine calcium, or age < 50 years
- Single adenoma- remove affected gland
- Four gland hyperplasia- remove 3 ½ gland or total parathyroidectomy with autotransplantation of ½ a gland
- Intraoperative PTH monitoring confirms successful gland removal
- Secondary HPT- nonoperative management includes use of bisphosphonates or cinacalcet in select patients

Acknowledgement The editors would like to acknowledge and thank the following authors for their contributions to the previous edition of the chapter: Paul N. Frank.

Suggested Reading

Bilezikian, et al. Evaluation and Management of Primary Hyperparathyroidism: Summary Statement and Guidelines from the Fifth International Workshop. J Bone and Miner Res. 2022;37(11):2293–2314.

Li S, et al. Trends in parathyroidectomy rates in US hemodialysis patients from 1992 to 2007. Am J Kidney Dis. 2011;57(4):602–11.

Schneider DF, et al. Predictors of recurrence in primary hyperparathyroidism: an analysis of 1386 cases. Ann Surg. 2014;259(3):563–8.

Stewart AF. Clinical practice. Hypercalcemia associated with cancer. N Engl J Med. 2005;352(4):373–9.

Wilheim SM, et al. The American Association of Endocrine Surgeons Guidelines for definitive management of primary hyperparathyroidism. JAMA Surg. 2016;151(10):959–68.

Yeh MW, et al. Surgery for primary hyperparathyroidism: are the consensus guidelines being followed? Ann Surg. 2012;255(6):1179–83.

Yeh MW, et al. Incidence and prevalence of primary hyperparathyroidism in a racially mixed population. J Clin Endocrinol Metab. 2013;98(3):1122–9.

Intermittent Episodes of Sweating, Palpitations, and Hypertension

Eugene J. Park, Masha J. Livhits, Areg Grigorian, and Michael W. Yeh

Contents

C. de Virgilio, A. Grigorian (eds.), *Surgery*, https://doi.org/10.1007/978-3-032-09799-6_13

Case Study

A 34-year-old woman presents with a chief complaint of what she calls "rushes," intermittent episodes of sweating, headaches, and palpitations lasting for a few minutes and occurring sporadically every few days. These episodes can occur at any time of day and have sometimes awakened her from sleep. She notes that exercise may provoke her symptoms. Past medical history is significant for newly diagnosed hypertension. Her physical exam is remarkable only for hypertension, with a blood pressure of 165/100 mmHg. Her biochemical workup reveals an elevated 24-hour urine metanephrine (1163 mcg/day; normal <400 mcg/day). A dedicated adrenal protocol CT scan shows a 4-cm mass in the right adrenal gland.

Diagnosis

What Is the Differential Diagnosis of Secondary Hypertension? (Table 13.1)

Table 13.1 Differential diagnosis of secondary hypertension

Diagnosis	History and physical	Comments
Pheochromocytoma	Episodic hyperadrenergic symptoms (5 P's): Pressure (hypertension), pain (headache), perspiration, palpitation, and pallor	Associated with MEN 2, neurofibromatosis-1, and VHL
Hypercortisolism (Cushing syndrome)	Weight gain, central obesity, muscle weakness, poor wound healing, hirsutism, amenorrhea, depression, hypertension, and diabetes mellitus	Exogenous glucocorticoids, ACTH-secreting pituitary adenoma (Cushing disease), ectopic source of ACTH production, and cortisol-secreting adrenal adenoma
Hyperaldosteronism (Conn's syndrome)	Muscle cramps, weakness, hypertension, and hypokalemia	Aldosterone-secreting adrenal adenoma and adrenal hyperplasia
Kidney disease	Decreased urine output, edema, fatigue, and muscle aches	Polycystic kidney disease, kidney failure, and diabetic nephropathy
Thyroid disease	Thyroid storm: Tachycardia, arrhythmias, fever, hypertension, tremor, lid lag, and altered mental status	Both hyperthyroidism and hypothyroidism may cause hypertension
Fibromuscular dysplasia	Severe hypertension in a young female	Renal artery has "string-of-beads" appearance due to medial thickening alternating with stenosis; it also affects the carotid, superior mesenteric, and external iliac arteries
Coarctation of the aorta	Hypertension in the arms but not the legs, weak femoral and pedal pulses	Turner syndrome, aortic valve pathology
Drug induced	Combination of MAOI with decongestants, sympathomimetics, and serotonin syndrome	Never give β-blockers to patients using cocaine (can lead to vasoconstrictive angina due to unopposed alpha-receptor stimulation)
	Illicit drugs, including phencyclidine, LSD, and cocaine	

VHL von Hippel-Lindau disease, *TSH* thyroid stimulating hormone, *MEN* multiple endocrine neoplasia, *MAOI* monoamine oxidase inhibitors

What Is the Most Likely Diagnosis?

The most likely diagnosis is pheochromocytoma. This is suggested by the patient's newly discovered hypertension, episodic symptoms of sweating, flushing, and palpitations, as well as elevated urine metanephrines, all indicative of catecholamine surges. The diagnosis is further supported by a CT scan revealing a mass in the right adrenal gland, a common location for pheochromocytoma.

History and Physical

What Is the Classic Triad of Symptoms in Pheochromocytoma?

The classic triad of symptoms is headache, flushing, and palpitations. Though only a minority of patients have all three of these symptoms, 90% have at least one.

What Are the Other Symptoms of Pheochromocytoma?

In addition to the classic triad, pheochromocytoma symptoms stem from the systemic effects of catecholamines released by the tumor. Most patients experience sustained or episodic hypertension, often resistant to standard therapies. Other symptoms include anxiety, impaired gastrointestinal motility, orthostatic hypotension, weight loss, and hyperglycemia. Significant cardiovascular complications can also arise, such as myocardial infarction, arrhythmias, stroke, and, less commonly, heart failure.

> **Watch Out**
> Hypertension associated with pheochromocytoma can be paroxysmal or can have fluctuations superimposed on *constantly* elevated blood pressure. This is dependent on whether catecholamines are released continuously or in shorter bursts.

Why Do Some Patients Have Orthostatic Hypotension?

Orthostatic hypotension is seen in up to 50% of pheochromocytoma patients, which may reflect a low intravascular volume due to persistent vasoconstriction. In addition, patients with pheochromocytoma may have desensitized adrenergic receptors from long-term exposure to large amounts of catecholamine. This can compromise the normal baroreceptor reflex responsible for vasoconstriction upon standing from a supine position, resulting in orthostatic hypotension.

Can Patients with Pheochromocytoma Be Asymptomatic?

With the increasing use of CT scans, upward of 25% of pheochromocytoma cases are now diagnosed incidentally during imaging for unrelated disorders. About 5% of incidentally discovered adrenal nodules are pheochromocytomas.

What Is the Average Age of Diagnosis? Is There a Gender Predisposition?

Patients are usually diagnosed at age 40–50 years. There is an equal incidence of cases in males and females.

What Is the "Rule of Tens," and Is It Still True?

The "rule of tens" regarding pheochromocytoma (10% bilateral, 10% extra-adrenal, 10% familial, 10% multifocal, 10% malignant) was taught to generations of medical students. It was ultimately disproved in the year 2000 after a series of reports described novel germline mutations causing pheochromocytoma. We now recognize that 20–40% of pheochromocytomas arise as a result of an underlying familial syndrome and that clear genotype-phenotype correlations exist (◘ Table 13.2).

Table 13.2 Hereditary syndromes associated with pheochromocytoma

Syndrome	Gene mutation (function)	Clinical phenotype	Pheo characteristics	Risk[a] (%)
MEN 2A	RET (proto-oncogene)	Medullary thyroid cancer, primary hyperparathyroidism	Benign, bilateral, or multicentric; intra-adrenal	50
MEN 2B	RET (proto-oncogene)	Medullary thyroid cancer, marfanoid habitus, mucosal neuromas	Benign, bilateral, or multicentric; intra-adrenal	50
NF type 1 (von Recklinghausen's disease)	NF1 (negative regulator of the RAS oncogene pathway)	Neurofibromas, café au lait spots, Lisch nodules (benign iris hamartomas)	15% malignant; intra-adrenal	1–5
von Hippel-Lindau (VHL)	VHL (tumor suppressor)	Retinal angioma, CNS hemangioblastoma, renal cell cancer, PNET, pancreatic and renal cysts	Benign, bilateral; younger age at diagnosis	10–20
Paraganglioma syndromes 1–5	SDHx (tumor suppressor)	Renal cell, thyroid carcinoma, gastrointestinal stromal tumor	Multiple, intra- and extra-adrenal, in SDHB 50% malignant	30–50

MEN multiple endocrine neoplasia, *NF* neurofibromatosis, *VHL* von Hippel-Lindau, *CNS* central nervous system, *PNET* pancreatic neuroendocrine tumor, *SDHx* succinate dehydrogenase
[a]lifetime risk of pheochromocytoma

Pathophysiology

What Is a Pheochromocytoma?

A pheochromocytoma is a catecholamine-producing tumor that is derived from chromaffin cells in the adrenal medulla or sympathetic ganglia. Extra-adrenal catecholamine-producing tumors are sometimes referred to as "paragangliomas."

What Are the Effects of Normal and Excessive Catecholamine Secretion? (Table 13.3)

Table 13.3 Physiological effects of catecholamine receptors

Receptor	Normal function	Excessive function
α_1	Smooth muscle contraction, gluconeogenesis, glycogenolysis	Hypertension, hyperglycemia
α_2	Smooth muscle contraction, platelet aggregation	Pallor
β_1	Chronotropic, inotropic, sweat glands	Tachycardia, sweating
β_2	Smooth muscle relaxation	Hypotension

Watch Out

Paragangliomas in the neck are very rarely biologically active. Those involving the carotid sinus are called carotid body tumors.

What Are the Predominant Catecholamines in Adrenal and Extra-Adrenal Tumors?

Norepinephrine, epinephrine, and dopamine are the three biologically active catecholamines produced by pheochromocytomas. The predominant catecholamine produced varies depending on the local expression of particular catecholamine synthesis enzymes. Most intra-adrenal pheochromocytomas produce both epinephrine and norepinephrine, with norepinephrine being the predominant catecholamine. Epinephrine-secreting pheochromocytomas can also arise extra-adrenally from the organ of Zuckerkandl, which is located near the aortic bifurcation or origin of the inferior mesenteric artery. Phenylethanolamine N-methyltransferase (PNMT), the enzyme that converts norepinephrine to epinephrine, is primarily present only in the adrenal medulla and organ of Zuckerkandl. Therefore, pheochromocytomas outside of these locations produce predominantly norepinephrine and little or no epinephrine.

Where Do Pheochromocytomas Develop?

Pheochromocytomas originate from chromaffin cells, primarily located in the adrenal medulla. However, they can also develop anywhere along the sympathetic nervous system from the skull base to the bladder. The most common extra-adrenal sites are in the abdomen (75% near the organ of Zuckerkandl), bladder or prostate (10%), thorax (10%), and head/neck region (5%).

Watch Out

The organ of Zuckerkandl is located along the abdominal aorta between the origin of the inferior mesentery artery and bifurcation of the aorta into the common iliac arteries.

What Can Trigger a Hypertensive Crisis in Pheochromocytoma?

Catecholamine release may be caused by changes in blood flow, physical stimulation, tumor necrosis, and certain drugs, including sympathomimetics and anesthetic agents. Endotracheal intubation, foods containing tyramine, abdominal trauma, surgical manipulation, emotional stress, urination (with bladder paragangliomas), and attempts at biopsy are all known to stimulate catecholamine release from pheochromocytomas. Biopsies of the adrenal gland are generally not recommended.

Why Do Patients with Pheochromocytoma Have Elevated Hematocrit Levels?

The chronic alpha constriction in patients with pheochromocytoma leads to volume depletion and hemoconcentration. Additionally, paraneoplastic production of erythropoietin (EPO) leading to high hematocrit levels may be associated with pheochromocytoma.

Why Do Patients with Pheochromocytoma Have Hyperglycemia?

In pheochromocytoma, catecholamines elevate blood glucose by stimulating hepatic glucose production and inhibiting insulin secretion and action. Specifically, catecholamines act on β_2-receptors in the pancreas, reducing insulin secretion, and on peripheral tissues, where they inhibit insulin's action on cells. This dual effect leads to reduced glucose uptake by tissues and increased circulating glucose levels, resulting in hyperglycemia.

What Defines a Malignant Pheochromocytoma?

The presence of local invasion into adjacent organs (e.g., kidney, liver, vessels) or distant metastases to nonchromaffin sites (liver, lungs, bone) defines a malignant pheochromocytoma. In contrast to most other tumor types, the determination of malignancy cannot be made by histopathologic analysis of the primary tumor, as cytologic atypia, high mitotic count, presence of necrosis, and even microscopic vascular invasion can occur in tumors with benign clinical behavior. Hence, the diagnosis of malignant pheochromocytoma rests on surgical assessment of invasion and radiologic identification of metastases or invasion.

Workup

What Laboratory Tests Can Help Establish the Diagnosis of Pheochromocytoma?

The diagnosis of pheochromocytoma begins with measuring plasma-free metanephrines, a highly sensitive screening test. Confirmatory testing is done with a 24-h urine collection for catecholamines and their metabolites (metanephrine, normetanephrine, and vanillylmandelic acid), which is the gold standard (high specificity). Urine values exceeding twice the upper limit of normal are considered diagnostic. Plasma chromogranin A, though nonspecific, is also elevated in most pheochromocytoma cases and can support the diagnosis.

What Medications Can Interfere with Urine or Plasma Testing?

The following medications can cause false elevations of catecholamines: beta-blockers, decongestants, antidepressants (notably tricyclics, monoamine oxidase inhibitors, and venlafaxine), and antipsychotics (notably clozapine). Whenever possible, interfering medications should be discontinued for 2 weeks prior to biochemical testing for pheochromocytoma.

What Imaging Studies Are Helpful in Making the Diagnosis?

First-line imaging consists of CT (◘ Fig. 13.1) or MRI with contrast, which have high sensitivity and can detect tumors as small as 1 cm. Nuclear imaging with iodine-metaiodobenzylguanidine (I-MIBG), a catecholamine precursor that is taken up by chromaffin cells, is highly specific for pheochromocytoma and may be useful in cases of suspected multifocal disease or when not well visualized on CT or MRI.

What Should Be Done If Imaging Demonstrates Bilateral Adrenal Gland Masses?

If imaging reveals bilateral adrenal gland masses and biochemical tests confirm the presence of a hormonally active tumor, adrenal vein sampling is recommended to determine the source of hormone excess. In this procedure, an interventional radiologist inserts catheters into the adrenal veins to collect blood samples directly from each adrenal gland. These samples are then analyzed to assess hormone levels and to identify whether one or both glands are hypersecreting.

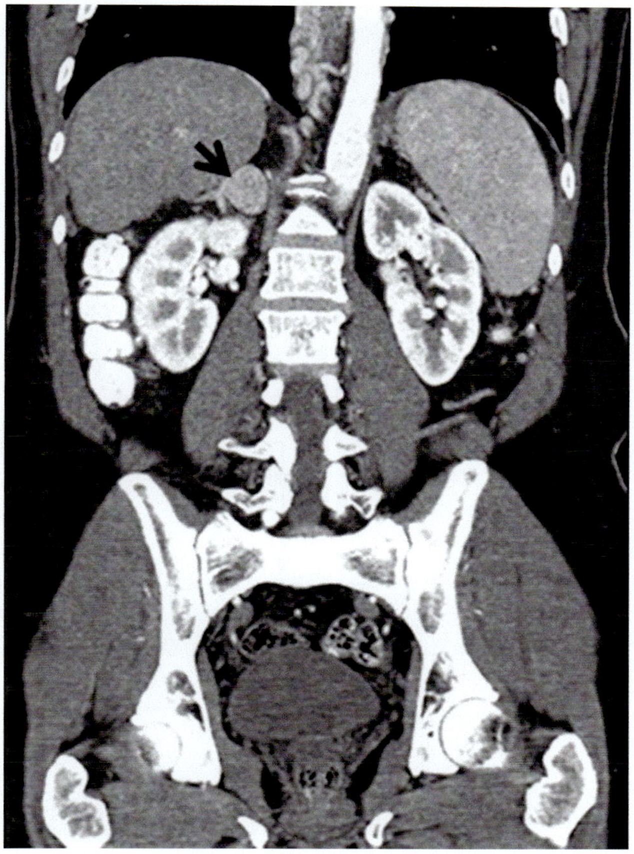

◘ **Fig. 13.1** Coronal CT with an enhancing adrenal nodule consistent with pheochromocytoma

Management

What Is the Treatment for Pheochromocytoma?

Treatment (◘ Fig. 13.2) should begin with medical optimization using alpha-blockers (i.e., phenoxybenzamine, doxazosin) and volume expansion. In refractory cases or for patients developing tachycardia, beta-blockers can be added after appropriate alpha-blockade. Medical therapy should continue for at least 2 weeks, followed by surgical resection (a.drenalectomy). Surgery is usually curative, except in malignant cases.

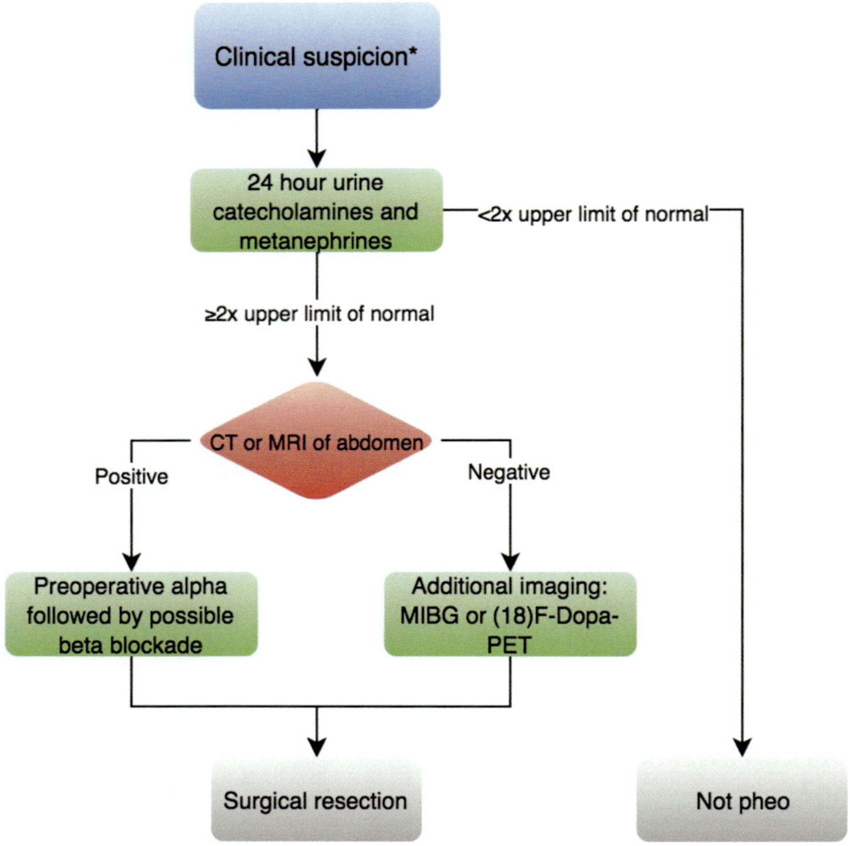

Fig. 13.2 Algorithm for diagnosis and treatment of pheochromocytoma (Paroxysmal symptoms, intermittent or sustained hypertension, family history, or adrenal mass seen on imaging)

Watch Out
Pheochromocytoma tumors need to be treated and removed first before addressing other simultaneous tumors in patients with MEN 2A/B. Remember, that the general anesthesia is a trigger for hypertensive crisis in pheochromocytoma.

What Are the Important Surgical Principles?

The laparoscopic approach is preferred for patients with adrenal pheochromocytomas that are less than 6 cm in size and have no malignant features on imaging. The operation can be performed either transabdominally or retroperitoneally. The arterial supply of the adrenal gland comes from the aorta, renal artery, and inferior phrenic artery. Venous drainage is generally from a single adrenal vein, which drains into the renal vein on the left side. On the right side, a short adrenal vein drains directly into the inferior vena cava. As such, ligation of the right adrenal vein is more difficult. The operation should be completed with minimal and very gentle handling of the tumor to avoid intraoperative catecholamine surges. Effective communication between the surgical team and the anesthesia team is essential. Ligation of the adrenal vein should be performed *early* and *prior* to ligation of the adrenal artery to prevent spillage of catecholamines during tumor manipulation and provide prompt resolution of hypertension. However, vein ligation may, in some cases, bring about some degree of hypotension, requiring isotonic fluids and/or vasopressin for blood pressure support.

How Do You Prepare a Patient for Surgery?

Alpha-blockade with doxazosin or phenoxybenzamine is initiated 2 weeks prior to surgery. It is titrated up until blood pressure is optimally controlled, resulting in mild orthostatic hypotension (endpoint of medical therapy to consider surgical resection). This allows time for patients to restore their preexisting contracted plasma volume, ensuring that patients are not volume depleted going into surgery. For the same reason, patients are encouraged to consume a high-salt and high-fluid diet to ensure adequate volume status. A beta-blocker can be added for patients who develop tachycardia after adequate alpha-blockade.

What Can Happen If a Beta-Blocker Is Given Prior to Adequate Alpha-Blockade?

The unopposed alpha-adrenergic stimulation from the pheochromocytoma can cause vasoconstriction and precipitate a hypertensive crisis. For this reason, alpha-blockers are always administered first.

When Is Genetic Testing Indicated?

Genetic testing is currently recommended for all patients with pheochromocytoma or paraganglioma. This can generally be performed after surgical treatment through referral to a genetic counselor.

What Are the Main Complications Specifically Associated with Adrenalectomy for Pheochromocytoma? (Table 13.4)

Table 13.4 Postoperative complications after adrenalectomy

Complication	Features
Hypertension	May be due to residual tumor, metastatic disease, or underlying essential hypertension
Hypotension	Loss of catecholamine-induced peripheral vasoconstriction, +/− residual effects of preoperative alpha-blockade; may require vigorous fluid hydration postoperatively
Hypoglycemia	Disinhibition of insulin secretion and peripheral action of insulin; symptoms may be masked by beta-blockade; monitor serum glucose closely
Arrhythmia	Can result from a hypertensive crisis

Watch Out

Patients undergoing bilateral adrenalectomy (typically due to malignancy) are at risk for Addisonian crisis and can develop severe postoperative hypotension, fever, and/or hypoglycemia. Check plasma ACTH and start IV dexamethasone.

How Often Should Plasma and Urinary Catecholamines Be Measured Postoperatively?

These should first be measured 2 weeks after surgery. If they remain high, the patient may have a residual or metastatic tumor present. Monitoring should be continued every 3 months for the first year and then annually afterward. This applies to normotensive and hypertensive patients.

Prognosis

What Is the Overall Prognosis for Pheochromocytoma?

Surgical resection is usually curative and results in normalization of blood pressure. The likelihood of malignant, multifocal, or recurrent disease varies largely as a function of the underlying genotype, since a large fraction of cases are syndromic.

What Is the Treatment for Malignant Pheochromocytoma?

Since malignant pheochromocytoma is defined by evidence of spread to other organs or distant metastasis, there is currently no cure, since there is no effective systemic therapy. Thus, treatment is mainly directed toward palliation of symptoms. Blood pressure is controlled with alpha-blockers. Surgical debulking is often performed and can help to ameliorate symptoms and reduce the toxic effects of high circulating catecholamines on the heart and other organs.

Key Areas Where You Can Get in Trouble

Do Not Biopsy a Pheochromocytoma

The discovery of an adrenal mass on cross-sectional imaging may tempt physicians to biopsy the mass. This is ill-advised, as biopsies of the adrenal gland are generally non-informative and may be dangerous (i.e., bleeding). Biopsy of an undiagnosed pheochromocytoma may result in a hypertensive crisis. The first step when an adrenal mass is found or pheochromocytoma is suspected is to perform a biochemical workup looking for elevated plasma-free metanephrines and elevated 24-hour urine levels of catecholamines and their metabolites.

Pheochromocytoma Along with MEN 2A

The diagnosis of MEN 2A may not be immediately apparent. If a patient presents with one of the three associated conditions, which are pheochromocytoma, primary hyperparathyroidism, or medullary thyroid carcinoma, it is important to evaluate for the others. For example, a patient with symptoms of pheochromocytoma such as episodic hypertension or palpitations, along with findings that suggest primary hyperparathyroidism such as hypercalcemia or kidney stones, should also be assessed for medullary thyroid carcinoma by measuring serum calcitonin. Recognizing this pattern is critical to making the diagnosis of MEN 2A.

Hypertensive Crisis During Surgery Due to Undiagnosed Pheochromocytoma

It is mandatory to work up any known adrenal nodule prior to elective surgery to rule out pheochromocytoma. If a patient has unexplained severe hypertension and tachycardia intraoperatively, the diagnosis of pheochromocytoma should be considered. Blood pressure should be managed with intravenous antihypertensive drips and volume repletion. In elective cases, the operation should be terminated after stabilizing the patient.

Summary of Essentials

History and Physical

- Look for episodic hyperadrenergic symptoms (5 P's): pressure (hypertension), pain (headache), perspiration, palpitation, and pallor
- Associated with the MEN 2A/B disorders, neurofibromatosis-1, VHL, and familial paraganglioma syndromes

Etiology/Pathophysiology

- Tumor derived from chromaffin cells in the adrenal medulla or sympathetic ganglia
- Norepinephrine is the predominant catecholamine (followed by epinephrine)
- Triggers of hypertensive crisis include changes in blood flow, physical stimulation, tumor necrosis, anesthetic agents, foods containing tyramine, and surgical manipulation
- Malignancy based on the presence of local invasion or metastasis, not cellular features

Diagnosis

- Urine and/or blood levels of catecholamines (epinephrine, norepinephrine, and dopamine) and their metabolites
- Plasma-free metanephrine is most sensitive but has higher false positives
- First-line imaging consists of CT or MRI with contrast
- Nuclear imaging with iodine-metaiodobenzylguanidine (I-MIBG) is highly specific for pheochromocytoma and may be useful in cases of suspected multifocal disease or those not visualized on CT or MRI

Management

- Medical conditioning with alpha-blockade for at least 2 weeks
- Volume and salt replacement
- Add beta-blockade for tachycardia and/or arrhythmia
- Surgical resection (adrenalectomy) is curative for benign lesions
- Laparoscopic approach is preferred for patients with adrenal pheochromocytomas that are less than 6 cm in size and have no malignant features on imaging

Watch Out

- Do not biopsy adrenal masses
- Never give a beta-blocker first (unopposed alpha constriction)

Suggested Reading

Brink I, Hoegerle S, Klisch J, Bley TA. Imaging of pheochromocytoma and paraganglioma. Fam Cancer. 2005;4(1):61–8.

Dluhy RG. Pheochromocytoma – death of an axiom. N Engl J Med. 2002;346(19):1486–8.

Hodin R, Lubitz C, Phitayakorn R, Stephen A. Diagnosis and management of pheochromocytoma. Curr Probl Surg. 2014;51(4):151–87.

Karasek D, Frysak Z, Pacak K. Genetic testing for pheochromocytoma. Curr Hypertens Rep. 2010;12(6):456–64.

Lenders JW, Duh QY, Eisenhofer G, et al. Pheochromocytoma and paraganglioma: an endocrine society clinical practice guideline. J Clin Endocrinol Metab. 2014;99(6):1915–42.
Lenders JW, Eisenhofer G, Mannelli M, Pacak K. Phaeochromocytoma. Lancet 2005;366(9486):665–75.
Neary NM, King KS, Pacak K. Drugs and pheochromocytom-don't be fooled by every elevated metanephrine. N Engl J Med. 2011;364(23):2268–70.
Plouin PF, Amar L, Dekkers OM, et al. European Society of Endocrinology Clinical Practice Guideline for long-term follow-up of patients operated on for a phaeochromocytoma or a paraganglioma. Eur J Endocrinol. 2016;174(5):G1–G10.
Ricketts CJ, Forman JR, Rattenberry E, et al. Tumor risks and genotype-phenotype-proteotype analysis in 358 patients with germline mutations in SDHB and SDHD. Hum Mutat. 2010;31(1):41–51.
Sawka AM, Jaeschke R, Singh RJ, Young WF. A comparison of biochemical tests for pheochromocytoma: measurement of fractionated plasma metanephrines compared with the combination of 24-hour urinary metanephrines and catecholamines. J Clin Endocrinol Metab. 2003;88(2):553–8.
Scholz T, Eisenhofer G, Pacak K, Dralle H, Lehnert H. Clinical review: current treatment of malignant pheochromocytoma. J Clin Endocrinol Metab. 2007;92(4):1217–25.

Neck Mass That Moves with Swallowing

James X. Wu and Michael W. Yeh

Contents

C. de Virgilio, A. Grigorian (eds.), *Surgery*, https://doi.org/10.1007/978-3-032-09799-6_14

Case Study

A 53-year-old woman is referred to our clinic with a chief complaint of a neck mass and a hoarse voice. She sought care after feeling a lump in the lower anterior neck, just right of the midline. She complains of a sensation of neck tightness, especially when lying supine. She denies any difficulty swallowing, or pain. She denies exposure to ionizing radiation. She takes no medications and has no known drug allergies. Her social history is negative for tobacco and alcohol use. She does not have a family history of neck tumors or thyroid problems. On physical exam, she is a well-nourished normal adult female with a solitary, 2-cm nodule in the right lobe of the thyroid that moves with swallowing. There is no associated cervical adenopathy. Laboratory tests demonstrate a thyroid-stimulating hormone (TSH) of 2 mIU/L (normal 0.4–4 mIU/L) and normal serum-free thyroxine (T4) and free triiodothyronine (T3) levels. An ultrasound confirms the presence of a roughly spherical, well-demarcated 2-cm nodule in the right lobe of the thyroid and normal cervical lymph nodes.

Diagnosis

What Is the Differential Diagnosis for a Thyroid Mass? (Table 14.1)

Table 14.1 Differential diagnosis for a thyroid mass

Diagnosis	Description	Characteristics
Thyroglossal duct cyst	Congenital persistence of thyroglossal duct	Well-defined, smooth neck mass located in the midline, above the cricoid cartilage; elevates with tongue protrusion (and swallowing)
Multinodular goiter	Multiple nodules distributed throughout the thyroid, can be toxic or nontoxic	Usually benign, may arise from iodine deficiency in childhood
Benign follicular nodule	Solitary nodule of follicular origin, may be solid or cystic *(colloid nodule)*	Common in the general population; prevalence increases with age, women > men
Toxic adenoma	Solitary nodule overproducing thyroid hormone	Almost always benign, appears as a "hot nodule" on thyroid scintigraphy; causes hyperthyroidism
Graves' disease	Autoantibodies that stimulate TSH receptor causing hyperthyroidism, diffuse enlargement, and hypervascularity of the thyroid	Ophthalmopathy (lid retraction, exophthalmos, extraocular muscle restriction, optic neuropathy) is present in half of patients
Hashimoto's thyroiditis	Chronic lymphocytic infiltration and autoimmune destruction of the thyroid; usually painless; thyroid may be shrunken and fibrotic at the end stage	Positive serum TPO antibodies; patient euthyroid in early stage, progressing to hypothyroid over years
Postpartum thyroiditis	Painless goiter, due to autoimmune thyroid disease following pregnancy	Patient initially hyperthyroid, followed by euthyroid state, and then hypothyroidism
Subacute thyroiditis	Painful, transient goiter; cause unknown, possibly viral	Typically preceded by URI; patient hyperthyroid, followed by hypothyroidism
Suppurative thyroiditis	Transient, painful goiter due to bacterial infection. Most commonly due to *Staph. aureus* or *Strep. Pyogenes*	Often preceded by URI; patient euthyroid
Riedel's thyroiditis	Painless, progressive, firm, or "woody" goiter; cause unknown; results in extensive fibrosis	Mainly affects women, may have positive thyroid antibodies; patient hypothyroid or euthyroid
Thyroid cancer (papillary, medullary, follicular, anaplastic lymphoma, metastases)	Typically nonfunctional, painless thyroid nodules occurring more often in females and extremes of age	Patient usually euthyroid; prognosis varies widely from extremely indolent (papillary) to highly lethal (anaplastic)

TPO thyroid peroxidase, *URI* upper respiratory infection

What Is This Patient's Diagnosis?

With an isolated nodule in the thyroid gland and symptoms of local invasion (e.g., hoarse voice), there is concern for thyroid cancer. However, there is insufficient information to make the diagnosis.

History and Physical

What Are the Common Symptoms of a Patient with a Thyroid Nodule?

Patients often appreciate a lump in the anterior neck. Some may complain of shortness of breath, sensation of neck tightness, voice changes, and/or dysphagia. It is important to also assess for symptoms of hyperthyroidism or hypothyroidism (discussed below).

How Common Are Thyroid Nodules, and How Often Are They Cancerous?

Thyroid nodules are common and are identified by palpation in approximately 5% of adults. However, with the widespread use of high-resolution ultrasonography, incidental thyroid nodules are detected in up to 50% of adults. The vast majority of these nodules (95%) are benign. In contrast, thyroid cancer is relatively uncommon, affecting about 0.2% of the adult population in the United States. Notably, the incidence of thyroid cancer has tripled over the past four decades, largely due to increased detection of small papillary carcinomas.

Describe the Different Types of Thyroid Cancer? (◘ Table 14.2)

◘ **Table 14.2** Types and characteristics of thyroid cancer

Type	Description	% of thyroid cancer	Characteristics
Papillary adenocarcinoma	Arises from follicular cells; presents as single nodule, often with internal calcifications, usually in early adulthood	~80%	*Slow growing*, excellent prognosis with overall survival rates ~95%; propensity to spread to regional lymph nodes; diagnosis established by characteristic nuclear features found on FNA
Follicular adenocarcinoma	Arises from follicular cells; occurs later in life than papillary; forms soft, rubbery, encapsulated tumors	10–20%	Good prognosis with overall survival rates ~85%; propensity *to spread hematogenously* to distant sites (most common is bone); *cannot be diagnosed on FNA* or frozen section; diagnosis rests on demonstration of capsular and/or vascular invasion on permanent section after thyroid lobectomy
Hurthle cell carcinoma	Subtype of follicular carcinoma; composed of Hurthle cells: large eosinophilic epithelial cells	5%	Similar to follicular carcinoma but with slightly worse prognosis (overall survival ~75%); most do not take up RAI
Medullary carcinoma	Arises from C (parafollicular) cells, secretes calcitonin; hard, solid, tumors containing amyloid	5–7%	Overall survival ~75%; commonly spreads to regional lymph nodes; miliary liver metastases also common; underlying germ line mutation exists in 25% of cases; associated with multiple endocrine neoplasia (MEN)-2A/B
Anaplastic carcinoma	Extremely aggressive cancer, likely dedifferentiated papillary or follicular thyroid cancer	1–2%	Median survival 6 months; uniformly lethal
Thyroid lymphoma	Typically, B-cell non-Hodgkin lymphoma	<5%	Usually develops in the setting of Hashimoto's thyroiditis
Metastases to the thyroid	Metastases from distant primary malignancy	<1%	Primary malignancy usually arises from the kidney, breast, lung, or skin (melanoma)

FNA fine-needle aspiration, *RAI* radioactive iodine

Watch Out
Although papillary thyroid carcinoma is known to *first* spread to the lymphatic system, the prognosis is based on the presence of local invasion.

What Are the Risk Factors for Thyroid Cancer?

Female gender, exposure to ionizing radiation, and family history of thyroid cancer are the risk factors for thyroid cancer. MEN-2A, MEN-2B, and familial medullary thyroid carcinoma account for 25% of medullary thyroid cancer cases and are all related to activating mutations in the RET proto-oncogene, a cell membrane tyrosine kinase. Papillary thyroid cancer is associated with Cowden syndrome, Gardner syndrome, and familial adenomatous polyposis. One-fifth of papillary thyroid cancers are due to RET/papillary thyroid carcinoma (PTC) rearrangements, which create a fusion gene comprised of PTC promoters and the RET tyrosine kinase. An estimated one-third or more are due to mutations in BRAF, a gene encoding a signal transduction protein kinase. Thyroid cancer occurs more frequently in women than men. However, nodules occurring in men and in children or the elderly are *more* likely to be malignant.

Watch Out
Childhood exposure to ionizing radiation, especially before age 15, significantly increases the risk of thyroid cancer. Common sources include prior radiation therapy and nuclear fallout.

What Are the Symptoms of Hyperthyroidism?

Nervousness, weight loss, heat intolerance, thirst, palpitations, pressured speech, and tremors are the symptoms of hyperthyroidism. Women may have irregular or absent menses. Thyroid storm, a severe type of hyperthyroidism, causes high-grade fever, arrhythmia, bloating, diarrhea, and high-output cardiac failure and can be fatal.

Watch Out
The most common cause of death in patients with thyroid storm is high-output cardiac failure. It typically occurs in postoperative patients with undiagnosed Graves' disease. First-line therapy includes beta-blockers and propylthiouracil. Aspirin can precipitate thyroid storm.

What Are the Symptoms of Hypothyroidism?

Fatigue, weight gain, lethargy, hair changes, cold intolerance, constipation, difficulty with memory/cognition, impaired libido, and impaired fertility.

How Should the Thyroid Be Examined?

To examine the thyroid, stand behind the patient and locate the cricoid cartilage. Palpate just below it for the isthmus, then move laterally to assess each lobe for asymmetry. Gently rotate each lobe forward and ask the patient to swallow to help reveal hidden nodules. Finish by checking along the sternocleidomastoid muscles for lymphadenopathy.

What Is the Significance of the Mass Moving Up and Down with Swallowing?

The ligament of Berry attaches the thyroid gland to the trachea, causing it to move cranially when a patient swallows. A mass that moves with swallowing is more likely to originate within the thyroid gland as opposed to some other part of the anatomy (lymph nodes, for instance). In rare circumstances, an aggressive thyroid cancer will become fixed due to local invasion of surrounding structures. This is a worrisome sign.

Watch Out
Ectopic thyroid tissue in the lateral position of the neck is a well-differentiated thyroid cancer that has metastasized to cervical lymph nodes, until proven otherwise.

What Is the Appearance of a Patient with Severe or Long-Standing Hyperthyroidism?

Flushed face, warm skin, tremor, weight loss with possible muscle wasting, tachycardia, widened pulse pressure, and hyperactive reflexes.

What Is the Appearance of a Patient with Severe or Long-Standing Hypothyroidism?

Periorbital swelling with puffy face and extremities, fine hair, loss of the outer aspects of the eyebrows, waxy or clammy skin, and weight gain.

Pathophysiology

What Is the Function of the Thyroid Gland?

The thyroid contains follicular cells and parafollicular C cells. Follicular cells of the thyroid produce, store, and secrete the thyroid hormones thyroxine (T4) and triiodothyronine (T3). Synthesis of T4 and T3 requires iodide, which the thyroid takes up and stores. T4 is a precursor to T3, and T3 is considered ten times more potent. The thyroid normally produces 20% of circulating T3; the rest is converted from T4 in peripheral tissues. These remain protein bound in the circulation, and only the free fraction is active. The parafollicular C cells of the thyroid secrete calcitonin.

> **Watch Out**
> Most patients with thyroid carcinoma are euthyroid.

What Is Thyroglobulin?

Thyroglobulin (Tg) is a glycoprotein housed within thyroid follicles that is a storage form/precursor of T4 and T3. Serum thyroglobulin levels correlate positively with the amount of thyroid tissue, thyroid injury/inflammation, and the TSH level. Thus, serum Tg can be used as a tumor marker during surveillance after initial treatment of papillary and follicular thyroid cancer but only if a *total* thyroidectomy has been performed. Anti-Tg autoantibodies are present in about 20% of thyroid cancer patients and can interfere with Tg testing.

What Are the Actions of Thyroid Hormones?

In general, T4 and T3 regulate basal metabolic rate, growth and development, and sensitivity to catecholamines with effects on many organ systems.

> **Watch Out**
> Metastatic medullary carcinoma frequently causes diarrhea and flushing, thought to be due to the high *calcitonin* level.

What Is the Embryologic Origin of the Thyroid?

The primitive thyroid gland arises from the medial pharynx, part of the embryologic endoderm. This tissue descends along the thyroglossal duct into the neck and ultimately gives rise to thyroid follicles and colloid. The rostral-most aspect of the thyroglossal duct is the foramen cecum. Parafollicular C cells, which produce calcitonin, arise from the fourth pharyngeal pouch and migrate from the neural crest into the thyroid gland.

> **Watch Out**
> Ectopic thyroid tissue may be found anywhere along the path of thyroglossal duct as well as in the anterior mediastinum. Additionally, the thyroglossal duct may not completely obliterate, leaving behind thyroglossal duct cysts.

Why Is Fine-Needle Aspiration (FNA) Unable to Diagnose Follicular Thyroid Carcinoma?

FNA cannot diagnose follicular thyroid carcinoma because the distinction between benign and malignant follicular neoplasms requires evidence of capsular or vascular invasion, which is a histologic rather than a cytologic feature. As FNA collects only cells, it cannot assess for these invasive features and therefore cannot confirm malignancy.

What Is Considered a Well-Differentiated Thyroid Cancer?

Tumors arising from follicular cells are categorized as well differentiated. This category includes papillary, follicular, and Hurthle cell carcinomas.

> **Watch Out**
> Thyroid cancer is considered the most common endocrine malignancy in the United States.

What Are Psammoma Bodies?

Microscopic findings of round, laminar collections of calcified tissue are known as psammoma bodies. It is seen in papillary thyroid cancer but also found in several malignant and benign lesions.

> **Watch Out**
> The cancers associated with psammoma bodies can be remembered by **PS**a**MM**oma: **p**apillary carcinoma of the thyroid, **s**erous cystadenocarcinoma of the ovary, **m**eningioma, and **m**esothelioma.

Workup

What Laboratory Tests Are Recommended for a Thyroid Mass?

The first test is a TSH level. It is the most sensitive measure of thyroid dysfunction and the only test indicated for screening or in the absence of symptoms of hyperthyroidism or hypothyroidism. T4 and T3 testing may be indicated if the TSH is abnormal. Thyroid function tests may be altered in the setting of severe illness. This is often due to decreased peripheral conversion of T4 to T3, resulting in low serum T3 with normal T4 and TSH levels. This pattern, often termed euthyroid sick syndrome, reflects an adaptive central hypothyroid state and should not be misinterpreted as primary thyroid dysfunction.

What Are the Appropriate Imaging Studies for a Thyroid Nodule?

Surgeon-performed bedside ultrasound is the preferred initial imaging for thyroid nodules. It identifies nodules, characterizes them as solid or cystic, detects suspicious features such as hypoechogenicity, irregular margins, or microcalcifications, and can guide FNA. If there is concern for local invasion into the aerodigestive tract or substernal extension, cross-sectional imaging with CT or MRI is indicated.

Is Routine Use of Nuclear Imaging Useful for an Isolated Thyroid Nodule?

Thyroid scintigraphy, performed with I^{123}, is rarely used today. Although iodine-avid (hyperfunctional or "hot") nodules are virtually all benign, "cold" nodules (with low or no uptake, meaning they are nonfunctional) are only malignant in about 5% of cases. As such, whether a nodule is hot or cold is not that discriminating and has largely been replaced by FNA. The rare situation where scintigraphy is useful in the setting where repeat FNA is indeterminate for malignancy. Rather than proceeding to open surgery, some advocate scintigraphy as it may obviate the need for biopsy if the nodule is hot.

What Nodules Should Undergo FNA?

FNA is recommended for thyroid nodules larger than 1 cm, nodules with ultrasound characteristics suggestive of malignancy (e.g., internal microcalcifications), nodules demonstrating interval growth, or any size nodule associated with abnormal cervical lymph nodes. Nodules smaller than 1 cm, purely cystic lesions, or those with clearly benign features on ultrasound do not require FNA.

What Is the Bethesda Reporting System for FNAs of Thyroid Nodules? (Table 14.3)

Table 14.3 Bethesda reporting system for thyroid FNAs

FNA result	Risk of malignancy (%)
Benign	0–3
Atypia of undetermined significance or follicular lesion of undetermined significance (AUS/FLUS)	5–15
Suspicious for follicular neoplasm	15–30
Suspicious for malignancy	60–75
Malignant	97–99
Inadequate/nondiagnostic	1–4

Management

What Is the Next Step in a Patient with an Inadequate/Nondiagnostic FNA?

An *inadequate* FNA is a technically failed biopsy which does not yield sufficient cells to establish a diagnosis. This must be distinguished from an *indeterminate* FNA, which is a technically successful biopsy with adequate cellular yield in which no definite diagnosis of a benign or malignant process can be made (corresponding to Bethesda categories AUS/FLUS and suspicious for follicular neoplasm). *Inadequate* biopsies should generally be repeated (Fig. 14.1).

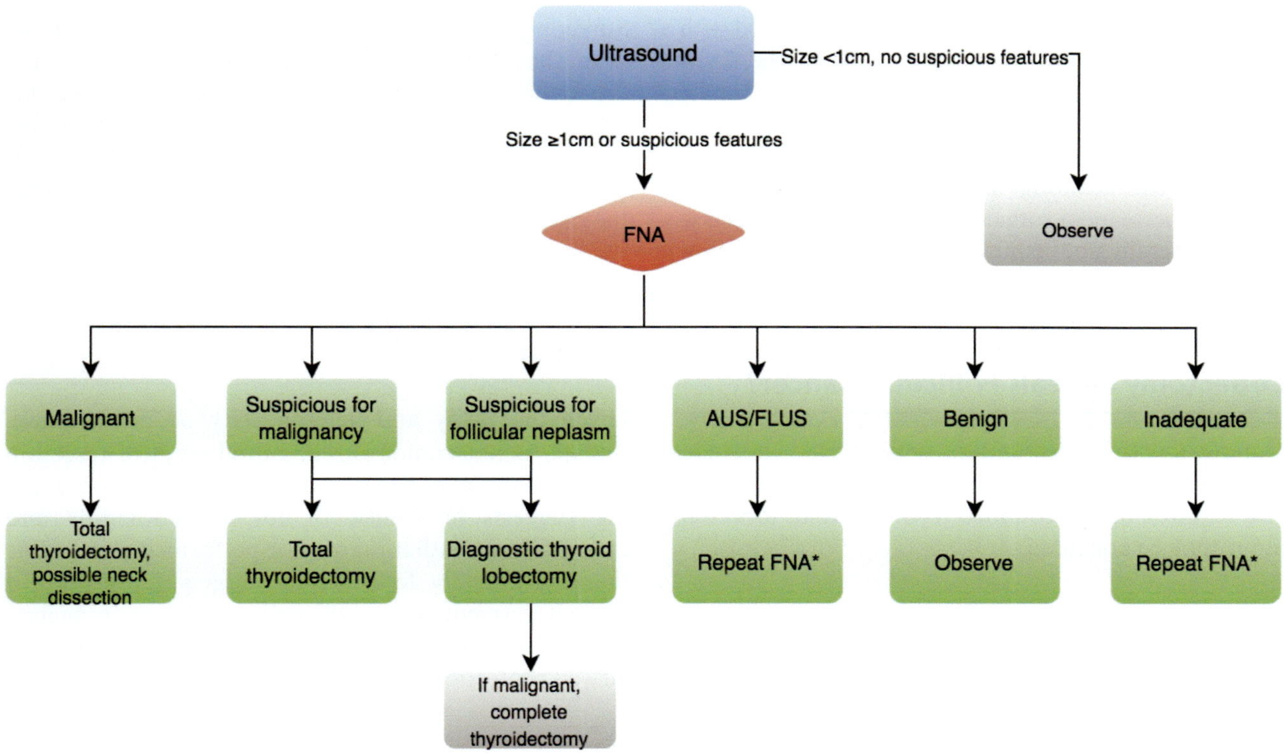

Fig. 14.1 Diagnostic algorithm for nonfunctioning solitary thyroid nodule found on examination or imaging

What Is the Next Step for a Benign FNA Result?

Annual follow-up with ultrasonography. Nodules that enlarge and/or develop suspicious sonographic features warrant repeat FNA or surgical excision.

What Is the Next Step for an FNA Which Reports AUS or FLUS?

The standard approach is to repeat FNA, as most nodules are benign on subsequent biopsy. If indeterminate again, molecular testing or diagnostic lobectomy may be considered based on clinical context and patient preference.

What Is the Next Step for an FNA Result of Suspected Follicular Neoplasm?

Perform a thyroid lobectomy (hemithyroidectomy). There are several reasons for performing a lobectomy instead of a simple biopsy: (a) the thyroid gland is extremely vascular, and a biopsy would carry a higher risk of hemorrhage, (b) tumor cells may be spilled with a simple biopsy, and (c) removing a lobe of the thyroid does not adversely affect thyroid function. Approximately 25% of these lesions are ultimately found to be malignant. Follicular thyroid carcinoma is indistinguishable from follicular adenoma on FNA and can only be diagnosed on permanent surgical histopathology. Frozen section is generally not helpful for these lesions (see below).

What Is the Next Step If the Thyroid Lobectomy Reveals Follicular Cancer?

Completion thyroidectomy is typically recommended. However, if the tumor is smaller than 4 cm, lacks high-risk features, and is confined to the thyroid, lobectomy alone may be adequate.

What Are the Advantages of Total Thyroidectomy in Thyroid Cancer Versus Lobectomy?

Removing the remainder of the thyroid allows for removal of any missed contralateral foci of thyroid cancer (present in up to 70% of cases). It also allows for using a radioactive iodine scan to detect/treat recurrence or metastases (otherwise the remaining thyroid lobe concentrates all the radioiodine). Finally, total thyroidectomy allows the use of serum thyroglobulin as a marker for recurrence.

What Thyroid Malignancy Is Amenable to Thyroid Lobectomy Alone? When Is Total Thyroidectomy Appropriate?

Small (<1 cm), unifocal, papillary thyroid carcinomas have such a favorable prognosis and low recurrence rates that total thyroidectomy is of little or no value. Hemithyroidectomy and total thyroidectomy are both considered appropriate for follicular and papillary thyroid cancers between 1 and 4 cm in size. Total thyroidectomy should be performed when tumors are larger than 4 cm, if extra-thyroidal extension is present, or if there is spread of disease to lymph nodes or distant sites.

Is It Ever Appropriate to Proceed Directly to Total Thyroidectomy without Performing a Lobectomy First?

Surgeons will proceed directly to total thyroidectomy when the FNA returns suspected follicular neoplasm in the following scenarios: bilateral nodules, index nodule >4 cm (higher rate of malignancy), preexisting hypothyroidism, family history of thyroid cancer, or history of exposure to ionizing radiation (the latter two increase the risk of multicentric cancer).

What Is the Management of Anaplastic Thyroid Cancer?

Given the rarity and heterogeneity of presentation, therapy is not standardized. Initial surgical resection or debulking may be considered if preoperative imaging suggests feasibility. If not, chemotherapy and external beam radiation may be performed as first-line therapy, possibly followed by surgery in responsive cases. Treatment is generally palliative (given its aggressive nature) and may include early tracheostomy for airway protection.

Watch Out

The most common complication following thyroid surgery is hypocalcemia.

When Should Central Lymph Node Dissection Be Done? Lateral Neck Dissection?

For medullary and some papillary cancers. All patients with medullary thyroid carcinoma should undergo initial central neck dissection. The indications for central neck dissection in papillary thyroid carcinoma are controversial and discussed below. Lateral neck dissection (modified radical neck dissection) is generally performed when palpable or sonographically abnormal lymph nodes are found in the lateral compartment (jugular chain, deep to the sternocleidomastoid muscle). Follicular cancer spreads hematogenously so there is no role for lymph node dissection.

What Is the Role of Intraoperative Frozen Section Pathology?

Frozen section is generally not useful in the diagnosis of follicular thyroid lesions, and its use should therefore be highly selective. Frozen section may be used to confirm the presence of thyroid cancer within the lymph nodes.

Which Thyroid Cancers Concentrate Radioactive Iodine?

Most papillary thyroid cancers (70%) and follicular thyroid cancers (80%) concentrate radioactive iodine. This has important implications in the use of postoperative radioactive iodine ablation. Only a minority of Hurthle cell carcinomas (5%) concentrate iodine. Medullary thyroid cancers do not.

What Are the Important Elements of Postoperative Management of Thyroid Cancer?

Radioactive Iodine Ablation

Radioactive iodine (RAI) ablation with I^{131} may improve survival and reduce recurrences in a follicular thyroid carcinoma and a subset of high-risk papillary thyroid carcinomas.

Suppressive Thyroxine Therapy

TSH promotes thyroid tissue growth, so postoperative TSH suppression with levothyroxine is indicated for all differentiated thyroid cancer.

Follow-Up

After total thyroidectomy, serum thyroglobulin and antithyroglobulin antibodies should be monitored every 6–12 months. In follicular and papillary thyroid cancers, rising or detectable thyroglobulin suggests recurrence. Neck ultrasound should also be performed annually. Medullary thyroid carcinomas should be followed with serum calcitonin.

> **Watch Out**
> Tg antibodies can falsely lower serum thyroglobulin levels. Always interpret Tg in the context of Tg antibody and TSH levels during thyroid cancer follow-up.

If You Suspect Recurrence, What Study Do You Perform?

If serum Tg levels increase on postoperative monitoring and there is concern for cancer recurrence, patients should first undergo neck ultrasound with a full lymph node survey by an experienced practitioner. This often demonstrates a target lesion that is amenable to FNA. Foci of thyroid cancer outside the neck may be detected by diagnostic I^{131} radionuclide scan or thin cut (noncontrast) chest CT.

Does External Beam Radiation Play a Role in Thyroid Cancer?

Yes, but it is only used in <5% of cases. External beam radiation is used for locally invasive tumors following incomplete resection (positive margins) or for palliation of bony metastases.

What Nonoperative Management Is Available for Thyroid Nodules?

Radioactive ablation with I^{131} can treat hyperfunctioning nodules, reducing tumor size and rendering patients euthyroid in 75% of cases. For nonfunctioning thyroid nodules, which are the great majority, the alternative is observation.

Complications

What Are the Major Structures That Can Be Injured During Thyroidectomy?

The recurrent laryngeal nerve, the external branch of superior laryngeal nerve, and the parathyroid glands. The recurrent laryngeal nerve, a branch off the vagus nerve, innervates all of the muscles of the larynx except the cricothyroid muscle. It also provides sensory innervation to the larynx below the vocal cords. Damage to the recurrent laryngeal nerve on one side results in a paralyzed vocal cord in a median or paramedian position. This manifests as hoarseness and sometimes aspiration. The rate of permanent unilateral recurrent laryngeal nerve injury during thyroidectomy should be less than 2% in expert hands. The external branch of the superior laryngeal nerve permits speaking or singing in a high pitch. This nerve may be injured in up to 25% of cases but is usually asymptomatic unless the patient is a singer or voice professional. Permanent hypoparathyroidism usually results from devascularization of the parathyroids and should occur in less than 2% of cases. It is treated with calcium and calcitriol supplementation.

What Should Always Be Assessed Preoperatively in Patients Undergoing Thyroid Surgery that Have Had Previous Neck Surgery?

Indirect or direct laryngoscope to identify bilaterally functioning recurrent laryngeal nerves. Bilateral recurrent laryngeal nerve injury causes airway obstruction and may necessitate urgent tracheostomy, and so if a unilateral injury exists, this should be discussed with the patient prior to surgery.

What Is the Next Step If a Postoperative Patient Develops Stridor in the Recovery Room and the Neck Wound Appears to Be Tense?

Emergent bedside decompression of the hematoma—cut the sutures and open the wound. This usually relieves the airway obstruction immediately. The patient should then return to the operating room for evacuation of the hematoma, irrigation, and careful hemostasis.

Key Areas Where You Can Get in Trouble

Incomplete Family History in Patient with Thyroid Mass

Family history must be carefully assessed in any patient with suspected medullary thyroid carcinoma, as 25% have a germline mutation associated with MEN-2A, MEN-2B, or familial medullary thyroid cancer. If medullary cancer is confirmed on FNA, biochemical testing for pheochromocytoma with 24-hour urine catecholamines and metanephrines is essential before surgery. Failing to exclude pheochromocytoma may result in catastrophic intraoperative hypertensive crisis. All patients with medullary cancer should undergo RET mutation testing, and if positive, first-degree relatives must be screened. Children with known RET mutations should undergo prophylactic thyroidectomy, with the timing based on genotype. MEN-2B requires the earliest intervention, ideally within the first year of life (**B** is **B**ad-er).

Obtaining CT with Iodinated IV Contrast in Patients with Thyroid Cancer

Prior to radionuclide imaging and ablation, patients are depleted of iodine by maintaining a low iodine diet for several weeks. This, combined with an elevated TSH (achieved by either thyroid hormone withdrawal or injection of recombinant human TSH), optimizes RAI uptake by thyroid cells. Iodinated contrast carries a large load of iodine and may suppress RAI uptake for up to 1 month.

Missing Postoperative Hypocalcemia

Postoperative hypoparathyroidism must be promptly recognized and treated in order to avoid hypocalcemic emergencies and near emergencies. Oral calcium supplementation is the preferred method of treatment. Because of the delayed action of oral calcium, an anticipatory rather than reactive protocol of managing postoperative hypoparathyroidism, aided by PTH measurement, is most effective.

Areas of Controversy

Role of Prophylactic Central Neck Dissection (CND) for Papillary Thyroid Cancer

Reoperation for lymphadenectomy is difficult, and pathology reveals central lymph node involvement in 40–60% of patients with papillary thyroid cancer with clinically negative nodes. Some surgeons advocate prophylactic central lymphadenectomy, citing the following benefits: improved staging, lower postoperative thyroglobulin levels, and a reduced need for reoperation. The effect of prophylactic CND on overall survival is unclear at this time. CND theoretically increases the risk of injury to the recurrent laryngeal nerve and the parathyroid glands; however, recent studies have shown no increase in the permanent complication rate within expert centers rate.

Summary of Essentials

History and Physical

- Thyroid nodules are common, most are benign, while thyroid cancer is relatively rare
- Risk factors for thyroid cancer include female sex, childhood exposure to ionizing radiation, and family history of thyroid cancer
- Hyperthyroidism: nervousness, fatigue, weight loss, thirst, and palpitations
- Hypothyroidism: fatigue, weight gain, constipation, and impaired cognition/libido

Diagnosis

- The most important initial test is TSH
- High-resolution neck ultrasound is the imaging study of choice to characterize thyroid nodules and guide FNA
- FNA is indicated for nodules >1 cm with suspicious ultrasound features, for enlarging nodules, and for any nodule with abnormal cervical lymph node

Pathophysiology

- Follicular cells produce thyroid hormones T4 and T3; parafollicular C cells secrete calcitonin
- Papillary and follicular thyroid cancers arise from follicular cells; they are considered "well differentiated" and a majority take up iodine
- Medullary thyroid carcinoma arises from parafollicular C cells and does not concentrate RAI
- Thyroglobulin serves as a tumor marker post-thyroidectomy in follicular and papillary cancers, but results may be falsely low if Tg antibodies are present

Management

- Benign FNA: surveillance with annual ultrasound
- AUS/FLUS: repeat FNA; consider lobectomy or molecular testing if indeterminate again
- Suspicious for follicular neoplasm: diagnostic thyroid lobectomy
- Suspicious for malignancy or malignant: lobectomy or total thyroidectomy based on tumor size, location, and risk factors
- RAI is used in follicular and select papillary cancers
- Medullary thyroid carcinoma requires calcitonin monitoring and genetic testing for RET mutations

Watch Out

- Twenty-five percent of patients with medullary thyroid carcinoma have an underlying germ line mutation.
- Pheochromocytoma must be excluded biochemically prior to surgery in all patients with an FNA diagnosis of medullary thyroid carcinoma.
- "Ectopic thyroid tissue" in the lateral neck usually metastasizes to cervical lymph nodes.
- Numbness and tingling in the lips and fingers after total thyroidectomy usually represent hypoparathyroidism and should be promptly treated with oral calcium.
- Postoperative neck swelling accompanied by stridor is a hematoma compressing the airway; this is a surgical emergency requiring bedside decompression.

Suggested Reading

Alexander EK, et al. Preoperative diagnosis of benign thyroid nodules with indeterminate cytology. N Engl J Med. 2012;367(8):705–15.

Barczynski M, et al. Prophylactic central neck dissection for papillary thyroid cancer. Br J Surg. 2013;100(3):410–8.

Bonnet S, et al. Prophylactic lymph node dissection for papillary thyroid cancer less than 2 cm: implications for radioiodine treatment. J Clin Endocrinol Metab. 2009;94(4):1162–7.

Broome JT, Solorzano CC. The impact of atypia/follicular lesion of undetermined significance on the rate of malignancy in thyroid fine-needle aspiration: evaluation of the Bethesda System for Reporting Thyroid Cytopathology. Surgery. 2011;150(6):1234–41.

Chen JC, et al. Yield of repeat fine-needle aspiration biopsy and rate of malignancy in patients with atypia or follicular lesion of undetermined significance: the impact of the Bethesda System for Reporting Thyroid Cytopathology. Surgery. 2012;152(6):1037–44.

Cibas ES, Ali SZ, N.C.I.T.F.S.o.t.S. Conference. The Bethesda System for Reporting Thyroid Cytopathology. Am J Clin Pathol. 2009;132(5):658–65.

Harvey AM, Mody DR, Amrikachi M. Thyroid fine-needle aspiration reporting rates and outcomes before and after Bethesda implementation within a combined academic and community hospital system. Arch Pathol Lab Med. 2013;137(11):1664–8.

Kouvaraki MA, et al. RET proto-oncogene: a review and update of genotype-phenotype correlations in hereditary medullary thyroid cancer and associated endocrine tumors. Thyroid. 2005;15(6):531–44.

Marotta V, et al. RET/PTC rearrangement in benign and malignant thyroid diseases: a clinical standpoint. Eur J Endocrinol. 2011;165(4):499–507.

Nikiforov YE, et al. Impact of mutational testing on the diagnosis and management of patients with cytologically indeterminate thyroid nodules: a prospective analysis of 1056 FNA samples. J Clin Endocrinol Metab. 2011;96(11):3390–7.

Nygaard B, et al. Long-term effect of radioactive iodine on thyroid function and size in patients with solitary autonomously functioning toxic thyroid nodules. Clin Endocrinol. 1999;50(2):197–202.

Popadich A, et al. A multicenter cohort study of total thyroidectomy and routine central lymph node dissection for cN0 papillary thyroid cancer. Surgery. 2011;150(6):1048–57.

Raffaelli M, et al. Prospective evaluation of total thyroidectomy versus ipsilateral versus bilateral central neck dissection in patients with clinically node-negative papillary thyroid carcinoma. Surgery. 2012;152(6):957–64.

Vaccarella S, et al. Worldwide thyroid-cancer epidemic? The increasing impact of overdiagnosis. NEJM. 2016;375:614–7.

VanderLaan PA, Marqusee E, Krane JF. Clinical outcome for atypia of undetermined significance in thyroid fine-needle aspirations: should repeated fna be the preferred initial approach? Am J Clin Pathol. 2011;135(5):770–5.

Wiseman JE, et al. An algorithm informed by the parathyroid hormone level reduces hypocalcemic complications of thyroidectomy. World J Surg. 2010;34(3):532–7.

Endocrine

Question Set: Endocrine

Questions

1. A 42-year-old woman presents to the emergency department with confusion, weakness, and vomiting. She underwent laparoscopic appendectomy 2 days ago. Her medical history is significant for rheumatoid arthritis, for which she takes chronic oral prednisone. Her temperature is 37.1 °C, blood pressure (BP) is 80/50 mmHg, heart rate is 110/min, and respiratory rate is 22/min. She appears lethargic and dry mucous membranes are noted. Initial intravenous (IV) fluids are administered, but her blood pressure remains low. Laboratory values reveal: sodium 128 mEq/L (135–145), glucose 62 mg/dL (70–110), potassium 4.9 mEq/L (3.5–5.0), and eosinophils 9% (normal <5%). What is the most appropriate next step in management?
   (A) CT scan of the abdomen and pelvis
   (B) IV broad-spectrum antibiotics
   (C) IV hydrocortisone
   (D) Vasopressin
   (E) Intravenous dextrose-containing fluids

2. A 45-year-old female presents to her physician complaining of abdominal pain. She has a history of recurrent kidney stones and was recently discharged from the hospital after undergoing ureteroscopic laser lithotripsy. Her laboratory examination is significant for calcium of 13.6 mg/dL (normal 8.5–10.2 mg/dL) and parathyroid hormone (PTH) of 112 pg/mL (10–55 pg/mL). She is scheduled for operative management of her underlying condition. At surgery, all four parathyroid glands are identified. Only one appears to be abnormally enlarged and is removed. Confirmation of curative resection is best achieved via:
   (A) Intraoperative ultrasound
   (B) Intraoperative frozen section
   (C) Intraoperative PTH levels
   (D) Immediate postoperative serum calcium level
   (E) Postoperative sestamibi scan

3. A 27-year-old woman has 3 months of intermittent spells of severe headache, heart palpitations, and sweating. A pregnancy test at her primary care doctor's office is positive. Further workup reveals that her plasma metanephrine level is 220 pg/mL (normal 12–60 pg/mL). What is the next step in establishing the diagnosis?
   (A) CT abdomen
   (B) Repeat plasma metanephrine level after the patient has delivered
   (C) MRI abdomen
   (D) I^{131}-MIBG scan
   (E) Reassure patient that symptoms are related to pregnancy

4. A 12-year-old boy presents to the doctor for a lump in his neck. He is healthy with no previous medical problems. On physical examination, he has a well-defined anterior neck mass, located in the midline and above the cricoid cartilage. The mother states that she has noted the lesion since he was about 2 years old. It does not bother him. On physical examination, the mass elevates with swallowing and is non-tender. He has no cervical adenopathy and no other complaints. The neck mass is described as a hypoechoic mass on ultrasonography. A subsequent thyroid scintogram is performed and confirms the thyroid gland is in its correct anatomic position. Which of the following would be recommended next for this mass?
(A) Fine-needle aspirate (FNA)
(B) Proceed to surgical excision
(C) Reassurance and observation
(D) Thyroid-stimulating hormone (TSH) and free T4
(E) CT scan

5. In addition to elevated plasma free metanephrine, a change in what other serum marker can help support the diagnosis of pheochromocytoma?
(A) Plasma chromogranin-A
(B) Plasma superoxide dismutase
(C) Malondialdehyde
(D) CA 19–9
(E) 5-Hydroxyindoleacetic acid (HIAA)

6. An elderly nursing home patient has been bedridden for several months due to a series of debilitating strokes. Past medical history is significant for hypertension, controlled with a diuretic, and Paget's disease. Recently, the patient has been complaining of vague abdominal pain, constipation, and depressed mood. On physical examination, the patient is alert and oriented. Abdominal examination is unremarkable. Which of the following electrolyte abnormalities would most likely explain her symptoms?
(A) Hyponatremia
(B) Hypernatremia
(C) Hyperphosphatemia
(D) Hypocalcemia
(E) Hypercalcemia

7. Which of the following is most consistent with an aldosterone-secreting adrenal adenoma?
(A) Hyperglycemia, hirsutism, and abdominal striae
(B) Hypertension and hyperkalemia
(C) Hypertension in a patient requiring potassium supplementation
(D) Elevated plasma metanephrine and hypertension
(E) Increased vanillylmandelic acid excretion and hypertension

8. A 35-year-old patient presents for a follow-up visit for an elevated serum calcium level of 12.8 mg/dL and an elevated parathyroid hormone (PTH). He is a thin man without a significant past medical history. He reports that for the past 2 weeks, he has been experiencing loose stools, polydipsia, and polyuria. On physical exam, he was found to have large erythematous erosions with blisters over the lower abdomen. Which tumor would best explain the patient's symptoms and rash?
(A) Insulinoma
(B) Prolactinoma
(C) VIPoma
(D) Glucagonoma
(E) Adrenal adenoma

9. A 32-year-old female patient arrives for follow-up for new-onset hypertension. She was started on hydrochlorothiazide 6 months ago. During her visit, she was found to have a blood pressure of 152/98 mmHg. She also complains of recent episodes where she experiences sudden palpitations, chest pain, diaphoresis, headache, and anxiety. Her laboratory exam demonstrates a calcium of 13.2 mg/dL (normal 8.5–10.2 mg/dL), parathyroid hormone (PTH) of 102 pg/mL (10–55 pg/mL), and an elevated plasma metanephrine. Which of the following would be an important additional component in the workup?
   (A) Fasting blood glucose
   (B) Prolactin level
   (C) MRI of the sella turcica
   (D) Serum calcitonin
   (E) Serum gastrin level

10. A 55-year-old otherwise healthy patient undergoes a non-contrast CT abdomen to evaluate for possible kidney stones and is incidentally noted to have a 8 cm mass in the left adrenal gland. The mass has irregular borders and high attenuation, suggesting a lipid-poor lesion, and appears to be adherent to the kidney. How should this patient be managed?
   (A) Observation with repeat CT scan in 3 months
   (B) Open adrenalectomy
   (C) Laparoscopic adrenalectomy
   (D) Radiation therapy
   (E) Percutaneous biopsy

11. A 50-year-old female has been recently diagnosed with primary hyperparathyroidism. She comes in to her doctor complaining of increased bone pain in her legs. She is found to have elevated serum calcium, alkaline phosphate, and parathyroid hormone (PTH). Her doctor decides to order plain films of her lower extremities. The radiographs show very thin bones with a stress fracture and bowing of both femur bones. She also has characteristic cysts with a moth-eaten appearance. What is the most likely diagnosis?
   (A) Osteoporosis
   (B) Osteopetrosis
   (C) Osteomalacia
   (D) Osteitis fibrosa cystica
   (E) Paget's disease of the bone

12. A 60-year-old man is found to have a 3 cm right adrenal mass on CT scan which was obtained a month earlier following a motor vehicle accident. He is asymptomatic, and does not report a history of hypertension or diabetes. What is the most appropriate next step in management?
   (A) Repeat CT scan in 6 months
   (B) Percutaneous needle biopsy
   (C) Biochemical workup for hormone excess
   (D) Laparoscopic adrenalectomy
   (E) No further follow-up is necessary

13. A 42-year-old man with a family history of endocrine tumors is diagnosed with MEN-2A after presenting with uncontrolled hypertension and subsequent genetic workup. He was found to have a right adrenal pheochromocytoma and asymptomatic hyperparathyroidism. What is the recommended surgical management for this patient?
   (A) Parathyroid surgery first, followed by adrenalectomy
   (B) Adrenalectomy first, followed by parathyroid surgery
   (C) Medical conditioning for 2 weeks prior to adrenalectomy, followed by parathyroid surgery

procedure, one well-known complication is airway obstruction following bleeding and hematoma formation which occurs within the first 24 h after thyroidectomy. Checking oxygen saturation or waiting for labs is never appropriate for a patient with a compromised airway (D–E).

21. Answer D

The superior laryngeal nerve lies adjacent to the superior thyroid artery and is thus at high risk of being injured during mobilization of the thyroid, particularly the superior pole. The external branch of the superior laryngeal nerve permits singing in a high pitch. This nerve may be injured in up to 25% of cases but is usually asymptomatic unless the patient is a singer or voice professional. Damage to the recurrent laryngeal nerve on one side results in a paralyzed vocal cord in a median or paramedian position. This manifests as hoarseness and sometimes aspiration (A). The rate of permanent unilateral recurrent laryngeal nerve injury during thyroidectomy should be less than 2% in expert hands. If both recurrent laryngeal nerves were injured during a total thyroidectomy, then both vocal cords could be paralyzed, and this may lead to a compromised airway which may necessitate a permanent tracheostomy (E). Therefore, it is imperative to perform a flexible laryngoscopy to visualize the vocal cords in a patient with previous neck surgery that is scheduled for parathyroid or thyroid surgery. A droop in the corner of the mouth results from injury to the marginal mandibular branch of the facial nerve (B). Swallowing is controlled by multiple nerves including the glossopharyngeal, vagus, and/or hypoglossal nerves (C).

22. Answer C

With the increasing use of routine laboratory testing, most patients with primary hyperparathyroidism are currently discovered incidentally in asymptomatic patients. Although the patients may be asymptomatic, long-standing hyperparathyroidism can lead to kidney injury and osteoporosis. Evidence of such should be sought out via bone mineral density testing as well as calculation of creatinine clearance. For patients with asymptomatic hyperparathyroidism diagnosed through laboratory screening, a 2013 consensus statement recommended the following indications for surgery:

1. Serum calcium level of 1.0 mg/dL greater than the upper limit of normal
2. Creatinine clearance reduced to <60 mL/min
3. Elevated 24-h urine calcium >400 mg/day AND increased risk for calcium stone formation on biochemical stone risk analysis
4. Presence of asymptomatic nephrolithiasis or nephrocalcinosis seen on imaging
5. Bone mineral density with T-score less than −2.5 at any site
6. Evidence of vertebral fracture
7. Age <50
8. Patients that do not desire or cannot undergo routine surveillance

The patient described meets the age criterion for surgical intervention. The surgical treatment of primary hyperparathyroidism due to four-gland hyperplasia is to remove 3.5 glands. An acceptable alternative is to remove all four glands and to reimplant half of a gland within the muscles of the forearm. That way if the patient develops recurrent hyperparathyroidism, additional parathyroid tissue can be removed from the forearm under local anesthesia as opposed to re-operative neck surgery with the attendant risk of cranial nerve injury. Removal of all four glands is not recommended as it will render the patient permanently hypocalcemic with a lifelong need for calcium supplementation (B). Observation would not be appropriate for patients meeting criteria for surgery (A). Patients not selected for surgical therapy require biochemical monitoring of serum calcium and serum creatinine annually (D). Bone mineral density should be measured every 1–2 years. Cinacalcet, a calcimimetic, is mainly used to treat secondary hyperparathyroidism (seen in patients with renal failure) (E). It may be considered to reduce the serum calcium in patients who are not candidates for surgery.

23. Answer A
A sudden rise in blood pressure after anesthetic induction raises concern for an undiagnosed pheochromocytoma, malignant hyperthermia, and thyrotoxicosis (thyroid storm). For each of these situations, cessation of anesthesia is recommended. There are several clues that point to pheochromocytoma as the cause. The administration of beta-blockers without alpha-blockade first leads to worsening hypertension due to unopposed alpha-mediated vasoconstriction as in the case above. Pheochromocytoma is associated with neurofibromatosis-1 which may present with skin neurofibromas (rubberlike discolored skin lesions) and cataracts (hazy vision). Malignant hyperthermia presents with muscle rigidity (most often the masseter), a rapid increase in core body temperature, a rise in end tidal CO_2, arrhythmia, and a mixed metabolic and respiratory acidosis at anesthetic induction (B). Treatment is immediate cessation of surgery and dantrolene. Thyrotoxicosis presents in a similar fashion to malignant hyperthermia (fever, hypertension, tachycardia); however, it is not associated with muscle rigidity or rising end tidal CO_2 (C). The associated hypertension and tachycardia respond to the administration of beta-blockade. It is due to a hypermetabolic state caused by excess thyroid hormone. Inadequate anesthetic agents may lead to hypertension and tachycardia but would not lead to high fevers (D). An undiagnosed pituitary tumor resulting in excess ACTH production can cause hypertension, but this will be accompanied with symptoms consistent with Cushing's disease (e.g., truncal obesity, abdominal striae, muscle wasting, hirsutism) (E).

24. Answer C
Patients with pheochromocytoma are volume depleted due to intense alpha-mediated vasoconstriction. Hypertension is controlled with alpha-blockade (e.g., phenoxybenzamine) for 10–14 days before surgery. This allows for volume expansion, and the patient is encouraged to liberally intake salt and fluids. The dose is titrated until hypertensive episodes are controlled, often resulting in *mild orthostatic hypotension*. Beta-blockers can be used to decrease reflex tachycardia once appropriate alpha-blockade has been established (B). Initiating beta-blocker therapy prematurely can precipitate a hypertensive crisis due to unopposed alpha-adrenergic vasoconstriction. Octreotide is a somatostatin analogue that may have minimal efficacy in the palliation of symptoms from malignant pheochromocytoma, but it has no role in preparing a patient for surgery (A). Metyrosine inhibits catecholamine production and is a secondary agent for pheochromocytoma, though now rarely used (D). Diuresis would be contraindicated as these patients are volume depleted (E). In fact, some patients may need to be admitted preoperatively for continuous maintenance fluids prior to surgery.

25. Answer C
Sestamibi scanning involves using a radioisotope, technetium-99m, which is taken up by cells with high mitochondrial activity. It is more accurate for single adenomas than for four-gland hyperplasia. Sestamibi scanning and to a lesser extent ultrasound are the most frequently used imaging tests to localize the involved gland(s) in primary hyperparathyroidism (B). Localizing studies are generally not indicated in secondary or tertiary hyperparathyroidism, since multiple-gland hyperplasia is the expected underlying pathology. Preoperative FNA is not helpful in the workup of primary hyperparathyroidism (D). In about 85% of patients, imaging will localize the abnormal parathyroid gland, and a great majority will have a single parathyroid adenoma. If localizing scans are negative, yet the diagnosis of primary hyperparathyroidism is clearly established, surgery is still performed at which time intraoperative exploration of all four glands is performed (E).

Head and Neck

Vishad Nabili

Contents

Progressively Hoarse Voice

Kevin A. Peng, Irene A. Kim, and Vishad Nabili

Contents

C. de Virgilio, A. Grigorian (eds.), *Surgery*, https://doi.org/10.1007/978-3-032-09799-6_15

Case Study

A 62-year-old male presents with a 2-month history of a progressively hoarse voice. Initially, his voice was only slightly raspy, but over time, he has lost the ability to project it and can now only speak in a loud whisper. He endorses blood-tinged sputum with coughing, which has occurred approximately twice a week for the past month. His social history is remarkable for a 40-pack-year smoking history, and he continues to smoke 1 pack per day. On review of systems, he denies dyspnea, dysphagia, and odynophagia. On physical examination, his voice is breathy and raspy. His oral cavity and oropharynx are remarkable only for caries, and his neck is supple, without lymphadenopathy. Flexible laryngoscopy performed in the clinic reveals friable masses on both vocal cords, with a widely patent airway but with impaired mobility of the left vocal cord.

Diagnosis

What Is the Differential Diagnosis for Hoarseness? (▫ Table 15.1)

▫ **Table 15.1** Differential diagnosis of hoarseness

Diagnosis	History and physical
Viral laryngitis	Acute onset of fever, sore throat, cough, and/or other symptoms consistent with upper respiratory tract infection
Vocal cord paralysis	Breathy voice, most commonly idiopathic or iatrogenic (e.g., injury to the recurrent laryngeal nerve during thyroid or thoracic surgery)
Vocal cord nodules, polyps, cysts, or granulomas	Unilateral or bilateral lesions usually result from trauma to the vocal cord (voice abuse, endotracheal intubation)
Recurrent respiratory papillomatosis	Benign, occasionally aggressive growths caused by HPV
Spasmodic dysphonia, Parkinson's disease, or other neurological disorder	Vocal tremors or an intermittently breathy or strained voice
Laryngeal cancer	Subacute to chronic onset of dysphonia, possibly with cervical lymphadenopathy (signifying cancer metastasis to regional lymph nodes); smoking is the single greatest risk factor

HPV human papillomavirus

15

What Is the Most Likely Diagnosis in This Patient?

The patient's age, male gender, history of smoking, subacute onset, progression of symptoms, hemoptysis, and friable mass on the vocal cords are all concerning for malignancy (most likely squamous cell carcinoma of the larynx). The absence of cervical lymphadenopathy does not rule out the possibility of laryngeal cancer.

Watch Out

Many lesions that cause hoarseness concomitantly narrow the airway. Be on the lookout for airway compromise and remember the ABCs: airway first, followed by breathing, circulation.

History and Physical Examination

What Information Can the Nature of Hoarseness Provide?

Hoarseness, more strictly termed "dysphonia," can be qualified specifically. In order to phonate (produce a sound), the vocal cords must move and oppose at the midline (adduction). To breathe, the vocal cords must open (abduction). A *breathy* voice is caused by incomplete closure, as seen with unilateral vocal cord paralysis. *Aphonia*, the inability to create any vocal sound, is usually due to vocal cords that remain abducted during attempted phonation. This can be due to mucosal swelling or irregularities precluding any vibration from occurring along the vocal cord. A *strained* voice usually implies a narrowing at the level of the vocal cords, as with a laryngeal mass such as papillomatosis or carcinoma. A *tremulous* voice may indicate a neurological disorder, such as spasmodic dysphonia or Parkinson's disease.

At What Point Should Hoarseness Warrant Consultation with an Otolaryngologist?

The most common cause of hoarseness is viral laryngitis, a self-limited condition that usually resolves within 1–2 weeks. Any hoarseness persisting for longer than 2 weeks necessitates timely otolaryngologic referral.

What Are the Risk Factors for Laryngeal Carcinoma?

Tobacco use, in both smoked and chewed forms, is the single greatest risk factor for squamous cell carcinoma of the upper aerodigestive tract. Alcohol use multiplies the risk of cancer in the presence of tobacco use. Human papillomavirus (HPV), particularly HPV-16, is strongly associated with cancers of the oropharynx.

What Is the Significance of Bloody Sputum?

The vast majority of noncancerous causes of hoarseness are not associated with bloody sputum. Hemoptysis, or bloody oral secretions, is a red flag for malignancy in the upper aerodigestive tract.

What Is the Most Common Type of Laryngeal Cancer?

The most common type of cancer found in the larynx, as well as in the entire upper aerodigestive tract, is *squamous cell carcinoma*. The pathogenesis is closely linked to tobacco use in any form.

Watch Out

The most common site of malignant lesions of the larynx is the glottis. However, the most common oral cavity cancer is on the tongue.

Pathophysiology

What Is the Innervation of the Larynx? (Table 15.2)

Table 15.2 Innervation of the laryngeal muscles

Nerve	Branch	Sensory	Motor
Superior laryngeal nerve (external branch)	Vagus	None	Cricothyroid
Superior laryngeal nerve (internal branch)	Vagus	Supraglottis	None
Recurrent laryngeal nerve	Vagus	Glottis and subglottis	All intrinsic laryngeal muscles except cricothyroid

What Are the Potential Consequences of Unrecognized Squamous Cell Carcinoma of the Upper Aerodigestive Tract?

Squamous cell carcinoma of the larynx, if diagnosed early, portends a favorable prognosis. A laryngeal ulcer, particularly in a smoker, is likely squamous cell carcinoma. However, other mucosal sites of the head and neck carry a worse prognosis. If the diagnosis is made late in the course of the disease, the cancer may lead to eventual mortality.

Do Laryngeal Papillomas Cause Cancer?

Though possible, papillomas rarely give rise to laryngeal carcinoma. Laryngeal papilloma, also known as recurrent respiratory papillomatosis, is a condition caused by HPV 6 and 11. These subtypes are also most likely to cause genital warts. Infection is often from vertical transmission during pregnancy. The virus can lead to benign papillary tumors of the larynx, which present primarily with hoarseness. Adults tend to have more limited papillomas, while children develop multiple lesions.

Workup

What Examination Should Be Performed to Evaluate the Vocal Cords?

A laryngoscopy (Fig. 15.1) can look for structural abnormalities, such as masses, ulcers, or mucosal irregu-

15

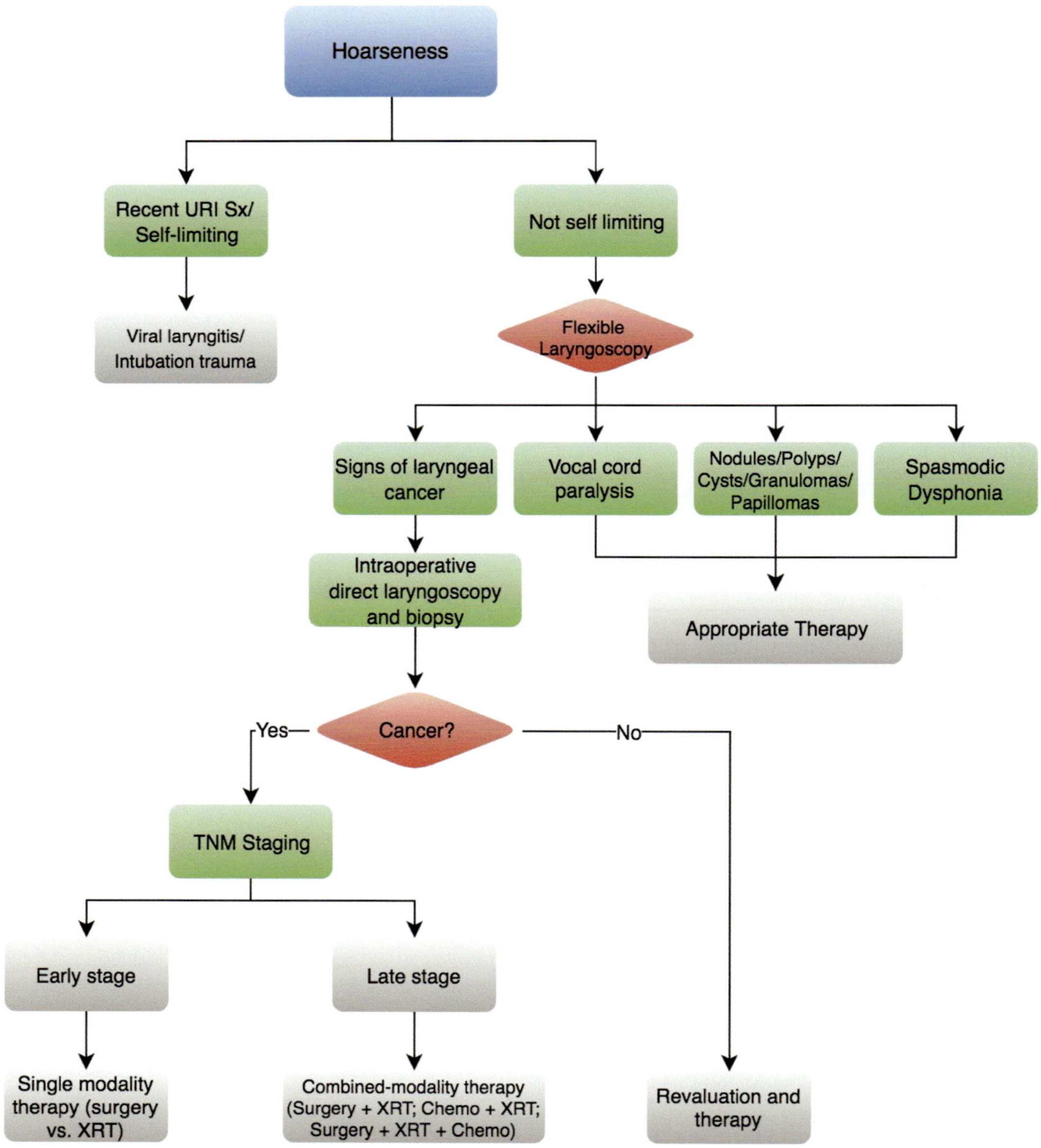

Fig. 15.1 Algorithm for diagnosis and management of hoarseness

larities. Functionally, the otolaryngologist will be able to assess the motion of the vocal cords, which are innervated by the recurrent laryngeal nerve.

If Laryngeal Cancer Is Suspected, What Additional Tests Are Warranted?

Persistent hoarseness should always be evaluated by laryngoscopy to ensure no delay in the diagnosis of possible cancer. A *chest X-ray* is also routinely performed to rule out a concurrent primary lung cancer or pulmonary metastases. This is important because a majority of laryngeal and lung cancers are attributed to smoking. In addition, the most common location for distant metastasis of head and neck squamous cell carcinoma is the lungs. CT of the neck can reveal metastases to cervical lymph nodes.

Management

What Treatments Are Available?

In early-stage laryngeal cancer, single-modality therapy—either surgery or radiation—is usually effective in eradicating the disease. In metastatic head and neck cancer, combined-modality therapy (surgery and radiation, chemotherapy and radiation, or a combination of all three) is often required to eradicate the disease.

What Variables Affect Prognosis for Laryngeal Cancer?

The TNM stage is the single most important prognostic indicator. The 5-year relative survival of stage I laryngeal cancer is 90%, while that of stage IV is approximately 45%.

Areas Where You Can Get in Trouble

Airway Compromise

The larynx is the narrowest segment of the human airway. An exophytic mass, such as a squamous cell carcinoma, can cause life-threatening airway obstruction. This may present in a chronic fashion, where a patient with known squamous cell carcinoma becomes increasingly short of breath, or it may present more acutely. In a patient with advanced laryngeal cancer, a tracheostomy may be necessary prior to initiating any treatment.

Summary of Essentials

History and Physical Examination

- Duration, progression, and quality of hoarseness
- Tobacco use, including smoking and chewing tobacco
- Alcohol use

Etiology/Pathophysiology

- Chronic inflammation and increased cellular turnover from toxic insults, such as tobacco smoke, lead to dysplasia and progression to invasive squamous cell carcinoma

Diagnosis

- Indirect laryngoscopy in the office, or direct laryngoscopy in the operating room setting, to visualize the larynx and to obtain biopsies
- Chest X-ray
- CT of the neck

Management

- Early stage
- Radiation
- Surgical resection
- Late stage
- Chemotherapy with radiation
- Surgery followed by radiation
- Tracheostomy may be necessary to secure the airway

Watch Out

- Hoarseness that persists longer than 2 weeks merits immediate referral to an otolaryngologist

Suggested Reading

Caudell JJ, Gillison ML, Maghami E, et al. NCCN Guidelines® Insights: Head and Neck Cancers, Version 1.2022. J Natl Compr Canc Netw. 2022;20(3):224–234. doi:https://doi.org/10.6004/jnccn.2022.0016

Forastiere AA, Goepfert H, Maor M, et al. Concurrent chemotherapy and radiotherapy for organ preservation in advanced laryngeal cancer. N Engl J Med. 2003;349(22):2091–8.

Hoffman HT, Porter K, Karnell LH, et al. Laryngeal cancer in the United States: changes in demographics, patterns of care, and survival. Laryngoscope. 2006;116(9 Pt 2 Suppl 111):1–13.

Lump on the Neck Increasing in Size

Jon Mallen-St. Clair, Aaron J. Feinstein, and Vishad Nabili

Contents

C. de Virgilio, A. Grigorian (eds.), *Surgery*, https://doi.org/10.1007/978-3-032-09799-6_16

Case Study

A 58-year-old man presents with a right-sided neck mass that has been increasing in size over the past 3 months. He denies fever, chills, or recent weight loss. He also denies sore throat, difficulty swallowing, changes in his voice, or difficulty breathing. Past medical history is significant for hypertension and gastroesophageal reflux disease (GERD). Social history is significant for 20 pack-years of smoking. He averages two alcoholic drinks every day. Physical exam of the oral cavity/oropharynx including close visualization of the tongue, tonsils, and floor of the mouth reveals no obvious lesions that are suspicious for malignancy. Examination of the neck reveals a 2 × 3-cm, firm, right-sided neck mass that is poorly mobile, nonerythematous, and not tender to palpation.

Diagnosis

What Is the Differential Diagnosis? (Apply the "KITTENS" Mnemonic) (Table 16.1)

Table 16.1 Differential diagnosis of clinical presentation

Condition	Comments
K—congenital	
Thyroglossal duct cyst	Midline mass, moves with tongue protrusion; may become infected; *most common* congenital neck anomaly
Branchial cleft cyst	Lateral to midline; at risk for infection
Dermoid cyst	Arises from entrapment of the epithelium during fetal midline closure
Laryngocele	Intermittent lateral neck swelling caused by herniation of a laryngeal diverticulum through the thyrohyoid membrane; may arise from chronic severe cough or sustained blowing into a musical instrument
Sebaceous cyst	Arises from obstruction of the sebaceous gland duct; may become infected
Lymphangioma	Lymphatic ducts that do not communicate with the internal jugular lymphatic system resulting in impaired drainage; also known as cystic hygroma
Thymic cyst	Only requires excision if causing compression of other structures; may occasionally be ectopic parathyroid tissue
I—infectious/inflammatory	
Lymphadenitis	Viral, bacterial, or fungal infection causing lymph node enlargement
Tuberculosis	Lymph nodes may be matted together and form draining sinus tract; also known as scrofula
Actinomycosis	Suppurative lymph nodes form sinuses with a bright-red color; pus contains sulfur granules
Deep neck abscess	Presents with fever, pain, stiffness, odynophagia, and purulent oral secretions; retropharyngeal infection may spread to the mediastinum
T—toxin	
Metals/drugs	Exposure to industrial fumes, nickel, cigarette smoke, and wood dust has been associated with head and neck cancers, which can metastasize to lymph nodes and present as a neck mass
T—trauma	
Hematoma	Contusion or vascular injury; may compromise airway, may require surgical exploration
Foreign body	Shrapnel or bullet
Aneurysm	Blunt or penetrating injury may cause pseudoaneurysm of the carotid artery
E—endocrine	
Thyroid hyperplasia	Graves' disease, goiter
Ectopic thyroid gland	May be found anywhere along the thyroglossal duct; beware of lateral ectopic thyroid tissue as this may be metastatic spread of malignancy
N—neoplastic	
Benign growths	Lipoma, neuroma, fibroma
Malignant growths	Thyroid carcinoma, lymphoma, salivary gland carcinoma, carotid body (paraganglioma)
Metastatic	Unknown primary, mucoepidermoid, adenoid cystic, lung, breast, kidney, GI
S—systemic	
Viral	Human immunodeficiency virus; increased susceptibility to infections
Kawasaki disease	Autoimmune disease associated with coronary artery abnormalities

Data from Stackler et al. (2014) and Eustermann (2005)

What Is the Most Likely Diagnosis for This Patient?

A neck mass in a patient over the age of 40 should be considered malignant until proven otherwise. The "rule of 80s" should be applied. A neck mass in an adult has an 80% chance of being neoplastic and 80% chance of being malignant. In contrast, >80% of pediatric neck masses are benign. Risk factors such as tobacco and alcohol use further increase the likelihood of head and neck cancer, particularly squamous cell carcinoma (SCC). A progressively enlarging, firm, painless neck mass without signs of infection (e.g., tenderness and erythema) or systemic symptoms (e.g., fever and weight loss) is suspicious for malignancy. The absence of B symptoms (fever, night sweats, and weight loss) and the unilateral nature of the mass argue against lymphoma. Infectious causes are less likely given the chronicity and lack of associated signs. The most likely diagnosis is a metastatic squamous cell carcinoma to a cervical lymph node from an unknown primary tumor. Further work-up is needed to confirm the diagnosis and identify the primary site.

What Risk Factors Are Associated with Head and Neck Cancer in General?

Alcohol and tobacco in combination confer a greater risk. Other risk factors include male gender, age > 40 years, poor dental hygiene, radiation exposure, and Black race.

What Risk Factors Are Associated with Specific Head and Neck Cancers? (Table 16.2)

Table 16.2 Risk factors for head and neck cancers

Risk factor	Type of cancer
HPV	Oropharyngeal cancer
EBV	Nasopharyngeal cancer, Burkitt's lymphoma
Chinese	Nasopharyngeal cancer
GERD	Laryngeal cancer
Plummer-Vinson syndrome[a]	Pharyngeal and upper esophageal cancer

HPV human papillomavirus; *EBV* Epstein-Barr virus; *GERD* gastroesophageal reflux disease

[a]Symptoms include glossitis, cervical dysphagia, iron deficiency anemia, and esophageal webs.

How Have the Demographics of Head and Neck Cancer Changed in the Last 10 Years?

Over the past decade, there has been a significant increase in oropharyngeal squamous cell carcinoma (SCC), particularly among White males aged 40 to 55. These patients often present with a neck mass and typically lack a history of significant tobacco or alcohol use. The rise in incidence is largely due to human papillomavirus (HPV)-associated SCC, which tends to occur in younger individuals with a history of multiple sexual partners. HPV-associated tumors differ from traditional alcohol- and tobacco-related SCC in their clinical behavior, with greater responsiveness to radiation therapy and improved overall prognosis.

What Premalignant Lesions Should Be Looked for on Physical Examination?

Look for leukoplakia (white patch or plaque) on the buccal mucosa or lower lip and for erythroplakia (red patch or lesion) on the floor of the mouth, tongue, or soft palate.

What Are Torus Palatinus and Mandibular Tori?

Torus palatinus and mandibular tori are benign bony outgrowths (exostoses) of the hard palate and mandible, respectively. They are often congenital or develop slowly and are typically asymptomatic. They are more common in adults and are usually found incidentally. No treatment is needed unless they interfere with speech, eating, or denture fitting.

What Symptoms Can Be Associated with Head and Neck Cancer, and What Are the Likely Sources? (Table 16.3)

Table 16.3 Symptoms of head and neck cancer

Symptom	Definition	Pathophysiology/possible malignant sources
Otalgia	Pain in the ear	Cranial nerves IX and X supply sensory innervation to both the tongue and floor of the mouth and also supply sensory innervation to the ear; pain can be referred to the ear from CN IX via Jacobson's nerve and CN X via Arnold's nerve; in addition, the lingual nerve (V3) supplies sensation to the tongue and floor of the mouth as well as the external auditory canal and tympanic membrane via the auriculotemporal nerve
Dysphagia	Difficulty in swallowing	Mass effect of tumor obstructing the path of food bolus (hypopharynx) versus interference with swallowing mechanism (common in the pharynx/tongue/hypopharynx)
Odynophagia	Pain with swallowing	Tumor-related inflammation can cause pain
Dysphonia	Impairment in producing voice sounds	Lesion on vocal cords blocking efficient phonation or vocal cord paralysis from neural involvement
Dyspnea	Difficulty breathing	Upper airway obstruction
Trismus	Limited opening of the jaw	Tumor invasion into pterygoid muscles
Stridor	High-pitched sound resulting from a narrowed or obstructed airway	Upper airway obstruction
Hemoptysis	Expectoration of blood-stained sputum	Ulceration of tumor into the blood vessel in the upper airway versus secondary pulmonary lesion

What Are the Key Aspects of the Head and Neck Exam in the Evaluation of a Solitary Neck Mass?

Although it is tempting to focus completely on examination of the neck, it is imperative that a full head and neck exam be performed. This should include careful inspection and palpation of the scalp, skin, parotids, ears, ear canals, nose, nasal cavity, oral cavity, and oropharynx. In particular, the base of the tongue and tonsillar fossa should be palpated for any evidence of firmness. Full characterization of the neck mass should be performed, with assessment of the size, location, mobility, consistency, fluctuance, overlying skin changes, and associated pain. A full cranial nerve exam should be performed to assess for deficits, which are often associated with advanced head and neck cancer.

What Is the Typical Presentation of Sialadenitis and What Is Its Most Common Cause?

Sialadenitis presents with painful swelling of the salivary gland, often triggered by eating, and may be associated with fever and purulent discharge from the duct. It is commonly caused by bacterial infection secondary to salivary stasis, which is frequently due to ductal obstruction from salivary stones (sialolithiasis). The submandibular gland is most often affected due to its thick mucus secretions and gravity-defying ductal anatomy.

Etiology

What Are Nonneoplastic Causes of Salivary Gland Enlargement?

Sialadenosis is a noninflammatory, nonneoplastic enlargement of the salivary glands, most often affecting the parotids. It is associated with chronic alcohol use, eating disorders (e.g., bulimia), malnutrition, diabetes, and liver disease. The enlargement is typically bilateral, painless, and without signs of infection.

What Is the Differential Diagnosis for Salivary Glands Tumors? What Is Their Malignant Potential?

The salivary glands include the parotid, submandibular, sublingual, and minor salivary glands. Masses in large salivary glands are more likely to be benign, while masses in smaller salivary glands are more likely to be malignant. However, the parotid glands (the largest salivary glands) are the most frequent site of malignant tumor. Refer to ◘ Table 16.4 for the common salivary gland tumors. Risk factors for malignant transformation include prior radiation exposure and clinical signs of neural invasion such as facial weakness (CN VII) or facial numbness (CN V). These findings warrant urgent evaluation for malignancy.

◘ **Table 16.4** Differential diagnosis for salivary glands tumors

Tumor	Comment
Pleomorphic adenomas (mixed tumor)	Most common benign salivary gland tumor
Papillary cystadenoma (Warthin's tumor)	Second most common benign salivary gland tumor; smokers, can be bilateral
Mucoepidermoid carcinoma	Most common malignant salivary gland tumor
Adenoid cystic carcinoma	Second most common malignant salivary gland tumor

What Is Virchow's Node? Why Is It Concerning?

Virchow's node is an enlarged left supraclavicular node. It occurs on the left as this is where the cisterna chyli (dilated lymph sac at the end of the thoracic duct) empties into the subclavian vein. Virchow's node is suggestive of metastatic lung or gastrointestinal malignancy.

What Are the Most Common Sites of Head and Neck Cancer?

The oral cavity (tongue most common), larynx, and pharynx represent 44%, 31%, and 25% of head and neck cancers, respectively.

What Is Meant by the Term "Primary Tumor"? What Is Meant by "Unknown Primary"?

A primary tumor refers to the original anatomic site of a tumor growth. An unknown primary tumor refers to a situation where a metastatic tumor such as a cancerous lymph node is discovered and the site of the original cancer is not evident.

What "Primary Tumors" Arise in the Neck?

Primary tumors of the neck include lymphoma, thyroid neoplasms, salivary neoplasms, schwannomas, paragangliomas, and lipomas, among others.

What Does a Newly Discovered Malignant Neck Mass Most Likely Represent?

Malignant neck masses represent spread of cancer via the lymphatic system (metastatic lymph node) until proven otherwise. In these cases, the primary site of cancer is unknown and thus represents an "unknown primary." The primary site is most frequently in the upper aerodigestive tract and must be found in order to appropriately treat the cancer. The unknown primary can also more rarely represent a distant metastasis from breast, lung, or renal cancer. There is a less than a 15% chance that a malignancy that is found in the neck represents a primary neck tumor.

What Types of Abscess Are in the Differential of a Neck Mass? (Table 16.5)

Table 16.5 Types of neck abscesses

Type of abscess	History and physical	Treatment
Peritonsillar	Older children (>10 years), fever, odynophagia, ear pain, muffled voice, trismus, uvula deviation; does not typically cause airway obstruction	Needle aspiration and drain through the tonsillar bed
Retropharyngeal	Younger children (<10 years), fever, odynophagia, drooling, can lead to airway obstruction	Calm the patient, intubate, drain through the posterior pharyngeal wall
Parapharyngeal	All age groups, associated with dental infections and tonsillitis	Drain through the lateral neck (to avoid damaging the carotid artery)

Watch Out

Fever, ear pain, muffled voice, and deviation of the uvula are highly suggestive of a peritonsillar abscess. This should be treated with needle aspiration and antibiotics.

Etiology/Pathophysiology

What Is the Pathophysiology of Head and Neck Cancer?

Most head and neck cancers arise from the mucosa of the upper aerodigestive tract after chronic exposure to carcinogens such as tobacco and alcohol. These exposures cause progressive genetic mutations that lead to malignant transformation. In some cases, histologically abnormal but grossly normal-appearing mucosa may be present adjacent to tumors, a phenomenon known as field cancerization. This may explain the tendency for multifocal tumors or local recurrence.

Work-Up

Is Observation an Acceptable Strategy for a Newly Discovered, Isolated, and Enlarged Cervical Lymph Node?

Observation is only appropriate for patients who do not present with any red-flag symptoms (e.g., dysphagia, odynophagia, dysphonia, hoarseness, and weight loss) and if the lymph node has been present for less than 2 weeks. Patients should be reexamined in 2 weeks. If the node disappears, it most likely was inflammatory in nature.

In Addition to the Physical Exam Mentioned in the Vignette, What Procedure Is Performed in the Office by the Head

and Neck Surgeon When a Metastatic Neck Lymph Node Is Suspected?

Flexible nasopharyngoscopy is used to evaluate the nasal cavities, nasopharynx, oropharynx, hypopharynx, and glottis to look for a site of primary tumor. If a suspicious lesion is identified, a biopsy is obtained to confirm the diagnosis.

What Laboratory Tests Should Be Obtained?

Complete blood count (CBC), coagulation profile, liver enzymes, chemistry panel with renal function, and thyroid-stimulating hormone level.

What Initial Imaging Modality Is the Diagnostic Test of Choice to Search for the Primary Tumor?

CT scan of the head and neck with contrast is the initial preferred imaging modality to look for the primary tumor in the presence of a solitary neck mass that is concerning for metastatic malignancy. A chest X-ray is also recommended. MRI is an acceptable alternative. Ultrasound would not be useful in this setting; however, it is particularly useful in the diagnosis of congenital neck masses.

What Is the Best Way to Obtain a Tissue Sample to Determine If the Neck Mass Is a Metastatic Lymph Node?

16

Fine-needle aspiration (FNA) is the procedure of choice for a solitary neck mass that is suspicious for being a metastatic lymph node. FNA is highly sensitive and specific and is diagnostic in the majority of cases with minimal morbidity. FNA is >95% sensitive and specific when diagnostic material is obtained. FNA can yield fluid for cytology to assess for malignancy. In addition, it can facilitate gram stain, acid fast stain, and cultures. A nondiagnostic FNA should often be repeated, with or without ultrasound guidance prior to proceeding to an open biopsy.

Watch Out

Lymphoma is difficult to diagnose via FNA. If lymphoma is suspected, core needle biopsy or open biopsy should be performed.

Once FNA Confirms that the Neck Mass Is a Metastasis, What Is the Next Step in Determining the Location of the Primary Tumor?

Panendoscopy (triple endoscopy) is performed in the OR under general anesthesia. This involves a complete endoscopic evaluation of the upper aerodigestive tract, including laryngoscopy, esophagoscopy, and bronchoscopy. This is performed after other less invasive imaging modalities if no primary site can be identified. Panendoscopy allows for biopsy of the upper aerodigestive tract, including the nasopharynx, tonsils, tongue base, valleculae, postcricoid region, and pyriform sinuses.

What Is the Role of an Open Neck Biopsy in the Evaluation of Solitary Neck Mass?

Open neck biopsies are only considered after a complete work-up has been performed with appropriate history and physical examination, imaging studies (CT vs. MRI), FNA (at least once), and panendoscopy (▫ Fig. 16.1). If the neck biopsy is positive for SCC on frozen section performed at the time of the biopsy, then it is imperative to proceed with a neck dissection. The reason is that open neck biopsies have been shown to be associated with increased morbidity and increased rates of local and distant recurrences, possibly from seeding tumor cells at the time of biopsy (although this dogma

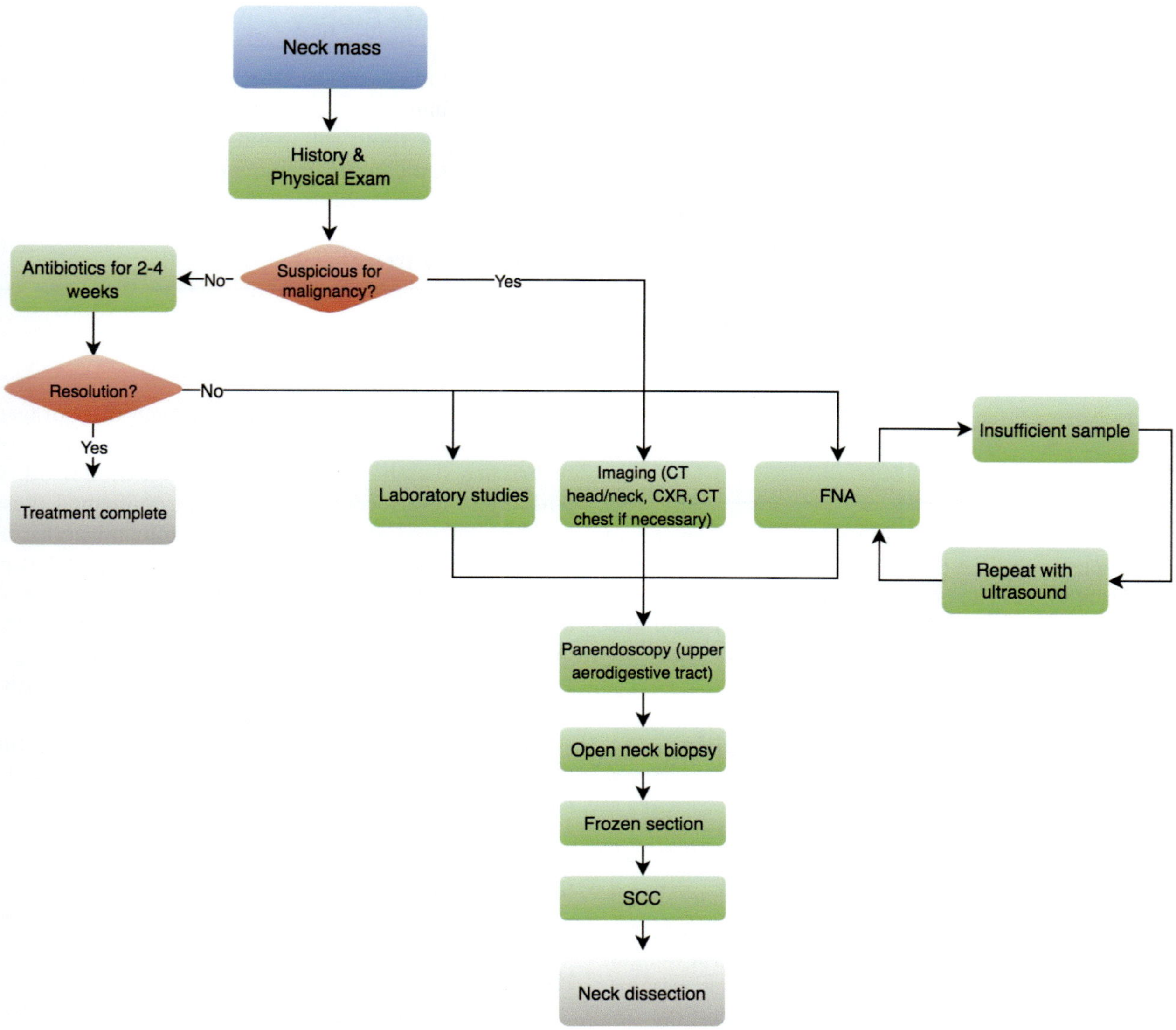

Fig. 16.1 Work-up of neck mass suspicious for malignancy: If at any point in the work-up the primary tumor is identified, treatment should be tailored to the specific site and type of the tumor. If at the end of the diagnostic work-up no primary tumor has been identified, all sites in the head and neck should be treated

has been questioned in recent studies as discussed in Areas of Controversy section).

What Laboratory Studies Can Be Utilized to Assess for Infectious and Inflammatory Causes of Neck Masses?

If the history and physical examination suggest an infectious etiology, laboratory tests are obtained that include CBC, purified protein derivative, rapid plasma reagin, toxoplasma, HIV, monospot, EBV, and *Bartonella* antibody.

Management

The management of head and neck cancer is dependent on the subsite and the extent of neck disease at the time of presentation. The management of head and neck malignancy is outside the scope of what medical students should be required to know for exams.

Areas Where You Can Get into Trouble

Missing a Cancer Diagnosis

Malignancy should be suspected for any unilateral neck mass that is progressively enlarging and in patients over 40 years. Other danger signs include unilateral otalgia, dysphagia, odynophagia, dysphonia, dyspnea, trismus, stridor, and hemoptysis, which are concerning for advanced head and neck cancer. Pain can be associated with neural spread.

Not Recognizing Potentially Life-Threatening Signs in Advanced Stages of Cancer

Any sign of dyspnea or stridorous breathing should prompt an immediate evaluation of the airway by an otolaryngologist. Similarly, any bleeding from the mouth or hemoptysis should prompt an evaluation of the airway, as erosion into large vessels in the neck can result in airway compromise and exsanguinating hemorrhage. The patient should also be evaluated for signs that would indicate difficulty obtaining an oropharyngeal airway including trismus and obstructing lesions in the oropharynx.

Inappropriate Biopsy

It is difficult to control bleeding in the oropharynx, so biopsies in clinic should be performed with caution. Open biopsy without ruling out tuberculosis (scrofula) can also lead to chronic draining fistulas to the skin.

Areas of Controversy

The Role of Open Biopsy

Open neck biopsy has traditionally been discouraged due to earlier studies suggesting increased risk of recurrence, distant metastasis, and surgical morbidity. Although more recent data have not confirmed these findings, current guidelines still recommend performing at least one FNA before open neck biopsy. Given the high sensitivity and specificity and minimal morbidity of FNA and the possible risks of open neck biopsy, it is also reasonable to perform an image-guided repeat FNA if the first FNA is nondiagnostic. If an open biopsy is truly necessary for diagnosis, completion of neck dissection in the event of the biopsy being positive for SCC is recommended to avoid morbidity.

Summary of Essentials

History and Physical

- A solitary neck mass in an adult over 40 is malignant until proven otherwise.
- Red flags for malignancy in head and neck include otalgia, dysphagia, odynophagia, dysphonia, dyspnea, trismus, stridor, and hemoptysis.
- Palpate the base of the tongue and the tonsillar fossa for firmness.
- Always perform a complete cranial nerve exam.

Etiology/Pathophysiology

- Risk factors for head and neck cancer include smoking, alcohol, age over 40 years, HPV, infection, EBV infection, GERD, Chinese ethnicity, and Plummer-Vinson syndrome.
- Primary tumors of the neck include lymphoma, thyroid carcinoma, salivary gland neoplasms, schwannoma, paragangliomas, and lipomas.

- Beware of deep neck abscesses: peritonsillar, retropharyngeal, and parapharyngeal.
- Consider sialadenosis, sialadenitis, and benign bony exostoses in the differential.

Diagnosis

- Start with physical exam and flexible nasopharyngoscopy.
- FNA biopsy and CT with contrast should be performed after flexible laryngoscopy.
- Further imaging such as chest CT scan, PET scan, or chest X-ray may be performed for further staging.
- If indicated, panendoscopy will be performed to identify the site of primary tumor.

Watch Out

- Missing diagnosis or failing to expedite work-up.
- Missing danger signals of advanced head and neck cancer.
- Referring for open biopsy without full work-up.

Suggested Reading

Amedee RG, Dhurandhar NR. Fine-needle aspiration biopsy. Laryngoscope. 2001;111(9):1551–7.

Ang KK, Harris J, Wheeler R, Weber R, et al. Human papillomavirus and survival of patients with oropharyngeal cancer. N Engl J Med. 2010;363:24–35.

Blot WJ, McLaughlin JK, Winn DM, et al. Smoking and drinking in relation to oral and pharyngeal cancer. Cancer Res. 1988;48:3282.

Califano J, van der Riet P, Westra W, et al. Genetic progression model for head and neck cancer: implications for field cancerization. Cancer Res. 1996;56:2488.

Chen A, Otto KJ. Differential diagnosis of neck masses. In: Flint P, Haughey B, Lund V, Niparko J, editors. Cummings otolaryngology—head and neck surgery. 5th ed. Philadelphia: Mosby Elsevier; 2010. p. 1636–42.

Ellis ER, Mendenhall WM, Rao PV, et al. Incisional or excisional neck node biopsy before definitive radiotherapy, alone or followed by neck dissection. Head Neck. 1991;13:177–83.

Eustermann VD. Tumors of the oral cavity and pharynx. In: Jafek BW, Murrow BW, editors. ENT secrets. 3rd ed. Philadelphia: Mosby Elsevier; 2005. p. 221–2.

Greven KM, Keyes JW Jr, Williams DW 3rd, McGuirt WF, Joyce WT 3rd. Occult primary tumors of the head and neck: lack of benefit from positron emission tomography imaging with 2-[F-18]fluoro-2-deoxy-D-glucose. Cancer. 1999;86(1):114–8.

Jungehulsing M, Scheidhauer K, Damm M, et al. 2[F]-fluoro-2-deoxy-D-glucose positron emission tomography is a sensitive tool for the detection of occult primary cancer (carcinoma of unknown primary syndrome) with head and neck lymph node manifestation. Otolaryngol Head Neck Surg. 2000;123(3):294–301.

Liu ES, Bernstein JM, Sculerati N, Wu HC. Fine needle aspiration biopsy of pediatric head and neck masses. Int J Pediatr Otorhinolaryngol. 2001;60(2):135–40.

McGuirt WF, McCabe BF, et al. Significance of node biopsy before definitive treatment of cervical metastatic carcinoma. Laryngoscope. 1978;88:594–7.

Mendenhall WM, et al. Squamous cell carcinoma metastatic to the neck from an unknown head and neck primary site. Am J Otolaryngol. 2000;22(4):261–7.

Miller FR, Hussey D, Beeram M, Eng T, McGuff HS, Otto RA. Positron emission tomography in the management of unknown primary head and neck carcinoma. Arch Otolaryngol Head Neck Surg. 2005;131(7):626–9.

Park R, Nabili V, Yoo GH, Golub JS, Pasha R. Head and neck cancer. In: Pasha R, Golub JS, editors. Otolaryngology-head and neck surgery: clinical reference guide. 4th ed. San Diego: Plural Publishing; 2014. p. 230–6.

Ridge, et al. Head and neck cancer. In: Cancer management. 13th ed. Goodhouse, New York, 2006.

Schwarz R, Chan NH, MacFarlane JK. Fine needle aspiration cytology in the evaluation of head and neck masses. Am J Surg. 1990;159(5):482–5.

Spitz MR. Epidemiology and risk factors for head and neck cancer. Semin Oncol. 1994;21:281.

Stackler RJ, Shibuya TY, Golub JS, Pasha R. General otolaryngology. In: Pasha R, Golub JS, editors. Otolaryngology-head and neck surgery: clinical reference guide. 4th ed. San Diego: Plural Publishing; 2014. p. 275–8.

Zanation AM, Sutton DK, Couch ME, Weissler MC, Shockley WW, Shores CG. Use, accuracy, and implications for patient management of [18F]-2-fluorodeoxyglucose-positron emission/computerized tomography for head and neck tumors. Laryngoscope. 2005;115(7):1186–90.

Aural Fullness, Hearing Loss, and Tinnitus

Andrew M. Vahabzadeh-Hagh, Edward C. Kuan, and Vishad Nabili

Contents

C. de Virgilio, A. Grigorian (eds.), *Surgery*, https://doi.org/10.1007/978-3-032-09799-6_17

Case Study

A 5-year-old boy is brought to the doctor by his mother because she is concerned that he may be experiencing hearing loss. Over the past several weeks, he has been turning the volume of his favorite television program louder and has been sitting closer to the television set. He has reached all his developmental milestones and is up to date with his immunizations. When asked, the child states that he feels that his ears are always "plugged up." His medical history includes recurrent episodes of acute otitis media. He is currently afebrile. On exam, his nasopharynx is clear, and he has no cervical lymphadenopathy. On otoscopic examination, his left tympanic membrane (TM) is immobile with an air-fluid level behind it and partial dependent opacification. It does not appear to be erythematous. A vibrating tuning fork placed in the middle of his forehead is appreciated as louder on the left side when compared to the right. The same tuning fork, when placed on the left mastoid bone, is appreciated as louder in comparison to when it is placed near the left external auditory meatus.

Diagnosis

What Is the Differential Diagnosis for Hearing Loss in a Child? (Table 17.1)

Watch Out

Cholesteatoma is a misnomer in that it does not contain fat or cholesterol but instead is secondary to desquamated keratinized epithelium. It can be very locally destructive but is not a tumor as its name suggests.

Table 17.1 Differential diagnosis of hearing loss in a child

Diagnosis	History and physical
Acute otitis media (AOM)	Otalgia, fever, bulging, and erythematous tympanic membrane (TM) with decreased mobility, poor light reflex; duration <3 weeks
Otitis media with effusion (OME)	Middle ear effusion without signs of acute infection; commonly follows an episode of AOM but may develop in isolation; children with OME may present with parental concerns about hearing, language development, behavior, or school performance; immobile, dull TM with air-fluid levels
Chronic otitis media (COM)	Recurrent or chronic ear infections that result in a perforation of the TM +/– otorrhea; higher incidence in children with cleft palate and Down's syndrome
Cholesteatoma	Often preceded by Eustachian tube dysfunction and COM, an expansile, often cystic, collection of keratinized, desquamated epithelium in the middle ear
Labyrinthitis	Often preceded by a viral infection, the acute onset of vertigo, gait instability, nausea, vomiting, and hearing loss; physical exam demonstrates nystagmus
Otitis externa or swimmer's ear	Recent contact with water; presents with a tender, swollen pinna (especially the tragus) and erythematous ear canal with possible malodorous discharge
Congenital	Hearing loss present at birth that may be hereditary or acquired; intrauterine (TORCH) infections
Miscellaneous	Cerumen impaction, foreign body, trauma

TORCH toxoplasmosis, other (syphilis, varicella-zoster, parvovirus B19), rubella, cytomegalovirus, and herpes infections and is seen most commonly with untreated otitis media (D). Patients will present with very tender ear canals, and otoscopy shows large red vesicles on the tympanic membrane.

12. Answer C
Croup, also known as *laryngotracheobronchitis*, is caused by the parainfluenza virus and primarily affects young children. The cough associated with this condition is described as a low-pitched seal-like bark. The diagnosis can be confirmed by looking for the classic "steeple sign" on posteroanterior X-ray of the neck, which is indicative of subglottic narrowing. Patients are at risk of airway obstruction and will require intubation if they appear to be in respiratory distress. Management includes steroids and aerosolized racemic epinephrine. Respiratory distress syndrome of the newborn is caused by surfactant deficiency (A). It occurs within 2 days of birth and presents with cyanosis, nasal flaring, crackles, and expiratory grunting. Epiglottitis is a rapidly progressive infection of the epiglottis, most commonly due to *Haemophilus influenzae type B* (B). Patients with epiglottitis may require intubation or even tracheostomy due to airway compromise from the swollen epiglottis. Bronchiolitis is characterized by a viral infection of the bronchioles and occurs most commonly in patients less than 2 years old (D). Laryngomalacia is a congenital abnormality of the laryngeal cartilage and can result in collapse of the supraglottic structures in newborns, leading to airway obstruction (E). Infants with laryngomalacia should be fed upright and remain in this position for at least 30 min after each feed.

13. Answer E
The larynx is the most common site for foreign body aspiration in children younger than one, while the trachea and right main stem bronchus are the most common sites in older children (A, C–D). The left main stem bronchus is a less frequent site for foreign body aspiration owing to its acute angle as it enters the lung versus an obtuse angle in the right (B). Patients with foreign body aspiration may have wheezing, but using a bronchodilator increases the risk of further pushing the foreign body down the airway. Order a chest X-ray if there is a suspicion for a foreign body obstruction. Bronchoscopy is recommended for definitive diagnosis. Extracting the foreign body requires a *rigid* bronchoscopy.

14. Answer C
Mastoiditis usually occurs days to weeks after an episode of acute otitis media. Patients present with fevers and complaints of a red, swollen, and tender area behind the ear (mastoid process). Physical exam may reveal a displaced ear on the affected side. The diagnosis can be confirmed with a CT scan of the mastoid process and is recommended for patients suspected of having mastoiditis. Patients with CT-confirmed acute surgical mastoiditis are candidates for mastoidectomy with insertion of a tympanostomy tube (E). Observation is not an appropriate management for patients suspected to have mastoiditis (A). Oral corticosteroids are not considered part of the management of acute mastoiditis (B). Augmentin would be an appropriate choice for patients with acute otitis media suspected of having a resistant strain (D).

15. Answer D
This patient most likely has torus palatinus, a bony benign mass located on the hard palate of the mouth. The cause is unknown. It occurs more frequently in women and those of Asian descent. There is no associated malignant transformation. Biopsy is not warranted, and patients only need reassurance (C). Operative management with surgical removal would be indicated only for symptomatic patients (e.g., interference with denture placements, pain, trouble swallowing) (A). There is no medical management

available for torus palatinus (B). Nasopharyngeal carcinoma, a rare tumor arising from the epithelium of the nasopharynx, occurs more frequently in patients of Asian descent and those infected with EBV (E). Early spread to cervical lymph nodes is common in patients with nasopharyngeal carcinoma, and so these patients often present with cervical adenopathy.

16. Answer B
This patient's presentation is concerning for mucormycosis, most commonly caused by *Rhizopus* or *Mucor* fungi. Patients with poorly controlled diabetes and/or neutropenia are the most common groups affected with mucormycosis. They most often present with local invasion of the fungi into the facial sinuses and eventually the brain (e.g., sudden onset or worsening of headache), as in this patient. Black eschar on the nose and discharge from the nares are characteristics of *mucormycosis*. Management consists of immediate antifungal therapy with liposomal amphotericin B and wide surgical debridement. Antifungal therapy alone would be inappropriate, as well as antibiotics (A, C–D). Hyperbaric oxygen is currently being investigated as an adjunctive therapy for select patients with mucormycosis (E). Mortality for mucormycosis ranges from 50 to 75%.

17. Answer D
The most appropriate recommendation for a young patient presenting with a newly discovered, isolated, and enlarged cervical node is observation with follow-up and reexamination in 3 weeks. If the node disappears, it most likely was inflammatory in nature. However, if this patient presented with any red-flag symptoms (e.g., dysphagia, odynophagia, dysphonia, hoarseness, and weight loss), additional workup would be required to rule out malignancy. FNA is indicated for neck masses that are persistent, enlarging, or suspicious for malignancy (A). CT scan with contrast is the initial preferred imaging modality for a solitary neck mass that is concerning for malignancy (following a careful head and neck examination) (B–C). Panendoscopy or triple endoscopy is performed in the operating room in the setting of a metastatic neck lymph node (when the primary is occult) (E).

Hepatopancreaticobiliary

Matthew Y. C. Lin

Contents

Postprandial Right Upper Quadrant Pain

Manan P. Shah, Matthew Y. C. Lin, and Christian de Virgilio

Contents

C. de Virgilio, A. Grigorian (eds.), *Surgery*, https://doi.org/10.1007/978-3-032-09799-6_18

Case Study

A 40-year-old, gravida six and para six, moderately obese Hispanic female presents to the emergency department with a one-day history of constant epigastric and right upper quadrant (RUQ) pain. She describes the severity of the pain as a 7 out of 10. The pain began after eating fried pork. She reports that the pain also seems to radiate to the right side of her back near her scapula. She feels nauseated and has vomited twice. She has had similar pain, but of lesser severity and duration, several times over the past year, usually after eating fatty, spicy foods. On physical examination, her temperature is 38 °C, heart rate is 110/min, and her blood pressure is 120/80 mmHg. She has marked tenderness to palpation in the RUQ of her abdomen. After being instructed to take a breath, deep palpation of her RUQ causes her to abruptly cease inspiration due to pain. The remainder of the abdominal examination is benign. Laboratory studies are remarkable for leukocytosis of $14 \times 10^3/\mu L$ (normal $4.1–10.9 \times 10^3/\mu L$), total bilirubin 1.0 mg/dL (0.1–1.2 mg/dl), alkaline phosphatase 70 u/L (33–131 u/L), amylase 60 u/l (30–110 u/L), and lipase 30 u/L (7–60 u/L).

Diagnosis

What Is the Differential Diagnosis? (Table 18.1)

Table 18.1 Differential diagnosis of clinical presentation

Diagnosis	History and physical
Symptomatic cholelithiasis	Postprandial RUQ pain radiating to the back; typically resolves within a few hours; common in obese, multigravida females
Acute cholecystitis	Persistent RUQ pain >4–6 hours, radiating to the back or scapula; fever, tachycardia, positive Murphy's sign
Choledocholithiasis	RUQ pain with jaundice but no systemic inflammatory signs (no fever or leukocytosis)
Sphincter of Oddi dysfunction	Episodic RUQ pain aggravated by opioids
Acute cholangitis	Persistent RUQ pain with fever and jaundice (*Charcot's triad*)
Acute pancreatitis	Severe epigastric pain radiating straight through to back; most often related to gallstones followed by alcohol use
Acute gastritis	NSAID use, steroid use, gnawing epigastric pain
Peptic ulcer disease	Intermittent burning epigastric pain that improves with meals (duodenal) or worsens with meals (gastric); associated with *H. pylori*, NSAIDs, or steroids
Malignancy	Gallbladder (*porcelain gallbladder*), pancreatic (*Courvoisier sign*), bile duct; chronic pain, weight loss, fatigue; +/– painless jaundice, pale stools, dark urine, pruritus
Fitz-Hugh-Curtis syndrome	RUQ pain; history of recent pelvic inflammatory disease (either *Chlamydia trachomatis* or *Neisseria gonorrhoeae*), fever, "violin string" adhesions between liver and diaphragm
Acute hepatitis	Hepatitis A (recent foreign travel, IVDU, raw shellfish, fecal-oral)
Hepatic abscess	RUQ pain, high fever, hepatomegaly; may be bacterial or amoebic in origin
Myocardial infarction	Epigastric pain (referred pain), diabetes, cardiovascular disease, and hypercholesterolemia
Acute pyelonephritis	Costovertebral angle tenderness, dysuria, hematuria

NSAID nonsteroidal anti-inflammatory drug, *IVDU* intravenous drug use

What Is the Most Likely Diagnosis?

With her history of severe, persistent abdominal pain following ingestion of fatty foods, nausea and vomiting, and associated RUQ tenderness to palpation, the etiology is most likely of biliary origin. The patient's prior history is consistent with symptomatic cholelithiasis. With a positive Murphy's sign, fever, tachycardia, and elevated white blood cell (WBC) count, the most likely diagnosis is acute cholecystitis. With normal total bilirubin and alkaline phosphatase, choledocholithiasis and acute cholangitis are less likely. Similarly, a normal amylase and lipase rule out gallstone pancreatitis.

History and Physical

Why Is the Term Biliary Colic a Misnomer? What Is a Better Term?

Colicky pain typically waxes and wanes, with periods of intense pain (such as from a ureter intermittently contracting in the presence of a renal stone) followed by relief. The pain from gallstones is constant, may last from minutes to hours, and then dissipates. A more correct term is symptomatic cholelithiasis.

Why Is It Important to Distinguish Between Symptomatic Cholelithiasis and Acute Cholecystitis?

Symptomatic cholelithiasis is usually managed as an outpatient, with eventual elective laparoscopic cholecystectomy. Acute cholecystitis requires hospital admission, IV antibiotics, and urgent cholecystectomy.

Pathophysiology

What Is the Significance of the Patient's Inspiration Stopping with RUQ Palpation?

This physical examination finding is called *Murphy's sign* and is thought to be specific to acute cholecystitis. It represents focal peritonitis of the anterior abdominal wall parietal peritoneum due to inflammation of the adjacent gallbladder. When the patient inspires, the diaphragm and therefore the gallbladder move caudad (inferiorly). Palpating deep in the RUQ causes the gallbladder to come into contact with the anterior abdominal wall, further irritating the inflamed parietal peritoneum and causing cessation of inspiration due to the sudden increase in pain.

What Is the Significance of Abdominal Pain After Eating Fatty Foods?

It suggests a biliary origin of the pain. Fatty food ingestion triggers the release of cholecystokinin (CCK), which leads to contraction of the gallbladder. Gallstones may obstruct the cystic duct so that the gallbladder is unable to empty bile as it attempts to contract. The ensuing distention of the gallbladder stretches the visceral peritoneum that surrounds it, leading to RUQ and/or epigastric pain that is vague and mild to moderate in severity (symptomatic cholelithiasis).

What Is the Significance of RUQ Pain Combined with Scapular Pain?

The scapula and the soft tissue surrounding the gallbladder receive sensory innervation from the same spinal cord levels. The scapula is innervated by the supraclavicular nerves, and the soft tissue surrounding the gallbladder is innervated by the phrenic nerve. Since the same spinothalamic pathways (pain and temperature) from both nerves travel to the same cervical cord levels, gallbladder distention/inflammation leads to referred scapular pain.

What Is the Difference Between Visceral and Somatic Pain?

Visceral pain tends to occur first. It is caused by stretching of the peritoneum surrounding an organ (or ischemia). It tends to be vague and less localizable. Somatic pain occurs when the inflammation extends to the adjacent peritoneum lining the abdominal wall. It is well localized and typically severe. Patients can often point to where it hurts, and it is elicited as guarding and rebound on physical examination.

How Does One Clinically Distinguish Between Symptomatic Cholelithiasis and Acute Cholecystitis? (Table 18.2)

Table 18.2 Differentiation between symptomatic cholelithiasis and acute cholecystitis

	Symptomatic cholelithiasis	Acute cholecystitis
History	RUQ pain usually resolves within minutes to 3–4 hours	Unremitting RUQ pain >6 hours, often with nausea/vomiting
Physical exam	Mild RUQ tenderness to palpation	Positive Murphy's sign
Vital signs	Normal	Fever, tachycardia
Laboratory values	Normal white blood cell count	Elevated white blood cell count with left shift
Ultrasound findings	Gallstones	Gallstones, gallbladder wall thickening >4 mm, pericholecystic fluid, sonographic Murphy's sign

What Is the Clinical Significance of the Patient's Low-Grade Fever, Tachycardia, and Leukocytosis?

The presence of a systemic inflammatory response, such as fever, tachycardia, and leukocytosis, suggests a more severe biliary disease such as acute cholecystitis, pancreatitis, or acute cholangitis. Symptomatic cholelithiasis (biliary colic) does not typically present with a systemic response.

What Is Chronic Cholecystitis?

Recurrent bouts of symptomatic cholelithiasis often lead to chronic inflammation of the gallbladder with fibrotic changes seen on histologic examination. As such, biliary colic, symptomatic cholelithiasis, and chronic cholecystitis are interchangeable terms.

What Exactly Causes Acute Cholecystitis?

Acute cholecystitis is caused by sustained obstruction (impaction) of the cystic duct, most often by a gallstone. This obstruction leads to inflammation and edema of the gallbladder wall and then eventually bacterial overgrowth and invasion of the gallbladder wall. This may lead to ischemia and necrosis (gangrenous cholecystitis), and rarely gallbladder perforation.

What Is Hydrops of the Gallbladder?

In some patients, chronic obstruction of the cystic duct does not lead to acute cholecystitis. In this setting, the gallbladder mucosa continues to secrete mucus, and the bile in the gallbladder eventually gets reabsorbed, leaving a glycoprotein-rich white fluid, sometimes called "white bile."

What Are the Typical Pathogens in Bile?

The most common organisms found in biliary cultures from patients with acute cholecystitis are, in order, *Escherichia coli*, *Klebsiella*, *Bacteroides fragilis*, *Enterobacter*, *Enterococcus*, and *Pseudomonas* species.

What Are the Components of Bile?

The three main components of bile are bile salts, cholesterol, and lecithin (a phospholipid). Bile also contains water, electrolytes, proteins, and bile pigments.

What Are the Two Main Types of Gallstones?

The two main types of gallstones are cholesterol (70–80% of gallstones in the USA) and pigmented.

What Are the Main Risk Factors for Developing Cholesterol Gallstones?

Cholesterol gallstones form in the setting of lithogenic bile, which is characterized by supersaturation of cholesterol and impaired gallbladder motility. Estrogen increases biliary cholesterol secretion and reduces gallbladder contractility, making females, pregnant patients, and those on oral contraceptives more susceptible. Obesity, hyperlipidemia, and high-fat diets contribute to increased cholesterol in bile, while Crohn's disease and terminal ileal resection reduce bile salt reabsorption, impairing cholesterol solubilization. Conditions that hinder gallbladder emptying, such as rapid weight loss after bariatric surgery, vagotomy, somatostatin therapy, or total parenteral nutrition, promote biliary stasis and sludge formation. Additionally, certain populations, including Hispanics and Pima Indians, have a genetic predisposition to gallstone disease.

How Do Cholesterol Gallstones Form?

Cholesterol gallstones form when the concentration of cholesterol in the bile exceeds its solubility, which causes precipitation of cholesterol crystals. The solubility of cholesterol is dependent on the concentration of cholesterol, bile salts, and lecithin in the bile. High concentrations of cholesterol or lower concentrations of bile salts or lecithin lead to precipitation of cholesterol stones.

How Do Pigmented Gallstones Form?

Pigmented stones are classified as black or brown and contain less than 30% cholesterol. The dark coloration is a result of the presence of calcium bilirubinate within the stones. *Black stones* are often associated with hemolytic diseases such as hereditary spherocytosis, sickle cell disease, or G6PD deficiency. The breakdown of red blood cells leads to an increase in unconjugated bilirubin, driving the formation of black stones. Black stones are most often found within the gallbladder. *Brown stones*, in comparison, are larger and softer and most often form within the bile ducts. They are usually associated with bacterial infection or parasites (e.g., *Clonorchis sinensis* or "Chinese liver fluke") and are more common in Asian countries.

Watch Out
Brown stones form from **B**acte**r**ia, while **Bl**ack stones form from the **Bl**ood.

What Are the Different Manifestations of Gallstone Disease? (Table 18.3)

Table 18.3 Manifestations of gallstone disease

Condition	Mechanism
Symptomatic cholelithiasis	Transient obstruction of the cystic duct → visceral peritoneal stretch → RUQ pain
Acute cholecystitis	Persistent obstruction of the cystic duct → visceral peritoneal stretch → inflammation of the gallbladder → bacterial overgrowth → infection of the gallbladder → parietal peritoneum inflammation
Choledocholithiasis	Obstruction of the common bile duct (CBD)
Cholangitis	Obstruction of the CBD → bacterial overgrowth → infection of the entire biliary tree → ascends into the liver
Acute gallstone pancreatitis	Obstruction of the CBD and pancreatic duct → pancreatic enzyme release
Gallstone ileus	Very large stone erodes into the duodenum → gallbladder-duodenal fistula → stone travels down the GI tract → small bowel obstruction (not ileus!)
Mirizzi's syndrome	Large gallstone impacted in the cystic duct → compresses the common hepatic duct

Watch Out
Gallstone ileus causes mechanical small bowel obstruction, often at the ileocecal valve. It presents in elderly women with a triad of air in the biliary tree, small bowel obstruction, and calcific mass (gallstone), usually in the right lower quadrant. It is due to a cholecystoduodenal fistula.

Work-Up

What Is the Next Step in the Work-Up? What Are the Specific Findings That Would Confirm the Diagnosis?

An RUQ ultrasound is the diagnostic test of choice. Gallstones appear as highly echogenic areas with acoustic shadows. The ultrasound should also note the thickness of the gallbladder wall (◘ Figs. 18.1, 18.2, and 18.3) and whether there is any fluid surrounding the gallbladder. These two findings, gallbladder wall thickening (>4 mm) and pericholecystic fluid, are diagnostic for acute cholecystitis. The ultrasound should make note of the diameter of the CBD as well as whether a stone is visualized within it.

> **Watch Out**
> Most gallstones are radiolucent, so a CT scan of the abdomen may be negative. Be sure to still order an RUQ ultrasound if biliary disease is suspected since ultrasonography has higher sensitivity in detecting gallstones.

What Is a Sonographic Murphy's Sign?

Instead of using the examiner's hand, direct pressure to the RUQ is applied by the ultrasound probe, under ultrasound guidance, while the patient inspires. The pain causes cessation of inspiration. This is thought to be more specific than a clinical Murphy's sign because the gallbladder can be directly visualized as coming in contact with the abdominal wall.

What Is the Normal CBD Diameter, and What Is the Implication of a Dilated CBD?

The normal common bile duct diameter is typically 4–5 mm, but it increases with age, approximately 1 mm per decade after age 40. In general, a CBD >6 mm is considered dilated in younger patients; however, a larger diameter may be normal in older individuals. A dilated CBD raises concern for obstruction, most commonly due to choledocholithiasis or malignancy.

How Accurate Is Ultrasonography in Detecting Gallstones Within the Gallbladder? Within the CBD?

Ultrasound is very sensitive (95%) and specific (97%) for gallstones (even as small as 1–2 mm) within the gallbladder. Conversely, it is very poor for detecting gallstones within the CBD (sensitivity of about 50%), as bowel gas interferes with the ultrasound waves.

What If the Ultrasound Demonstrates Gas Bubbles in the Gallbladder Wall?

This would be concerning for emphysematous cholecystitis, an infection due to gas-forming organisms. This diagnosis is common in older men, often with diabetes

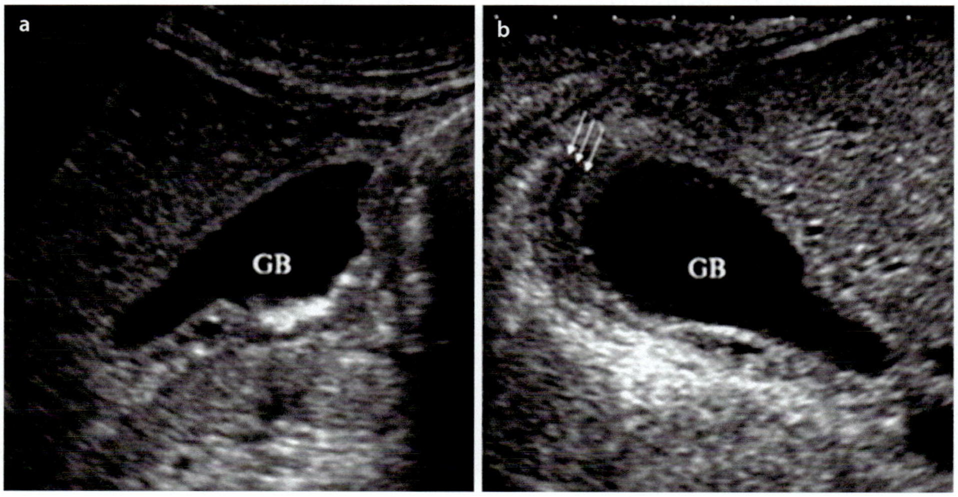

◘ **Fig. 18.1** Thickened gallbladder wall on ultrasound. (From Kimura Y et al. TG13 current terminology, etiology, and epidemiology of acute cholangitis and cholecystitis. J Hepatobiliary Pancreat Sci. 2013;20:12. ©Japanese Society of Hepato-Biliary-Pancreatic Surgery. Reprinted with permission.)

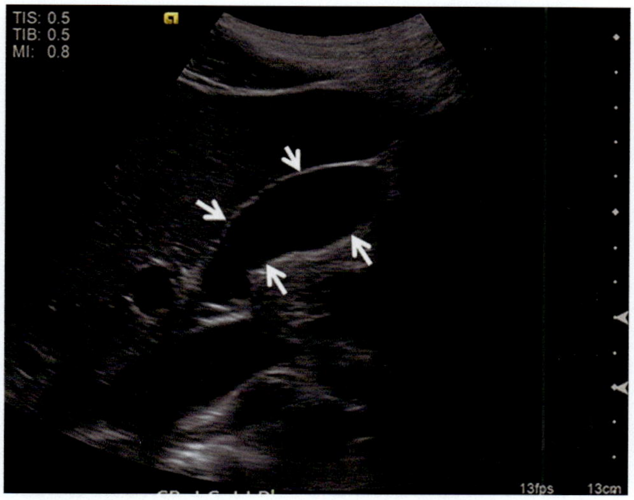

Fig. 18.2 RUQ abdominal ultrasound of a normal thin-walled gallbladder

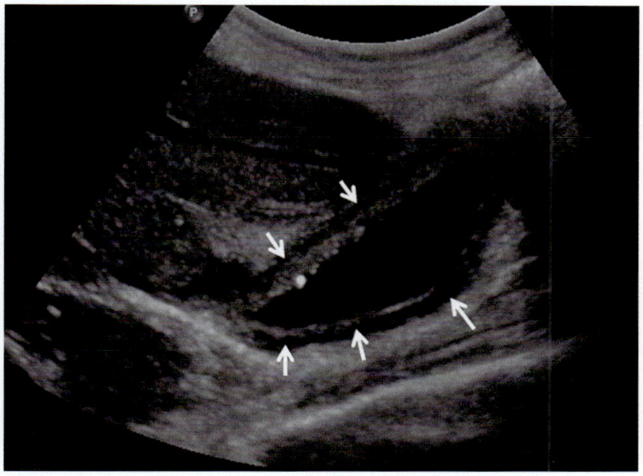

Fig. 18.3 RUQ ultrasound showing thickened, edematous gallbladder wall consistent with acute cholecystitis

mellitus. Bile cultures will often grow *Clostridium* or *E. coli*. This can progress to gallbladder perforation, intra-abdominal abscess, sepsis, and death if cholecystectomy is not performed emergently, along with administration of broad-spectrum antibiotics (that must also cover *Clostridia*).

Watch Out

Do not confuse pneumobilia (Fig. 18.4), which is air in the biliary tree secondary to recent biliary instrumentation or gallstone ileus, with air in the gallbladder wall, a hallmark of emphysematous cholecystitis caused by gas-forming bacteria (Figs. 18.5 and 18.6).

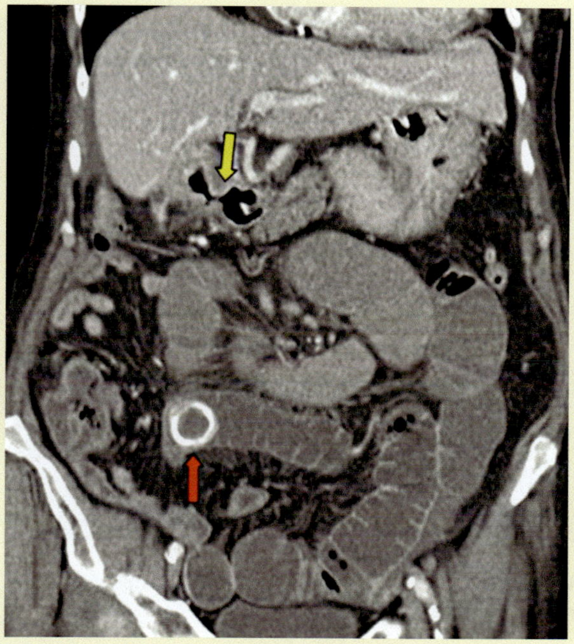

Fig. 18.4 Gallstone ileus. (From Liau et al. A case of gallstone-induced small bowel necrosis masquerading as clinical appendicitis. Clin J Gastroenterol. 2009;2:239. Reprinted with permission)

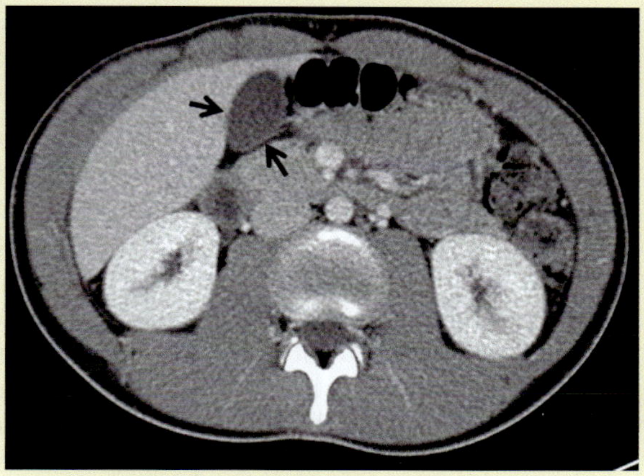

Fig. 18.5 Axial CT of a normal thin-walled gallbladder

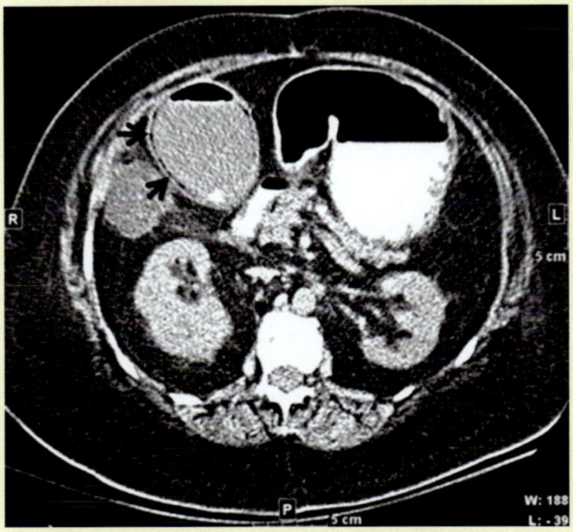

Fig. 18.6 Axial CT showing air in the gallbladder wall, known as emphysematous cholecystitis

Why Should Liver Tests, Amylase, and Lipase Always Be Sent in the Presence of RUQ and Epigastric Pain? What Is the Significance of Abnormalities?

A liver panel should include total and direct bilirubin, aspartate (AST) and alanine (ALT) aminotransferase, alkaline phosphatase (AP), and gamma-glutamyl transferase (GGT). In a patient who only has symptomatic cholelithiasis, all of these should be normal. Mild elevations can be seen in acute cholecystitis. Significantly elevated AP and GGT out of proportion to AST and ALT suggest cholestasis or biliary obstruction and are often related to choledocholithiasis. In contrast, marked elevations in AST or ALT, out of proportion to the AP and GGT, indicate hepatocellular damage and a primary hepatic pathology such as viral or alcoholic hepatitis or any other condition in which hepatocyte necrosis is occurring.

Is Amylase or Lipase Better to Rule Out Pancreatitis?

Lipase has a much higher sensitivity for pancreatitis than amylase. Lipase is the test of choice to rule out pancreatitis.

Watch Out

Liver tests such as AST, ALT, and AP do not actually reflect the synthetic function of the liver (thus the term "liver function test" is a misnomer). Better tests of the liver's synthetic function include serum albumin, prothrombin time (PT), and international normalized ratio (INR), as the liver synthesizes albumin and clotting factors. Even these tests, however, can be affected by extrahepatic disease.

What If Acute Cholecystitis Is Suspected but the Ultrasound Does Not Demonstrate Gallstones?

One possible explanation is the rare false-negative ultrasound (<5%). This may occur if gallstones are very small (≤1 mm) or if there are very few gallstones. Another possibility is acalculous cholecystitis. If an abdominal ultrasound is negative for gallstones, a hepatobiliary iminodiacetic acid (HIDA) scan is done. In this test, radiolabeled hepatic iminodiacetic acid is given intravenously, and then imaging is performed. This compound is absorbed by hepatocytes and then excreted into bile and seen within 30–60 min in the gallbladder, bile ducts, and small bowel in a normal patient. If the cystic duct is obstructed, as in acute cholecystitis, no uptake will be seen within the gallbladder, and the HIDA scan is considered positive. This test has a sensitivity of 97% and a specificity of 90%.

Watch Out

HIDA scans may yield false-positive results in patients with cirrhosis due to impaired hepatic uptake and excretion of the tracer. In this setting, HIDA is not a reliable test for diagnosing acute cholecystitis.

Can You Develop Acute Cholecystitis Without Gallstones?

Yes, acalculous cholecystitis (cholecystitis in the absence of gallstones) can occur, though it is very rare. This typically occurs in critically ill patients who are hospitalized for other reasons, have fasted for prolonged periods, and/or are receiving total peripheral nutrition. It is thought to be a combination of bile stasis and gallbladder ischemia from hypoperfusion. Ultrasound will typically demonstrate a thickened gallbladder wall or pericholecystic fluid without stones. If the ultrasound is completely negative, a HIDA scan is obtained. Treatment includes IV antibiotics and emergent intervention. If the patient is stable, an emergent cholecystectomy is performed. If the patient is unstable, percutaneous cholecystostomy (tube to drain the gallbladder) is performed, followed by cholecystectomy once the patient is medically stable.

Watch Out
Common settings for acalculous cholecystitis include critically ill patients on ventilators and post cardiopulmonary bypass. The low-flow state leads to gallbladder ischemia, stasis, and inflammation.

Management

What Is the Next Step in the Management of a Patient with an Ultrasound Demonstrating Gallstones, Pericholecystic Fluid, Gallbladder Wall Thickening of 5 mm, and a Positive Sonographic Murphy's Sign?

This ultrasound is diagnostic for acute cholecystitis. Management includes hospital admission, NPO status, IV fluids, and IV antibiotics with gram-negative and anaerobic coverage. Early laparoscopic cholecystectomy within 48–72 hours of presentation is recommended, as it reduces surgical complications and shortens hospital stay in medically stable patients.

What Is the Ideal Choice of Antibiotics?

Antibiotics must be tailored to the most likely organisms (enteric). Second-generation cephalosporins (e.g., cefoxitin) are considered first line. An alternative would be broad-spectrum penicillin/β-lactamase inhibitors such as piperacillin/tazobactam or ampicillin/sulbactam. In severe cases, third- and fourth-generation cephalosporins may be used.

What If Gallstones Are Discovered Incidentally? Do They Require a Cholecystectomy?

There is no benefit for cholecystectomy for asymptomatic gallstones. Up to 20% of Americans >60 years old have asymptomatic gallstones.

How Should Symptomatic Cholelithiasis Be Managed?

A patient with symptomatic cholelithiasis should undergo elective laparoscopic cholecystectomy. In patients who are poor surgical candidates, conservative management with dietary modification and symptom control is preferred. Ursodeoxycholic acid, which dissolves gallstones, may be considered in select cases, but it is rarely used due to limited efficacy and high recurrence rates.

Postoperative

What Is a Major Complication of Laparoscopic Cholecystectomy That Is More Common in the Setting of Acute Cholecystitis?

CBD injury is one of the most feared complications of laparoscopic cholecystectomy. There is a higher risk of CBD injury in men and during surgery for acute cholecystitis as compared to symptomatic cholelithiasis. The injury often occurs when the CBD is mistaken for the cystic duct, and thus, the CBD is inadvertently divided. Bile duct injuries can lead to strictures, resulting in recurrent cholangitis and eventually cirrhosis and liver failure requiring transplantation.

What Is the Differential Diagnosis and Work-Up for Abdominal Pain That Develops Soon After Cholecystectomy?

The work-up for patients who present postoperatively with abdominal pain, bloating, and anorexia soon after cholecystectomy is demonstrated in ◘ Fig. 18.7. Work-up includes liver function tests, an ultrasound,

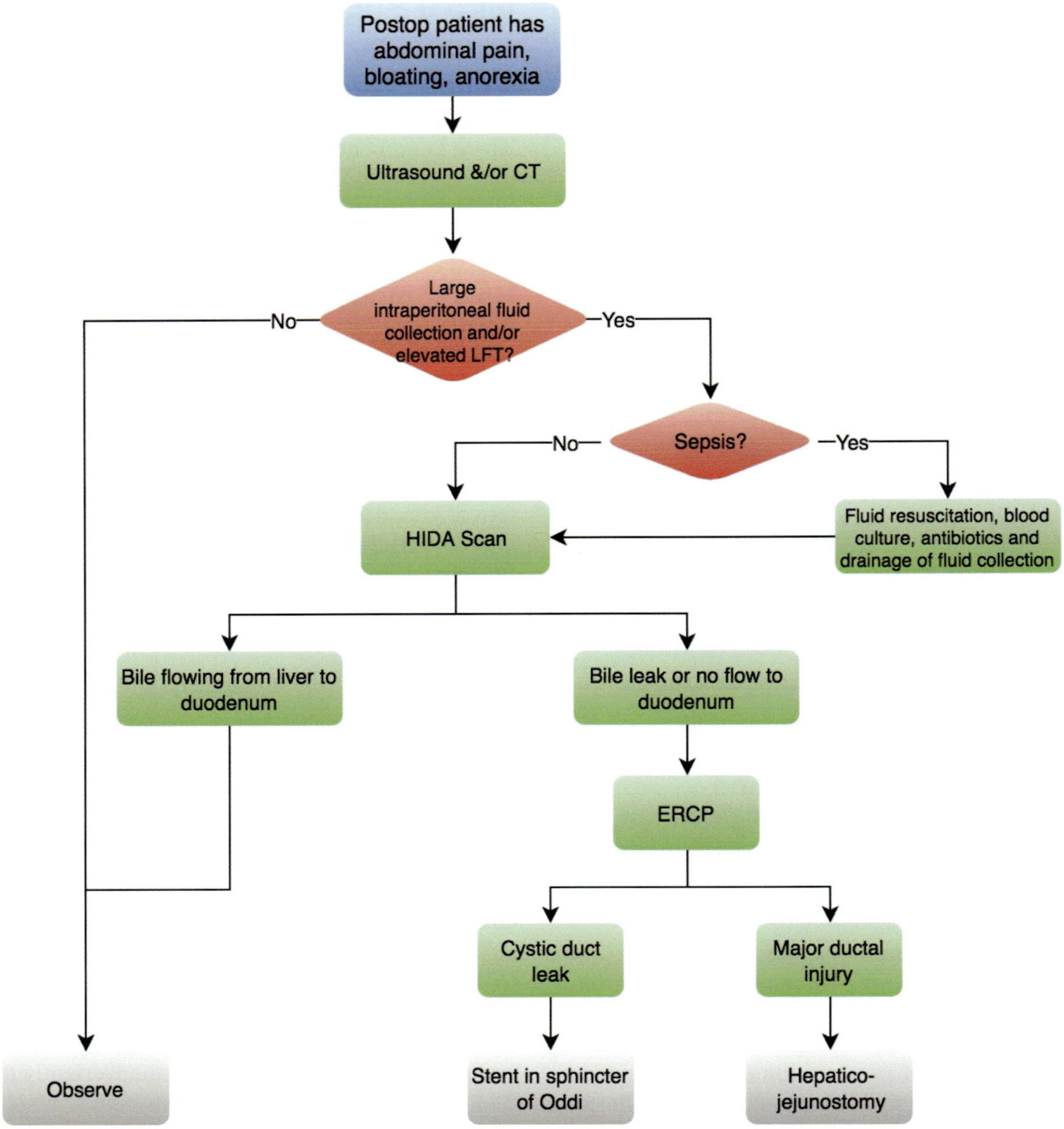

Fig. 18.7 Work-up for delayed recognition of CBD injuries

18

and/or a CT scan of the abdomen/pelvis to look for an intraperitoneal fluid collection. Such a fluid collection after cholecystectomy represents either blood (from a liver injury or cystic artery bleed) or bile leaking.

What Is a Biloma? How Is It Diagnosed? Treated?

A biloma is a collection of bile in the right upper quadrant after a cholecystectomy. It is usually caused by bile leaking from either a liver injury (if the liver was entered when removing the gallbladder), a cystic duct stump leak (if the clip inadvertently comes off), or a CBD injury. Bilomas are usually detected on CT. If a fluid collection is found, it should be percutaneously drained. If bilious drainage continues, the options are to either obtain a HIDA scan to rule out a bile leak and/or a bile duct injury or to go directly to an endoscopic-retrograde cholangiopancreatography (ERCP). A cystic duct stump leak is treated with stenting of the sphincter of Oddi via ERCP. However, a CBD injury may require hepaticojejunostomy. Liver injuries usually stop leaking on their own.

What Is the Differential Diagnosis If the Patient Develops RUQ Pain Several Weeks or Months After Cholecystectomy?

Recurrent RUQ/epigastric pain that develops weeks or months after cholecystectomy is referred to as postcholecystectomy syndrome (PCS) and is detailed in ◘ Table 18.4. Work-up should begin with a complete blood count and liver function tests, followed by a RUQ ultrasound. If ongoing pathology in the biliary tree is suspected, an ERCP would be the next test of choice.

What Is Sphincter of Oddi Dysfunction (SOD)?

SOD is a rare functional biliary disorder due to either stenosis or dyskinesia of the sphincter of Oddi. It is most commonly recognized in patients who have recently undergone laparoscopic cholecystectomy and continue to have episodic RUQ pain, particularly when they receive opioids (e.g., morphine). It can also occur in patients with an intact gallbladder, in which case ultrasonography generally shows moderate distension of the gallbladder and common bile duct (CBD). Mildly elevated liver enzymes corresponding with episodic pain are also seen. Further management may include sphincter of Oddi manometry or endoscopic sphincterotomy. Of note, SOD has also been implicated in recurrent acute pancreatitis.

◘ **Table 18.4** Postcholecystectomy Syndrome (PCS)

Etiology	Features
Residual stone in CBD	This can lead to pancreatitis, cholangitis, or biliary obstruction
Gallstone in cystic duct stump	Patients with anatomically longer cystic ducts are at risk for retained gallstones
Sphincter of Oddi dysfunction	Increased pressure at the sphincter of Oddi can lead to impaired function of the biliary tree
Other	Gastritis, peptic ulcer disease

Area of Controversy

When Should Acute Cholecystitis Be Managed Nonoperatively?

Critically ill patients with acute cholecystitis may have an unacceptable amount of operative risk. In a high-risk surgical patient, occasionally, acute cholecystitis can be managed initially with antibiotics alone. Some will resolve with this approach. If the patient does not improve and is a prohibitive operative risk, a percutaneously placed cholecystostomy tube is used to decompress the infected gallbladder. This approach is often used for acute acalculous cholecystitis. The problem with percutaneous cholecystostomy is that it is associated with increased complications and may not represent a permanent solution to acute cholecystitis, so it may require interval cholecystectomy anyway, depending on the patient's clinical status.

What Is the Role of Robot-Assisted Laparoscopic Cholecystectomy?

Robot-assisted laparoscopic cholecystectomy offers wristed instruments, tremor filtration, and an ergonomically superior console. Large database studies and several randomized trials show equivalent overall morbidity and length of stay when robot-assisted cholecystectomy is compared with conventional laparoscopy. However, some studies suggest that in addition to longer operative times and higher direct costs, robotic cholecystectomy may have a higher bile duct injury rate. Conversion to open surgery is slightly less common in some series, likely because improved dexterity helps in dense inflammation, yet this has not produced clearly superior clinical outcomes. Compared with open cholecystectomy, both minimally invasive approaches yield less postoperative pain, earlier return to work, and fewer wound complications. Because robot-assisted cholecystectomy requires expensive capital equipment and trained staff, access is still concentrated in high-volume centers; consequently, laparoscopic cholecystectomy remains the current standard of care, with robotic platforms best reserved for surgeons and institutions where resources, case volume, and expertise justify the added expense.

Gallstones (◘ Figs. 18.8 and 18.9)

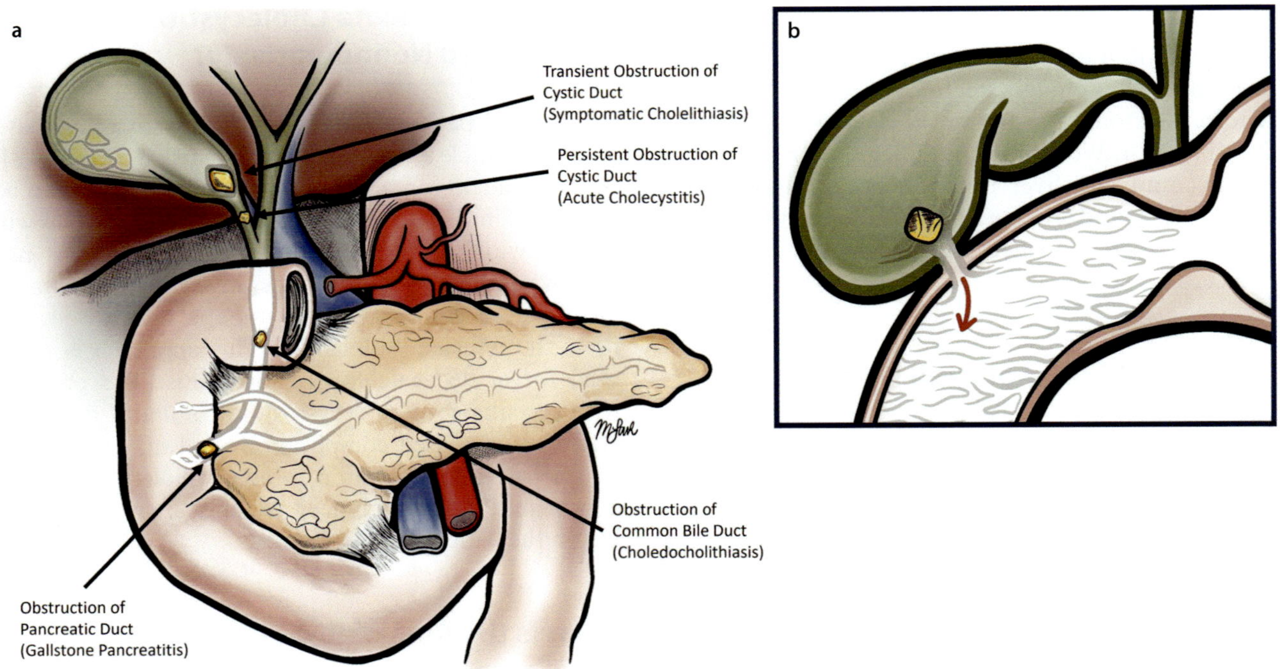

◘ **Fig. 18.8** **Gallstones:** Clinical scenarios (**a**) in which gallstones can cause significant problems within the biliary and gastrointestinal systems, including: **Symptomatic cholelithiasis:** Transient obstruction of the cystic duct causing intermittent biliary colic. **Acute cholecystitis:** Persistent obstruction of the cystic duct, leading to inflammation and infection of the gallbladder. **Choledocholithiasis:** Obstruction of the common bile duct, potentially causing jaundice and cholangitis. **Gallstone pancreatitis:** Obstruction of the pancreatic duct, resulting in inflammation of the pancreas. **Gallstone fistula to duodenum:** Formation of a fistula (**b**) between the gallbladder and duodenum, leading to the passage of gallstones into the gastrointestinal tract

◘ **Fig. 18.9** **Critical view of safety:** A key step in laparoscopic cholecystectomy to prevent bile duct injury. It is achieved when the hepatocystic triangle is cleared of tissue, the lower third of the gallbladder is dissected off the cystic plate, and only two structures (the cystic duct and artery) are seen entering the gallbladder

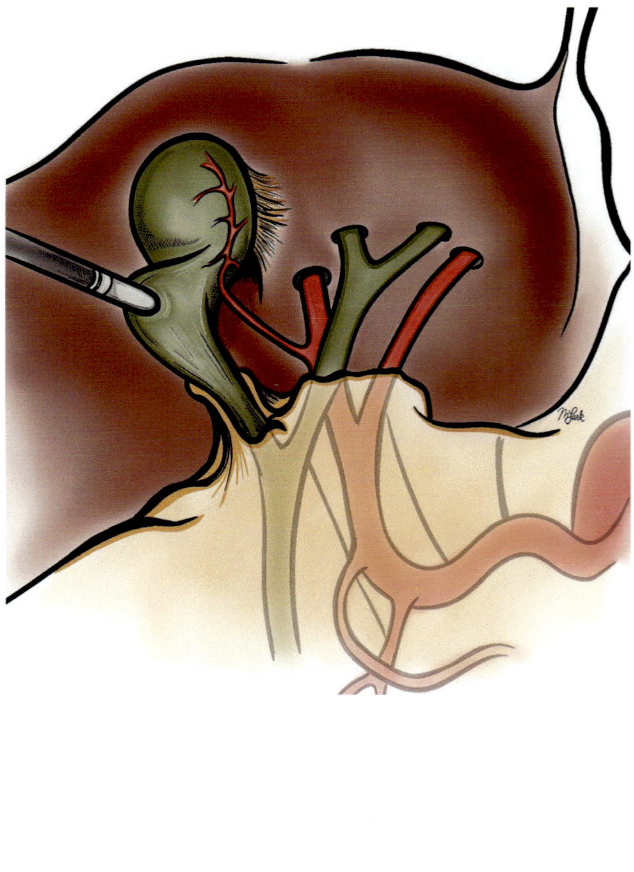

Summary of Essentials

History

- Postprandial RUQ pain, especially in obese, multiparous females
- Pain after fatty meals suggests gallbladder dysfunction

Physical Exam

- Murphy's sign: inspiratory arrest with deep palpation of the RUQ, specific for acute cholecystitis

Pathology/Pathophysiology

- Acute cholecystitis: cystic duct obstruction by gallstone → gallbladder wall inflammation and infection

Diagnosis

- RUQ US: gallstones, pericholecystic fluid, thickened gallbladder wall, and sonographic Murphy's sign
- HIDA scan: used when ultrasound is equivocal; avoid in cirrhosis due to false positives
- Lipase is preferred over amylase to rule out gallstone pancreatitis
- CT scan: used to evaluate complications or alternative diagnoses; can detect pneumobilia in gallstone ileus

Management

- Asymptomatic gallstones: cholecystectomy not indicated
- Symptomatic cholelithiasis (biliary colic): elective lap cholecystectomy
- Acute cholecystitis: early (within 48–72 hours) lap cholecystectomy
- Acute acalculous cholecystitis: percutaneous cholecystostomy tube if critically ill
- Emphysematous cholecystitis: emergent cholecystectomy
- Gallstone ileus: remove a large impacted gallstone from the terminal ileum (leave the gallbladder alone)

Postoperative

- If a patient presents within the first week after cholecystectomy with abdominal pain, distention, and anorexia, consider a biloma (cystic duct stump leak, CBD injury).
- Cystic duct stump leak readily treated with ERCP and stenting of the sphincter of Oddi.
- CBD injury may require hepaticojejunostomy.

Additional Important Facts

- Calcified gallbladder (porcelain) (Fig. 18.10): increased risk of malignancy (especially if scattered calcification), perform cholecystectomy
- Choledochal cysts are congenital dilations of the biliary tree; they are prone to cholangitis, have a risk of associated malignancy, and need to be excised (if intrahepatic ducts are involved (Caroli's disease), liver transplantation may be needed)
- Gallbladder cancer: associated with gallstones (always check final path)
- Gallbladder polyps: >1 cm suspicious for cancer; >2 cm high likelihood of cancer

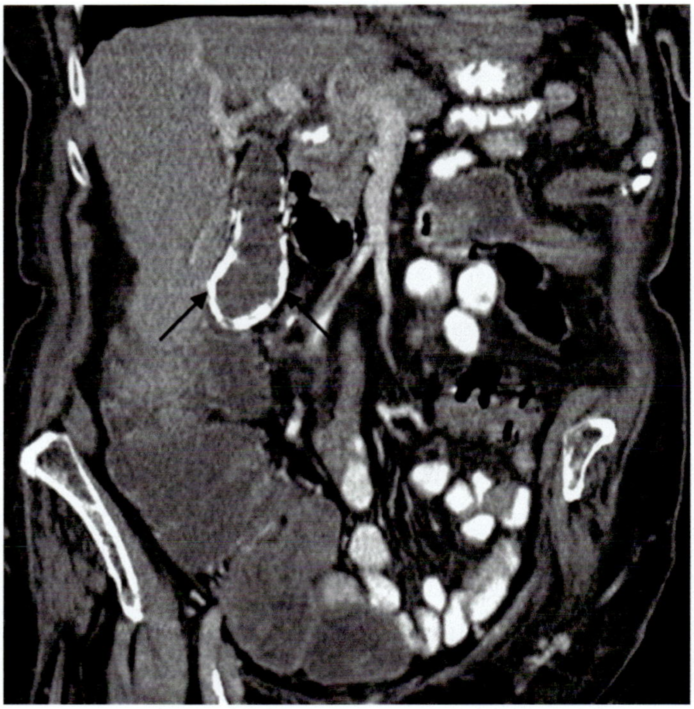

Fig. 18.10 Porcelain gallbladder on coronal CT. (From Amorosa JK, et al. GastroIntestinal radiology. In: Pitchumoni C, Dharmarajan T, editors. Geriatric gastroenterology. New York: Springer; 2012. Reprinted with permission)

Suggested Reading

Falor AE, Zobel M, Kaji A, Neville A, de Virgilio C. Admission variables predictive of gangrenous cholecystitis. Am Surg. 2012;78(10):1075–8.

Gutt CN, Encke J, Köninger J, Harnoss JC, Weigand K, Kipfmüller K, Büchler MW. Acute cholecystitis: early versus delayed cholecystectomy, a multicenter randomized trial (ACDC study, NCT00447304). Ann Surg. 2013;258(3):385–93.

Right Upper Quadrant Pain, Fever, Nausea, and Vomiting

Areg Grigorian, Matthew Y. C. Lin, and Christian de Virgilio

Contents

C. de Virgilio, A. Grigorian (eds.), *Surgery*, https://doi.org/10.1007/978-3-032-09799-6_19

Case Study

A 40-year-old female presents with a 24-hour history of right upper quadrant (RUQ) and epigastric pain associated with nausea and vomiting. She has had similar pain in the past, particularly after eating greasy foods. According to her family, over the last few hours, the patient has become slightly confused. She has also noticed dark urine today. Past medical history is negative. Physical examination reveals a temperature of 39.1 °C, a heart rate of 110 beats/min, respiratory rate of 16/min, and a blood pressure of 90/60 mmHg. Her RUQ is moderately tender to deep palpation. She has slight scleral icterus. The remainder of her abdominal exam is negative. Laboratory examination is significant for a white blood count of 15 × 10^3/μL (normal 4.1–10.9 × 10^3/μL), a total bilirubin of 4.0 mg/dl (0.1–1.2 mg/dL), alkaline phosphatase (ALP) of 350 μ/L (33–131 μ/L), aspartate aminotransferase (AST) of 44 μ/L (5–35 μ/L), alanine aminotransferase (ALT) of 65 μ/L (7–56 μ/L), gamma-glutamyl transpeptidase (GGT) of 330 μ/L (8–88 μ/L), and an amylase of 100 μ/L (30–110 μ/L). Urine is positive for bilirubin.

Diagnosis

What Is the Differential Diagnosis? (◘ Table 19.1)

◘ Table 19.1 Differential diagnosis of clinical presentation

Disease	Pathophysiology
Acute cholecystitis	Obstruction of cystic duct by gallstone → cholestasis and inflammation of the gallbladder
Choledocholithiasis	Obstruction of common bile duct (CBD) by gallstone
Gallstone pancreatitis	Obstruction of the CBD distal to pancreatic duct, often at the ampulla of Vater → inflammation of pancreas
Cholangitis	Obstruction of the CBD → ascending bacterial infection of the biliary system, cholestasis
Sphincter of Oddi dysfunction	Dyskinesia or stenosis of the sphincter of Oddi leading to cholestasis, worsened with opioids
Mirizzi's syndrome	Large stone lodged in the neck of the gallbladder causing external compression of the common hepatic duct
Viral hepatitis	Viral infection of the liver; can be acute or chronic
Pyogenic (bacterial) liver abscess	Hematogenous infection (e.g., endocarditis, IV drugs) or local spread from biliary disease
Amoebic liver abscess	*Entamoeba histolytica* enters portal system from the colon via ulceration; history of travel to endemic region

What Is the Diagnosis for This Patient?

The most likely diagnosis in a patient with a 1-day history of RUQ pain worsened with greasy foods, nausea, altered mental status, jaundice, and fever is acute cholangitis secondary to gallstone impaction in the distal common bile duct (CBD). Additionally, she has leukocytosis, hypotension, hyperbilirubinemia, and elevated ALP, all of which are consistent with acute cholangitis.

What Are the Diagnostic Criteria for Cholangitis?

The Tokyo guidelines have proposed diagnostic criteria for acute cholangitis. Acute cholangitis should be suspected in patients who show evidence of systemic inflammation (fever, chills, leukocytosis) and cholestasis (jaundice or elevated bilirubin). The diagnosis is confirmed by imaging that shows evidence of biliary obstruction such as dilation of the CBD and/or intrahepatic bile ducts.

History and Physical

What Are the Causes of Obstructive Jaundice that Lead to Cholangitis?

Gallstones are the most common cause. Other causes of obstruction include bile duct strictures, parasites (such as *Ascaris lumbricoides* and *Clonorchis sinensis* [Chinese liver fluke]), instrumentation of the biliary system (such as during endoscopic retrograde cholangiopancreatography [ERCP]), and occluded biliary stents.

Why Does the Patient Have Dark Urine but Not Pale Stools?

Pale or acholic stools are a result of prolonged biliary obstruction, so this would not be expected in patients with acute biliary obstruction. However, acute biliary obstruction can lead to an increased level of conjugated bilirubin, which may be excreted by the kidneys making the urine appear dark ("Coca-Cola-colored urine").

At What Level of Bilirubin Will Jaundice First Be Visible?

Jaundice may be visible when the total bilirubin level exceeds 2.5 mg/dL. The normal total bilirubin level is up to 1.0 mg/dL. Jaundice will manifest first in the sclerae of the eyes and under the tongue as the blood vessels there are more superficial. It will then descend down toward the chest, abdomen, and legs.

What Is Charcot's Triad?

Charcot's triad consists of fever, RUQ pain, and jaundice (or hyperbilirubinemia). This cluster of symptoms is classically associated with cholangitis. This presentation is found in only about 40–50% of patients with cholangitis. Thus, Charcot's triad is not very sensitive. Jaundice is not always clinically obvious.

What Is Reynolds' Pentad? What Percent of Patients with Cholangitis Have All Components?

Reynolds' pentad implies cholangitis with septic shock. It includes Charcot's triad plus hypotension and altered mentation. It is present in a minority of patients with cholangitis (5%).

> **Watch Out**
> Elderly patients with cholangitis may remain asymptomatic until they develop septic shock.

Pathophysiology

Why Are Gallstones the Most Common Cause of Obstructive Jaundice with Cholangitis?

Cholangitis arises from a combination of biliary obstruction and bacterial contamination of the bile. Gallstones are the most common cause because they can migrate from the gallbladder and become impacted in the distal

CBD, the narrowest segment of the biliary tree. This obstruction results in stasis, which impairs the normal flushing action of bile and facilitates bacterial overgrowth. Normally, bacteria are cleared from the biliary system by secretory IgA and Kupffer cells. However, in the setting of obstruction, reduced IgA secretion and Kupffer cell dysfunction allow bacterial proliferation. Additionally, gallstones themselves may harbor bacterial biofilms, and up to 90% of patients with gallstones have bacteria in their bile. Once infection is established, it can spread via the portal system and involve the liver.

What Are Potential Consequences of Unrecognized Acute Cholangitis?

Severe untreated cholangitis can give rise to severe sepsis, hepatic microabscesses, and death. If the patient with acute cholangitis develops hepatic microabscesses, AST and ALT will markedly increase as a result of direct hepatocyte damage and necrosis.

Is Clinical Jaundice Always a Sign of Biliary Disease?

No. Jaundice can be divided into prehepatic, hepatic (such as hepatitis), and posthepatic causes. Gilbert syndrome, an inherited disorder of bilirubin glucuronidation affecting about 5% of the population, is a common non-biliary cause of prehepatic clinical jaundice. These patients can present with clinical jaundice shortly after stressors such as intense sports activities or even after surgery. Unlike biliary obstruction, which causes increased total and conjugated (direct) bilirubin levels, Gilbert syndrome causes an isolated increase in unconjugated (indirect) bilirubin.

Watch Out
Patients presenting with postoperative jaundice secondary to unconjugated hyperbilirubinemia shortly after a relatively minor surgery (e.g., laparoscopic appendectomy, skin surgery) may have Gilbert syndrome.

How Does *Entamoeba Histolytica* Infection Lead to RUQ Pain?

Entamoeba histolytica is a parasitic amoeba that is endemic to areas of Mexico, Africa, India, and Central and South America. It is transmitted via the fecal-oral route, typically after ingestion of food or water contaminated with cysts. After ingestion of cysts, trophozoites form and invade the intestinal mucosa, leading to diarrhea (often bloody), abdominal pain, and weight loss. Infection may spread hematogenously to the liver, resulting in an amoebic liver abscess. Stool antigen testing and microscopy are used for the diagnosis. Treatment is with metronidazole to eradicate the trophozoites, followed by paromomycin to eradicate the cysts.

Watch Out
Pyogenic liver abscess and amebic abscess from *Entamoeba histolytica* both present with fever, RUQ pain, and elevated liver enzymes. CT typically shows solitary right-lobe lesions in amebic abscesses, while pyogenic abscesses are often multiple. Both appear as well-defined, hypoattenuating lesions with peripheral enhancement. Travel to endemic areas suggests amebic etiology.

Are there Any Congenital Conditions that Can Lead to Obstructive Jaundice and/or Cholangitis?

Worsening obstructive jaundice, pale stool, hepatosplenomegaly, or dark urine in a neonate is suggestive of congenital biliary atresia. This is a failure of the normal development of the biliary tree, leading to fibrosis and obliteration of the bile ducts and obstruction of bile flow. Early surgical intervention is required and may involve a hepaticoportoenterostomy (Kasai procedure) or liver transplant. Following this procedure, they are at risk for recurrent cholangitis.

Workup

How Can LFTs Help Distinguish Between Hepatic and Posthepatic Causes of Jaundice?

LFTs are important in differentiating hepatic from posthepatic causes of jaundice due to their distinct enzyme patterns. In hepatic injury, AST and ALT—enzymes within liver cells—rise significantly, often into the thousands, and are disproportionately higher than ALP, indicating hepatocellular damage (e.g., viral hepatitis or liver trauma). In contrast, posthepatic causes, such as biliary obstruction from choledocholithiasis or cholangitis, typically show a marked elevation in ALP, equal to, or higher than AST and ALT. To confirm that ALP elevation is liver-specific, GGT is assessed; a corresponding increase in GGT alongside ALP suggests a biliary obstruction.

Watch Out

Global hypoperfusion causing transaminitis >1000s and delayed hyperbilirubinemia (days postinsult) suggests ischemic hepatitis or "shock liver." Look for histology showing zone 3 necrosis. Transaminitis typically resolves within 7 days, but hyperbilirubinemia can persist for weeks. Distinguish from acalculous cholecystitis, also linked to hypoperfusion, which presents with mild LFT elevations but lacks the extreme transaminitis seen in shock liver.

What Imaging Is the Diagnostic Test of Choice? Does the Test Provide Direct or Indirect Evidence for the Diagnosis?

The first-line diagnostic test is RUQ ultrasound (US), which is excellent in terms of visualizing gallstones within the gallbladder and in demonstrating dilation of the CBD due to obstruction. However, US is poor at detecting stones within the CBD as a single stone doesn't cause the same acoustic shadowing as multiple ones in the gallbladder, and gas in the adjacent duodenum obscures the view. Thus, RUQ US provides only indirect evidence (dilated CBD) for cholangitis.

Management

What Are the Most Important Immediate Management Steps Once a Patient Develops Fever and Leukocytosis?

19

When sepsis is suspected, a sepsis bundle should be initiated and completed within one hour (◘ Fig. 19.1). Immediate steps include obtaining blood cultures and measuring serum lactate. Intravenous fluid resuscitation with normal saline or lactated Ringer's solution should be started, titrated to maintain a mean arterial pressure of at least 65 mmHg and a urine output of at least 0.5 mL/kg/h. A Foley catheter may help guide resuscitation. Broad-spectrum IV antibiotics should be administered as soon as possible, ideally within one hour. If hypotension persists after fluid administration, vasopressors such as norepinephrine should be started to maintain adequate perfusion.

What Is the Antibiotic Treatment for Acute Cholangitis?

In the case of suspected cholangitis, antibiotics should cover enteric organisms (Gram-negative rods, enterococci, and anaerobes). The most common bacteria causing biliary infection are *Escherichia coli*. Additionally, at least two sets of *blood cultures* should be obtained, ideally before the administration of antibiotics, but only if this does not cause delay.

Once the Patient Is Resuscitated, Antibiotics Started, and the Diagnosis Is Established, What Intervention Is Recommended? What Is the Goal of that Intervention?

Once the patient has been resuscitated, and the vital signs stabilized, the next step in treatment is to drain the infected bile, termed biliary decompression. This is best accomplished by ERCP. During ERCP, a scope is inserted through the mouth to the ampulla of Vater. The ampulla is cannulated, the stone can be extracted, the sphincter of Oddi is cut (sphincterotomy) to allow drainage of the bile into the duodenum, and a stent is often placed. If ERCP is unsuccessful, percutaneous transhepatic drainage (PTC) is the next choice. In this procedure, the bile is drained via a catheter inserted directly into the liver. Very rarely, if both of these options fail, the bile may need to be decompressed operatively by placing a drain (called a T-tube) directly into the CBD.

Watch Out

ERCP has a 5% chance of causing ERCP-induced pancreatitis.

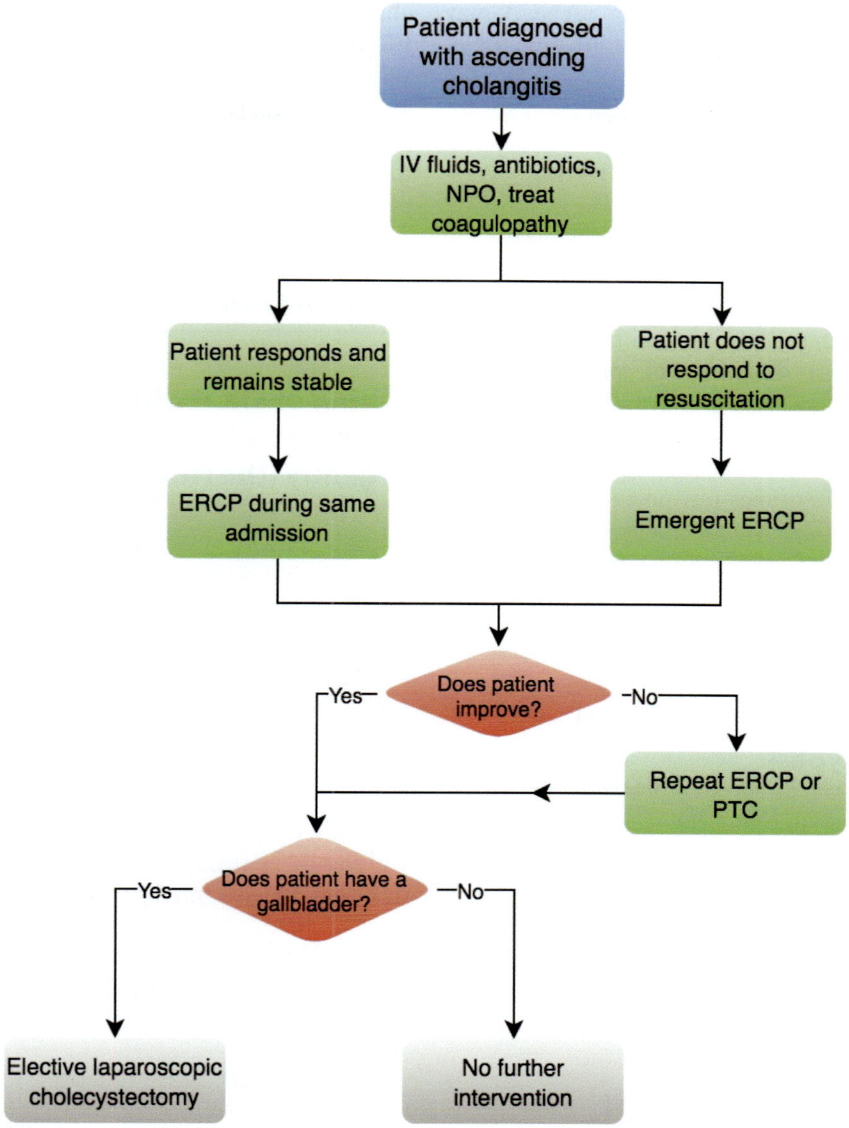

Fig. 19.1 Overall treatment algorithm

Following Successful ERCP, What Is the Next Step in Management?

Once the patient's sepsis has completely resolved, if the cause is gallstones, they should undergo laparoscopic cholecystectomy (Fig. 19.1). Cholecystectomy will prevent additional complications from gallstones, such as recurrent choledocholithiasis and cholangitis. Several randomized controlled trials have confirmed this by demonstrating significantly lower risk of biliary complications in patients who undergo elective laparoscopic cholecystectomy after bile duct clearance. Cholecystectomy should be done during the same admission.

Areas Where You Can Get in Trouble

A History of Bloody Diarrhea in a Patient Who Presents with Cholangitis

A history of bloody diarrhea in a patient who presents with cholangitis is suggestive of inflammatory bowel disease (IBD) with primary sclerosing cholangitis (PSC). This occurs more commonly in patients with ulcerative colitis (vs. Crohn's disease) and is characterized by inflammation and fibrosis of the intrahepatic and extrahepatic bile ducts. Cholangiography typically reveals multifocal stricturing and dilation, giving a "beaded" appearance to the bile ducts. Testing for pANCA may support an associated diagnosis of ulcerative colitis in IBD-related PSC.

A Middle-Aged Woman with Pruritus, Fatigue, and Normal RUQ US

If a patient (generally a middle-aged woman) presents with pruritus, fatigue, mildly elevated AP, normal transaminases, and a normal RUQ US (no bile duct dilatation), then suspect a diagnosis of primary biliary cholangitis (PBC). Most patients are often diagnosed while asymptomatic with incidentally discovered elevation of ALP. PBC is a rare, autoimmune disorder of the bile ducts. Patients oftentimes test positive for the anti-mitochondrial antibody. Management often includes ursodeoxycholic acid. Complications of PBC include cirrhosis, hepatobiliary cancers, malabsorption, and osteopenia.

Biliary Decompression in a Patient with a Gastric Bypass

Bariatric procedures, particularly gastric bypass, are increasingly common. Some patients with gastric bypass may later develop conditions requiring ERCP, such as choledocholithiasis or cholangitis. However, in patients with a gastric bypass, the altered anatomy (with separation of the remnant stomach and duodenum from the alimentary tract) often prevents the use of a standard ERCP approach. In these cases, advanced endoscopic skills and specialized equipment are typically required, and even then, the procedure may be challenging. A surgeon may need to assist by providing operative access to the remnant stomach, allowing the gastroenterologist to perform ERCP through this route.

Areas of Controversy

Timing of ERCP with Severe Cholangitis: Emergently (in the Middle of the Night) or Urgently (the Next Morning)?

In patients with severe cholangitis, the initial management should focus on IV fluids, antibiotics, and, if needed, vasopressors (norepinephrine is the first-line agent). In general, a hemodynamically unstable and under-resuscitated patient should not be rushed to ERCP (as it requires deep sedation that may cause further hypotension). However, if the patient fails to improve, ERCP should be performed expeditiously. Current guidelines suggest that emergent, middle-of-the-night ERCP does not consistently improve outcomes and should be reserved for the rare cases of rapidly deteriorating patients unresponsive to initial stabilization.

Endoscopic Retrograde Cholangiopancreatography (▣ Fig. 19.2)

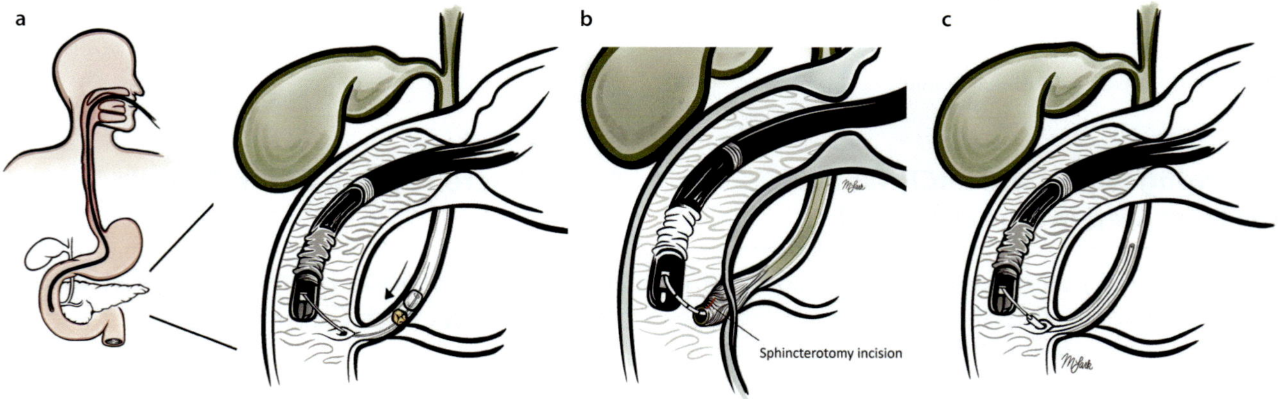

▣ **Fig. 19.2** **ERCP Procedure:** During an ERCP, an endoscope is advanced into the duodenum to cannulate the ampulla of Vater. The procedure can be used for stone extraction (**a**), performing a sphincterotomy (**b**), and placing a biliary stent (**c**) to prevent further obstruction

Summary of Essentials

History and Physical

- Charcot's triad: fever, RUQ pain, and jaundice (or hyperbilirubinemia).
- Reynolds' pentad: Charcot's triad plus hypotension and altered mentation.
- Look for evidence of systemic inflammation (fever, tachycardia, leukocytosis).
- Elderly patients may be hypothermic and have leukopenia (are relatively immunosuppressed).

Etiology/Pathophysiology

- Biliary obstruction with ascending bacterial infection.
- Gallstones may harbor bacterial biofilms; obstruction causes biliary stasis, allowing bacterial overgrowth and entry into the liver via the portal vein.
- Most commonly caused by gallstone obstruction of the distal CBD.
- Other causes: biliary stricture, obstructed stent, parasites, cancers.
- Suppurative cholangitis: acute cholangitis complicated by septic shock.

Diagnosis

- Elevated white blood cell count
- ALP elevated equal to or above AST/ALT, elevated GGT
- US: dilated CBD

Management

- Aggressive IV fluids, blood cultures, broad-spectrum antibiotics.
- Biliary decompression via ERCP.
- PTC if ERCP fails.
- Cholecystectomy after sepsis resolves to prevent further biliary complications.

Watch Out

- The diagnosis of acute cholangitis may be missed in the elderly and immunosuppressed (e.g., steroids).
- Think sclerosing cholangitis if also having symptoms of IBD.
- Suspect PSC in a patient with ulcerative colitis.
- Suspect PBC if there is pruritus, elevated AP, no duct dilatation, and positive AMA.

Acknowledgment The editors would like to acknowledge and thank the following authors for their contributions to the previous edition of the chapter: Manan P. Shah, Paul N. Frank.

Suggested Reading

Kiriyama S, Kozaka K, Takada T, et al. Tokyo Guidelines 2018: diagnostic criteria and severity grading of acute cholangitis (with videos). J Hepatobiliary Pancreat Sci. 2018 Jan;25(1):17–30. doi: https://doi.org/10.1002/jhbp.512. Epub 2018 Jan 5. PMID: 29032610.

Schwed A, Boggs M, Pham XD, Watanabe DM, et al. Association of admission laboratory values and the timing of endoscopic retrograde cholangiopancreatography with clinical outcomes in acute cholangitis. JAMA Surg. 2016;151(11):1039–45.

Severe Epigastric Pain with Nausea and Vomiting

Areg Grigorian, Matthew Y. C. Lin, and Christian de Virgilio

Contents

C. de Virgilio, A. Grigorian (eds.), *Surgery*, https://doi.org/10.1007/978-3-032-09799-6_20

Case Study

A 41-year-old woman presents to the emergency department complaining of severe and continuous epigastric pain for the past 24 hours. The pain radiates straight through to her back. She has had progressive nausea with vomiting. The vomit is bile-stained and without blood. She has had similar but less severe episodes of abdominal pain in the past, usually after eating heavy meals, but they always resolved within a few hours. She is gravida two, para two, with last menses two weeks ago, and does not consume any alcohol. On examination, she is afebrile, heart rate is 115 beats/min, blood pressure is 128/86 mmHg, and respiratory rate is 18/min. Her abdomen is not distended. She has no surgical scars on her abdomen, and no obvious masses are visible. She has no bruising around her umbilicus or along her flank. Bowel sounds are hypoactive. She has marked tenderness to palpation in her epigastrium, without guarding or rebound. The remainder of her abdomen is soft and nontender to palpation. No masses or organomegaly is appreciated. Laboratory examination reveals a white blood cell count of 17.2×10^3 cells/μL (normal $4.1–10.9 \times 10^3$ cells/uL), amylase of 1545 u/L (30–110 u/L), lipase of 1134 u/L (7–60 u/L), ALT of 245 u/L (7–56 u/L), AST of 263 u/L (5–35 u/L), serum glucose of 156 mg/dl (65–110 mg/dL), total bilirubin of 1.1 mg/dL (0.2–1.2 mg/dL), and LDH of 180 u/L (0–250 u/L). An abdominal series demonstrates gas throughout the small and large bowel and a focal dilated loop of proximal small bowel without air-fluid levels. There is no free air under the diaphragm.

Diagnosis

What Is the Differential Diagnosis for Epigastric Abdominal Pain? (Table 20.1)

Table 20.1 Differential diagnosis of epigastric abdominal pain

Condition	History and physical
Gastroenteritis	Nausea, vomiting, diarrhea, myalgias, fever, mild abdominal tenderness
Acute gastritis	Burning/gnawing epigastric pain, NSAID use, mild abdominal tenderness
Acute cholecystitis	Right upper quadrant/epigastric pain radiating to around the right back, nausea, vomiting, fever, *Murphy's sign*
Peptic ulcer disease (PUD)	Intermittent burning epigastric pain that is better (duodenal ulcer) or worse (gastric ulcer) with food intake, nausea, *Helicobacter pylori infection*, NSAID use, steroids
Perforated ulcer	Initial epigastric pain, followed by diffuse tenderness, abdominal rigidity, rebound tenderness
Pancreatitis	Epigastric pain radiating to the back, nausea, vomiting, anorexia, fever, tachycardia, cholelithiasis, alcohol use disorder
Appendicitis	Periumbilical pain migrating toward the right lower quadrant (*McBurney's point*), associated with nausea, vomiting, anorexia, fever, Rovsing's sign, psoas sign
Small bowel obstruction	Crampy pain, vomiting, distension; dilated loops with air-fluid levels, no colonic gas, prior abdominal surgery
Acute mesenteric ischemia	"Severe abdominal pain out of proportion to physical exam," nausea, irregularly irregular rhythm (most often cardiac embolus to superior mesenteric artery from atrial fibrillation), bloody diarrhea in severe cases
Ruptured AAA	Sudden back or flank pain, hypotension, pulsatile abdominal mass; elderly male smoker
Referred pain from myocardial infarction	Atypical presentation more common in women and diabetics, cardiovascular disease, obesity, hypercholesterolemia

NSAID nonsteroidal anti-inflammatory drugs

What Is the Diagnosis for this Patient?

Acute pancreatitis is most likely secondary to cholelithiasis. This patient has the classic presentation which consists of epigastric abdominal pain radiating straight through to the back with nausea and vomiting. She has had prior episodes of pain, which have resolved within a few hours, after eating heavy meals, which is characteristic of symptomatic gallstones. Since the vast majority of pancreatitis cases are due to gallstones or alcohol use and this patient does not consume alcohol, we can conclude that her symptoms are most likely related to gallstones. Finally, the amylase and lipase are elevated.

How Do You Diagnose Acute Pancreatitis?

Acute pancreatitis is considered a clinical diagnosis. The Atlanta criteria were created for the diagnosis of acute pancreatitis. They require two of the following three:

1. Sudden, severe, persistent epigastric pain radiating to the back
2. Elevated lipase or amylase to three times greater than the upper limit of normal
3. Characteristic findings of acute pancreatitis on imaging (i.e., enlarged pancreas, sentinel loops [dilated small bowel], colon cutoff sign)

History and Physical

What Nonsurgical Conditions Can Mimic an Acute Abdomen?

Gastroenteritis, acute adrenal insufficiency, sickle cell crisis, diabetic ketoacidosis, acute porphyria, pelvic inflammatory disease, kidney stones, pyelonephritis, and acute pancreatitis.

What Is the Significance of Bruising Around the Umbilicus, Flank, and Inguinal Ligament?

They are all signs of retroperitoneal hemorrhage in association with acute hemorrhagic pancreatitis where methemalbumin formed from digested blood tracks subcutaneously to different parts of the abdominal wall. *Grey Turner's sign* refers to a blue-black discoloration in the flanks. *Cullen's sign* is a blue-red discoloration at the umbilicus, and *Fox's sign* is bruising over the inguinal ligament.

> **Watch Out**
> Only about 10% of gallstones are radiopaque (visible on plain radiographs) versus 90% of kidney stones. An abdominal ultrasound is the first step in the evaluation for gallstones.

What Are the Signs, Symptoms, and Findings of Acute Pancreatitis?

Epigastric pain radiating to the back worsened with food, nausea/vomiting (90% of cases), anorexia, or decreased oral intake. Physical examination frequently reveals fever, tachycardia, epigastric tenderness with localized guarding, and hypoactive bowel sounds secondary to reactive ileus. Rarely, severe pancreatitis can present with diffuse tenderness and peritoneal signs mimicking an acute abdomen.

What Structures Are in the Retroperitoneum?

One can remember these structures with the following mnemonic: "SAD PUCKER": suprarenal (adrenal) glands, aorta/IVC, duodenum (2nd and 3rd part), pancreas (except tail), ureters, colon (ascending and descending), kidneys, esophagus, and rectum.

Pathophysiology

What Is the Pathophysiology of Pancreatitis?

It initially occurs as a result of inappropriate activation of pancreatic enzymes leading to peripancreatic inflammation. Intraparenchymal extravasation of enzymes causes autodigestion of pancreatic parenchyma but primarily damages the peripancreatic tissues and vasculature. The inflammatory response is out of proportion to the insult and, with time, potentiates further damage leading to fluid sequestration, fat necrosis, vasculitis, and hemorrhage.

What Are the Etiologies for Pancreatitis?

- "*GET SMASHED*" will help you remember the causes of acute pancreatitis
- *G*—gallstones (40%)

- *E*—ethanol (30%)
- *T*—tumors
- *S*—scorpion stings
- *M*—mycoplasma or mumps
- *A*—autoimmune (lupus or polyarteritis nodosa)
- *S*—surgery or trauma
- *H*—hyperlipidemia/hypercalcemia
- *E*—ERCP or embolic/ischemic
- *D*—drugs or toxins

Watch Out

Almost 40% of acute pancreatitis cases are caused by gallstones. However, only about 5% of patients with gallstones develop acute pancreatitis.

What Medications Can Cause Pancreatitis? (Table 20.2)

Table 20.2 Common etiologies of acute pancreatitis

Disease treated	Medications
Cardiovascular disease	Furosemide, thiazides
Inflammatory bowel disease	Sulfasalazine, 5-ASA
Immunosuppression	Azathioprine
Seizures	Valproic acid
Diabetes	Exenatide
Human immunodeficiency virus (HIV)	Didanosine, pentamidine

How Do Gallstones Cause Acute Pancreatitis?

Gallstones can cause acute pancreatitis by transiently obstructing the ampulla of Vater as they pass through the common bile duct (CBD). This obstruction impedes the outflow of pancreatic secretions, as the CBD and the pancreatic duct usually meet and end in a short common channel, leading to a sudden increase in intraductal pressure. The resulting stasis and activation of pancreatic enzymes within the pancreas initiate autodigestion and inflammation.

In Patients with Gallstone Pancreatitis, How Often Does the Gallstone Remain Impacted in the Distal Common Duct?

The gallstones that cause pancreatitis are usually small, and as such, in the majority of cases, the stone remains impacted very briefly, only transiently obstructing the ampulla of Vater, and soon after passes into the duodenum. As such, persistence of a CBD stone is uncommon, and therefore, ERCP is not usually needed. This differs from gallstones that cause acute cholangitis, where the stones are usually large and usually need ERCP for removal.

What Are the Differences Between Acute and Chronic Pancreatitis? (Table 20.3)

Table 20.3 Acute vs. chronic pancreatitis

	Acute pancreatitis	Chronic pancreatitis
Onset	Severe and sudden	Recurrent episodes
Etiology	Gallstone (40%), alcohol (30%)	Alcohol (90%), anatomic defects (pancreas divisum), hereditary
Presentation	Epigastric pain radiating to the back, nausea, vomiting anorexia	Recurrent epigastric pain, weight loss, diabetes, steatorrhea
Labs	High amylase and lipase (more sensitive)	Low fecal elastase levels
Radiology	Dilated loops of bowel near pancreas (*sentinel loop*) on plain films	*Pancreatic calcifications* on plain films

How Is the Severity of Pancreatitis Classified?

The severity of pancreatitis is classified as mild, moderately severe, and severe. Mild pancreatitis is the most common form and is defined by the absence of organ failure and local or systemic complications; it typically resolves within 2 to 5 days. Moderately severe complications include transient organ failure lasting less than 48 hours, and/or local or systemic complications. Severe pancreatitis is defined by organ failure that persists for more than 48 hours (worst prognosis).

Watch Out
The first stage of pancreatitis involves the premature activation of trypsin within the pancreatic acinar cells.

How Is Organ Failure Defined?

Organ failure in acute pancreatitis is defined by the Modified Marshall Scoring System, which evaluates three organ systems: respiratory, renal, and cardiovascular. Organ failure is present if any of the following criteria are met:

- Respiratory: PaO_2/FiO_2 ratio < 300 (with or without mechanical ventilation)
- Renal: serum creatinine >1.9 mg/dL
- Cardiovascular: systolic blood pressure < 90 mmHg despite fluid resuscitation or the need for vasopressors

Organ failure is considered persistent if it lasts more than 48 hours, which defines severe pancreatitis.

What Is the Mechanism of Hypotension in Pancreatitis?

Inflammation and cytokine storm cause endothelial injury and increased permeability in the peripancreatic vasculature, leading to fluid leaking into the retroperitoneal space (known as third spacing). The cytokine storm also causes massive vasodilation, which along with a shrunken intravascular volume can cause severe hypotension.

What Are the Main Pulmonary Complications of Acute Pancreatitis?

Pleural effusions (the majority on the left side) and acute respiratory distress syndrome (ARDS) (◘ Fig. 20.1).

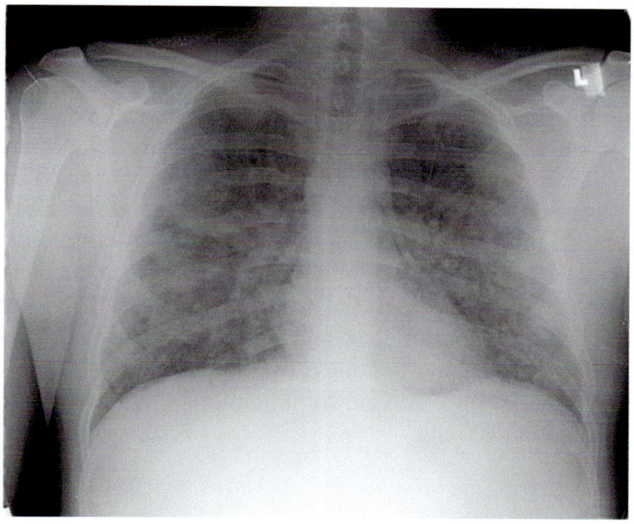

◘ **Fig. 20.1** Chest X-ray showing diffuse bilateral pulmonary infiltrates characteristic of ARDS

These complications are thought to be due to cytokine-mediated vasodilation and pancreatic enzyme (e.g., phospholipase-A2)–mediated lung injury.

What Are the Different Histopathologic Types of Acute Pancreatitis? What Are the Important Differences?

The majority of patients (>80%) develop *acute interstitial edematous pancreatitis*, characterized by an enlargement of the pancreas due to inflammatory edema. Such patients have no inflammation or destruction of pancreatic cells. Less than 20% develop *necrotizing pancreatitis* characterized by necrotic pancreatic parenchyma which can lead to sepsis in over half the cases. *Hemorrhagic pancreatitis* is a type of necrotizing pancreatitis in which there is extensive bleeding into the pancreatic parenchyma and surrounding tissues. The type of pancreatitis is important because it determines both prognosis and management.

Prognosis

How Is the Severity of Pancreatitis Determined?

Severity of acute pancreatitis is determined using clinical scoring systems or by identifying local or systemic complications. Several scoring systems exist, including the Ranson criteria, APACHE II, and the Bedside Index for Severity in Acute Pancreatitis (BISAP) score. The BISAP score is commonly used due to its simplicity and similar predictive accuracy to APACHE II. One point is assigned for each of the following present within the first 24 hours: blood urea nitrogen (BUN) greater than 25 mg/dL, impaired mental status, presence of systemic inflammatory response syndrome (SIRS), age over 60 years, and the presence of a pleural effusion. The Ranson criteria, although more complex, remain widely known and involve five variables assessed at admission and six assessed after 48 hours. Mnemonics such as "GA LAW" for the initial values and "CHOBBS" for the 48-hour parameters may aid recall. Ultimately, severity may also be gauged by the presence of persistent organ failure or local complications such as necrosis or fluid collections.

Watch Out

In adults, the degree of amylase and lipase elevation does *not* correlate with the severity of acute pancreatitis and should not be used to influence management (i.e., timing of surgery).

Why Does One Get Hypocalcemia with Severe Pancreatitis?

With severe pancreatitis, free fatty acids are generated by the action of pancreatic lipase. The free fatty acids chelate calcium salts that are present in the pancreas, leading to saponification (the deposition of calcium soaps in the retroperitoneum).

What Is the Natural Disease Course of Acute Pancreatitis?

The majority of patients with acute pancreatitis recover in less than five days without any complications. Close to 20% of patients have a severe presentation with local or systemic complications (including organ failure).

What Is the Most Common Cause of Mortality in the First Week of Severe Acute Pancreatitis? Beyond the First Week?

20

In the first week, death is most often due to multiorgan failure as a result of severe systemic inflammatory response. After the first week, mortality is most commonly due to sepsis secondary to pancreatic necrosis and peripancreatic abscesses (these most often develop in the third and fourth week of hospitalization). If a pancreatic abscess is not drained, mortality approaches 100%.

Workup

What Are the Most Important Laboratory Tests to Order When Suspecting Acute Pancreatitis?

Serum amylase, lipase, liver enzymes (AST, ALT, AP), total bilirubin, electrolytes, complete blood count, and a lipid panel. Amylase and lipase should be elevated. Amylase levels tend to be much higher (often >1000 u/L) in patients with gallstone pancreatitis as compared to other etiologies. Similarly, the elevated ALT greater than three times the upper limit of normal is highly suggestive of gallstone pancreatitis. However, close to 20% of patients will have normal liver enzymes. A lipid panel is important to rule out hyperlipidemic pancreatitis, usually due to hypertriglyceridemia (must be >1000 mg/dl).

Which Laboratory Test Is Most Specific for Acute Pancreatitis?

Lipase is most specific (and sensitive). Numerous other diseases can cause hyperamylasemia (◘ Table 20.4).

◘ **Table 20.4** Hyperamylasemia

Conditions	Specific diseases
Pancreatic disease	Pancreatitis, pancreatic pseudocyst, trauma, ERCP, pancreatic carcinoma, cystic fibrosis
Salivary disease	*Parotitis*, radiation, ductal obstruction
Gastrointestinal disease	Peptic ulcer disease, perforated bowel, mesenteric ischemia, appendicitis, cholecystitis, celiac disease, small bowel obstruction
Other	Ruptured ectopic pregnancy, alcohol use disorder, *renal failure* (amylase is renally cleared)

Watch Out

In patients with hemorrhagic pancreatitis, the initial hematocrit is *not* a good indicator of blood loss. The hematocrit may take 1–2 days to equilibrate. In addition, if the patient is severely volume-depleted, it may lead to hemoconcentration, giving a falsely elevated or normal hematocrit.

What Is the Diagnostic Imaging of Choice on Admission for Acute Pancreatitis?

Right upper quadrant ultrasound. Since the most common cause of acute pancreatitis is gallstones, this is the first etiology that should be ruled out.

What Are the Classic Abdominal X-Ray Findings in Acute Pancreatitis?

A sentinel loop (dilated loops of proximal small bowel in the left upper quadrant near the pancreas) and colon cutoff sign (distended proximal colon with abrupt collapse in the left upper quadrant at the splenic flexure). Both are due to local ileus (paralyzed, nonmotile bowel) as a result of the pancreatic inflammation.

Watch Out

The delayed development of an ileus in a patient with pancreatitis or following trauma may indicate retroperitoneal bleeding.

What Is the Classic Chest X-Ray Finding in Acute Pancreatitis? How Does This Finding Influence Prognosis?

A pleural effusion, classically on the left side. In patients with severe pancreatitis, nearly 85% have evidence of pleural effusion on admission. In contrast, only 15% of patients with mild pancreatitis have a pleural effusion on plain films upon admission. This finding is strongly associated with severe pancreatitis.

What Is the Role of Abdominal CT Scan on Admission?

A routine CT scan is not generally necessary on admission in most patients with pancreatitis. The Atlanta criteria establish the diagnosis without the need for imaging, and the initial CT scan does not change management in the vast majority of cases. Though CT scan can help distinguish between mild and severe pancreatitis, clinical criteria are equally useful in making this distinction. One exception is the patient who presents with diffuse peritonitis. Severe pancreatitis can mimic an acute surgical abdomen, so a CT is useful to rule out other etiologies.

What Is the Role of Abdominal CT Scan during Subsequent Hospitalization?

If the patient is not clinically improving after several days of conservative management, CT scan is helpful as it may explain the lack of improvement (such as whether there is pancreatic necrosis). Beyond the first week, CT scan is helpful in the situation where a patient develops worsening abdominal pain, fever, and sepsis, as it may demonstrate a pseudocyst or a pancreatic abscess (these local complications do not manifest on admission) (Figs. 20.2, 20.3, and 20.4).

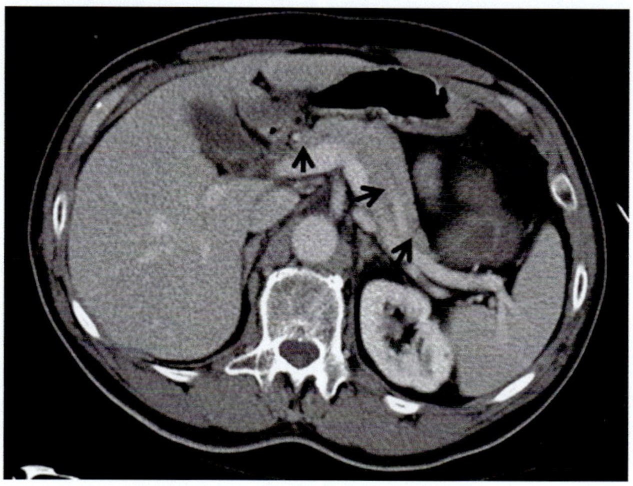

Fig. 20.2 Axial CT with a normal-appearing pancreas (*black arrows: normal pancreas*)

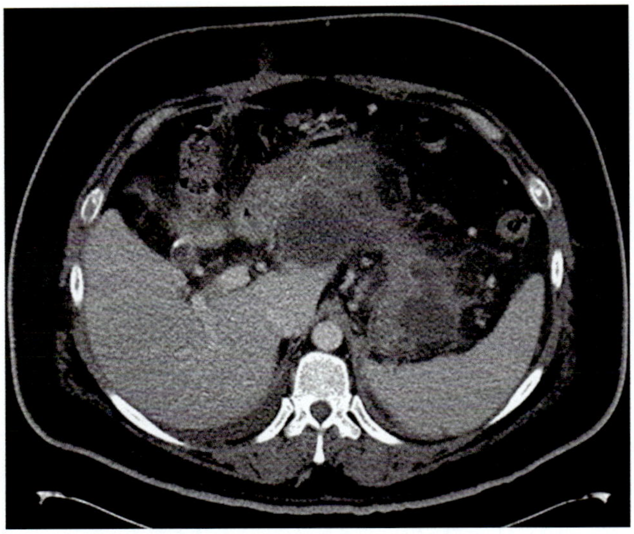

Fig. 20.3 Axial CT scan with peripancreatic fluid collections exhibiting thick irregular walls and marked fat stranding, consistent with abscesses

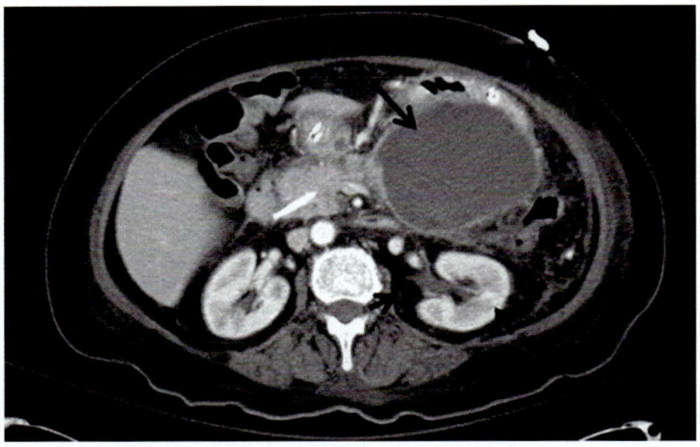

Fig. 20.4 Axial CT scan showing a thin-walled peripancreatic fluid collection consistent with pancreatic pseudocyst

What Is the Role of Urgent ERCP in Gallstone Pancreatitis?

Urgent ERCP is not routinely indicated in gallstone pancreatitis and is reserved for cases where there is clinical suspicion of concomitant acute cholangitis, such as the presence of fever, jaundice, and abnormal liver function tests. In the absence of cholangitis or ongoing biliary obstruction (as defined by a total bilirubin >4 mg/dL and a dilated CBD), ERCP offers no benefit and may increase the risk of procedure-related complications, including pancreatitis. When ERCP is necessary, administration of rectal indomethacin prior to the procedure has been shown to reduce the risk of post-ERCP pancreatitis.

Management

What Is the Initial Treatment for Acute Pancreatitis?

Treatment is supportive, and patients are managed conservatively with vigorous intravenous fluid resuscitation, NPO, and analgesics. Routine nasogastric tube decompression is not recommended (only if there is ongoing vomiting). Similarly, routine use of antibiotics is not recommended as pancreatitis is an inflammatory response, not an infection. The majority of patients' symptoms resolve within 3–5 days with this management.

What Is the Subsequent Management Plan? And How Does This Differ Between Gallstone and Alcoholic Pancreatitis?

If gallstones were found on presentation (and there is no history of alcohol abuse), a cholecystectomy should be performed during the same hospitalization because recurrent gallstone pancreatitis risk is high within 30 days. The timing of surgery depends on pancreatitis severity. Amylase and lipase levels should *not* influence timing of surgery. If alcohol is the etiology, counsel the patient on alcohol cessation, and provide referral for support groups.

How Does the Severity of Acute Pancreatitis Affect Management?

Pancreatitis severity assists in triage to a ward (mild pancreatitis) or monitored step-down or ICU bed (moderately severe or severe pancreatitis). If severe pancreatitis is predicted, it raises awareness to monitor the patient closely for local and/or systemic complications. For gallstone pancreatitis, it assists in determining timing of cholecystectomy: early (within 48–72 hours) for mild pancreatitis versus delayed (weeks later after complete resolution) for moderately severe or severe pancreatitis.

What Is the Management Algorithm for Acute Pancreatitis? It Is Shown in ◘ Fig. 20.5

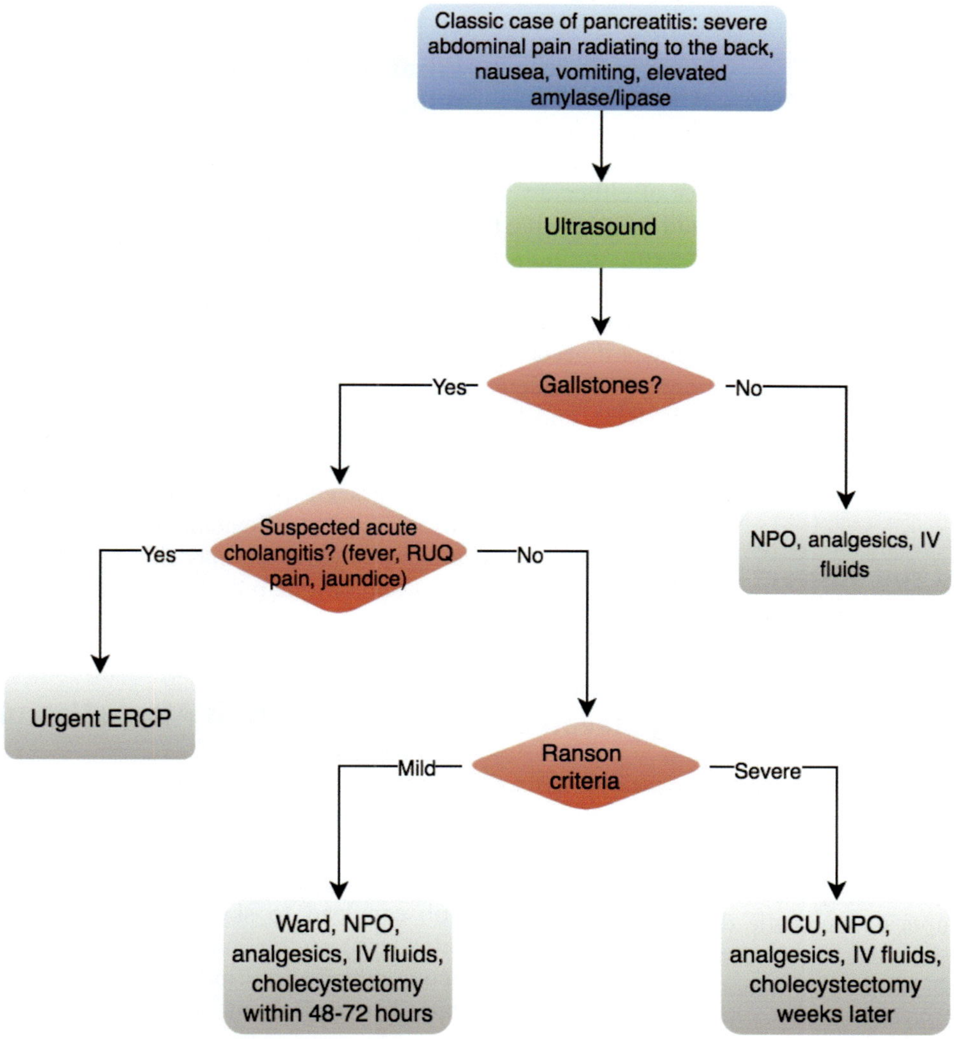

◘ **Fig. 20.5** Management algorithm for acute pancreatitis (based on the practice guidelines from the American College of Gastroenterology)

Special Situations

What Should You Suspect If a Patient with Severe Acute Pancreatitis Develops a Fever and Leukocytosis 4 Weeks into the Hospitalization?

This presentation is concerning a pancreatic abscess. The first step is to order a CT scan with contrast looking for necrotic tissue (i.e., areas that do not enhance) or a pancreatic abscess. If you find evidence of either, a CT or ultrasound-guided aspiration should be performed and sent for culture. If infection is present, antibiotics are administered. Infected pancreatic necrosis and pancreatic abscesses require surgical debridement using a step-up approach (sequential additional steps if needed): (1) percutaneous or endoscopic drainage, (2) video-assisted retroperitoneal debridement (VARD), and (3) open necrosectomy. These procedures are termed external drainage.

What Should You Suspect If a Patient with a Recent Hospitalization for Pancreatitis Comes in 6 Weeks Later with Vague Abdominal Pain, a Palpable Epigastric Mass, and Persistently Elevated Serum Amylase?

A pancreatic pseudocyst, a collection of pancreatic fluid surrounded by a wall without epithelium. It results from pancreatic injury such as pancreatitis or trauma, which essentially disrupts a pancreatic duct. The pancreatic enzymatic fluid that leaks out is contained by surrounding fibrotic tissue. Although this most commonly appears in patients with chronic pancreatitis, it can also occur in the weeks following resolution of an acute pancreatitis. Patients often present with vague abdominal pain, elevated serum amylase, and possibly a palpable epigastric mass. The diagnostic test of choice is a CT scan, and most can be managed conservatively. Predictors of failure for conservative management include pseudocysts larger than 6 cm or those that have persisted for more than 6 weeks. Treatment of a symptomatic, noninfected pseudocyst that fails to resolve is usually via *internal drainage*, by creating a connection between the cyst and the adjacent intestinal organ, usually the stomach (endoscopic cystogastrostomy). External drainage is not recommended as this may create a pancreatico-cutaneous fistula. A pseudocyst can erode into arteries, leading to a pseudoaneurysm and upper GI bleed (managed with angiographic embolization).

> **Watch Out**
> Pancreatic cysts in the absence of a history of pancreatitis should raise suspicion for a neoplasm; biopsy should be considered.

What Are the Complications of Chronic Pancreatitis?

Patients may develop *diabetes mellitus* secondary to the destruction of beta-islet insulin-producing cells in the pancreas caused by chronic inflammation. This type of diabetes is termed *type-3 diabetes* and is very difficult to treat, and most patients require insulin. Patients may also develop *steatorrhea* due to poor absorption (particularly of fats and fat-soluble vitamins) from the digestive tract. These patients require pancreatic enzyme supplementation. Most patients also complain of severe and persistent *chronic pain*. Cross-sectional imaging such as CT often reveals pancreatic atrophy and parenchymal calcifications. MR cholangiopancreatography (MRCP) may show a nondilated pancreatic duct and can help exclude intraductal stones or strictures.

Acute Pancreatitis After a Vascular Procedure

Although rare, patients who undergo an endovascular procedure are at risk of atheroemboli (cholesterol embolism) dislodged by wires or stents. Cholesterol atheroemboli can lead to skin changes (e.g., blue toe, livedo reticularis) and/or gastrointestinal complications (e.g., acute pancreatitis, mesenteric ischemia). Pancreatitis can also result from ischemia (such as after being on heart bypass). Acute pancreatitis that results from uncorrectable causes such as atheroembolism and ischemia should be managed with supportive treatment (e.g., IV fluids, analgesia).

What Is the Most Common Indication for Surgical Management in Chronic Pancreatitis?

The most common indication for surgical intervention is *persistent and severe pain*. The reason why chronic inflammation leads to constant pain is not fully understood, but the mechanism proposed includes nerve injury in the pancreatic head. Nonoperative management, providing temporary pain relief, includes placement of a stent in the pancreatic duct, allowing for improved anterograde flow of pancreatic juices. For definitive treatment, the Puestow procedure (lateral pancreaticojejunostomy) is performed, in which the pancreatic duct is opened all the way from the head to the tail and sutured into the jejunum, allowing the free flow of pancreatic juices into the small intestine.

What Are Less Common Vascular Complications of Pancreatitis?

One uncommon complication of pancreatitis is splenic vein thrombosis, which occurs due to local inflammation and compression by surrounding pancreatic edema or pseudocyst. Diagnosis is typically made by contrast-enhanced CT or MR venography. Management is based on symptoms; anticoagulation is controversial and typically reserved for patients with thrombus extension. Splenic vein thrombosis in the long term leads to impaired venous drainage of the spleen which is forced to drain via the short gastric veins. This in turn causes gastric varices to form which may cause upper gastrointestinal bleeding. Such GI bleeding may be treated with splenectomy which removes the pressure on the short gastric veins.

Areas of Controversy

Is Urgent ERCP Beneficial for Severe Pancreatitis?

Only if there is suspicion of concomitant cholangitis. Studies have failed to consistently show benefit in using urgent ERCP in the absence of cholangitis. This may be a result of ERCP having a 5% risk of causing pancreatitis, related to overinjection of contrast medium into pancreatic ducts, and due to the fact that the majority of gallstones pass into the duodenum spontaneously.

Should Prophylactic Antibiotics Be Administered for Severe Acute Pancreatitis?

There is no role of antibiotics for mild pancreatitis, as the disease is due to inflammation, not infection. Patients with severe pancreatitis have increased mortality as a result of subsequent infections, justifying a possible role of prophylactic antibiotics, anecdotally supported by its use in clinical practice over the past several decades. However, its role has been scrutinized by multiple studies in recent years, with most concluding that there is no decrease in mortality with prophylactic antibiotics.

Areas Where You Can Get in Trouble

Missing Hypercalcemia as the Cause of Pancreatitis

In the absence of gallstones and alcohol abuse, the etiology of acute pancreatitis may be elusive. In a patient with hyperparathyroidism or hypertension controlled with hydrochlorothiazide, consider hypercalcemia as the etiology. Hydrochlorothiazide increases calcium reabsorption in the distal convoluted tubule. Hypercalcemia leads to a secretory block in the pancreatic duct. While *hyper*calcemia can cause pancreatitis, pancreatitis can cause *hypo*calcemia. Inflammation generates free fatty acids that avidly chelate insoluble calcium salts in the pancreatic bed, resulting in hypocalcemia. Thus, the predisposing hypercalcemia may be missed.

Pseudohyponatremia in Pancreatitis

In cases of hyperlipidemic pancreatitis, pseudohyponatremia may be observed. This occurs due to displacement of plasma water by elevated lipids, resulting in an artifactually low sodium measurement. True serum sodium is usually normal.

Nutritional Support

If patients require being NPO greater than 7 days, nutritional support is needed. *Enteral nutrition* (not parenteral) is preferred, with the feeding tube placed past the ligament of Treitz to avoid activation of the pancreas.

Whipple (Pancreaticoduodenectomy)

It is shown in ◘ Fig. 20.6,

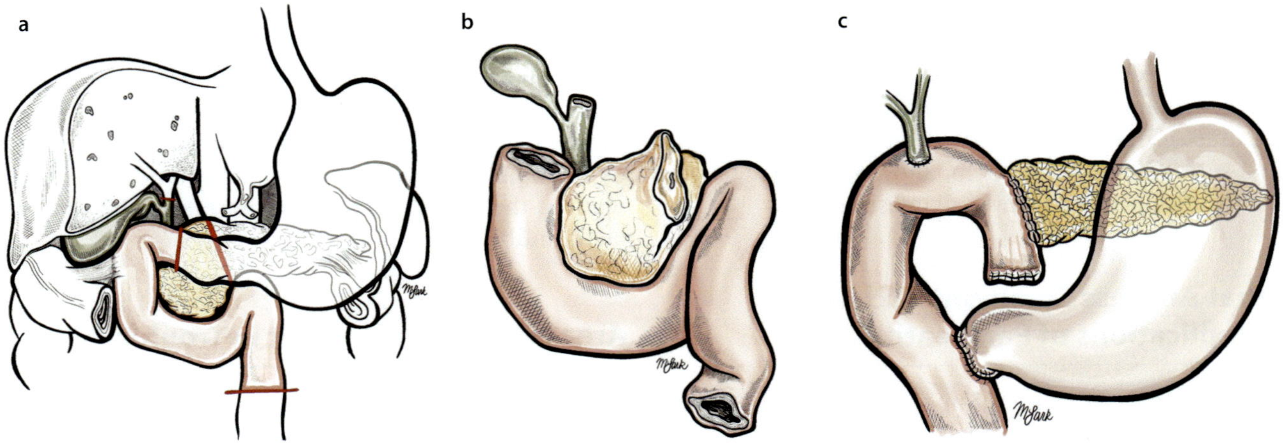

Fig. 20.6 **Whipple procedure:** This procedure involves the division of four structures: the stomach/duodenum, CBD, pancreatic neck, and jejunum (**a**). The surgical specimen contains the duodenum, gallbladder, CBD, and the head of the pancreas (**b**). Reconstruction involves three new connections: a pancreaticojejunostomy, a gastrojejunostomy, and a hepaticojejunostomy (**c**)

Summary of Essentials

History and Physical

- Epigastric pain radiating to the back, often worsened by food, is the hallmark of acute pancreatitis.
- Nonsurgical conditions that mimic an acute abdomen: gastroenteritis, acute adrenal insufficiency, sickle cell crisis, diabetic ketoacidosis, acute porphyria, pelvic inflammatory disease, kidney stones, acute pancreatitis, and pyelonephritis.
- Patients with pancreatitis typically present with epigastric pain radiating to the back, nausea, vomiting, anorexia, fever, and tachycardia.

Pathophysiology

- Pancreatitis begins with inappropriate activation of pancreatic enzymes causing autodigestion, inflammation, and vascular injury.
- Gallstones and alcohol are the most common causes. Other etiologies can be remembered with the mnemonic "GET SMASHED."

20

Diagnosis

- Most cases can be diagnosed with just a history, physical, and abnormal amylase/lipase.
- Most cases do not require CT imaging on admission if the diagnosis is clear clinically and with labs.
- Elevated ALT >3× normal is highly suggestive of gallstone pancreatitis.

Workup

- Amylase/lipase levels do not correlate with severity of pancreatitis.
- Right upper quadrant ultrasound is the initial imaging test of choice to evaluate for gallstones.

Management

- Patients should initially be managed conservatively with IV fluids, NPO, and narcotic analgesia.
- Cholecystectomy is indicated for gallstone pancreatitis: early for mild disease, delayed for moderately severe or severe disease.
- ERCP is only indicated for suspected cholangitis or persistent biliary obstruction.

Complications

- Early (first week): systemic inflammatory response, multiorgan failure.
- Late (after three weeks): pancreatic necrosis, abscess, or pseudocyst.
- Pseudocysts that are large (>6 cm), persistent (>6 weeks), or symptomatic may require endoscopic drainage.
- Chronic pancreatitis may result in exocrine insufficiency (steatorrhea), diabetes mellitus (type 3c), and chronic pain.

Suggested Reading

Aboulian A, Chan T, Yaghoubian A, Kaji AH, Putnam B, Neville A, de Virgilio C. Early cholecystectomy safely decreases hospital stay in patients with mild gallstone pancreatitis: a randomized prospective study. Ann Surg. 2010;251(4):615–9.

Banks PA, Bollen TL, Dervenis C, Gooszen HG, et al. Classification of acute pancreatitis—2012: revision of the Atlanta classification and definitions by international consensus. Gut. 2013;62(1):102–11.

Chang L, Lo S, Stabile BE, Lewis RJ, Toosie K, et al. Preoperative versus postoperative endoscopic retrograde cholangiopancreatography in mild to moderate gallstone pancreatitis: a prospective randomized trial. Ann Surg. 2000;231(1):82.

Uhl W, Warshaw A, Imrie C, Bassi C, et al. IAP guidelines for the surgical management of acute pancreatitis. Pancreatology. 2003;3(2):565–73.

McDermott, J., Kao, L.S., Keeley, J.A., Nahmias, J. and de Virgilio, C., 2024. Management of gallstone pancreatitis: a review. JAMA surgery, 159(7), pp.818–825.

New Onset of Painless Jaundice

James McDermott, James X. Wu, Christian de Virgilio, Matthew Y. C. Lin, and Danielle M. Hari

Contents

C. de Virgilio, A. Grigorian (eds.), *Surgery*, https://doi.org/10.1007/978-3-032-09799-6_21

Case Study

A 68-year-old woman presents to the emergency department, complaining of fatigue and intermittent vague abdominal pain. She denies nausea or vomiting but "does not have much of an appetite these days." She reports unintentionally losing almost 20 lbs. in the past two months. She was recently diagnosed with type 2 diabetes, but she had no other medical problems and no previous surgeries. Her stools have become lighter in color, and her urine is much darker than before. Her social history is negative for alcohol use, but she had a 50+ pack-year smoking history before quitting last year. She has no significant family history. On exam, she has a yellow hue to her eyes and tongue, along with scratch marks on her skin. A non-tender mass is palpated in the right upper quadrant (RUQ) of the abdomen. Laboratory testing reveals total and direct bilirubin of 18 mg/dl (normal 0.2–1.3 mg/dl) and 9.2 mg/dl (<0.3 mg/dl), respectively, and alkaline phosphatase (ALP) of 215 μ/L (33–131 μ/L). Aspartate aminotransferase (AST) and alanine aminotransferase (ALT) are mildly elevated. CA 19-9 and CEA levels are normal.

Diagnosis

What Is the Differential Diagnosis of Jaundice? (Table 21.1)

Table 21.1 Differential diagnosis of painless jaundice

Condition		Comments
Prehepatic (hemolytic)	Hemolytic anemia	Pallor, fatigue, shortness of breath
	Gilbert's syndrome	Benign condition triggered by overexertion, dehydration, menstruation, concurrent illness, surgery; decreased activity of the enzyme UDP-glucuronyl transferase
	Crigler–Najjar syndrome	Absent (type 1) or severely decreased (type 2) activity of the enzyme UDP-glucuronyl transferase; type 1 associated with kernicterus; requires phototherapy, early referral for liver transplant
Hepatic (hepatocellular)	Ischemic liver injury	May result from transient hypotension and hypoxia, or trauma, or in a transplanted donor liver; marked rise in ALT and AST
	Viral	Virus infects hepatocytes; anorexia, nausea, vomiting; aminotransferases >25× upper limit of normal; may progress to acute liver failure, become a chronic infection, or completely resolve
	Toxic ingestion	Acetaminophen, alcohol (AST:ALT ratio > 2), and iron overload can cause acute liver failure
	Nonalcoholic fatty liver disease	Often asymptomatic; hepatic steatosis, metabolic syndrome, AST:ALT ratio < 1
	Primary biliary cirrhosis	Autoimmune process, skin xanthomas, associated with rheumatoid arthritis or Sjogren's syndrome; antimitochondrial antibody
	Primary sclerosing cholangitis	Associated with ulcerative colitis, fatigue, pruritus, p-ANCA
	Hepatolenticular degeneration (Wilson's disease)	Autosomal recessive, retention of copper, Kayser-Fleischer ring (brown ring on the edge of the iris), cirrhosis, and neurologic manifestations, including parkinsonism
	Cirrhosis	Hyperestrinism (gynecomastia, testicular atrophy, decreased body hair, spider angiomas, palmar erythema), portal hypertension (esophageal varices, splenomegaly, ascites, caput medusae, anorectal varices), hepatic synthetic dysfunction (ecchymoses, edema, hydrothorax)
	Rotor syndrome	Benign condition of decreased bile transport and uptake by the liver; otherwise normal LFTs; manifests after birth or childhood
	Dubin Johnson	Benign condition of decreased hepatic bile excretion; associated with black liver pigmentation; manifests in adolescents or young adults

(continued)

Table 21.1 (continued)

Condition		Comments
Posthepatic	Choledocholithiasis	Gallstone (from the gallbladder) enters the common bile duct (CBD), causing obstruction, RUQ pain, and nausea
	Acute cholangitis	Ascending infection of the CBD often caused by gallstone obstruction; fever, jaundice, RUQ pain, ± hypotension, ± altered mental status
	Chronic pancreatitis	May cause biliary stricture, recurrent epigastric pain, and malabsorption
	Mirizzi syndrome	RUQ pain due to external compression of the common hepatic duct by a large gallstone in the gallbladder or cystic duct
	Pancreatic carcinoma	Painless jaundice is more common in carcinomas arising from the head of the pancreas; new onset diabetes may precede diagnosis of cancer; poor prognosis
	Ampullary carcinoma	Malignancy arising from the ampulla of Vater; the most common presentation is painless obstructive jaundice
	Cholangiocarcinoma	Associated with sclerosing cholangitis, chronic parasitic infections, and malignancy of the bile ducts, usually present at an advanced stage, highly lethal
	Biliary atresia	Obstructive jaundice, pale stool, hepatosplenomegaly, dark urine in a neonate; failure of the normal development of the biliary tree; surgical treatment with hepaticoportoenterostomy (Kasai procedure) or liver transplant

What Is the Most Likely Diagnosis?

In a former smoker presenting with new onset of painless jaundice accompanied by constitutional symptoms of malignancy (e.g., weight loss), pancreatic cancer is the most likely diagnosis. This is further supported by Courvoisier's sign. New onset of type 2 diabetes in an older patient is associated with pancreatic cancer. Additionally, elevated levels of direct bilirubin and alkaline phosphatase further support the diagnosis.

History and Physical

What Is Courvoisier's Sign?

It is the presence of a palpable RUQ mass, which represents a non-tender, chronically enlarged gallbladder. It signifies obstruction, most often of the distal common bile duct, causing the biliary tree and the gallbladder to markedly distend slowly over time, and is most commonly seen with malignancy (pancreatic, ampullary, or biliary).

What Is the Implication of Painful Versus Painless Jaundice?

Painful jaundice is usually due to gallstones. Painless jaundice suggests a malignancy or autoimmune disease of the biliary system.

What Is Migratory Thrombophlebitis?

Also called Trousseau's sign, migratory thrombophlebitis is the development of superficial vein thromboses in multiple extremities. It results from the hypercoagulable state associated with malignancy, most often pancreatic adenocarcinoma (as well as lung cancer). It involves localized tenderness and subsequent erythema along superficial veins of the trunk and extremities. This should not be confused with *necrolytic migratory erythema,* which is a rash on the lower abdomen or perineum and is associated with glucagonomas.

Watch Out

Trousseau's sign is also a term used to describe an exam finding for hypocalcemia (tetany in the hand with inflation of a blood pressure cuff above systolic pressure for 3 minutes).

What Are the Risk Factors for Pancreatic Cancer? Cholangiocarcinoma? Gallbladder Carcinoma?

Risk factors for pancreatic cancer include chronic pancreatitis (the strongest risk factor), smoking, tobacco, high-fat diet, obesity, male sex, and family history. While the recent onset of type 2 diabetes is also associated with pancreatic cancer, it is difficult to discern whether it is a risk factor or an early symptom of the disease. Patients with ulcerative colitis, especially with primary sclerosing cholangitis, are at increased risk for developing bile duct malignancy. Choledocholithiasis, particularly when associated with parasites, is considered a risk factor for bile duct cancer. Long-standing gallstone disease is associated with carcinoma of the gallbladder.

What Is a Sister Mary Joseph Nodule? And What Is the Implication?

This is an umbilical nodule suggestive of carcinomatosis and is most commonly associated with gastric cancer but may represent any metastatic lesion from an intra-abdominal cancer. It was named after Dr. William Mayo's surgical assistant, who noted the nodes when prepping the abdomen of patients with gastric cancer who were found to have widespread metastasis once the abdomen was explored.

Pathophysiology

What Causes Jaundice?

Jaundice can be caused by excess serum bilirubin due to hemolysis or impaired metabolism/excretion from the liver into the intestines. Jaundice becomes apparent at approximately bilirubin >2.5 mg/dl.

Why Is some Jaundice Painless and some Painful?

In cases of chronic obstruction of the distal common bile duct or pancreatic duct (malignancy), back-pressure gradually dilates the proximal biliary tree and slowly stretches bile ducts, the gallbladder, and Glisson's capsule, which encases the liver. This gradual stretching allows the capsule to accommodate the distention without causing pain, resulting in painless jaundice. In contrast, with acute obstruction, such as from a gallstone, the sudden stretching of bile ducts, the gallbladder, and/or Glisson's capsule triggers pain, combined with the associated infection/inflammation.

What Is the Metabolism of Bilirubin?

Bilirubin is the product of heme degradation. Breakdown of red blood cells occurs in the spleen, liver, and intravascular space. Initially, bilirubin is unconjugated (hydrophobic) and bound to albumin. Bilirubin is conjugated in the liver, becoming water-soluble, and excreted into the duodenum. Intestinal bacteria convert conjugated bilirubin into urobilinogen, which can be reabsorbed into the systemic circulation, converted to urobilin, and excreted in the urine. Urobilin gives urine its yellow color. The remaining intestinal urobilinogen is converted to stercobilin and excreted in the stool. In direct hyperbilirubinemia, the bilirubin is excreted in the urine, making it appear much darker or "Coca-Cola colored."

What Is the Mechanism behind "Clay-Colored" Stools?

Stool derives its brown color from stercobilin, a final product of bilirubin metabolism in the intestine. Biliary obstruction decreases bilirubin in the intestines, decreasing stercobilin and resulting in the "clay-colored" stool.

Workup

In a Patient with Obstructive Jaundice, What Would the Typical Laboratory Findings be?

Conjugated/direct bilirubin, and consequently total bilirubin, will be increased in obstructive jaundice. Oftentimes unconjugated/indirect bilirubin will also be elevated in obstructive jaundice, as the impaired forward flow limits hepatic uptake and glucuronidation of indirect bilirubin. Urine urobilinogen is decreased. ALP level will also be elevated, indicating bile duct obstruction.

> **Watch Out**
> Obstructive jaundice will often present with increased conjugated and unconjugated bilirubin. If conjugated bilirubin is greater than 20% of total bilirubin, suspect a posthepatic cause of jaundice.

How Do you Distinguish Between Jaundice from Biliary Obstruction (Posthepatic) and Hepatocellular Damage?

Hepatic causes of jaundice (such as hepatocellular injury from hepatitis) are usually nonsurgical problems, whereas posthepatic causes (such as biliary obstruction from acute cholangitis) are typically surgical. Distinguishing between the two is not always straightforward. Both will have some degree of elevation in total bilirubin, AST, ALT, gamma-glutamyl transpeptidase (GGT), and ALP. AST and ALT are enzymes within the liver cells (though AST is also found in muscle and other cells). With hepatocellular injury, these enzymes are released. As such, with hepatic causes, the AST and ALT (transaminases) can sometimes reach into the thousands and rise out of proportion to the ALP. Such a disproportionate rise in the transaminases is indicative of hepatocellular damage, as seen in acute viral hepatitis, ischemic liver injury, or toxic insult. ALP is present in the cells that line the bile ducts. A marked rise in ALP, out of proportion to the AST and ALT, is therefore indicative of posthepatic (biliary obstruction) pathology such as tumors or choledocholithiasis. Since ALP levels increase with many other diseases (such as bone pathology), a concomitant and proportionate rise in GGT is helpful, as it is more specific to liver disease.

What Initial Imaging Is Recommended?

The initial test (◘ Fig. 21.1) should be an RUQ ultrasound. Ultrasound is useful to detect dilation of the biliary tree, which, combined with the appropriate laboratory values, confirms the presence of obstructive jaundice. It will also detect gallstones. If gallstones are found in the presence of painful jaundice, ultrasound is more likely to be the definitive study. With painless jaundice, further imaging is needed, as an ultrasound may not detect or adequately delineate the tumor.

What Is the Next Recommended Imaging Choice for Painless Jaundice?

For painless jaundice, since the suspicion for malignancy is high, the next study of choice is a "triple-phase" abdominal CT scan, which includes (1) arterial phase, (2) early venous phase, and (3) late venous phase. A classic imaging finding for pancreatic head cancer is the "double duct sign," which refers to the simultaneous dilatation of both the pancreatic duct and the common bile duct, as the cancer obstructs both. CT imaging not only detects pancreatic/periampullary masses, but importantly, it identifies whether the mass is invading adjacent arteries and veins, which determines the resectability of the mass.

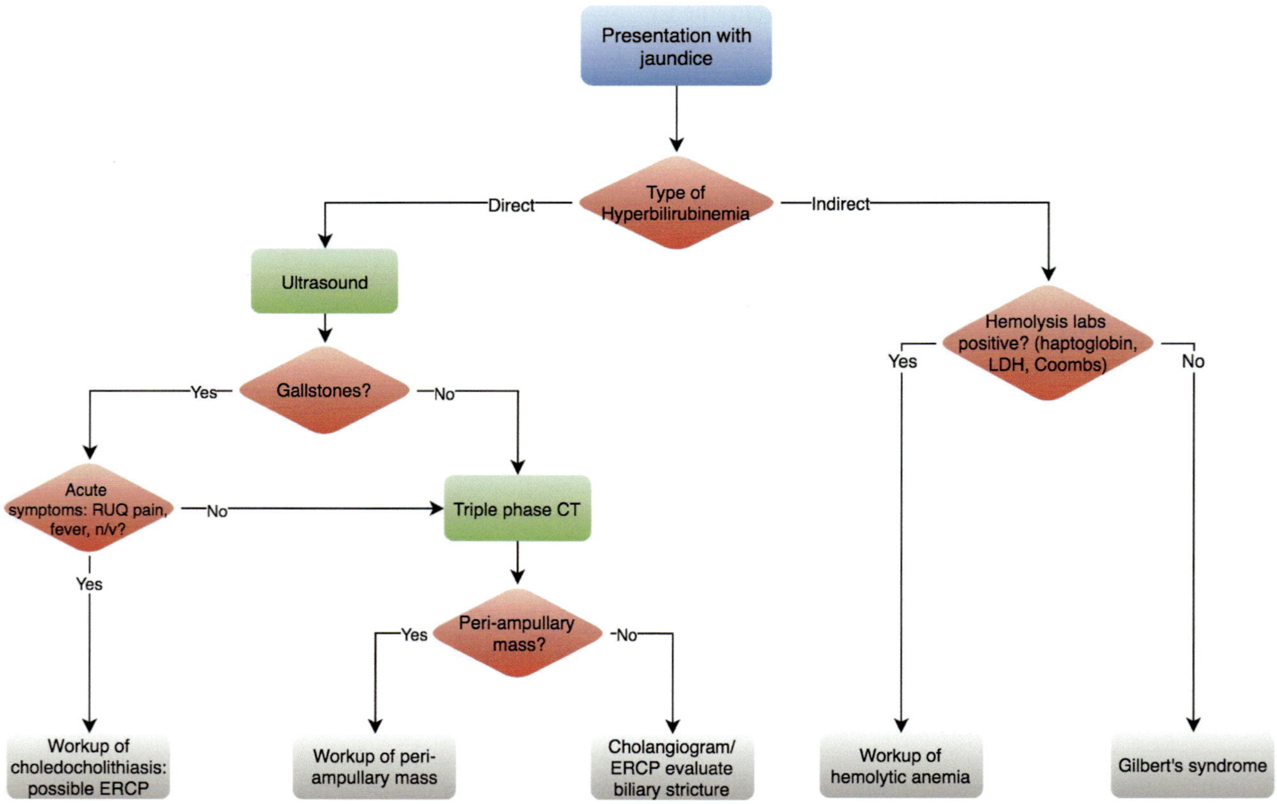

◘ **Fig. 21.1** Algorithm for presentation of jaundice

21

What Three Categories Are Used with Respect to the Resectability of Pancreatic Cancer?

There are three surgical categorizations for pancreatic cancer: resectable, borderline resectable, and unresectable. Only about 15–20% of patients present with surgically resectable disease. It is considered unresectable if there is distant metastasis or it is locally invading or encasing local arteries (superior mesenteric artery, hepatic artery, or celiac trunk). Partial invasion of the veins (portal or superior mesenteric vein) is still potentially resectable (with partial vein excision and vein grafting). Differentiating further between these three categories is beyond the scope of this book.

Is a Biopsy of a Suspected Pancreatic Cancer Necessary in all Cases?

It depends on whether the tumor is thought to be clearly resectable or not. In cases where it is resectable, surgery is generally pursued without a confirmatory tissue biopsy, as (1) biopsies can have false negatives due to sampling error, and (2) the fact that the tumor is obstructing the bile duct means that resection is required and that it is highly likely to be cancer. If the tumor is borderline resectable, a tissue biopsy is required, as neoadjuvant therapy is typically given first. This biopsy not only confirms the diagnosis but also provides important information for oncology and radiology teams to determine the optimal treatment regimen based on molecular and genetic testing. A tissue biopsy is generally performed with endoscopic ultrasound (EUS) guidance using a core needle, which offers superior diagnostic accuracy compared to fine-needle aspiration (FNA), though FNA remains an acceptable alternative when necessary.

What Is the Role of Magnetic Resonance Cholangiopancreatography (MRCP) and/or Endoscopic Retrograde Cholangiopancreatography (ERCP)?

MRCP and ERCP are not routinely needed. They are used selectively to further assess the biliary tree when a mass is not visualized, and the cause of biliary obstruction remains unclear. ERCP can also provide therapeutic intervention, such as stent placement or biliary decompression, if needed. In cases where the clinical history, physical examination, and initial CT imaging indicate resectable pancreatic cancer with no local or distant metastasis, no additional diagnostic workup is required.

What Is the Role of Tumor Markers CA 19-9 and Carcinoembryonic Antigen (CEA)?

CA 19-9 and CEA are not suitable as screening tools for the early detection of pancreatic cancer due to insufficient sensitivity and specificity. However, both markers can be elevated in pancreatic cancer, so they are measured when a pancreatic mass is identified. CEA may also be elevated in other malignancies, including colorectal, breast, lung, ovarian, and prostate cancers, as well as in certain benign conditions like smoking and inflammatory bowel disease. CA 19-9 levels may rise in benign biliary obstruction as well. Extreme elevation of these tumor markers may be associated with advanced disease, and a decline in the markers can indicate a response to treatment.

Management

What Is the Role of Preoperative Stenting in the Presence of a Pancreatic Mass with Obstructive Jaundice?

The need for biliary stenting depends on the planned oncologic treatment approach. For patients with pancreatic or periampullary cancers who are candidates for upfront surgery, routine biliary decompression (via ERCP and stenting) is not recommended, as it does not provide additional benefit and is associated with a higher rate of postoperative infectious complications. Stenting should be reserved for patients with severe symptoms of obstructive jaundice (e.g., intense pruritus) or evidence of sepsis from cholangitis. Stenting is also performed when neoadjuvant therapy is planned, as the hepatotoxic effects of chemotherapy are exacerbated with obstructive jaundice.

What Is the Role of Neoadjuvant Therapy for Pancreatic Adenocarcinoma?

Neoadjuvant chemoradiation can make as many as one-third of initially "borderline resectable" pancreatic cancers resectable, with the same expected survival as patients with initially resectable disease.

What Is the Surgical Management of Pancreatic Head (or Periampullary) Cancer?

The traditional surgical intervention for pancreatic head cancer has been a pancreaticoduodenectomy, also known as the Whipple procedure. This is best thought of in two stages: resection and re-anastomosis. The first stage involves resection of the head of the pancreas (pancreatectomy), duodenum (duodenectomy), proximal jejunum (jejunectomy), distal stomach (partial gastrectomy), gallbladder (cholecystectomy), and distal common bile duct. The second stage involves three anastomoses to the jejunum: pancreas to jejunum (pancreaticojejunostomy), common hepatic duct to jejunum (hepaticojejunostomy), and proximal stomach to jejunum (gastrojejunostomy).

Why Must the Duodenum Be Removed When Surgically Resecting a Pancreatic Head Tumor?

The pancreas and the duodenum share the same blood supply (the pancreaticoduodenal arteries). Failure to remove the duodenum would lead to ischemic necrosis of that portion of the intestinal tract.

In Addition to Pancreatic Cancer, for What Other Conditions Is a Whipple Performed?

Cancer of the duodenum, cholangiocarcinoma, and ampullary carcinoma.

What Are the Options for Palliation in Patients Who Are Not Candidates for Pancreatic Resection? (Table 21.2)

Table 21.2 Palliative options

Condition	Options
Chronic abdominal pain	Celiac axis block, palliative external beam radiation
Gastric outlet obstruction	Gastrojejunostomy (allows oral feeding), open gastrostomy tube placement, or percutaneous gastrostomy tube
Symptomatic biliary obstruction	ERCP with biliary stenting (preferable), percutaneous cholecystostomy (may not adequately drain the biliary tree), or hepaticojejunostomy (most invasive)

What Is the Most Common Complication that Is Specific to a Whipple/Pancreatectomy? What Are Some Other Pancreas Surgery Specific Complications?

Up to 40% of patients suffer a complication after the Whipple procedure. Apart from wound infection, the most common complication is a pancreatic fistula, followed by delayed gastric emptying (gastroparesis) that is best treated with metoclopramide. Other postoperative complications include biliary leaks or fistulas, hemorrhage, malabsorption (loss of pancreatic enzymes), weight loss, and marginal ulceration.

Is There a High Risk of Diabetes After a Whipple Procedure?

The risk of postoperative diabetes is related to preoperative glucose levels. If the patient does not have diabetes preoperatively and has normal glucose levels, the risk of postoperative diabetes is low, as only the pancreatic head is removed.

How Do You Suspect/Diagnose a Postoperative Pancreatic or Biliary Leak?

Patients who undergo resection of the pancreatic head commonly have postoperative drains left in place. Normal drainage is serosanguinous or straw yellow-red in color. High hourly outputs of sanguineous drainage are concerning for hemorrhage. Green fluid suggests a biliary leak. Milky, gray-white fluid with a sheen on the drain bulb suggests a pancreatic leak. To confirm the diagnosis of a pancreatic leak, drain fluid can be sent for fluid amylase, which would be significantly higher than serum levels (drain amylase must be >3x the serum amylase). Most pancreatic leaks stop on their own, provided the collection is adequately drained. Octreotide may assist by reducing pancreatic secretion.

Areas Where You Can Get in Trouble

Increased INR (PT) with Pancreatic Cancer

Bile is necessary for the absorption of vitamin K in the GI tract. Any disease process that leads to prolonged biliary obstruction (such as pancreatic cancer) will cause vitamin K deficiency and therefore a prolonged INR. This can be treated with parenteral vitamin K (if the patient is not actively bleeding) or fresh frozen plasma (if the patient is actively bleeding or needs immediate correction). Keep an eye out for fat-soluble vitamin (A, D, E, K) deficiencies in all patients with prolonged biliary obstructive disease.

Incidental Liver Findings on CT Scan

Hemangioma is the most common benign tumor of the liver and is often asymptomatic. Large (>10 cm) tumors can result in consumptive thrombocytopenia and high-output cardiac failure, particularly in children. *Focal nodular hyperplasia* is found in the periphery of the liver, and the hallmark feature on CT imaging is a hypodense central stellate scar that enhances with contrast. It is often asymptomatic with no risk of rupture or subsequent malignancy. As such, resection is only indicated if a hemangioma or focal nodular hyperplasia is symptomatic (e.g., mass effect). *Hepatic adenomas* typically present in young women taking oral contraceptives. Due to a potential malignant transformation and risk of rupture, most clinicians recommend resection for all hepatic adenomas in males and those greater than 5 cm in females. Acute episodes of bleeding secondary to a ruptured hepatic adenoma should be managed with angioembolization.

Summary of Essentials

History and Physical

- Malignant biliary obstruction suggested by:
  - Insidious onset of jaundice
  - Painless jaundice
  - Tea-colored urine
  - Clay-colored stool

Etiology/Pathophysiology

- Three categories of jaundice:
  - Prehepatic
    - Hemolytic anemia
    - Gilbert's syndrome
  - Hepatic
    - Ischemic liver injury
    - Hepatic viral infection
    - Toxic ingestion
    - Nonalcoholic fatty liver disease
    - Primary biliary cirrhosis
    - Primary sclerosing cholangitis (mixed hepatic and posthepatic)
    - Hepatolenticular degeneration (Wilson's disease)
    - Cirrhosis
  - Posthepatic
    - Choledocholithiasis
    - Acute cholangitis
    - Chronic pancreatitis
    - Mirizzi syndrome
    - Malignant biliary obstruction
  - Most common causes of malignant biliary obstruction:
    - Pancreatic cancer
    - Cholangiocarcinoma
    - Ampullary carcinoma

Diagnosis

- LFTs (total bilirubin [direct/indirect], AST, ALT, ALP)
  - Amylase/lipase to rule out pancreatitis
- Imaging to evaluate for mass/stricture:
  - RUQ ultrasound
  - Triple-phase abdominal CT
  - EUS
- EUS-guided biopsy of mass
  - If planned neoadjuvant chemotherapy
  - Not needed if immediate surgery is planned in the presence of a mass causing obstructive jaundice
- Stenting of the CBD for neoadjuvant chemotherapy or intractable itching from obstructive jaundice
- If a stricture is present in the CBD with no mass
  - +/– FNA, biopsy, ERCP brushings.
- CEA/CA 19-9 if malignancy is suspected; the role is controversial for periampullary and biliary malignancies

Management

- Periampullary masses:
  - Resectable: pancreaticoduodenectomy (pylorus sparing versus traditional)
  - Borderline resectable: consider neoadjuvant chemotherapy and repeat imaging to assess for surgical intervention
  - Unresectable: in the absence of distant metastasis, consider neoadjuvant chemotherapy and repeat imaging to assess for surgical intervention
    - Biliary stent and palliative chemotherapy
    - Palliative surgical bypass (biliary and intestinal)

Watch Out

- Biliary obstruction associated with fever and pain may require urgent/emergent biliary decompression due to concern for cholangitis

Suggested Reading

Ballehaninna UK, Chamberlain RS. The clinical utility of serum CA 19-9 in the diagnosis, prognosis and management of pancreatic adenocarcinoma: an evidence based appraisal. J Gastrointest Oncol. 2012 Jun;3(2):105–93.

Gillen S, et al. Preoperative/neoadjuvant therapy in pancreatic cancer: a systematic review and meta-analysis of response and resection percentages. PLoS Med. 2010;7(4):e1000267.

Kimura Y, et al. Definitions, pathophysiology, and epidemiology of acute cholangitis and cholecystitis: Tokyo guidelines. J Hepato-Biliary-Pancreat Surg. 2007;14(1):15–26.

Maithel SK, et al. Preoperative CA 19–9 and the yield of staging laparoscopy in patients with radiographically resectable pancreatic adenocarcinoma. Ann Surg Oncol. 2008;15(12):3512–20.

Narang AK, et al. Evaluation of adjuvant chemoradiation therapy for ampullary adenocarcinoma: the Johns Hopkins Hospital-Mayo Clinic collaborative study. Radiat Oncol. 2011;6:126.

Neoptolemos JP, et al. Adjuvant chemoradiotherapy and chemotherapy in resectable pancreatic cancer: a randomised controlled trial. Lancet. 2001;358(9293):1576–85.

Neoptolemos JP, et al. Effect of adjuvant chemotherapy with fluorouracil plus folinic acid or gemcitabine vs observation on survival in patients with resected periampullary adenocarcinoma: the ESPAC-3 periampullary cancer randomized trial. JAMA. 2012;308(2):147–56.

Oettle H, et al. Adjuvant chemotherapy with gemcitabine vs observation in patients undergoing curative-intent resection of pancreatic cancer: a randomized controlled trial. JAMA. 2007;297(3):267–77.

Smeenk HG, et al. Long-term survival and metastatic pattern of pancreatic and periampullary cancer after adjuvant chemoradiation or observation: long-term results of EORTC trial 40891. Ann Surg. 2007;246(5):734–40.

Hepatopancreaticobiliary

Question Set: Hepatopancreaticobiliary

Questions

1. A 29-year-old woman is evaluated for intermittent right upper quadrant (RUQ) pain. She has no history of liver disease. She takes oral contraceptive pills and does not drink alcohol. She is afebrile with stable vital signs. Physical exam is unremarkable. Laboratory studies show a normal complete blood count (CBC) and liver panel. An abdominal ultrasound (US) reveals a solitary 6 cm heterogeneously echogenic lesion in the right hepatic lobe. Subsequent contrast-enhanced MRI shows a well-demarcated lesion with early arterial enhancement and washout in the portal venous phase. What is the most appropriate next step in management?
   (A) Discontinue oral contraceptive pills and observe with serial imaging
   (B) Surgical resection of the mass
   (C) Percutaneous biopsy of the lesion
   (D) Begin antiviral therapy and screen for hepatocellular carcinoma
   (E) Measure serum CA 19-9 and CEA levels

2. Which of the following is a risk factor for pancreatic cancer?
   (A) Alcohol
   (B) Smoking
   (C) Prostate cancer in the family
   (D) Malabsorption
   (E) Pancreatic enzyme supplementation

3. A 60-year-old woman arrives to the emergency department with bloody emesis. She has a past medical history significant for hypertension and an episode of severe pancreatitis due to alcohol abuse 1 year ago complicated by splenic vein thrombosis (SVT), and has since developed chronic pancreatitis. Her temperature is 38.5 °C, blood pressure is 110/88 mmHg, and pulse is 88/min. Esophagogastroduodenoscopy (EGD) shows bleeding coming from isolated gastric varices. Which of the following is most likely to successfully treat the bleeding?
   (A) Liver transplantation
   (B) Endoscopic banding of the varices
   (C) Endoscopic sclerotherapy
   (D) Transjugular portosystemic shunt (TIPS)
   (E) Splenectomy

4. A 40-year-old female presents with moderate epigastric abdominal pain. She has a history of intermittent right upper quadrant (RUQ) pain after eating fatty foods. She is afebrile with a heart rate of 100/min and blood pressure of 110/70 mmHg. She has moderate epigastric tenderness to palpation. Laboratory values are significant for a white blood cell (WBC) of $11 \times 10^3/\mu L$ (normal $4.1–10.9 \times 10^3/\mu L$) with 3% bands, total bilirubin of 1.2 mg/dL (0.1–1.2 mg/dL), aspartate transaminase (AST) of 250 μ/L (5–35 μ/L), alanine transaminase (ALT) of 300 μ/L (7–56 μ/L), alkaline phosphatase of 150 μ/L (33–131 μ/L), amylase of 1300 μ/L (30–110 μ/L), and lipase of 1100 μ/L (7–60 μ/L). RUQ ultrasound shows numerous small gallstones, normal gallbladder wall, and a normal common bile duct diameter. On the second hospital day, her pain has resolved; she is afebrile and has a normal heart rate, and her WBC count has normalized. The amylase has decreased to 350 μ/L. Optimal management consists of:
   (A) Proceed with laparoscopic cholecystectomy with intraoperative cholangiogram (IOC)
   (B) Wait until amylase has completely normalized, and then proceed to laparoscopic cholecystectomy with IOC
   (C) Endoscopic retrograde cholangiopancreatography (ERCP), followed by laparoscopic cholecystectomy during the same hospitalization
   (D) Schedule for elective outpatient laparoscopic cholecystectomy with IOC
   (E) ERCP only

5. A 50-year-old diabetic male presents with severe right upper quadrant (RUQ) pain and fevers. On physical examination, his temperature is 38.9 °C, blood pressure is 100/60 mmHg, and heart rate is 120/min. He has severe tenderness to palpation in the RUQ. WBC is $20 \times 10^3/\mu L$ (normal $4.1–10.9 \times 10^3/\mu L$) with 10% bands, total bilirubin is 1.0 mg/dL (0.1–1.2 mg/dL), amylase is 90 μ/L (30–110 μ/L), alkaline phosphatase is 90 μ/L (33–131 μ/L), AST is 110 μ/L (normal 5–35 μ/L), and ALT is 140 μ/L (7–56 μ/L). RUQ ultrasound shows gallstones, a normal common bile duct diameter, and a few gas bubbles within the wall of the gallbladder. Intravenous (IV) fluids and antibiotics are administered. The next step in the management consists of:
   (A) Immediate cholecystectomy
   (B) Admit to ICU for 24–48 h of IV antibiotics and careful monitoring
   (C) Percutaneous cholecystostomy tube
   (D) CT scan of the abdomen
   (E) Endoscopic retrograde cholangiopancreatography (ERCP)

6. A 30-year-old man is admitted to the hospital for severe acute pancreatitis due to alcohol use disorder. His hospital course is complicated by transient renal insufficiency. On hospital day 20, the patient complains of increasing epigastric abdominal pain, nausea, and vomiting. On physical examination, he has a fever of 38.6 °C and a heart rate of 110/min. Abdominal examination reveals marked epigastric tenderness. His lungs are clear bilaterally. WBC count is $14.5 \times 10^3/\mu L$ (normal $4.1–10.9 \times 10^3/\mu L$) with 10% bands. Blood cultures are sent, and fluid bolus is given. What is the next step in management?
   (A) Start IV antibiotics
   (B) CT scan of the abdomen with contrast
   (C) ERCP with sphincterotomy
   (D) Exploratory laparotomy for pancreatic debridement
   (E) Video-assisted retroperitoneal debridement

7. A 65-year-old man presents to the emergency department with RUQ pain. He is diagnosed with acute cholecystitis and undergoes a cholecystectomy the following day. He is discharged shortly after his procedure. Five days later, he arrives back to the emergency department with abdominal pain and low-grade fevers. On physical examination, his blood pressure is 120/70 mmHg, heart rate is 90/min, and temperature is 37.8 °C. He has diffuse mild abdominal tenderness to palpation. His laboratory examination is significant for white blood count of $16.9 \times 10^3/\mu L$ (normal $4.1–10.9 \times 10^3/\mu L$). What is the next best step?
(A) Endoscopic ultrasound
(B) Exploratory laparotomy
(C) CT scan of the abdomen
(D) ERCP with stenting
(E) Hepatobiliary iminodiacetic acid (HIDA) scan

8. A 63-year-old man is admitted to the hospital for alcohol pancreatitis. At 48 h after admission, he manifested four of Ranson's criteria. On hospital day 6, he has increasing epigastric abdominal pain. He denies any vomiting. His temperature is 37.9 °C, blood pressure is 134/74 mmHg, pulse is 89/min, and respirations are 16/min. The abdomen is distended but soft, and there is still significant epigastric tenderness. CT scan is obtained and shows diffuse edema surrounding the pancreas with a pancreatic phlegmon, but no evidence of necrosis. What is the most appropriate approach to his nutritional management?
(A) Continue nothing by mouth (NPO) and intravenous normal saline
(B) Clear liquid diet
(C) Enteral nutrition via nasojejunal feeding tube placed past ligament of Treitz
(D) Parenteral nutrition via central line
(E) Parenteral nutrition via peripheral line

9. A 52-year-old insulin-dependent diabetic man is evaluated for vague epigastric pain, is diagnosed with gastroesophageal reflux disease (GERD), and is treated with proton pump inhibitors with resolution of symptoms. In the course of the workup, however, an abdominal ultrasound was performed. No gallstones were seen, but an incidental single 12 mm polyp was found within the gallbladder. What is the next best step in management?
(A) Laparoscopic cholecystectomy
(B) Open cholecystectomy
(C) Percutaneous gallbladder drainage
(D) Endoscopic ultrasound
(E) Repeat ultrasound in 6 months

10. A 41-year-old man with alcohol use disorder is admitted to the ICU with a diagnosis of severe acute pancreatitis. He requires aggressive fluid resuscitation to maintain his blood pressure in the first 24 h, but over the next 3 days, his blood pressure stabilizes. On the third day of admission, he develops tachypnea, tachycardia, and hypoxia with oxygen saturation to 89%. Central venous pressure (CVP) is 8 mmHg. The patient is placed on nasal cannula, but the oxygen saturation remains the same. His temperature is 37.6 °C, pulse is 104/min, and blood pressure is 129/73 mmHg. A chest X-ray is obtained and shows bilateral infiltrates. Labs are drawn and shown below. What is the most likely diagnosis?
AST: 75 μ/L (normal 5–35 μ/L)
ALT: 92 μ/L (7–56 μ/L)
WBC: $11 \times 103/\mu L$ (normal $4.1–10.9 \times 103/\mu L$)
Arterial blood gas: pH 7.44, $PaO2$ 66 mmHg, $PaCO2$ 36 mmHg
(A) Acute respiratory distress syndrome (ARDS)
(B) Pulmonary embolism

cholangitis). For this reason, the vast majority of asymptomatic gallstones should not receive prophylactic cholecystectomy (A). Prophylactic cholecystectomy might be considered in patients who are planning extended travel to areas without healthcare access (Antarctica in the winter). Even in the diabetic population, it is reasonable to wait to see if symptoms develop. Ursodeoxycholic acid can dissolve gallstones. However, it is completely successful in only about one-third of cases, only for cholesterol stones, is associated with side effects (diarrhea), and is costly (B). In addition, the stones may recur once the medication is stopped. ERCP is an invasive procedure utilized for choledocholithiasis and acute cholangitis (C). Extracorporeal shock wave lithotripsy is effective in breaking the stones into small particles but does not prevent stone recurrence (E). This is more useful in patients presenting with nephrolithiasis (kidney stones).

19. Answer C

A calcified gallbladder is termed *porcelain gallbladder* and is most often found incidentally on imaging for unrelated reasons. Patients are frequently asymptomatic. Porcelain gallbladder has historically been associated with an increased risk of gallbladder adenocarcinoma, but more recent studies suggest that the risk is primarily associated with mucosal or incomplete calcification. In contrast, diffuse intramural calcification may carry a lower risk. Because the imaging often cannot reliably distinguish between mucosal and mural calcification, most clinicians still recommend laparoscopic cholecystectomy for patients with porcelain gallbladder, especially if the calcification is scattered or incomplete. Reassurance or observation with serial imaging is not generally recommended, even in asymptomatic patients, due to the potential for missed malignancy (A–B). There is no role for serum calcium or parathyroid hormone testing (D), and ERCP with brushings is useful for bile duct lesions, not gallbladder pathology (E).

20. Answer C

White opaque drainage from an abdominal drain following a pancreatic resection is concerning for a pancreatic fistula. The first step in working up a postoperative pancreatic fistula is to test the drained fluid for amylase. In addition, serum amylase level should be checked as well. Pancreatic fistula is highly suggested if the drain fluid volume is >50 mL/day and the amylase content is more than three times the normal serum amylase level. In this case, the patient should be made NPO to decrease secretion of pancreatic fluid that accompanies oral intake. Imaging can be done at a later time to evaluate adequacy of drainage (A–B). Octreotide can be given to decrease pancreatic secretions, but it is not used routinely, and there is no evidence-based data that demonstrate cost-effective efficacy of octreotide use in this setting (D). TPN is not routinely needed in this setting (E).

Lower Gastrointestinal

Beverley A. Petrie

Contents

Bright Red Blood per Rectum

Tracey D. Arnell and Beverley A. Petrie

Contents

C. de Virgilio, A. Grigorian (eds.), *Surgery*, https://doi.org/10.1007/978-3-032-09799-6_22

Case Study

A 72-year-old female presents to the emergency department reporting an episode of a large volume of bright red blood per rectum four hours earlier. She states that the toilet was filled with blood. The patient reports that the bleed was painless and was not associated with a bowel movement, and she thinks it stopped about two hours ago. She has never had rectal bleeding before. She denies fevers and chills. A colonoscopy two years ago only demonstrated a few diverticula but no polyps. She has not lost weight recently. Her past medical history is significant for hypertension and chronic constipation. She has had no prior surgery. On physical examination, her blood pressure is 135/88 mmHg, and her heart rate is 80/min. She is afebrile and has a normal respiratory rate. She appears to be pale and anxious. Cardiac and lung examinations are normal. Abdominal examination reveals no surgical scars and no masses. Her abdomen is nondistended, has normal bowel sounds, and is nontender to palpation, without rebound tenderness or guarding. Digital rectal examination reveals gross blood in the rectal vault but no masses. Anorectal examination shows no fissures, and anoscopy shows no internal hemorrhoids. Laboratory values reveal hemoglobin of 8 g/dL (normal 12–15.2 g/dL), hematocrit of 24% (37–46%), and normal mean corpuscular volume (MCV).

Diagnosis

What Is the Differential Diagnosis of a Lower GI Bleed (LGIB)? (▫ Table 22.1)

▫ **Table 22.1** Differential diagnosis of LGIB

Disease	Etiologies	Risk factors	Clinical presentation
Diverticulosis (30–50%)	Arterial bleed from vasa recta at the base of diverticula 90% of diverticula in sigmoid colon but 60% of diverticular bleeds from right colon	Advanced age, lack of fiber, obesity	Painless bright red blood per rectum (hematochezia)
Neoplastic (10–20%)	Colorectal adenocarcinoma may erode or ulcerate	Age > 50, Black race, IBD, family history, sedentary lifestyle, smoking, obesity, diabetes	Large LGIB is rare; iron-deficiency anemia and/or change in bowel habits
Iatrogenic	Up to 2 weeks postpolypectomy or biopsy	History of recent colonoscopy	Variable amount of bleeding occurring either immediately or days to weeks after the procedure (likely due to sloughing off of eschar)

(continued)

Table 22.1 (continued)

Disease		Etiologies	Risk factors	Clinical presentation
Colitis (10–20%)	Infectious	CMV, Kaposi's enteroinvasive organisms: *Salmonella*, *Campylobacter*, *Shigella*, *EHEC*, *Entamoeba histolytica*	History of eating undercooked or contaminated foods or drinks Immunosuppression Travel history	Bloating, crampy abdominal pain and tenderness, fever, chills, bloody diarrhea
	Ischemic	Secondary to low-flow state	Hypoperfusion secondary to hypotension, pressors, extreme exercise, hemodialysis, postaortic surgery	Acute abdominal pain and tenderness; bloody diarrhea; chronic ischemia can result in stricture formation
	Inflammatory	Ulcerative colitis or Crohn's disease	Family history of IBD	Bloody diarrhea and mucus in stool; abdominal pain and cramping; previous episodes
	Radiation	Direct mucosal damage from radiation exposure resulting in arteriolitis	History of pelvic radiation	Bloody diarrhea, tenesmus (feeling of incomplete defecation), mucus discharge
Angiodysplasia (5–10%)		Aberrant blood vessels in the GI tract; venous in origin; usually right-sided (cecum or ascending colon)	Advanced age; associated with von Willebrand's disease, CKD, aortic stenosis	Painless, often presents with iron-deficiency anemia
Anorectal (5–10%)		Internal hemorrhoids—bleeding from the hemorrhoidal venous plexus within the anus	Pregnancy, constipation, straining; 4.4% of US population	Painless bright red blood with straining at bowel movement
		Anal fissures	Constipation, trauma, IBD, malignancies	Minimal blood usually on toilet paper; tear most commonly posterior midline; severe pain with defecation
		Rectal varices—Bleeding is more proximal (within the rectum)	Portal hypertension	Massive painless bright red blood per rectum
		Rectal ulcers	Advanced age, debilitation, constipation; history of Crohn's disease	Anterior location; blood and mucus per rectum, sense of incomplete evacuation

LGIB lower GI bleed; *IBD* inflammatory bowel disease; *CMV* cytomegalovirus; *CKD* chronic kidney disease; *EHEC* enterohemorrhagic *Escherichia coli*

Watch Out

LGIB can be due to a large upper GI bleed (UGIB). If the patient is having a massive LGIB, or is unstable, an upper endoscopy should be performed to rule out an UGIB.

Watch Out

Diverticulosis is the most common cause of LGIB.

What Is the Most Likely Diagnosis?

An elderly patient with a recent colonoscopy showing colonic diverticula who presents with a large volume of bright red blood per rectum most likely has a LGIB from diverticular hemorrhage. Diverticulosis is the most common cause of acute LGIB in adults, particularly in the elderly. These bleeds are typically arterial in origin and painless, and may present with significant hematochezia. While often self-limited, they can be brisk and lead to hemodynamic instability. The differential diagnosis for LGIB can be remembered using the mnemonic

H-DRAIN: hemorrhoids, diverticular bleeding, radiation colitis, angiodysplasia, infectious/ischemic/inflammatory bowel disease, and neoplasms or polyps. Hemorrhoids usually cause minor, painless bleeding. Radiation colitis should be considered in patients with a history of pelvic radiation. Angiodysplasia is more common in the elderly and may cause intermittent bleeding. Inflammatory, infectious, and ischemic colitis typically present with additional symptoms such as abdominal pain or diarrhea. Neoplasms or polyps may result in chronic or intermittent bleeding and warrant evaluation for malignancy.

Why Is Age an Important Factor in a Patient with a LGIB?

Acute LGIB in patients over age 50 is more likely to be diverticulosis, angiodysplasia, or malignancy, whereas in younger patients, the most common causes are infectious, hemorrhoids, anal fissures, and IBD.

Why Are the Onset and Duration of Bleeding Important?

Diverticular bleeding is arterial and as a result tends to present acutely with relatively large amounts of blood. Angiodysplasia and cancer are more chronic and more likely to present with anemia or dark stools.

What Do the Color and Amount of Blood Tell Us About the Source of Bleeding? (◘ Table 22.2)

◘ **Table 22.2** Localization of bleeding based on stool characteristics

Color, amount of bleeding	Possible source(s)
Dark maroon, mixed with stools	Upper GI, small intestine, right colon
Copious bright red blood (hematochezia)	Right colon (e.g., diverticulum), rectum, anus, massive UGIB with rapid transit
Spots of blood on toilet paper, dripping after defecation	Rectum, anus
Scant, dark red blood	Angiodysplasia
Occult	Polyp, colorectal cancer

Watch Out

Right colonic diverticula are more likely to bleed, while left colonic diverticula are more likely to get infected.

What Is an Occult Bleed?

Occult bleeding means that the patient does not see any blood per rectum. The bleeding is only detected by fecal occult blood testing/fecal immunochemical testing or by finding iron-deficiency anemia. Occult bleeding (particularly in older patients) raises suspicion for malignancy (especially colorectal cancer), and in younger patients, it may be due to inflammatory bowel disease (IBD) or due to familial cancer syndromes (e.g., familial adenomatous polyposis, hereditary nonpolyposis colorectal cancer).

What Associated Symptoms Are Important to Look for, and How Do They Help in the Differential Diagnosis?

Systemic symptoms such as fever and bloody diarrhea may indicate an infectious or inflammatory cause. Recurrent symptoms in younger patients are suspicious for IBD. Weight loss should raise suspicion for malignancy, especially in older patients who have changes in bowel habits and/or iron-deficiency anemia. Bleeding that follows straining at stool suggests an anorectal cause. In this latter setting, painless bleeding suggests internal hemorrhoids, whereas anal pain is suggestive of anal fissures (bleeding with fissures is usually minimal). Tenesmus, a sense of incomplete evacuation of stool, is most often seen with ulcerative colitis and infectious etiologies. Bleeding from diverticulosis and angiodysplasia tends to be painless. Abdominal pain (especially in elderly patients) should raise suspicion for ischemic colitis (particularly in the setting of low-flow states). Hemorrhoids result from enlargement and distal displacement of the normal anal cushions, which contain vascular and connective tissue that contributes to continence. Diagnosis is clinical and may be aided by anoscopy.

Watch Out

Bloody diarrhea following recent travel to endemic areas raises suspicion for infectious causes. Patients with watery, progressing to bloody, diarrhea, and no fever should always be evaluated for *EHEC*.

Why Is a History of Pelvic Radiation or Prior Aortic Surgery Important?

Radiation can cause damage to the rectal mucosa, leading to radiation proctitis. There are two forms. *Acute radiation proctitis* occurs in days to weeks after pelvic radiation treatment and presents with rectal bleeding and pain secondary to ulceration and sloughing of the rectal mucosa. This is often a self-limiting condition and resolves with discontinuation of radiation therapy. *Chronic radiation proctitis* occurs years after radiation therapy, and unlike acute radiation proctitis, rectal bleeding is less common. Patients with chronic radiation proctitis may develop strictures, fistulas, and bowel obstruction. Acute radiation proctitis does not increase risk for the development of chronic radiation proctitis. Aortic surgery rarely results in erosion of the aortic graft into the duodenum, leading to an aortoduodenal fistula.

Why Should One Inquire About Alcohol History and Look for Stigmata of Liver Cirrhosis?

Liver disease can lead to coagulopathy and portal hypertension. Although portal hypertension most commonly causes esophageal varices and upper GI bleeding, varices can also form in the rectal veins of the lower GI tract due to their systemic and mesenteric connections.

What Is the Implication of Abdominal Tenderness on Physical Examination?

Abdominal tenderness is highly suggestive of colitis such as from IBD, ischemic colitis, or infectious diarrhea. Abdominal tenderness is unusual with bleeding from diverticulosis and angiodysplasia.

Can Upper and LGIB Be Distinguished Based on History and Physical Examination?

Sometimes. Vomiting of blood or coffee grounds, in conjunction with maroon or black stools, is indicative of an UGIB. Bright red blood per rectum is usually a LGIB (the exception is the patient with massive UGIB). Maroon stools, in the absence of vomiting, can be either an upper or lower GI source. Anoscopy/proctoscopy should be part of the initial physical examination.

What Is the Significance of Finding Iron-Deficiency Anemia in Association with a LGIB?

Iron-deficiency anemia in a man or a postmenopausal woman should raise suspicion for malignancy (especially right-sided colorectal cancer, particularly if the patient has never had screening). Although colorectal cancer usually causes occult bleeding, it may manifest as a larger, acute bleed when the cancer causes erosion through or ulceration of the bowel wall.

How Does Ischemic Colitis Classically Present?

Ischemic colitis typically presents with left-sided abdominal pain and bloody diarrhea in elderly patients with low-flow states, such as those with severe volume depletion, heart failure, and shock. Certain drugs (e.g., digitalis, vasopressors, cocaine) can also increase risk for ischemic colitis. These symptoms are most often localized to colonic watershed areas such as Griffith's and Sudeck's points, which are more susceptible to hypoperfusion due to limited collateral circulation.

What Are the Risk Factors for Diverticulosis?

Older individuals (60% of people over age 60 have diverticulosis) from Western countries or those who consume diets that are low in fiber, high in fat, and high in red meat are at risk. Obese individuals are also at increased risk. Inherited connective tissue disorders, such as Marfan's syndrome and Ehlers-Danlos syndrome, can also increase the likelihood of diverticulum formation.

Etiology/Pathophysiology

What Is a Diverticulum?

A diverticulum is defined as a saclike protrusion through the colonic wall. The presence of diverticula is known as diverticulosis or diverticular disease. As a diverticulum herniates, the vasa recta become draped over the dome of the diverticulum, at which point it is only separated from the lumen by mucosa. Chronic damage and stress on the luminal side of the vasa recta lead to weakness of the arterial walls, eventually resulting in rupture.

What Causes a Diverticulum?

High intraluminal pressure in the colon can cause the mucosa and submucosa to herniate through the muscular layer of the intestinal wall. Since not all layers are included, this is considered a false diverticulum.

What Is the Difference Between Diverticulum, Diverticulosis, and Diverticulitis? (Table 22.3)

Table 22.3 Terminology related to diverticular disease

Name	Features
Diverticulum	Saclike protrusion through the colonic wall
Asymptomatic diverticulosis	No symptoms in a patient with diverticula
Symptomatic diverticulosis	Bleeding diverticula
Diverticulitis	Microperforation or macroperforation of inflamed diverticula

What Is the Most Common Site of Diverticula? Why?

Ninety percent of diverticula occur in the sigmoid colon. As stool moves distally through the colon, water is reabsorbed, and it becomes harder. The left colon must contract more to get the stool to pass. The combination of harder stool and thickened muscular wall causes increased pressure and makes diverticulum formation more likely. The muscular layers (taenia) splay out at the rectosigmoid junction covering all of the rectum which is why diverticula do not appear in the rectum.

How Common Is a Diverticular Bleed?

Although a diverticular bleed is the most common cause of an acute LGIB in patients over 50, it occurs in only a small percentage (3–5%) of patients with diverticulosis.

What Is the Natural History of a Diverticular Bleed?

Seventy percent stop bleeding spontaneously. Each episode of a diverticular bleed increases the risk of a future bleed.

Watch Out
Significant GI bleeding from a diverticulum is from diverticul*osis*. Diverticul*itis* is not usually associated with bleeding.

What Is Angiodysplasia? What Are the Risk Factors?

Angiodysplasia refers to focal submucosal areas of thin, weak, and dilated (ectatic) vessels in the GI tract, most commonly in the cecum and right colon in individuals over age 60. It is the most common vascular abnormality of the GI tract. Incidence increases with age, likely due to degeneration of the vascular walls. Bleeding is typically small in quantity or occult, often resulting in iron-deficiency anemia and intermittently heme-positive stools but may present with larger bleeds. Unlike diverticular bleeds, which are arterial in origin, acute angiodysplasia bleeds generally produce less bleeding because their origin is venous. Angiodysplasia is associated with von Willebrand's disease, aortic stenosis, and chronic kidney disease. It is a common cause of gastrointestinal bleeding when no obvious lesion is seen on endoscopy, particularly in elderly patients. In those with aortic stenosis, high shear stress across the valve degrades von Willebrand factor multimers, impairing hemostasis. Although angiodysplasia may resemble telangiectasia on endoscopy, it lacks the mucosal pallor and friability is seen in radiation proctitis.

What Causes Ischemic Colitis?

The pathophysiology is decreased blood flow to the colon, causing nonocclusive (meaning not due to arterial thrombosis or embolism) ischemic colitis. The mucosa is affected first, and depending on the severity of the ischemia, progression may occur through all layers of the colon. The most common areas to be affected are "watershed" areas which have relatively poor perfusion as they are in between two areas of the colonic blood supply. In most cases, the ischemia is not transmural, meaning it does not affect the entire bowel wall, and most patients will recover after correction of their "low-flow" state.

What Are the Primary Watershed Areas of the GI Tract?

The most commonly affected watershed area in low-flow states is *Griffith's point* located at the splenic flexure where collaterals are present between the superior mesenteric and inferior mesenteric arteries. *Sudeck's point* is located at the rectosigmoid junction where collaterals are present between the sigmoid and superior rectal artery.

Watch Out

The rectum has a dual blood supply, so rectal mucosal ischemia is very rare.

What Is the Natural History of Ischemic Colitis?

Most cases of ischemic colitis will resolve with supportive measures, while a minority of cases will require resection for transmural (i.e., full thickness of the colonic wall) infarction.

What Are the Differences Between Ischemic Colitis and Acute Mesenteric Ischemia? (Table 22.4)

Table 22.4 Comparison of ischemic colitis and acute mesenteric ischemia

	Ischemic colitis	Acute mesenteric ischemia
Pathophysiology	Hypoperfusion due to low-flow state; ↓BP, ↓CO; due to volume depletion, heart failure, extreme exercise, vasoconstricting drugs, or recent aortic surgery	Arterial embolus to SMA (usually from atrial fibrillation) or thrombosis (from underlying atherosclerosis in SMA)
Natural history	80% resolve spontaneously with supportive care (e.g., fluids, IV antibiotics, blood pressure management)	Usually leads to bowel necrosis requiring resection; high mortality
Most commonly affected territories	Segment of colon between arterial supplies, known as watershed areas	Small bowel (from ligament of Treitz) to mid-transverse colon
Layers of bowel affected	Usually mucosa only	Often transmural (i.e., all layers)
Diagnosis	Colonoscopy often shows mucosal changes	CT scan often shows small bowel wall thickening, occlusion of SMA, and gas in the intestinal wall (known as pneumatosis)

BP blood pressure; *CO* cardiac output; *SMA* superior mesenteric artery; *IMA* inferior mesenteric artery

Initial Management

What Are the Initial Steps in the Management of a LGIB?

The first step is to place two large-bore IVs and send laboratory tests including a type and cross, complete blood count, chemistry, and INR/PTT. If the patient demonstrates evidence of significant blood loss, resuscitation should be instituted with crystalloid (normal saline or lactated Ringer's solution) followed by packed red blood cells as needed. A microcytic anemia raises suspicion for an underlying iron-deficiency anemia due to occult blood loss from colorectal cancer but may also indicate a chronic bleed from angiodysplasia. Leukocytosis is often seen in infectious or inflammatory etiologies.

What Is the Next Step?

In an unstable patient with a large volume LGIB, an UGIB source needs to be ruled out. This should be done expeditiously via upper endoscopy. Up to 10% of cases of hematochezia are due to massive UGIBs.

How Does the Hemodynamic Stability of the Patient Affect the Subsequent Management and Diagnostic Workup?

A hemodynamically unstable patient needs admission to the ICU for careful monitoring. In addition, further workup to find the source of bleed needs to be performed expeditiously. Most LGIB stop spontaneously. Thus, the need for urgent intervention as well as mortality is significantly less than for an UGIB.

What Is the First Diagnostic Test of Choice? How Effective Is This Test in Visualizing the Source of LGIB in the Acute Setting?

Colonoscopy is the first test of choice. Ideally, the patient should first undergo a rapid bowel prep to cleanse the bowel, in which a liter of polyethylene glycol solution is given every 45 minutes until the rectal effluent is clear. This allows colonoscopy to be performed in a few hours. However, if the patient is rapidly bleeding, colonoscopy is done urgently without the bowel prep. Sometimes, if the bleeding is brisk, the blood itself can act as a cathartic, allowing visualization. Often though, the colon is filled with blood and stool so that colonoscopy may fail to adequately visualize the bleeding site. However, one benefit of colonoscopy is that it can generally determine whether the bleed is coming from proximal to the ileocecal valve (and therefore from the small bowel) versus somewhere within the colon. This determination has important diagnostic and therapeutic implications. Colonoscopy cannot visualize the small bowel.

What If This Diagnostic Test Is Not Able to Visualize the Bleeding? What Are Other Options for Localizing the Source of Bleed? What Are the Advantages/Disadvantages of Each Modality?

If the patient is continuing to bleed, other modalities include formal arteriography and a tagged red cell scan (nuclear scintigraphy). The advantage of the arteriography is that the study can be both diagnostic and therapeutic (the area of bleeding can be embolized). However, arteriography is invasive, and bleeding must be brisk (about 0.5–1 ml/min) to see it. It is also not feasible to repeatedly perform arteriography if the patient stops bleeding and then rebleeds. Another option is a tagged red blood cell scan (nuclear scintigraphy) using technetium-99 m. The decision to choose one over the other depends on the suspected rate of bleeding and the availability of these modalities. Nuclear scanning detects bleeding at a much slower rate (only 0.1 ml/min), and since the radioactive agent remains labeled on the red blood cell for some time, repeat images can be obtained for up to 24 hours. Nuclear scanning does not permit therapy and is not able to pinpoint the exact vessel/location of the bleed but rather the general area. More recently, CT angiogram is being used. It may demonstrate a blush of contrast and therefore help localize the bleeding. If a blush is seen, a formal arteriography can then be performed to embolize the site of bleeding.

What Is the Next Step If These Modalities Fail to Identify the Exact Source of Bleeding?

If diagnostic tests fail to identify the source of lower gastrointestinal bleeding, the next step depends on whether the bleeding has stopped and whether the patient is hemodynamically stable. In a stable patient whose bleeding has ceased and in whom the source is suspected to be the small bowel, further evaluation includes a Meckel scan to assess for a Meckel diverticulum, capsule endoscopy to visualize the small intestine, or enteroscopy to directly examine the proximal small bowel. If the bleeding has stopped but the source remains unclear or is suspected to be within the colon, repeat colonoscopy, radionuclide scan, or angiography can be performed if the patient experiences recurrent bleeding. In contrast, if the patient remains unstable with ongoing hemorrhage and the bleeding has been localized to the colon, emergent surgical intervention is indicated. In this setting, exploratory laparotomy with subtotal colectomy and end ileostomy is recommended, provided that the source of bleeding has been confirmed to be between the ileocecal valve and the rectum either before surgery or during the operation using intraoperative endoscopy.

What If Arteriography Localizes the Source of Bleeding but Is Unable to Stop the Bleeding with Embolization?

If bleeding is ongoing, surgery is recommended. Resection is determined by the localization (i.e., right colectomy for bleeding localized to the right colon).

What Is the Pathophysiology and Management of Hemorrhoids?

Hemorrhoids result from the enlargement and distal displacement of the normal anal cushions, which are vascular structures composed of connective tissue, smooth muscle, and blood vessels. These cushions play a role in maintaining continence, but with increased venous pressure, such as from constipation, straining, or pregnancy, they can become symptomatic. Internal hemorrhoids originate above the dentate line and are typically painless, while external hemorrhoids arise below the dentate line and may cause pain if thrombosed. Diagnosis is clinical and often aided by anoscopy. Management depends on the severity and type. Conservative treatment includes increased dietary fiber, stool softeners, modification of toilet habits, and warm sitz baths. Symptomatic internal hemorrhoids may require rubber band ligation, while external hemorrhoids that are thrombosed and acutely painful can be excised if symptoms began within 72 hours. Surgical hemorrhoidectomy (removal of internal hemorrhoids) is reserved for patients with refractory or advanced disease.

Perianal Masses

The differential diagnosis for anal or perianal masses includes rectal prolapse, internal and external hemorrhoids, perianal abscess, anorectal cancer, anogenital warts, and skin tags. Rectal prolapse typically presents as a concentric, circular mass protruding from the anus, often during defecation or with straining. It is more common in elderly women and in those with chronic constipation, pelvic floor dysfunction, or a history of multiple vaginal deliveries. Unlike prolapsed internal hemorrhoids, which appear as discrete mucosal bulges, rectal prolapse involves full-thickness protrusion of the rectal wall and may be associated with fecal incontinence or mucous discharge. Management of rectal prolapse depends on the severity and degree of functional impairment. Initial treatment includes addressing constipation and pelvic floor strengthening. Definitive treatment is surgical, with options including perineal or abdominal rectopexy procedures. Surgical repair is especially indicated in patients with full-thickness prolapse or significant symptoms.

Areas Where You Can Get in Trouble

Bleeding After Colonoscopic Biopsy or Polypectomy

Bleeding after a colonoscopic biopsy can occur even several weeks later. It is important to obtain this history. Initial treatment consists of endoscopic injection of vasoconstrictive agents (e.g., epinephrine), cauterization, or clipping.

Pneumoperitoneum After Colonoscopy

Pneumoperitoneum, or free air under the diaphragm, typically suggests bowel perforation and often warrants urgent surgical intervention. However, in the setting of a recent colonoscopy, the presence of pneumoperitoneum does not always indicate a surgical emergency. Insufflation during the procedure can lead to minor, self-limited microperforations of the colon. In a patient who is hemodynamically stable, without fever, abdominal pain, or peritoneal signs, conservative management may be appropriate. This includes bowel rest, administration of broad-spectrum antibiotics, and close clinical monitoring with serial abdominal examinations. A CT scan should be obtained to assess for a contained perforation, which is defined by the absence of free fluid, lack of diffuse inflammation, and localization of air or contrast extravasation to a confined area without evidence of ongoing contamination. In such cases, the risk of generalized peritonitis is low, and nonoperative management is often successful.

Failure to Perform Anoscopy/Proctoscopy

Rarely, internal hemorrhoids can cause massive lower GI bleeding, particularly in the elderly who are receiving oral anticoagulants. Similarly, rectal varices may be a source of massive LGIB in patients with cirrhosis and portal hypertension. These may be missed on colonoscopy.

Large Intestine Pathologies (Fig. 22.1)

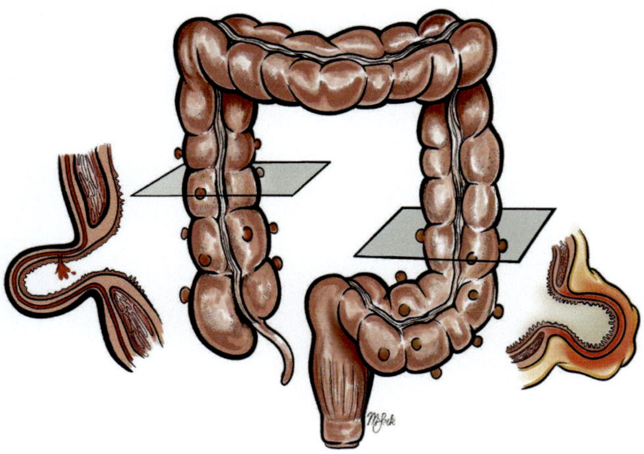

Fig. 22.1 **Diverticular disease:** The illustration depicts two forms of diverticular disease: a bleeding diverticulum in the right colon and diverticulitis in the left colon, which is characterized by inflammation that can lead to abscess or perforation.

Summary of Essentials

History and Physical

- Color, quantity, and duration of bleeding are important.
- Ask about anticoagulants and antiplatelet agents.
- Right colon diverticulosis, most common cause of LGIB.
- Hematemesis/coffee ground emesis indicates UGIB.
- Digital rectal examination, anoscopy/proctoscopy.

Pathophysiology

- Diverticulosis
  - Increased intraluminal pressure (low-fiber diet).
  - Most common cause of LGIB.
  - Right colon diverticula bleed (brisk and arterial).
  - Left colon diverticula get infected.
- Angiodysplasia
  - Associated with aortic stenosis and kidney disease.
  - Bleeding is slower (venous).
- Colon Cancer
  - Iron-deficiency anemia in males or postmenopausal females should raise suspicion for colon cancer (particularly right-sided cancers).
  - Massive LGIB is rare.
- Colitis
  - Inflammatory
  - Infectious
  - Ischemic

Management

- Fluid resuscitation, if there is a large bleed, admit to ICU
- Diagnostic studies
  - Upper endoscopy if massive LGIB (to rule out UGI source)
  - Colonoscopy
  - Nuclear-tagged RBC scan
  - Arteriography
  - CTA
- Most cases of LGIB will stop spontaneously
- Indications for surgery
  - Hemodynamically unstable despite resuscitation
  - Massive bleeding >6 units PRBC
  - Active bleeding with failure of embolization

Suggested Reading

Alonso-Coello P, Guyatt G, Heels-Ansdell D, et al. Laxatives for the treatment of hemorrhoids. Cochrane Database Syst Rev. 2005;4:CD004649.

Barnert J, Messmann H. Management of lower gastrointestinal tract bleeding. Best Pract Res Clin Gastroenterol. 2008;22:295–312.

Becquemin JP, Majewski M, Fermani N, et al. Colon ischemia following abdominal aortic aneurysm repair in the era of endovascular abdominal aortic repair. J Vasc Surg. 2008;47:258.

Peery AF, Barrett PR, Park D, et al. A high-fiber diet does not protect against asymptomatic diverticulosis. Gastroenterology. 2012;142:266.

Perry RJ, Martin MJ, Eckert MJ, et al. Colonic ischemia complicating open vs endovascular abdominal aortic aneurysm repair. J Vasc Surg. 2008;48:272.

Ruiz-Tovar J, Morales V, Hervas A, et al. Late gastrointestinal complications after pelvic radiotherapy: radiation enteritis. Clin Transl Oncol. 2009;11(8):539–43.

Touzios JG, et al. Diverticulosis and acute diverticulitis. Gastroenterol Clin N Am. 2009;38(3):513–25.

Vernava AM, Longo WE, Virgo KS. A nationwide study of the incidence and etiology of lower gastrointestinal bleeding. Surg Res Commun. 1996;18:113–20.

Right Lower Quadrant Abdominal Pain

Christian de Virgilio, Areg Grigorian, Beverley A. Petrie, and Tracey D. Arnell

Contents

C. de Virgilio, A. Grigorian (eds.), *Surgery*, https://doi.org/10.1007/978-3-032-09799-6_23

Case Study

A 25-year-old male presents to the emergency department with a 1-day history of periumbilical abdominal pain, which has now shifted to the right lower quadrant. He describes the pain as constant and a 7/10. After the onset of pain, he developed nausea and vomited twice. He has not eaten for 24 h due to a lack of appetite. Physical examination is significant for a temperature of 38 °C, absent bowel sounds, and marked tenderness to palpation at 1/3 the distance from the anterior superior iliac spine to the umbilicus. When palpating in the left lower quadrant (LLQ), he reports pain in the right lower quadrant (RLQ). Active flexion of his right hip and internal rotation of the right leg reproduce the pain. His skin in the RLQ is hypersensitive to touch. There is no rebound tenderness. Laboratory values are significant for a white blood cell (WBC) count of $13.5 \times 10^3/\mu L$ (normal $4.1–10.9 \times 10^3/\mu L$), with 15% bands. The urinalysis demonstrates 1+ WBCs without bacteria.

Diagnosis

What Is the Differential Diagnosis for Right Lower Quadrant Pain in an Adult? (Table 23.1)

Table 23.1 Differential diagnosis for RLQ pain in an adult

Diagnosis	History and physical
Appendicitis	Anorexia, vomiting, vague periumbilical pain shifting to localized RLQ pain (*McBurney's point*), Rovsing's, psoas, and obturator signs (see below)
Inflammatory bowel disease (IBD)	Abdominal pain, severe cramps, weight loss, bloody diarrhea, anemia, enterocutaneous fistula/anal fissures (Crohn's), toxic megacolon (ulcerative colitis); Crohn's can present with RLQ pain due to inflammation at the ileocecal region
Gastroenteritis	Nausea, vomiting, watery diarrhea (viral), bloody diarrhea (certain bacteria), myalgia, fever
Nephrolithiasis	Colicky flank pain that may radiate to the inner thigh or genitals, nausea, vomiting, dysuria, hematuria
Pyelonephritis	Costovertebral angle (CVA) tenderness, fever, pain on urination, vomiting
Cecal diverticulitis	Congenital solitary diverticulum
Meckel's diverticulitis	"Rule of 2's": Males get complications 2× more commonly than females, occur within 2 ft. of the ileocecal valve, two types of tissue (pancreatic, gastric), found in 2% of the population, can present at 2 years of age (with *painless rectal bleeding*)

What Other Conditions Should You Consider in the Differential Diagnosis for Right Lower Quadrant Pain in Women? (Table 23.2)

Table 23.2 Differential diagnosis for RLQ pain in women

Diagnosis	History and physical
Pelvic inflammatory disease	*Neisseria gonorrhoeae* or *chlamydia* infection, purulent cervical discharge, cervical motion tenderness, adnexal tenderness, dysuria
Ovarian torsion	Acute onset of severe pelvic pain, adnexal mass, history of ovarian cysts
Mittelschmerz	Physiologic recurrent mid-cycle pain, mild and unilateral, duration ranges from a few hours to a few days, normal pelvic exam
Ruptured ectopic	Typically presents 6–8 weeks after the last normal menstrual period, abdominal pain, amenorrhea, vaginal bleeding, breast tenderness, anemia (rarely hemorrhagic shock)

What Other Conditions Should You Consider in the Differential Diagnosis for Right Lower Quadrant Pain in a Child? (Table 23.3)

Table 23.3 Differential diagnosis for RLQ pain in a child

Diagnosis	History and physical
Mesenteric lymphadenitis	Concomitant or recent upper respiratory infection; high fever; enlarged, inflamed, and tender lymph nodes in the small bowel mesentery; generalized abdominal pain
Yersinia enterocolitica (pseudoappendicitis)	RLQ pain, fever, vomiting, bloody diarrhea, history of sick contacts (e.g., infected children at daycare)
Gastroenteritis	Nausea, vomiting, watery diarrhea (viral), bloody diarrhea (certain bacteria), myalgia, fever
Intussusception	Nausea, vomiting, crampy abdominal pain, "*red currant jelly*" stool, "sausage-shaped mass" in abdomen (12-month-old infant)

What Is the Most Likely Diagnosis?

Given the history of initial periumbilical pain that is now localized to the RLQ and subsequently followed by nausea/emesis and leukocytosis with increased bands, the most likely diagnosis is acute appendicitis.

Watch Out
Don't forget to rule out an ectopic pregnancy with a beta-hCG pregnancy test for *all* women of childbearing age presenting with abdominal pain.

History and Physical

What Is Usually the First Symptom of Appendicitis, and What Is the Classic Sequence of Symptoms?

In >95% of cases of acute appendicitis, anorexia is the first symptom. The classic sequence of symptoms is anorexia, vague periumbilical abdominal pain, nausea, vomiting, and then a shift to localized RLQ pain.

Watch Out
Nausea preceding abdominal pain is more consistent with gastroenteritis.

What Is the Hamburger Sign?

The majority of patients with acute appendicitis will have anorexia. If the patient is hungry, acute appendicitis is less likely. Inquire about the patient's favorite food (e.g., hamburger, pizza), and ask if the patient would like to eat it. Patients with true anorexia will decline their favorite food (positive hamburger sign). Children may not follow this sign.

What Are Rovsing's, Psoas, and Obturator Signs and McBurney's Point Tenderness?

Appendicitis creates an inflammatory response in the adjacent retroperitoneum and parietal peritoneum. These are signs (◘ Table 23.4) of localized peritonitis in the RLQ due to inflammation. *Rovsing's sign* is right lower quadrant pain with palpation of the left lower quadrant. Compression in the LLQ stretches the abdominal wall, triggering pain in the inflamed underlying RLQ parietal peritoneum. Appendicitis can also inflame the adjacent psoas or obturator muscles. The *psoas sign* is RLQ pain on passive extension of the right hip or active flexion of the right hip. *Obturator sign* is RLQ pain on internal rotation of the hip, which can occur with a pelvic appendix. *McBurney's point* (◘ Fig. 23.1) is located at one-third of the distance along an imaginary line drawn from the anterior superior iliac spine to the umbilicus and marks the incision site for open appendectomies. *McBurney's sign* is maximal tenderness at McBurney's point. In most clinical scoring systems for appendicitis, tenderness at McBurney's point is the most important finding supporting the diagnosis.

◘ **Table 23.4** Signs of appendicitis

Sign	Description	Appendix location
Rovsing's	RLQ pain with palpation of LLQ	Normal (intraperitoneal)
Psoas	RLQ pain on passive extension of the right hip or active flexion of the right hip	Retrocecal
Obturator	RLQ pain on internal rotation of the hip, typical of a pelvic appendix	Pelvic
Mcburney's	Tenderness to palpation at McBurney's point	Any

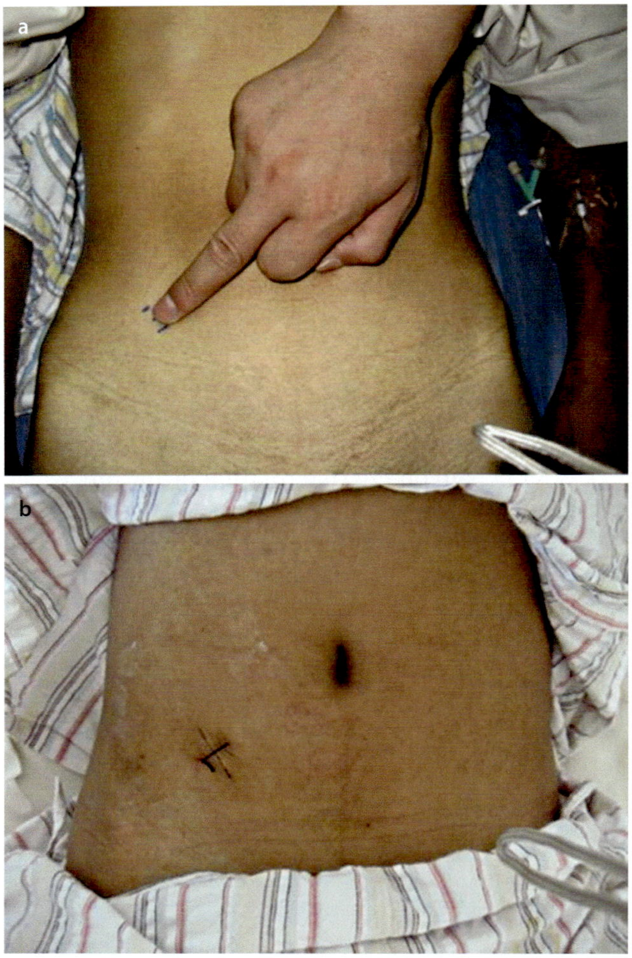

Fig. 23.1 McBurney's point. **a** McBurney's point marked for mini incision. **b** Incision appearance on postoperative day 4. The procedure began by making a small incision, 1.5–1.8 cm in length, according to the thickness of the abdominal wall, at McBurney's point. (From Chen D, et al. Gasless single-incision laparoscopic appendectomy. Surgical Endoscopy. 2011;25:1473. Reprinted with permission from Springer Nature)

Pathophysiology

What Explains the Transition from Periumbilical Pain to Right Lower Quadrant Pain in Appendicitis?

Autonomic nerves (sympathetic and parasympathetic) supply the visceral peritoneum, while the parietal peritoneum has somatic innervation derived from spinal nerves. The visceral peritoneum senses pain when stretched or distended, and results in dull, poorly localized pain associated with nausea. Often in the early hours of appendiceal inflammation, only the visceral peritoneum is affected. The patient perceives a vague type of abdominal pain in the periumbilical region. In contrast, as the inflammation progresses, the parietal peritoneum becomes affected, resulting in a sharp, severe type of pain localized to the region of appendiceal inflammation at the RLQ.

What Is a Closed-Loop Obstruction?

A closed-loop obstruction occurs when a segment of bowel is obstructed at two points, creating a closed loop with no outlet for bowel contents or gas. As intraluminal pressure builds, the bowel distends, eventually exceeding venous pressure and leading to venous congestion. This congestion further compromises arterial inflow, resulting in ischemia and infarction. The infarction typically occurs at the antimesenteric border, where the blood supply is most vulnerable.

How Does a Closed-Loop Obstruction Pertain to Acute Appendicitis?

In acute appendicitis, a commonly accepted etiology involves obstruction of the proximal appendiceal lumen by a *fecalith* (in adults) or *lymphoid hyperplasia* (in children). Since the appendix is a blind loop, this creates a closed-loop obstruction. The appendiceal mucosa continues to secrete mucus. Bacteria in the appendix begin to multiply rapidly. Consequently, the appendix distends, and intraluminal pressure exceeds venous pressure. Vascular congestion ensues until arteriolar supply is compromised as well. Ischemia and gangrene occur first in areas with the poorest blood supply, resulting in a weakened wall. Perforation eventually occurs at the antimesenteric border just beyond the point of obstruction, where the tension is high. Increased luminal pressure alone is not directly responsible for the perforation.

What Are Some Other Examples of a Closed-Loop Obstruction?

Obstructing colon cancer with a functioning ileocecal valve, diverticulitis, incarcerated hernia, volvulus, acute cholecystitis, and Richter's hernia (only part of the circumference of the bowel wall is trapped within the hernia sac).

What Are Other Causes of Appendiceal Obstruction?

Other causes of appendiceal obstruction include tumors (adenocarcinoma of the appendix), ingested seeds, and parasites (*Ascaris lumbricoides* is the most common).

Workup

What Are the Critical Laboratory Values Utilized in the Workup of Acute Appendicitis?

The most important laboratory value is leukocytosis with a left shift. Elevated C-reactive protein (CRP), a marker for inflammation, has been shown to be useful in the diagnosis of acute appendicitis in children. All women of childbearing age presenting with abdominal pain should receive a beta-hCG pregnancy test to rule out an ectopic pregnancy.

What Is the Significance of WBCs in the Urine Without Bacteria? How Might This Mislead the Clinician?

A few WBCs can be seen in the urine (sterile pyuria) with appendicitis as a result of ureteral or bladder irritation by the inflamed appendix. This laboratory finding may mislead the clinician into believing the patient may have cystitis. However, bacteriuria (bacteria in urine) should not be present in an uncontaminated urine specimen. Epithelial cells present in the urinalysis are suggestive of a contaminated sample.

What Imaging Is Used in Diagnosing Appendicitis?

Ultrasonography is used as an imaging modality for suspected appendicitis, particularly in women and children. In women, ultrasound helps to rule out gynecologic pathology such as ovarian torsion, tubo-ovarian abscess, or an ectopic pregnancy. In children, there is a heightened desire to avoid the radiation exposure of CT. Also, because children have less periappendiceal fat, the appendix is not as readily visualized on a CT scan. Ultrasound, on the other hand, can identify a thick-walled, noncompressible tubular structure (dilated appendix) in the right lower quadrant. Peritoneal fluid and/or an abscess can sometimes be seen in advanced cases. If ultrasound is not diagnostic but suspicion of appendicitis remains high, contrast-enhanced CT of the abdomen and pelvis is the preferred next imaging modality. CT findings consistent with acute appendicitis include periappendiceal fat stranding and an enlarged appendiceal diameter >6 mm (◻ Figs. 23.2, 23.3, and 23.4).

If Symptoms and Signs of Appendicitis Are Classic, Is Imaging Necessary?

Imaging is recommended in patients with atypical symptoms, which often occur in infants and small children, young women, and the elderly. If the history and physical exam are classic, imaging is not necessarily needed, particularly in young adult men. That being said, most adults undergo a CT scan to confirm the diagnosis. CT also helps confirm if the appendicitis is complicated (abscess, perforation), which may alter the management.

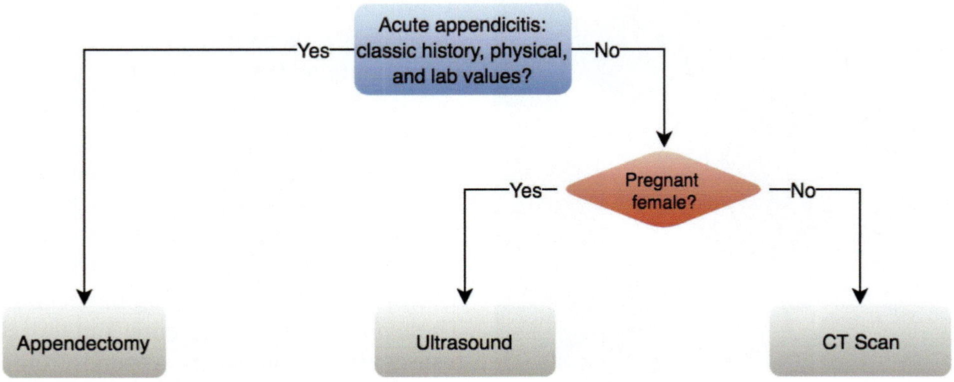

◻ **Fig. 23.2** Algorithm for acute appendicitis

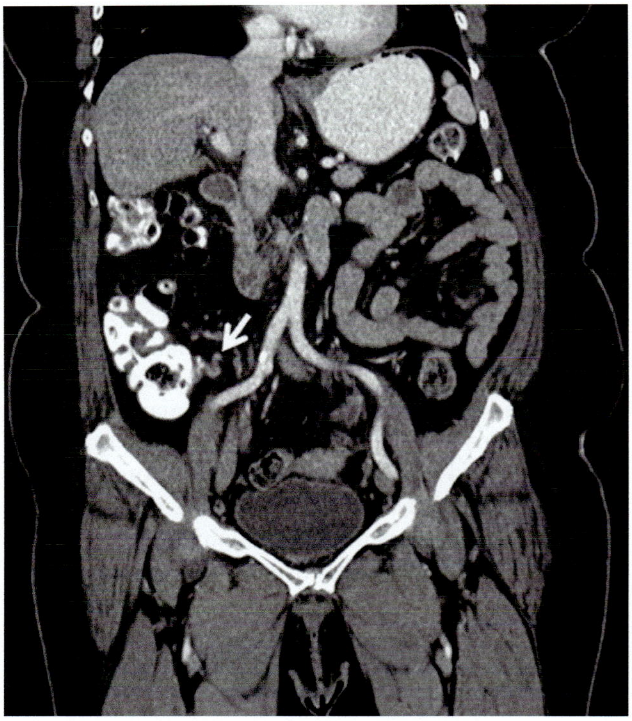

■ Fig. 23.3 Coronal CT showing the normal appendix (*white arrow*) as a thin tubular structure arising from the base of the cecum

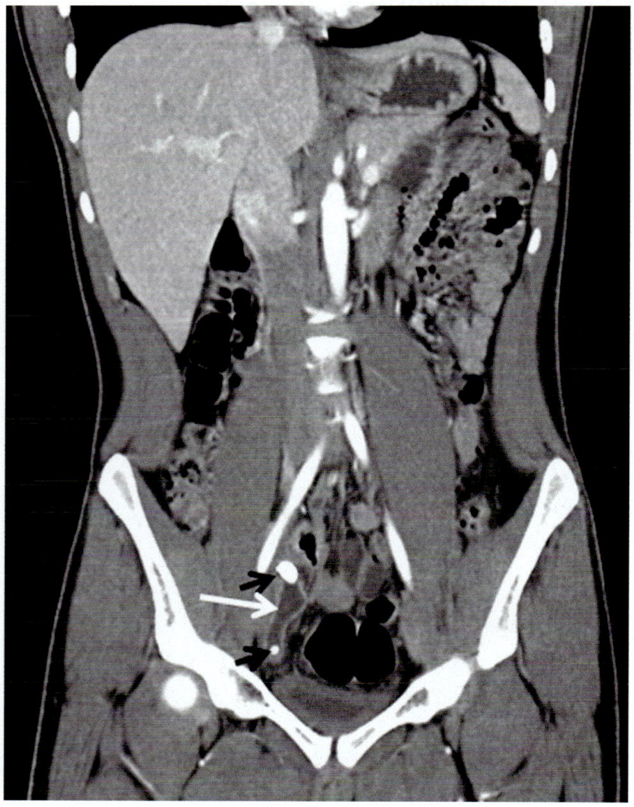

■ Fig. 23.4 Coronal CT showing a dilated, thick-walled, fluid-filled appendix containing appendicoliths, indicating acute appendicitis. *White arrows, dilated appendix*; *black arrows, appendicoliths*

Management

What Is the Surgical Treatment for Appendicitis?

The gold standard for treating appendicitis is surgical removal of the appendix with a laparoscopic approach (laparoscopic appendectomy).

Is Appendicitis a True Surgical Emergency?

Uncomplicated (non-perforated) acute appendicitis has traditionally been treated as a surgical emergency to prevent perforation. However, the risk of rupture in adults is low in the first 36 h, with a 5% risk of rupture in each subsequent 12-h period. Therefore, appendicitis is considered an urgent condition that should be treated within 24 h of diagnosis but does not always require immediate surgery, such as during nighttime hours, unless the patient shows signs of worsening sepsis.

What Is the Role of Pre- and Postoperative Antibiotics for Acute Non-perforated Appendicitis?

A single dose of preoperative antibiotics has been shown to reduce infectious complications and should be given to patients with both acute non-perforated and perforated appendicitis. In simple non-perforated appendicitis, antibiotics are usually not required postoperatively.

How Is Perforated or Gangrenous Appendicitis Generally Treated?

Approximately 15–20% of cases of appendicitis are associated with perforation. Most commonly, perforation is contained or "walled off" by surrounding abdominal structures. Similar to uncomplicated appendicitis, patients with a small appendiceal abscess and short duration of symptoms can be safely managed with a laparoscopic appendectomy. For perforated or gangrenous appendicitis, antibiotics are continued for 4 days after source control. In rare circumstances, there may be a "free" perforation resulting in generalized peritonitis. These patients are often septic and unstable and require resuscitation, emergency appendectomy vs ileocecectomy, and washout of the abdomen.

What if the CT Shows an Abscess or a Phlegmon?

Occasionally, patients with perforated appendicitis will develop a large abscess (which may instead require percutaneous drainage during the index hospitalization) or phlegmon (an inflammatory mass without pus). Proceeding with immediate surgery in the setting of an abscess or a phlegmon increases the risk of requiring a more extensive procedure for source control, such as removing the ileum and cecum (ileocecectomy), since the appendiceal base may not be suitable for a stapled resection. These are best managed nonoperatively with IV while keeping the patient NPO. There is controversy regarding whether a planned elective appendectomy should be performed on an outpatient basis 6–8 weeks after recovery. Prior to an interval appendectomy, a colonoscopy is recommended in adults to rule out cancer.

How Should You Proceed if You Are Performing a Laparoscopic Appendectomy and You Discover That the Appendix Appears to Be Normal? Do You Remove the Appendix Anyway? Are There Circumstances Where an Appendectomy Is Contraindicated?

In about 10% of cases, the appendix will appear normal during laparoscopic appendectomy. A negative appendectomy occurs more commonly in the elderly, infants, and young women. In general, if the appendix appears normal during surgery, it should still be removed to prevent future diagnostic uncertainty. That way, if the patient develops RLQ pain in the future, acute appendicitis is effectively ruled out. It is also important to intraoperatively search for other causes that can mimic appendicitis (e.g., inflammatory bowel disease, Meckel's diverticulitis, pancreatitis, cholecystitis, or perforated duodenal ulcer). In the case of regional enteritis (Crohn's) *involving* the cecum (as evident by inflammation/thickening of this area), the appendix should not be removed because of the high risk of developing an enterocutaneous fistula. Similarly, a biopsy should be avoided for the same reason, but the patient should be scheduled for a colonoscopy in 2–4 weeks. However, if the cecum does not appear to be inflamed, performing an appendectomy is the appropriate management.

Are There Long-Term Consequences to Removing the Appendix?

Potentially. The appendix does provide some immune function and stores healthy bacteria. Recent studies suggest that removal of the appendix increases the risks of inflammatory bowel disease, *Clostridium difficile* colitis, and colorectal cancer.

Areas Where You Can Get in Trouble

Pseudoappendicitis

Pseudoappendicitis refers to a disease which presents exactly like appendicitis but is due to another cause. The classic cause is a *Yersinia enterocolitica* infection, which presents with RLQ pain, fever, vomiting, and, in severe cases, bloody diarrhea. Patients may have sick contacts (e.g., a teacher at a daycare center). It is usually self-limited, but in immunosuppressed patients, it can result in fatal sepsis. Treatment consists of doxycycline.

Missing Ovarian Torsion: A Surgical Emergency

Right-sided ovarian torsion can be mistaken for acute appendicitis, given similar symptoms such as RLQ pain, fever, and leukocytosis. Transvaginal ultrasound and/or CT scanning can help with diagnosis. Ovarian torsion is a surgical emergency, and delays can result in necrosis of the ovary. In fact, salvage of the ovary is only about 10% in adults, due to delays in diagnosis.

Misdiagnosing Acute Appendicitis During Pregnancy

Acute appendicitis is the most common surgical emergency in pregnancy. Historically, diagnosing appendicitis in pregnant women was considered challenging due to the belief that advancing pregnancy distorts normal anatomy, causing the appendix to shift and pain to localize atypically in the upper quadrants. However, most pregnant patients with appendicitis still report pain in the RLQ across all three trimesters. Delayed diagnosis increases the risk of appendiceal perforation, which significantly raises the likelihood of fetal loss and preterm delivery. Establishing an accurate and early diagnosis with either ultrasound or MRI is crucial. If these imaging modalities are not available or are nondiagnostic, a low-dose CT scan should be performed.

Watch Out

Appendiceal perforation is the most significant risk factor for fetal mortality in a pregnant woman with acute appendicitis.

Under Age 5: Harder to Get History and Examine and More Prone to Early Rupture

Diagnosis of appendicitis is challenging in young children due to their inability to give an accurate history and frequent GI upset. Children under 5 years of age more frequently present with perforated appendicitis (45%) due to an underdeveloped omentum that is less capable of containing the rupture.

Elderly: More Prone to Rupture

Elderly patients tend to present later in their course of appendicitis, have an atypical presentation, and have a higher rate of rupture (>50%). The higher rate of morbidity and mortality associated with perforated appendicitis means that the index of suspicion for appendicitis should be higher in the elderly. Incidence of colon cancer increases with age. Perforated colon cancer can mimic appendicitis in the elderly. Advanced age or the presence of microcytic anemia should prompt a workup for colon cancer after recovering from the appendicitis.

Immunosuppressed Patient

The incidence of acute appendicitis is higher in patients with human immunodeficiency virus (HIV). Presenting symptoms are similar to those of non-infected patients; however, these patients manifest only relative leukocytosis. There is an increased risk of perforation secondary to low CD4 count and delay in presentation. HIV is not a risk for adverse surgical outcomes.

Areas of Controversy

Should Acute Non-perforated Appendicitis be Managed Nonoperatively?

The gold standard for managing acute appendicitis remains laparoscopic appendectomy. However, several studies support nonoperative management with antibiotics as an option for uncomplicated cases. A relative contraindication is the presence of an appendicolith. The CODA trial, one of the most comprehensive studies, found that antibiotics alone provided comparable quality of life and symptom resolution as surgery, with about 70% of patients successfully avoiding surgery in the first year. However, around 30% eventually required appendectomy, particularly among those with an appendicolith, who showed higher failure rates with antibiotic therapy. The APPAC study and similar trials also support nonoperative management, showing that recurrence rates hover between 15% and 30%. Despite these results, patients should be advised of a potentially higher risk of subsequent emergency visits and hospitalizations with nonoperative management compared to surgery.

After Nonoperative Management of an Appendiceal Abscess or Phlegmon, Is Interval Appendectomy Necessary?

Following successful nonoperative management of perforated appendicitis with abscess or phlegmon, the role of an interval appendectomy (performing appendectomy 6–8 weeks later) to prevent a future attack is controversial. The recurrence risk of appendicitis post-abscess is low, estimated at 5–25%, with most recurrences occurring within 6 months. As such, the majority of experts' opinion is that interval appendectomy is unnecessary. Oftentimes, in an interval appendectomy, the residual appendix is scarred and involuted. However, in patients over 40, most would recommend performing a colonoscopy 6–8 weeks after recovery to rule out colon cancer.

Acute Appendicitis (Fig. 23.5)

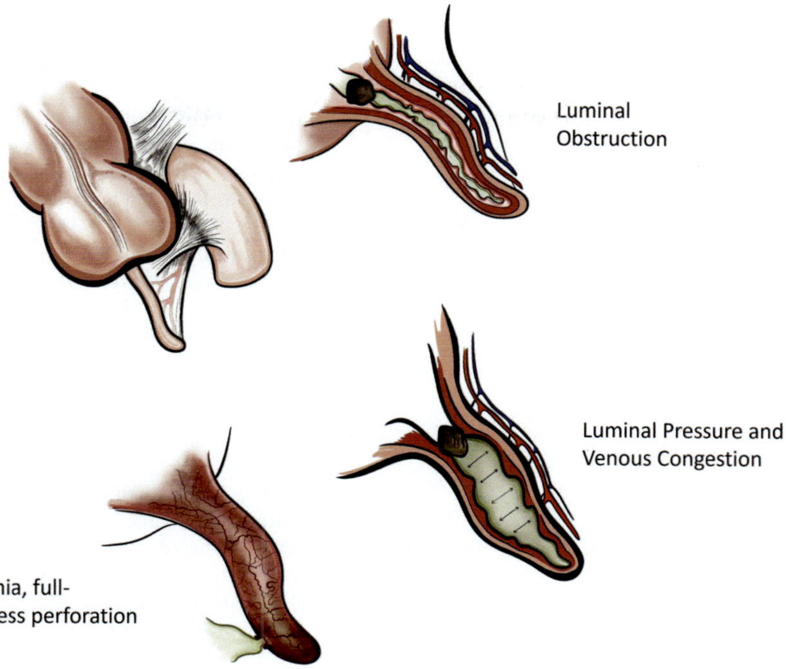

Fig. 23.5 Progression of Appendicitis: This figure shows the progression of appendicitis, which begins with luminal obstruction. This leads to increased pressure and venous congestion, followed by ischemia and full-thickness perforation of the appendix wall

Summary of Essentials

History

- Anorexia (hamburger sign), nausea, vomiting
- Vague periumbilical pain that shifts to the RLQ

Physical Exam

- McBurney's point tenderness
- Rovsing's, psoas, and obturator signs

Laboratory

- Elevated WBC with left shift
- C-reactive protein is more helpful for children
- Pregnancy test should be ordered for all women of childbearing age with abdominal pain
- Urinalysis: sterile pyuria

Diagnosis

- A clinical diagnosis of classic history, physical, and elevated WBC

Imaging

- Though none were needed with classic H&P and leukocytosis, imaging was usually obtained to confirm
- US: women and children
- Avoid CT in children (increased risk of malignancy) and pregnancy (risk to fetus)
- CT: if the diagnosis is equivocal in men and non-pregnant women
- MRI: pregnant women

Pathophysiology

- Closed-loop obstruction
- Fecalith in adults, lymphoid hyperplasia in children

Management

- Gold standard: Laparoscopic appendectomy
- Conservative management with antibiotics is an option in uncomplicated appendicitis

Special Situations

- CT is the most sensitive test for appendicitis and may show fecalith, periappendiceal fat stranding, free fluid, or phlegmon
- Perforated appendicitis is a result of a closed-loop obstruction, creating an ischemic mucosal wall and not a direct result of increased intraluminal pressure
- Most common cause of appendicitis is a fecalith in adults
- Consider pseudoappendicitis in a patient with a history suggestive of appendicitis + extensive diarrhea

Suggested Reading

Bonomo RA, Chow AW, Edwards MS, et al. 2024 Clinical Practice Guideline Update by the Infectious Diseases Society of America on Complicated Intra-abdominal Infections: Risk Assessment, Diagnostic Imaging, and Microbiological Evaluation in Adults, Children, and Pregnant People. *Clin Infect Dis.* 2024;79(Supplement_3):S81–S87. https://doi.org/10.1093/cid/ciae346

CODA Collaborative, Flum DR, Davidson GH, et al. A Randomized Trial Comparing Antibiotics with Appendectomy for Appendicitis. *N Engl J Med.* 2020;383(20):1907–1919. https://doi.org/10.1056/NEJMoa2014320

Di Saverio S, Podda M, De Simone B, et al. Diagnosis and treatment of acute appendicitis: 2020 update of the WSES Jerusalem guidelines. *World J Emerg Surg.* 2020;15(1):27. Published 2020 Apr 15. https://doi.org/10.1186/s13017-020-00306-3

Di Saverio S, Sibilio A, Giorgini E, Biscardi A, et al. The NOTA Study (Non Operative Treatment for Acute Appendicitis): prospective study on the efficacy and safety of antibiotics (amoxicillin and clavulanic acid) for treating patients with right lower quadrant abdominal pain and long-term follow-up of conservatively treated suspected appendicitis. Ann Surg. 2014;260(1):109–17.

Lee S, Jang EJ, Jo J, et al. Long-term impacts of appendectomy associated with increased incidence of inflammatory bowel disease, infection, and colorectal cancer. Int J Colorectal Dis. 2021 Aug;36(8):1643–1652. https://doi.org/10.1007/s00384-021-03886-x. Epub 2021 Feb 16. PMID: 33594506.

McCutcheon BA, Chang DC, Marcus LP, Inui T, et al. Long-term outcomes of patients with nonsurgically managed uncomplicated appendicitis. J Am Coll Surgeons. 2014;218(5):905–13.

O'Leary DP, Walsh SM, Bolger J, et al. A Randomized Clinical Trial Evaluating the Efficacy and Quality of Life of Antibiotic-only Treatment of Acute Uncomplicated Appendicitis: Results of the COMMA Trial. *Ann Surg.* 2021;274(2):240–247. https://doi.org/10.1097/SLA.0000000000004785

Podda M, Poillucci G, Pacella D, et al. Appendectomy versus conservative treatment with antibiotics for patients with uncomplicated acute appendicitis: a propensity score-matched analysis of patient-centered outcomes (the ACTUAA prospective multicenter trial) [published correction appears in Int J Colorectal Dis. 2021 Mar;36(3):599. doi: 10.1007/s00384-021-03862-5]. *Int J Colorectal Dis.* 2021;36(3):589–598. https://doi.org/10.1007/s00384-021-03843-8

Rushing A, Bugaev N, Jones C, et al. Management of acute appendicitis in adults: A practice management guideline from the Eastern Association for the Surgery of Trauma. *J Trauma Acute Care Surg.* 2019;87(1):214–224. https://doi.org/10.1097/TA.0000000000002270

Salminen P, Paajanen H, Rautio T, Nordström P, et al. Antibiotic therapy vs appendectomy for treatment of uncomplicated acute appendicitis: the APPAC randomized clinical trial. JAMA. 2015;313(23):2340–8.

Smith MC, Chung PJ, Constable YC, Boylan MR, Alfonso AE, Sugiyama G. Appendectomy in patients with human immunodeficiency virus: not as bad as we once thought. Surgery. 2017 Apr;161(4):1076–82.

Pencil-Thin Stools and Intermittent Constipation

Areg Grigorian, Christian de Virgilio, Tracey D. Arnell, and Beverley A. Petrie

Contents

C. de Virgilio, A. Grigorian (eds.), *Surgery*, https://doi.org/10.1007/978-3-032-09799-6_24

Case Study

A 57-year-old obese woman with diabetes visits her primary care physician for her annual examination. She reports an unintentional 20-lb weight loss over the past few months, without despite no changes in her diet or physical activity. She also describes experiencing pencil-thin stools, intermittent constipation, and a sensation of incomplete bowel evacuation. She also reports that there was no blood or mucus in her stool. Her medical history includes a 20 pack-year smoking history, and she has never undergone a colonoscopy. There is no family history of cancer. On physical examination, she is afebrile with a heart rate of 78 beats per minute and blood pressure of 132/74 mmHg. Her abdomen is soft, non-tender, and non-distended, with no palpable masses. Rectal examination shows no masses or visible blood. Laboratory studies reveal a hematocrit of 37% (normal range: 40–52%).

Diagnosis

What Is the Differential Diagnosis for a Change in Bowel Habits? (Table 24.1)

Table 24.1 The differential diagnosis for a change in bowel habits

Condition	Change in bowel habits	Other characteristics
Colorectal cancer	Diarrhea, constipation, decreased stool caliber (left colon)	Iron deficiency anemia (more right colon), fatigue, weight loss, bright red blood per rectum (rectal cancer)
Irritable bowel syndrome (IBS)	Diarrhea alternating with constipation, +/– mucus, no blood	Symptom-based diagnosis, chronic abdominal pain relieved by BM, bloating, tenesmus, depression/anxiety common
IBD (ulcerative colitis or Crohn's)	Diarrhea +/– blood, mucus	Abdominal pain, severe cramps, weight loss, anemia
Celiac disease	Pale, loose, and greasy stool (steatorrhea), diarrhea	Weight loss, failure to thrive (in children), malabsorption, anemia, *dermatitis herpetiformis* (autoimmune maculopapular rash)
Intestinal pseudo-obstruction (Ogilvie's)	Constipation	Bowel distention (especially cecum) in the absence of anatomic lesions, severely ill hospitalized patients, nausea, vomiting, electrolyte imbalance, opioid use
Thyroid disease	Diarrhea (hyperthyroid) or constipation (hypothyroid)	Anxiety, tremor, palpitations, heat intolerance (hyperthyroidism); fatigue, cold intolerance (hypothyroidism)
Drugs (laxatives, antidiarrheal)	Diarrhea or constipation	Medication-induced change in bowel habits, *melanosis coli*, weight loss, psychosocial comorbidities
Infectious	Diarrhea	Viral, bacterial, or parasitic infection

BM bowel movement, *IBD* inflammatory bowel disease

What Is the Most Likely Diagnosis?

Given the patient's bowel symptoms, anemia, weight loss, and age, the most likely diagnosis is colon cancer until proven otherwise. The predominant symptoms are those of a slowly obstructing lesion, as evidenced by a change in bowel habits with pencil-thin stools, which is most suggestive of a left-sided lesion.

Screening

What Screening Is Recommended for Colorectal Cancer?

The U.S. Preventive Services Task Force (USPSTF)) recommends that all average-risk adults begin colorectal cancer screening at age 45 and contine through age 75. For adults aged 76–85, the decision to continue screening should be individualized based on overall health, previous screening history, and personal preferences. Screening is not recommended for individuals older than 85 years.

What Are the Recommended Colorectal Cancer Screening Guidelines for Individuals Who Have a First-Degree Relative Diagnosed with Colorectal Cancer or Those with Inflammatory Bowel Disease (IBD)?

For individuals with a first-degree relative diagnosed with colorectal cancer before the age of 60, screening should start at **age 40** *or* **10 years earlier than the relative's age at diagnosis**, whichever comes first. Screening should be repeated every 5 years. Patients with IBD should begin screening 8–10 years after their initial diagnosis. If primary sclerosing cholangitis is present at the time of IBD, a screening colonoscopy should be performed immediately. Subsequently, surveillance colonoscopies are generally recommended every 1–2 years.

What Are the Differences Between the Various Screening Modalities?

The decision to use a particular screening tool needs to be made by the patient after discussing the benefits, risks, and financial considerations imposed on the patient. ◘ Table 24.2 goes over the key differences.

◘ **Table 24.2** Screening for colorectal cancer

Screening	USPSTF	Interval	Features
Colonoscopy	Yes	Every 10 years	Visualizes the entire rectum and colon, can detect lesions less than 0.5 cm, able to remove polyps and obtain biopsies, used as a follow-up test if other tests are equivocal, sedation required, 0.2% perforation risk
Fecal immunochemical test (FIT)	Yes	Annually	Detects human hemoglobin; no dietary restrictions; can be done at home; positive result requires colonoscopy
Fecal occult blood test (gFOBT)	Yes	Annually	Less specific than FIT; requires dietary and medication restrictions; positive result requires colonoscopy
Stool DNA test (FIT-DNA)	Yes	Every 1–3 years	Combines FIT with DNA markers for neoplasia; can be done at home; higher false-positive rate; positive result requires colonoscopy
Flexible sigmoidoscopy	Yes	Every 5 years	Limited to only the lower third of the colon, able to remove polyps and obtain biopsies, sedation required; if abnormal, must undergo colonoscopy
CT colonography	Yes	Every 5 years	Similar sensitivity to colonoscopy for large adenomas; no sedation; requires bowel prep; cannot biopsy or remove polyps; may identify incidental extracolonic findings (e.g., AAA); if abnormal, must undergo colonoscopy

Watch Out
In elderly patients, any new onset changes in stool frequency or consistency should raise concern and prompt screening for colon cancer. In both younger and older individuals, the presence of red flag features—such as unexplained weight loss, iron deficiency anemia, or blood in the stool (hematochezia)—also requires early diagnostic evaluation.

History and Physical

What Is the Significance of the Patient's Unintended Weight Loss?

Unintentional weight loss is a concerning sign that may indicate an underlying malignancy. In patients with colorectal cancer, it may signify the presence of **metastatic** disease. Although the pathogenesis of cancer-related cachexia is not fully understood, tumor necrosis factor-alpha (*TNF-α*) seems to play a key role due to its direct catabolic effects on skeletal muscle. Other causes of unexplained weight loss include depression, celiac disease, Addison's disease, chronic obstructive pulmonary disease, IBD, peptic ulcer disease, tuberculosis, and hyperthyroidism.

What Are the Risk Factors for Colon Cancer?

Risk factors for colorectal cancer include advancing age, African American or Ashkenazi Jewish heritage, a personal or family history of colorectal cancer or adenomatous polyps, and the presence of inflammatory bowel disease. Certain genetic disorders, such as Lynch syndrome and familial adenomatous polyposis, significantly increase the risk. Modifiable risk factors include a diet rich in red or processed meats, lack of physical activity, obesity, smoking, heavy alcohol consumption, type 2 diabetes, and a history of pelvic radiation.

Where Does Colon Cancer Rank in Terms of the Most Common Cancers in the United States? In Terms of the Highest Overall Mortality? (Table 24.3)

Table 24.3 The most frequently diagnosed cancers and its overall cancer-related mortality

	Incidence (in order of frequency)	Mortality (highest first)
Men	Prostate, lung, and colon	Lung, prostate, and colon
Women	Breast, lung, and colon	Lung, breast, and colon

Are Right- or Left-Sided Colon Cancers More Common, and How Do the Presentations Differ?

Most colon cancers develop on the left side, particularly near the rectosigmoid junction. Left-sided colon cancers are more likely to cause a change in bowel habits and symptoms of obstruction. When stool reaches the sigmoid, it is often dense and devoid of excess fluid. The caliber of the lumen is also narrower on the left side, and with a circumferential tumor causing partial obstruction, patients report pencil-thin stools, often tinged with blood. Bowel habits can alternate between constipation and diarrhea. Patients report distention with lower abdominal colicky pain. Patients with lesions that are closer to the anal orifice may report bright red blood per rectum (hematochezia). A smaller number of colon cancers are right-sided, and the most common finding is an insidious onset of iron deficiency anemia secondary to chronic GI blood loss. Because the cecum has the largest diameter, a change in stool caliber is uncommon. Rarely, if the tumor is rapidly growing, patients can experience severe pain, and an RLQ mass may be appreciated on exam.

Watch Out
Melena is more common in right-sided colon cancers.

Why Is the Rectal Examination Important in Suspected Colorectal Cancer?

The digital rectal exam (DRE)) is often overlooked by the novice, yet it is of critical importance in the evaluation of a patient with possible colorectal cancer. A DRE by itself is not a good test for detecting colon cancer because its reach is limited. However, the value of the DRE lies in its ability to detect low rectal cancers because it allows the examiner to feel a mass, which is suggestive of malignancy. In addition, distance from the anal verge, mobility, and anatomic relation to other pelvic structures can be assessed. A fixed mass is more likely to be locally advanced, and relation to the prostate, vagina, and sacrum is important for surgical planning.

Pathophysiology

What Is a Polyp, and How Are They Generally Classified?

A polyp is a mass that protrudes into the lumen of the GI tract and can either be pedunculated (with a stalk) or sessile (flat). Nonneoplastic polyps can arise from abnormal mucosal maturation, inflammation, or colonic architecture. However, polyps arising from epithelial proliferation and dysplasia are true neoplasms and may have malignant potential. They are collectively known as adenomatous polyps or adenomas.

What Is the Difference between Different Colonic Polyps? (Table 24.4)

Table 24.4 Adenomatous polyps/Adenomas

Adenoma type	Features	Malignancy potential
Tubular	The *most common type* with the majority occurring in the rectosigmoid but can be found anywhere in the colon	Low
Tubulovillous	Composed of both tubular and villous features; can be pedunculated or sessile	Moderate
Villous	Less common; tend to be larger and occur in older persons, typically in the rectum; more commonly sessile, and with cauliflower-like projections;	High
Sessile serrated adenoma	Flat, broad-based polyps that can be mistaken for hyperplastic polyps; have a "sawtooth" appearance under the microscope	High

What Is Juvenile Polyposis Syndrome?

Juvenile polyposis syndrome is a hereditary condition characterized by multiple hamartomatous polyps, most commonly in the colon and stomach. It typically presents in childhood or adolescence with painless, intermittent hematochezia. The polyps are 1–2 cm, mucus-filled, and histologically show dilated glands in the lamina propria. The syndrome is inherited in an autosomal dominant pattern, most often due to mutations in *SMAD4* or *BMPR1A*. Associated findings may include mucocutaneous telangiectasias and iron deficiency anemia from chronic GI bleeding. Surveillance colonoscopy is recommended every 1–3 years starting at diagnosis due to increased risk of colorectal cancer.

How Is Juvenile Polyposis Syndrome Distinguished from Other Syndromes with Hamartomatous Polyps?

Juvenile polyposis, Peutz-Jeghers Syndrome (PJS), and Cronkhite-Canada syndrome involve hamartomatous polyps. Unlike juvenile polyposis, in PJS the polyps are more common in the small bowel. PJS includes mucocutaneous pigmentation. Both have an increased risk of colon cancer, but PJS also has a broader cancer risk. Cronkhite-Canada syndrome features alopecia and nail dystrophy and is not inherited.

How Do You Distinguish the Adenomatous Polyposis Syndromes?

Familial adenomatous polyposis (FAP) features hundreds to thousands of adenomatous polyps. On the other hand, Lynch syndrome patients only have a few scattered adenomatous polyps. This makes Lynch syndrome harder to recognize without a careful family history.

What Is the Relationship of Colon Cancer with Lynch Syndrome?

Lynch syndrome, formerly known as hereditary nonpolyposis colorectal cancer (HNPCC), is an autosomal dominant disorder caused by germline mutations in DNA mismatch repair (MMR) genes, including MLH1, MSH2, MSH6, PMS2, and EPCAM. It was called nonpolyposis because it is not associated with hundreds of polyps like the polyposis syndromes. Rather, patients only have a few polyps, similar to patients who develop sporadic cancer. However, colorectal cancers in Lynch syndrome are more likely to arise from right-sided adenomatous polyps, are more likely to be flat, and progress to carcinoma more rapidly than sporadic adenomas. It accounts for approximately 3–5% of all colorectal cancers. Individuals with Lynch syndrome have a significantly increased lifetime risk of colorectal cancer, often developing right-sided tumors at a younger age, typically in the fourth or fifth decade of life. In addition to colorectal cancer, Lynch syndrome predisposes individuals to various extracolonic malignancies, notably endometrial cancer, as well as cancers of the ovary, stomach, small intestine, hepatobiliary tract, urinary tract, pancreas, brain (usually glioblastoma), and skin (sebaceous neoplasms).

What Are the Modified Amsterdam Criteria for Lynch Syndrome?

They are diagnostic criteria to help clinicians identify families that are more likely to have Lynch syndrome. The *3-2-1-1-0* rule can help you remember the requirements and are intended to prompt consideration of genetic testing for DNA mismatch repair gene mutations:

- *3* or more relatives with histologically verified cancers in the colon, endometrium, small intestine, or pelvis.
- *2* or more successive generation affected.
- *1* or more relatives diagnosed prior to age 50.
- *1* should be a first-degree relative of the other two.
- *0* familial adenomatous polyposis.

What Is the Relationship of Colon Cancer with FAP?

FAP is an autosomal dominant condition that, if left untreated, will develop into cancer. The mutation is in the adenomatous polyposis coli (APC) gene on chromosome 5 (remember, five letters in colon). Polyps begin on average in the mid-teens but can appear as early as age 7. Screening with flexible sigmoidoscopy should begin at age 10. Prophylactic colectomy is often recommended by age 20 to prevent the development of cancer. If left untreated, 100% of patients develop cancer by the fourth or fifth decade of life.

What Are the Two Variants of FAP?

Gardner's syndrome is an autosomal dominant condition with variable penetrance, characterized by osteomas and colonic polyps. If left untreated, all patients develop colon cancer by the fourth or fifth decade of life. *Turcot syndrome* is characterized by café au lait spots, malignant brain tumors (often glioblastoma multiforme), and neoplastic colon polyps that progress to cancer.

How Do Colon Cancers Develop?

The majority of colon cancers arise from the adenoma-carcinoma sequence (Fig. 24.1). This is also known as the chromosome instability pathway because there is a stepwise accumulation of mutations leading to carcinoma. The sequence begins with a loss of the APC tumor suppressor gene, resulting in decreased intercellular adhesion and increased proliferation. A subsequent activating mutation in the KRAS oncogene promotes adenoma formation through unregulated intracellular signaling. Adenomatous polyps are considered premalignant, with approximately 20% progressing to carcinoma. The malignant potential of an adenomatous polyp is related to the age of the patient, the size of the polyp, and the villous component. Finally, loss of

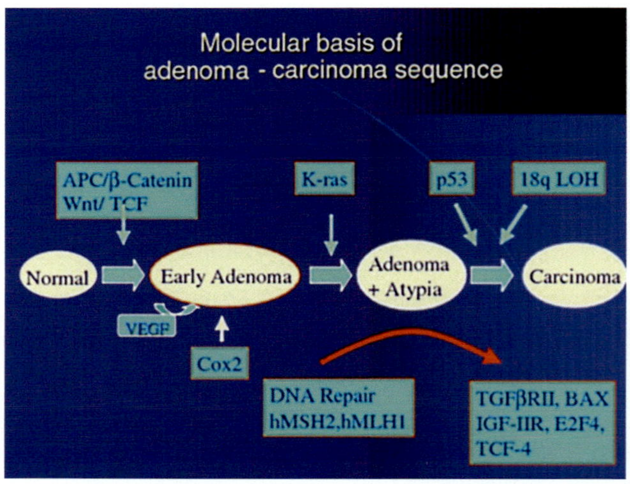

Fig. 24.1 Adenoma-carcinoma sequence (From Chu DZJ, et al. The Surgeon's Role in Cancer Prevention. The Model in Colorectal Carcinoma. Annals of Surgical Oncology 2007;14(11):3058. Reprinted with permission from Springer Nature)

the p53 tumor suppressor gene will increase tumorigenesis in an adenoma and result in carcinoma. A minority of colorectal cancers arise via the microsatellite instability pathway, in which defective DNA mismatch repair leads to accumulation of replication errors, increasing the risk of tumor development.

What Features of an Adenoma Are Associated with an Increased Malignant Risk?

There are four subtypes of adenomas (Table 24.5) that are based on their epithelial architecture. Their risk of malignancy is dependent on polyp size, architecture, and severity of dysplasia. Larger adenomas are more ominous, with a 40% chance of cancer in adenomas >4 cm. Disarrangements in architecture and severe dysplasia can also increase the risk of cancer.

Why Screen Every 10 Years When Using Colonoscopy?

The majority of adenocarcinomas arise from adenomatous polyps. Observational studies have suggested that the sequence from adenoma to carcinoma takes about 10 years. Visualizing the entire colon with a colonoscopy every 10 years is sufficient to catch the majority of these cancers. In patients with other risk factors, screening may need to occur more frequently.

Why Is Colonoscopy Superior to Flexible Sigmoidoscopy for Screening?

Flexible sigmoidoscopy is only able to visualize the rectum and the distal third of the colon, so polyps in the proximal colon will be missed. A complete colonoscopy is defined by the endoscope reaching the cecum and visualizing the ileocecal valve. Thus, colonoscopy can adequately visualize the entire colon.

Where Are the Most Common Metastatic Sites for Colorectal Cancer?

Regional metastases are to the mesenteric lymph nodes (the N in the TNM system). The *liver* is the most common location of distant metastasis, owing to the venous drainage of the colon to the liver via the mesenteric veins draining to the portal system and the tendency for these cancers to spread hematogenously. Rectal cancers may have atypical locations for metastasis because they drain into both the portal and systemic venous circulations. They first metastasize to the *lungs* because the inferior rectal veins drain into the inferior vena cava via the internal iliac veins. Via the systemic veins, rectal cancers may also metastasize to the inguinal lymph nodes. Additionally, via sacral veins, rectal cancers may result in spine and brain metastasis. Other locations for metastasis include the peritoneum, supraclavicular lymph node, and bones.

Watch Out

The most common site of metastasis for colon cancer is the liver, whereas the most common site for rectal cancer is the lung.

Watch Out

Individuals with first-degree family members with FAP should begin screening with a flexible sigmoidoscopy by age 10.

Watch Out

FAP needs to be ruled out prior to establishing a diagnosis of Lynch syndrome.

Watch Out

FAP patients are also at risk for the development of adenomas throughout the GI tract, particularly the duodenum with a malignant transformation such as periampullary carcinoma. As such, FAP patients should undergo surveillance with upper endoscopy every 1–3 years starting at age 25.

What Is the Difference Between Synchronous and Metachronous Tumors?

In some cases, patients may develop colon cancer in two separate locations simultaneously, a condition known as a synchronous tumor. Therefore, it is important to examine the entire colon via colonoscopy, even if a colon cancer is discovered in the sigmoid colon. Metachronous tumors are primary cancers that develop elsewhere in the colon at least 6 months after the primary resection. This should be distinguished from recurrent cancer, in which the colon cancer returns at the margins of the surgical resection in the colon or mesentery.

Workup

For the Patient Described Above, What Would Be the Next Steps in the Workup?

Given that the patient is manifesting symptoms that are highly concerning for colon cancer, colonoscopy is recommended, with biopsy of any suspicious lesions.

Is There Any Role for Testing His Stool for Blood?

In the case presented, there is sufficient suspicion for colon cancer and thus a strong indication for additional workup, such that testing for blood in the stool is not important. An error would be to test the stool for blood and, if negative, assume there is no colon cancer. Additionally, if a patients has a history of rectal bleeding, there is no value in Hemoccult testing because bleeding can be intermittent, and thus, the test may be a false negative. Evaluation should be based on their complaint.

Once a Diagnosis of Colon Cancer Is Established, What Laboratory Tests Are Recommended?

Carcinoembryonic antigen (CEA)) level and liver enzyme tests are recommended. Elevation of liver enzymes (particularly alkaline phosphatase) is suggestive of possible liver metastasis.

Is CEA Useful for Screening? How Is it Used?

No. CEA is not recommended for colorectal cancer screening due to low sensitivity and specificity. It is primarily used to monitor treatment response and detect recurrence. A decline in CEA after surgery suggests effective treatment. In patients with elevated preoperative CEA, levels should be checked every 3–6 months for the first 2 years postoperatively, along with periodic physical exams and imaging.

What Other Conditions Can Elevate the CEA Level?

Gastritis, peptic ulcer disease, hepatic disease, pulmonary disease (i.e., COPD), diabetes, visceral cancers (e.g., gastric or pancreatic cancers), IBD, chronic inflammatory conditions (e.g., rheumatoid arthritis), and smoking can elevate the CEA level.

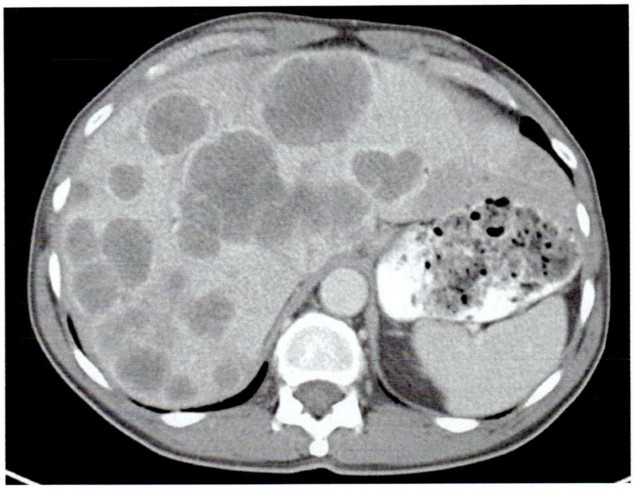

Fig. 24.2 Axial CT of hypoenhancing liver masses consistent with metastases

What Is Additional Imaging, if Any, Is Recommended Once a Diagnosis of Colon Cancer Is Established?

CT scans of the chest, abdomen, and pelvis are recommended to detect metastasis. Nearly 20% of patients initially present with metastatic spread. CT of the abdomen and pelvis may identify distant metastasis to the liver (Fig. 24.2). Additionally, the primary tumor may be visualized, and its relationship to surrounding structures, including possible extracolonic invasion, can be evaluated. However, CT has poor sensitivity and specificity for identifying metastasis to regional lymph nodes. Chest imaging is done to look for pulmonary spread of disease. Routine use of PET scans does not add significant information, and as such, is not recommended.

How Is the Workup of Colon and Rectal Cancers Different?

The evaluation of rectal cancer differs significantly from that of colon cancer due to the need for precise local staging and the potential impact on sphincter preservation. The rectum's confined pelvic position makes it more challenging to achieve adequate resection margins, and tumors close to the anal sphincter may compromise continence. For these reasons, high-resolution pelvic MRI is the preferred modality for local staging. MRI accurately assesses tumor depth, mesorectal involvement, and proximity to the sphincter complex. Patients with locally advanced disease or suspected nodal involvement are typically treated with neoadjuvant chemoradiation to shrink the tumor, improve resectability, and increase the likelihood of sphincter-sparing surgery. In contrast, colon cancer staging primarily relies on CT imaging, as local staging is less critical for surgical planning.

Watch Out

Adjuvant therapy is a planned addition of therapeutic agents (i.e., chemotherapy, radiation, or hormone therapy) following surgery in an attempt to treat advanced disease. *Neoadjuvant therapy* is administered prior to surgery and often done to shrink or debulk tumors to make resection more amenable. *Salvage therapy* is an unplanned addition employed when standard therapy fails.

How Do You Stage Colon Cancer?

The most commonly used staging system is the one described by the American Joint Committee on Cancer (AJCC). *T* (tumor) describes the size of the tumor and/or its depth of invasion. *N* (node) describes spread to regional lymph nodes. *M* (metastasis) indicates if the tumor has metastasized remotely.

Management

How Are Polyps That Are Found During Colonoscopy Managed?

Polyps can be removed with polypectomy and surveyed 1 to 5 years after for recurrence depending on the number, type, and size of polyps. Any identified polyp must be removed in its entirety if possible. If this cannot be done endoscopically, a biopsy should be obtained, and future surgical excision will likely be warranted.

What Is a "Bowel Prep," and Why Is it Done?

A "bowel prep" essentially prepares the colon for surgery. Its main purpose is to eliminate stool from the intestines, allowing for improved visualization of polyps and reducing the risk of postoperative infection. During colon surgery, when the bowel is cut, a clean colon helps minimize the chance of stool leakage into the peritoneal cavity. Most bowel preps involve the oral intake of polyethylene glycol the day before the operation to flush out the colon. Some clinicians also use an oral, nonabsorbable antibiotic prior to surgery to decrease the colonic bacterial levels.

Watch Out

Bowel prep should not be utilized in patients suspected of having an obstructing cancer or bowel perforation.

What Are the Recommended Operations in Colon Cancer?

The location (◘ Table 24.5) of the primary cancer is the main determinant for what procedure is most appropriate.

◘ **Table 24.5** Location of colon cancer and procedure

Location of cancer	Operation
Right-sided colon	Right colectomy with ligation of the ileocolic artery
Transverse colon	Extended right colectomy with ligation of the ileocolic and middle colic artery
Descending colon	Left colectomy with ligation of IMA
Sigmoid colon	Left colectomy with ligation of IMA

IMA inferior mesenteric artery

Watch Out

Intraoperatively, the large bowel can be identified by the taenia coli (longitudinal white line) and taenia epiploica (fat appendages). The taenia disappear at the transition from the colon to the rectum. In contrast, the small bowel does not have these features and is much smoother than the large bowel.

What Operations Are Typically Offered to Patients with Rectal Cancer?

If the tumor is more than 2 cm proximal to the dentate line, a low anterior resection (LAR)) is performed. LAR is done by removing part of the rectum through the abdomen and reconnecting the proximal colon with the distal rectum. If the tumor is within 2 cm of the dentate line, an abdominoperineal resection (APR)) is more likely to be needed. An APR involves removing the entire distal rectum and anus, including the sphincters, leaving a permanent colostomy.

How Many Lymph Nodes Should Be Resected?

A minimum of 12 lymph nodes should be resected, allowing for more accurate staging and improved prognosis.

Why Is Neoadjuvant Therapy Used for Rectal Cancer and Not Colon Cancer?

Neoadjuvant therapy is used in rectal cancer to reduce tumors size before surgery, improving resectability and increasing the chances of sphincter preservation. This is particularly important given the rectum's location in the narrow pelvis and its proximity to the sphincter complex. Standard neoadjuvant treatment consists of chemoradiation, as chemotherapy sensitizes tumor cells to radiation. In select cases, total neoadjuvant therapy (TNT), which delivers both chemotherapy and radiation before surgery, is used to further optimize outcomes. Immunotherapy is emerging as a nonoperative alternative in patients with mismatch repair-deficient (dMMR) or microsatellite instability-high (MSI-H) rectal cancers, where it may induce complete clinical responses. However, this approach remains investigational and is not yet standard care. In contrast, neoadjuvant therapy is not typically required for colon cancer, as tumors are more easily resectable. Adjuvant chemotherapy is reserved for patients with node-positive disease or high-risk stage II tumors.

Why Is Radiation Therapy Used for Rectal Cancer and Not Colon Cancer?

Radiation therapy is used in rectal cancer to reduce local recurrence rates and facilitate achieving complete tumor removal within the confined pelvic space. In contrast, radiation is not routinely used for colon cancer because the mobile position of the colon makes targeted delivery difficult, and the risk of small bowel toxicity is high. Irradiating a large intra-abdominal field would expose the small intestine to radiation, increasing the risk of acute and chronic radiation enteritis. The fixed location of the rectum allows for a more focused radiation field, minimizing exposure to surrounding organs.

What Are the Major Complications Specific to Colon Surgery?

Major complications unique to colon surgery include injury to the ureters (which can occur during either right or left colectomy), duodenum injury (during right colectomy), spleen injury (during left colectomy), and anastomotic leak. Careful dissection and identification of structures during surgery is important for avoiding intraoperative injuries. Approximately 6% of patients will develop an anastomotic leak, which usually manifests in the first week after surgery with fever, abdominal pain and tenderness, ileus, and leukocytosis. In some cases, *tachycardia* may be the only presenting symptom of an anastomotic leak. Depending on the patient's clinical status, this may require urgent return to the operating room for exploration or additional imaging such as a CT scan. Patients with clinical signs of infection and a confirmed anastomotic leak should be taken to the operating room for exploration, washout, and ostomy diversion. Wound infections occur in up to 25% of patients and are usually managed conservatively by opening the incision to allow for drainage of the infection.

How Is Surveillance Performed After Resection of Colon Cancer?

Postoperative surveillance following curative colon cancer resection depends on the stage at diagnosis. For stage I disease, a colonoscopy shoud be performed 1 year after surgery, then repeated every 3–5 years thereafter. For stages II and III, follow-up includes CEA measurement every 3–6 months for first 2 years, then every 6 months for a total of 5 years. Annual CT scans of the chest, abdomen, and pelvis are recommended for up to 5 years to detect recurrence or metastasis. Colonoscopy should be repeated at 1 year postoperatively; if normal, subsequent intervals are based on findings. The primary goal of ongoing follow-up is the early detection of recurrence and identification of new primary lesions.

Areas of Controversy

Treatment of Stage-IV (Metastatic) Colon Cancer

For patients with stage-IV colon cancer, there has been debate as to whether the appropriate primary treatment is surgery with chemotherapy or chemotherapy alone. Some retrospective studies suggest a survival benefit with resection of the primary tumor in select patients, particularly those with limited metastatic burden and satisfactory performance status. However, randomized trials have not consistently demonstrated a clear advantage over systemic chemotherapy alone. Current guidelines recommend individualized decision-making based on symptomatology, tumor characteristics, and patient factors.

Is it Useful to Follow CEA Levels After Surgery?

CEA monitoring is commonly employed postoperatively to detect recurrence in patients with initially elevated CEA levels. Guidelines suggest checking CEA every 3–6 months for the first 2 years, then every 6 months for a total of 5 years. However, the utility of CEA monitoring is limited in patients whose tumors did not produce CEA preoperatively. Additionally, factors like smoking and other benign conditions can influence CEA levels, potentially leading to false positives. Emerging modalities like circulating tumor DNA (ctDNA) assays are under investigation for their potential to provide more precise surveillance, but they are not yet standard practice.

Summary of Essentials

History and Physical

- Pencil-thin stools, change in bowel habits, weight loss, and iron deficiency anemia in an adult are concerning for colorectal cancer until proven otherwise.
- Right-sided colon cancer classically presents with iron deficiency anemia; left-sided colon cancer presents with obstructive symptoms (pencil-thin stools, constipation), and rectal cancer with hematochezia.
- Colon cancer is the third most frequent cause of cancer-related deaths in men and women.
- New onset bowel changes in elderly patients, or red flag symptoms (e.g., weight loss, anemia, hematochezia) in both older and younger patients, warrant evaluation for colorectal cancer.

Screening

- Average-risk individuals should begin screening at age 45 and continue until age 75; individualized decision-making for ages 76–85.
- Individuals with a first-degree relative diagnosed with colorectal cancer before age 60 should begin screening at age 40 or 10 years prior to the diagnosis, whichever comes first, and repeat every 5 years.
- Screening modalities include colonoscopy (every 10 years), FIT (annually), stool DNA testing, flexible sigmoidoscopy, and CT colonography.

Pathophysiology

- Adenomatous polyps are precursors to colorectal cancer and progress through the adenoma-carcinoma sequence.
- Hyperplastic polyps are the most common type and almost always benign.
- Villous histology, size >1 cm, and high-grade dysplasia increase malignant potential.
- Lynch syndrome, FAP, Gardner's syndrome, and Turcot syndrome are inheritable conditions of colon cancer.

Diagnosis

- Diagnosis confirmation involves colonoscopy and tissue biopsy of suspicious lesions.
- CEA is not useful for screening but may assist in monitoring treatment response and recurrence.

Workup

- All patients with suspected or confirmed colon cancer should undergo CT of the chest, abdomen, and pelvis to evaluate for metastases.
- High-resolution pelvic MRI is preferred for local staging in rectal cancer.
- CEA is used postoperatively for monitoring, not for initial diagnosis.

Management

- Polypectomy is appropriate for benign polyps; surgical resection is required when polyps are not fully removable endoscopically.
- Bowel prep is used prior to colonoscopy or surgery but should be avoided in patients with suspected obstructing cancer.
- Surgical resection is determined by tumor location: right or left colectomy, LAR, or APR.
- Rectal cancer often requires neoadjuvant chemoradiation for locally advanced disease.
- Immunotherapy is an emerging option for MSI-H or dMMR rectal cancer.
- At least 12 lymph nodes should be removed during surgery for accurate staging.
- Postoperative chemotherapy is used for node-positive or high-risk stage II disease.

Complications

- Major surgical risks include injury to adjacent organs (ureters, spleen, duodenum), wound infections, and anastomotic leak.
- Anastomotic leak typically presents within the first postoperative week and may require reoperation.

Suggested Reading

Amri R, Bordeianou LG, Sylla P, Berger DL. Impact of screening colonoscopy on outcomes in colon cancer surgery. JAMA Surg. 2013;148:747.

Cercek A, Lumish MA, Sinopoli J, et al. PD-1 Blockade in Mismatch Repair–Deficient, Locally Advanced Rectal Cancer. *N Engl J Med*. 2022;386(25):2363–2376

Chu DZJ, et al. The Surgeon's role in cancer prevention. The model in colorectal carcinoma. Ann Surg Oncol. 2007;14(11):3058.

Hamilton W, Round A, Sharp D, Peters TJ. Clinical features of colorectal cancer before diagnosis: a population-based case-control study. Br J Cancer. 2005;93:399.

NCCN Clinical Practice Guidelines in Oncology: Colon Cancer, Version 2.2024. *National Comprehensive Cancer Network*. Accessed April 2024.

Shaukat A, Kahi CJ, Burke CA, Rabeneck L, Sauer BG, Rex DK. ACG Clinical Guidelines: Colorectal Cancer Screening 2021. *Am J Gastroenterol*. 2021;116(3):458–479

USPSTF. Screening for Colorectal Cancer: US Preventive Services Task Force Recommendation. *JAMA*. 2021;325(19):1965–1977

Chronic Constipation Presenting with Severe Abdominal Pain

Beverley A. Petrie and Tracey D. Arnell

Contents

C. de Virgilio, A. Grigorian (eds.), *Surgery*, https://doi.org/10.1007/978-3-032-09799-6_25

Case Study

An 80-year-old male presents with severe abdominal distention and, no bowel movements or passage of gas for 3 days, and recent onset of vomiting. He has a history of Parkinson's disease and chronic constipation and lives in a nursing home. His medications include levodopa and benztropine, both of which he has been taking for several years. On examination, his temperature is 37 °C, heart rate 90/min, blood pressure 116/70 mmHg, and respiratory rate 22/min. He appears tachypneic but not acutely ill, and his mental status is unaltered from baseline. Lung examination reveals clear breath sounds bilaterally. His abdomen is severely distended and tympanitic without tenderness, surgical scars, or palpable hernias. Rectal examination demonstrates no stool, palpable masses, or strictures. Laboratory studies reveal a metabolic panel with BUN 26 mg/dL (normal 7–21 mg/dL), creatinine 1.4 mg/dL (0.5–1.4 mg/dL), electrolytes within normal limits, white blood cell (WBC) count $6.8 \times 10^3/\mu L$ ($4.1–10.9 \times 10^3/\mu L$), and lactate 0.9 mmol/L (0.5–2.2 mmol/L). Arterial blood gas (ABG) shows pH 7.48, $PaCO_2$ 30 mmHg, PaO_2 80 mmHg, HCO_3 24 mEq/L, and oxygen saturation (SpO_2) 99%. A plain upright abdominal radiograph shows a massively dilated loop of sigmoid colon with the apex pointing toward the right upper quadrant, consistent with the "coffee bean" or "bent inner tube" sign. An upright chest radiograph shows no free air under the diaphragm.

Diagnosis

What Is the Differential Diagnosis? (Table 25.1)

Table 25.1 Differential diagnosis of clinical presentation

	Pathophysiology leading to obstruction	Comments
Colorectal cancer	Mass (usually in sigmoid) causes mechanical LBO	History of weight loss; change in bowel habits, bloody stools, anemia
Sigmoid volvulus	Stretching and redundancy of sigmoid colon leads to twisting around mesentery	Elderly patients; debilitated or institutionalized patients with chronic constipation
Cecal volvulus	Congenital partial malrotation, in which the cecum and right colon are not fixed, leads to twisting around mesentery	Younger patients (30–60 years of age); may have history of cyclic recurring abdominal pain
Midgut volvulus	A closed-loop SBO secondary to congenital malrotation	Usually presents within first year of life with bilious emesis
Gastric volvulus	Stomach twists around its mesentery	Associated with paraesophageal hiatal hernia; may lead to gastric outlet obstruction
Diverticulitis	Severe bowel wall edema may lead to LBO	Acute diverticulitis: Pain and tenderness in LLQ
Stricture	Inflammation and scarring cause mechanical LBO	IBD, chronic diverticulitis, malignancy, abdominal/pelvic radiation; endoscopy can help identify cause
Fecal impaction	Inspissated stool in rectum or sigmoid causes mechanical LBO	Firm stool in rectal vault on exam
Ogilvie's syndrome (pseudo-obstruction)	Marked colonic distention (most notable in cecum) without mechanical obstruction can lead to perforation	Debilitated, hospitalized patients, electrolyte imbalances, may decompress with colonoscopy or neostigmine
SBO	Most common cause in the USA is adhesions from prior surgery; hernias are the most common cause worldwide	Nausea, extensive vomiting, abdominal surgical scar, hernia bulge
Toxic megacolon	Transmural infection of a markedly dilated colon, associated with ulcerative colitis, pseudomembranous colitis, other bacterial colitis	High fever, tachycardia, abdominal tenderness, acidosis, leukocytosis

IBD inflammatory bowel disease, *LBO* large bowel obstruction, *LLQ* left lower quadrant, *SBO* small bowel obstruction.

What Is the Most Likely Diagnosis?

The massive, slowly progressive abdominal distention, combined with obstipation and x-ray findings, is consistent with a large bowel obstruction (LBO). The radiologic appearance is most consistent with a sigmoid volvulus.

History and Physical

What Is the Difference Between Obstipation and Constipation?

Constipation implies infrequent stools (<3 per week), usually associated with hard stools. Obstipation implies a *complete* absence of gas or stool per rectum, which is highly suggestive of a bowel obstruction.

What Are the Classic Physical Exam Findings in Bowel Obstruction?

In uncomplicated bowel obstruction, the abdomen is generally not tender. The abdomen is typically distended and tympanic. A rectal exam must be performed to rule out fecal impaction, rectal neoplasm, or stricture. Tachypnea is common with LBO, as diaphragm excursion is impaired. The presence of fever or tachycardia in association with an intestinal obstruction suggests strangulation with bowel ischemia or perforation. On exam, check the abdomen and groins for irreducible hernias (the leading cause of small bowel obstruction [SBO] worldwide).

What Findings from History and Physical Examination Can Help Distinguish Between Small and Large Bowel Obstruction?

SBO tends to be associated with more pronounced and earlier-onset vomiting. In an early SBO, bowel sounds are hyperactive, with "rushes and tinkles" (high-pitched sounds of hyperperistaltic small bowel). However, it is important to note that while this finding is frequently emphasized in teaching, it is not particularly specific or clinically reliable. LBO is more likely to be associated with more pronounced distention, less or late-onset vomiting, and decreased bowel sounds.

Why Is a History of Neurologic or Psychiatric Disorders Important?

Drugs used to treat neurologic diseases (e.g., Parkinson's) or psychiatric conditions can affect colonic motility and predispose patients to chronic constipation, stretching of the sigmoid, and volvulus, as well as colonic pseudo-obstruction. It is also important to evaluate for fecal impaction as a potential cause of constipation.

> **Watch Out**
> The most common *symptom* of sigmoid volvulus is lower abdominal pain. The most common *sign* is abdominal distention.

What Is the Classic Presentation for Ogilvie's Syndrome?

Ogilvie's syndrome, or acute colonic pseudo-obstruction, typically occurs in critically ill or elderly patients or those recovering from non-abdominal surgeries such as orthopedic or cardiothoracic procedures. It mimics the presentation of an LBO but lacks a mechanical cause, hence "pseudo-obstruction." The etiology is multifactorial and often related to conditions that impair colonic motility, such as electrolyte imbalances, particularly hypokalemia, hypomagnesemia, and hypophosphatemia. These imbalances may arise postoperatively, in patients with diarrheal illness, or from the use of diuretics. Initial management in stable patients involves supportive care, including correction of fluid and electrolyte imbalances, nasogastric decompression, discontinuation of narcotics or antimotility medications, and addressing predisposing factors. If these measures are ineffective, pharmacologic treatment with neostigmine, an acetylcholinesterase inhibitor, may be used, but cardiac monitoring is required. If pharmacologic therapy fails or is not appropriate, colonoscopic decompression, which removes excess air from the colon, can be performed.

> **Watch Out**
> Neostigmine is contraindicated in pregnancy and in patients with heart block, as it can cause significant bradycardia. Atropine should always be available in the room when patients are receiving neostigmine.

Etiology/Pathophysiology

What Are the Most Common Causes of LBO?

In the United States, malignancy (primarily colon cancer) is the most common cause of LBO (more than half of cases), followed by diverticulitis (either acute or chronic with a stricture) and then volvulus.

> **Watch Out**
> Volvulus is a closed-loop obstruction that, if left untreated, will progress to intestinal ischemia, necrosis, and perforation. It requires urgent intervention.

Where in the Colon Is a Cancer Most Likely to Cause an LBO?

Left-sided colon (smaller diameter) cancers (most commonly sigmoid) are more likely to cause LBO, whereas right-sided colon cancers are more likely to present with iron deficiency anemia. The cecum has the largest diameter, so the tumor would need to become very large to cause an LBO.

What Is the Difference Between Malrotation and Volvulus?

Malrotation is a congenital condition in which the bowel fails to rotate and fixate in its normal anatomic position during fetal development. This abnormal positioning leaves the bowel and its mesentery improperly attached, making them susceptible to twisting and obstruction. Malrotation itself is asymptomatic unless twisting occurs. Volvulus refers to twisting of the bowel resulting in a closed-loop obstruction. It may occur as a manifestation of malrotation, such as midgut volvulus, which involves the small bowel. Midgut volvulus typically presents within the first year of life with bilious emesis. However, volvulus can also occur without malrotation, such as in cases of sigmoid volvulus, due to the sigmoid colon slowly becoming elongated and redundant.

> **Watch Out**
> Serum lactate is a poor marker for intestinal ischemia. For levels to rise, the amount of lactate released by the ischemic bowel needs to exceed the capacity to metabolize it. Additionally, circulation within the ischemic segment of bowel may cease, preventing the release of lactate.

How Does the Etiology Differ Between Sigmoid and Cecal Volvulus?

Cecal volvulus is thought to be due to a congenital partial malrotation, in which the cecum and right colon are not fixed. This predisposes the cecum to twist, leading to obstruction. It generally presents in younger patients. Patients may report intermittent, self-resolving episodes of abdominal symptoms caused by intermittent twisting and untwisting prior to the acute volvulus. In contrast, sigmoid volvulus is an acquired condition resulting from progressive stretching and redundancy of the sigmoid colon over time. This elongation allows the colon to twist around its narrow mesentery, often occurring in older patients or those with chronic constipation or a history of motility disorders.

What Are the Risk Factors for Sigmoid Volvulus?

Factors contributing to stretching and redundancy of the sigmoid include the use of anticholinergic drugs (which impair motility), neurologic and psychiatric diseases (likely due to chronic constipation with stool retention), cystic fibrosis, and Chagas' disease. Interestingly, a high-fiber diet is a risk factor too, as such a diet tends to create large, bulky stools that stretch out the sigmoid colon. Sigmoid volvulus is seen more commonly in regions that are part of the so-called volvulus belt, which includes Brazil, sub-Saharan Africa, and the Middle East, where diets are high in vegetables and fruits.

> **Watch Out**
> Low-fiber diet increases risk for diverticula, while a high-fiber diet increases risk for sigmoid volvulus.

What Is Meant By the Term Complicated Volvulus?

A complicated volvulus implies that there is bowel ischemia and its sequelae, such as gangrenous bowel, perforation, and sepsis. This can be recognized on history and physical by the following: severe diffuse abdominal pain, fever, tachycardia, altered mental status, marked tenderness to palpation with peritoneal signs, and laboratory evidence of bowel ischemia such as leukocytosis, hyponatremia, and metabolic acidosis. The distinction between uncomplicated and complicated volvulus is important, as it has therapeutic implications.

Workup

What Are the First Steps in the Workup of a Suspected Large Bowel Obstruction?

The initial evaluation should include obtaining laboratory studies, such as a complete blood count, serum lactate (or alternatively, bicarbonate), and serum electrolytes, to assess for electrolyte imbalances and evidence of volume depletion. The first steps are to obtain laboratory values and to include complete blood count, serum lactate (alternatively, bicarbonate), and serum chemistries to determine electrolyte abnormalities and the presence of volume depletion. Leukocytosis with a left shift, along with hyponatremia and lactic acidosis, is concerning for the presence of bowel obstruction with ischemia or complicated volvulus. Though these laboratory values alone lack sensitivity or specificity, they can be used as part of the broader clinical picture. In addition, the physical exam should evaluate for peritoneal signs, such as rebound or rigidity, indicative of an acute abdomen.

What Is the First Imaging Recommended for a Suspected Large Bowel Obstruction?

Plain abdominal (supine and upright) and upright chest radiographs (to look for free air under the diaphragm) should be obtained. Plain abdominal x-rays can generally distinguish between an SBO (dilated loops of small bowel with multiple air-fluid levels) and an LBO. Radiographs can also distinguish small and large bowel based on anatomical features: the small bowel has plicae circulares that traverse the entire lumen, whereas the large bowel exhibits haustra, which are spaced more widely and do not extend across the lumen.

Watch Out

If the ileocecal valve is competent, a sigmoid colon obstruction can result in a closed-loop obstruction, as the colonic contents are unable to flow back into the small intestine for decompression.

How Is Cecal Volvulus Differentiated from Sigmoid Volvulus on X-Ray?

Because cecal volvulus involves the proximal colon, these patients are more likely to have radiographic evidence of small bowel obstruction compared to sigmoid volvulus. They also will have a distended large bowel with the apex pointing toward the *left upper quadrant*. Sigmoid volvulus will have the apex pointing toward the *right upper quadrant*. ◘ Figure 25.1 demonstrates the classic x-ray finding of a "coffee bean" sign for sigmoid volvulus.

What Additional Imaging Is Recommended?

If the plain films are diagnostic of a volvulus, no further imaging is necessary. CT with oral and IV contrast is recommended if the diagnosis of large bowel obstruction is

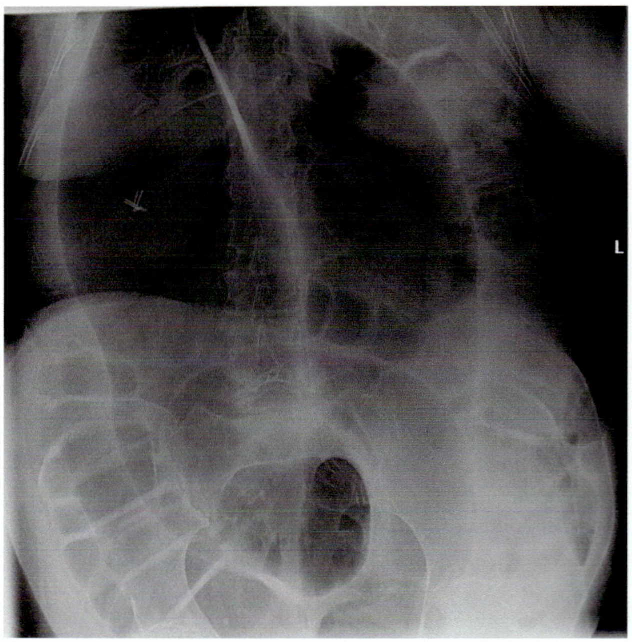

◘ **Fig. 25.1** Abdominal x-ray showing the "coffee bean" or "bent inner tube" sign of sigmoid volvulus

unclear. For volvulus it often demonstrates a "whirl" sign indicative of mesenteric twisting and dilated colon.

Management

What Are the Initial Steps in the Management of a Large Bowel Obstruction?

The initial management of an LBO involves resuscitating the patient with IV fluids and electrolyte repletion.. In patients experiencing vomiting, a nasogastric tube may be inserted to provide symptomatic relief and decompress the gastrointestinal tract.

> **Watch Out**
> Volvulus is a closed-loop obstruction. As such, NG tube decompression alone is not therapeutic.

What Is the Subsequent Treatment for a Sigmoid Volvulus?

In uncomplicated sigmoid volvulus, the first-line treatment is endoscopic detorsion (untwisting) of the affected bowel. This can be performed using a flexible sigmoidoscopy, rigid proctoscopy, and colonoscopy. The endoscope is advanced to the point of obstruction, and then gradually advanced through the twisted loop, allowing decompression as gas and stool are released. Care is then taken to inspect the mucosa for any signs of ischemia before removing the endoscope. A rectal tube can be placed for prevention of retorsion and continued decompression. If detorsion fails, the patient must undergo urgent surgery.

Following Successful Detorsion of Uncomplicated Sigmoid Volvulus, What Is the Next Step in the Management?

The recurrence rate after endoscopic detorsion of sigmoid volvulus is quite high. Therefore, in most cases, patient should undergo a semi-elective sigmoid resection within the same hospitalization. The advantage of first performing endoscopic detorsion is that it addresses the acute problem, allowing time for fluid resuscitation, optimization of comorbid conditions, and adequate bowel preparation before surgery. This approach also may prevent the need for a colostomy, as the ends of the colon can be anastomosed primarily. However, some studies indicate that elderly patients with significant comorbidities who are poor candidates for surgery may be managed nonoperatively.

How Is Complicated Sigmoid Volvulus Managed?

A complicated sigmoid volvulus suggests the presence of colonic ischemia or perforation, which needs surgical resection of the affected bowel. Thus, endoscopic detorsion and contrast enemas should be avoided. Intraoperatively, if the volvulized bowel is confirmed to be ischemic, it should not be detorsed but instead resected to prevent entry of bacteria and toxins into the systemic circulation. The colon is resected to viable margins. The proximal end of the colon is brought out as a colostomy, as the surrounding inflammation and infection will prevent appropriate healing of an anastomosis. The distal colon is closed and left in the pelvis.

What Is the Treatment for a Cecal Volvulus?

Cecal volvulus is not treated similarly to sigmoid volvulus. It is associated with a higher rate of bowel necrosis, failure of endoscopic detorsion, and recurrence. Thus, endoscopic detorsion is not recommended. The recommended management is an emergency laparotomy followed by a right colectomy.

Area Where You Can Get in Trouble

LBO in Pregnancy

LBO may not be readily recognized in pregnant patients, yet colonic volvulus is the second most common cause of intestinal obstruction in pregnancy (after SBO due to adhesions). For an uncomplicated sigmoid volvulus, detorsion is indicated. Resection may be delayed until after delivery to improve surgical risk for the fetus and mother, especially given that most cases occur in the third trimester and thus may not result in a significant delay.

Summary of Essentials

History and Physical

- LBO—gradual and severe abdominal distention, obstipation, and vomiting.
- Uncomplicated volvulus—normal vitals, normal mental status, and non-tender abdomen.
- Complicated volvulus—severe abdominal pain, fever, tachycardia, toxic appearance, peritoneal signs, acidosis, and leukocytosis.
- Look for abdominal scars and hernias and perform a rectal exam to assess other differential diagnoses.

Etiology/Risk Factors

- Most common causes of LBO:
  - Cancer
  - Diverticulitis
  - Volvulus
- Sigmoid volvulus—acquired stretching of the sigmoid
- Ogilvie's syndrome—Neuropsychiatric disease, institutionalization, chronic constipation, long-term anticholinergic use, high-fiber diet, and pregnancy.
- Cecal volvulus—congenital failure of fixation of the cecum.

Diagnosis

- Compared to LBO, SBO has a faster onset and is more likely to cause vomiting and high-pitched bowel sounds.
- Patients with Ogilvie's syndrome are more likely to be already hospitalized and bedridden, often in the postoperative setting.
- Abdominal x-ray:
  - Sigmoid volvulus—"coffee bean sign" in right upper quadrant, "omega," or "bent inner tube," "kidney bean" sign.
  - Cecal volvulus—"comma" or "kidney bean" sign, "coffee bean" sign in left upper quadrant.
- CT scan if equivocal x-ray findings:
- Swirl sign.
- Bowel wall thickening, mesenteric edema, pneumatosis, and portal venous gas suggest ischemic bowel.

Management

- Therapy differs based on the location and severity of the complication.
  - Uncomplicated sigmoid volvulus—endoscopic detorsion with rectal tube placement followed by semi-elective resection.
  - Complicated sigmoid volvulus—no detorsion attempted; emergent laparotomy with sigmoid colectomy and colostomy (in most cases).
  - Cecal volvulus—no detorsion attempted; take to OR for right colectomy.
- Complications of surgery—wound infection, anastomotic leak, and recurrence. Without detorsion or resection—ischemia, perforation, and sepsis.

Suggested Reading

Alavi K, Poylin V, Davids JS, et al. The American Society of Colon and Rectal Surgeons Clinical Practice Guidelines for the Management of Colonic Volvulus and Acute Colonic Pseudo-Obstruction. *Dis Colon Rectum*. 2021;64(9):1046–1057. https://doi.org/10.1097/DCR.0000000000002159

Arnell TD. Core subjects: colonic volvulus. Am Soc Colon Rectal Surg. 2002:29–41.

Dayton MT, Isenberg GA, Rakinic J, Thomas JS, Trudel JL. Colon, rectum, and anus. In: Lawrence PF, editor. Essentials of general surgery. 5th ed. Baltimore: Lipincott, Williams and Wilkins; 2013. p. 313–4.

Glasgow SC. Core subjects: colonic volvulus. Am Soc Colon Rectal Surg. 2012:352–68.

Schroeppel TJ, Fabian TC. The Colon. In: Gracias VH, Reilly PM, McKenney MG, Velhamos GC, editors. Acute care surgery: a guide for general surgeons. 1st ed. New York: McGraw-Hill Inc; 2008. p. 82–5.

Tian, B.W.C.A., Vigutto, G., Tan, E. *et al.* WSES consensus guidelines on sigmoid volvulus management. *World J Emerg Surg* 18, 34 (2023). https://doi.org/10.1186/s13017-023-00502-x

Vogel JD, Feingold DL, Stewart DB, Turner JS, Boutros M, Chun J, Steele SR. Clinical practice guidelines for colonic volvulus and acute colonic pseudo-obstruction. Dis Colon Rectum. 2016;59(7):589–600.

Left Lower Quadrant Pain and Fever

Christian de Virgilio, Tracey D. Arnell, and Beverley A. Petrie

Contents

C. de Virgilio, A. Grigorian (eds.), *Surgery*, https://doi.org/10.1007/978-3-032-09799-6_26

Case Study

A 55-year-old obese female presents with a two-day history of left lower quadrant (LLQ) pain, nausea, anorexia, and low-grade fevers. The pain is constant, moderately severe, and non-radiating, with no clear precipitating factor. She has not eaten in 24 h due to poor appetite and reports no bowel movement for 48 h. She denies vomiting or bloody or black stools and has no recent change in bowel habits, though she has a long history of constipation. She has noted similar pain in the past, but never this severe, and has never sought medical attention before. She has never had a screening colonoscopy. Her past medical history includes hypertension and diabetes, with no prior surgeries. On physical examination, blood pressure is 130/70 mmHg, heart rate 110/min, temperature is 38.2 °C, and respiratory rate is 16/min. Abdominal exam reveals mild distention, no surgical scars, and no masses. Bowel sounds are absent. The LLQ is moderately tender to palpation with guarding and no rebound tenderness. The remainder of the abdomen is nontender. Rectal exam is unremarkable. Pelvic exam reveals no cervical motion tenderness and no adnexal masses. Laboratory examination demonstrates a white blood cell (WBC) count of $16 \times 10^3/\mu L$ (normal $4.1–10.9 \times 10^3/\mu L$) with a left shift, hemoglobin of 13 g/dL (12–15 g/dL), hematocrit 39% (35–46%), normal electrolytes, and a normal urinalysis.

Diagnosis

What Is the Differential Diagnosis? (Table 26.1)

Table 26.1 Differential diagnosis of clinical presentation

Condition	Comments
Acute diverticulitis	Inflammation of diverticula, most commonly affecting the sigmoid colon, presenting with left lower quadrant pain, fever, and leukocytosis
Pelvic inflammatory disease	Infection of the upper genital tract characterized by cervical motion tenderness, adnexal tenderness, and foul-smelling vaginal discharge, typically occurring in sexually active, premenopausal women
Acute appendicitis	RLQ pain, fever, anorexia, and leukocytosis
Sigmoid volvulus	Twisting of the sigmoid colon around its mesentery, leading to large bowel obstruction; more common in elderly patients and presents with abdominal distension and constipation
Ischemic colitis	Mucosal ischemia due to hypoperfusion, most often affecting the splenic flexure, typically presents with crampy abdominal pain and bloody diarrhea
Acute mesenteric ischemia	Sudden onset of severe diffuse abdominal pain out of proportion to examination, acute occlusion of SMA (often embolus from atrial fibrillation), ischemia to the entire small bowel
Inflammatory bowel disease	History of abdominal cramps, bloody diarrhea, and acute abdominal pain
Colon cancer	Malignancy of the colon often presents insidiously with changes in bowel habits, weight loss, and occult or gross blood in the stool

LLQ left lower quadrant, *RLQ* right lower quadrant, *SMA* superior mesenteric artery

What Is the Most Likely Diagnosis?

Given the patient's age, LLQ pain and tenderness on exam, associated fever, and leukocytosis, acute diverticulitis is the most likely diagnosis.

> **Watch Out**
> In women of reproductive age presenting with acute lower abdominal pain, serum beta-hCG testing should be obtained to exclude pregnancy-related emergencies such as ectopic pregnancy.

History and Physical

What Are the Risk Factors for Diverticulosis?

Obesity, low-fiber and high-fat diets, red meat, constipation, opiate abuse, and advanced age. Approximately 5–15% of patients with diverticulosis will develop diverticulitis.

Pathophysiology

Where in the Colon Do Diverticula Occur Most Frequently? Which Diverticula Are More Prone to Infection? Bleeding?

The vast majority of diverticula occur in the sigmoid colon. Diverticula in the left or sigmoid colon are more likely to become infected (diverticulitis). Diverticula in the right colon are more likely to bleed (diverticulosis).

Do Diverticula Occur in the Rectum? Why or Why Not?

Rectal diverticula are extremely rare. It is hypothesized that they almost never occur because the taenia coli, the longitudinal bands of smooth muscle along the colon, coalesce into a circumferential band around the rectum, thereby eliminating points of weakness that predispose to diverticula.

What Are True and False Diverticula? Which Type Are Sigmoid Diverticula?

There are four layers of the intestinal wall: the mucosa, submucosa, muscularis propria, and serosa. In a true diverticulum (congenital), all layers are part of an outpouching of the intestine. In a false diverticulum (acquired), only the mucosa and submucosa are part of the outpouching. The most common diverticula are acquired (such as those causing sigmoid diverticulitis).

What Are the Main Complications of Diverticulitis? How Would They Present? (▫ Table 26.2)

▫ **Table 26.2** Complications of diverticulitis

Complication	Presentation
Abscess	Fever, localized pain, ileus, leukocytosis
Perforation	May seal spontaneously via the omentum (microperforation); can progress to purulent or feculent peritonitis (free perforation); diffuse abdominal tenderness, rebound, guarding, ileus, leukocytosis, fever
Fistula	Colovesical (refractory multi-organism urinary tract infection, pneumaturia, fecaluria); colovaginal (feculent vaginal discharge)
Stricture	Partial large bowel obstruction; abdominal distention, constipation, bloating
Large bowel obstruction	Feculent vomiting, abdominal distention, obstipation, crampy abdominal pain

What Are the Main Etiologies for a Colovesical Fistula? Colovaginal Fistula?

The most common cause for a colovesical fistula is diverticulitis. Other causes are colon cancer, IBD, bladder cancer, radiation injury, trauma, or foreign body. Although diverticulitis can also lead to a colovaginal fistula, nearly 80% of all colovaginal fistulas are due to obstetric injury.

How Does a Colovesical Fistula Present?

Patients with colovesical fistula may present with fecaluria (feces in the urine), pneumaturia (air in the urine), recurrent urinary tract infections that are refractory to treatment, or a urinary tract infection caused by multiple enteric organisms or anaerobes (most routine urinary tract infections are single organism and aerobes). Diagnosis can be confirmed with an abdominal CT scan using oral or rectal contrast, which may demonstrate contrast material in the bladder along with thickening of the colonic and bladder walls. Intravenous contrast alone is insufficient for diagnosis.

What Is Meant by Complicated Versus Uncomplicated Diverticulitis? What Is the Implication?

Diverticulitis that occurs with abscess formation, colonic obstruction, diffuse peritonitis, or fistulization is considered complicated diverticulitis, whereas diverticulitis without these sequelae is known as uncomplicated diverticulitis.

What Is the Hinchey Staging System?

This is a grading schema to describe the severity of complicated diverticulitis. Stage I involves pericolonic inflammation with a pericolic abscess. Stage II is characterized by a pelvic, retroperitoneal, or distant intra-abdominal abscess. Stage III represents generalized purulent peritonitis, while stage IV involves fecal peritonitis. Most surgeons consider stages II–IV as complicated diverticulitis.

Workup

What Imaging Is Recommended?

CT scan (Figs. 26.1 and 26.2) is recommended in patients suspected of having diverticulitis.

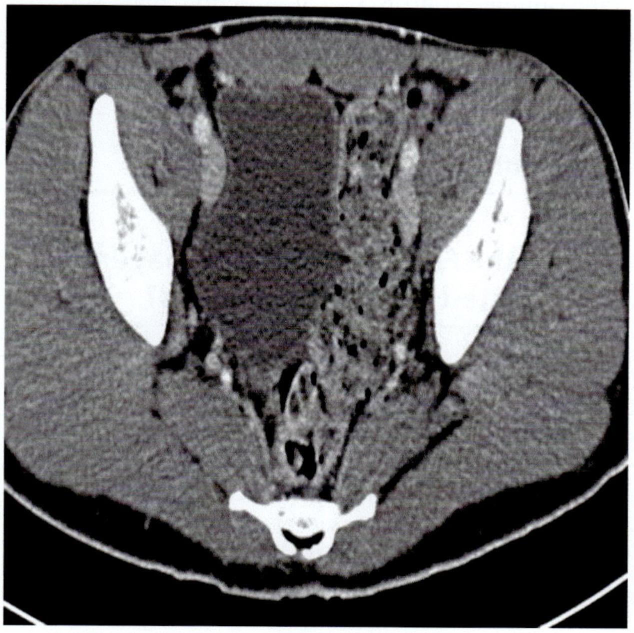

Fig. 26.1 Axial CT of the pelvis showing a normal sigmoid colon with thin walls and filled with stool. There are no diverticula

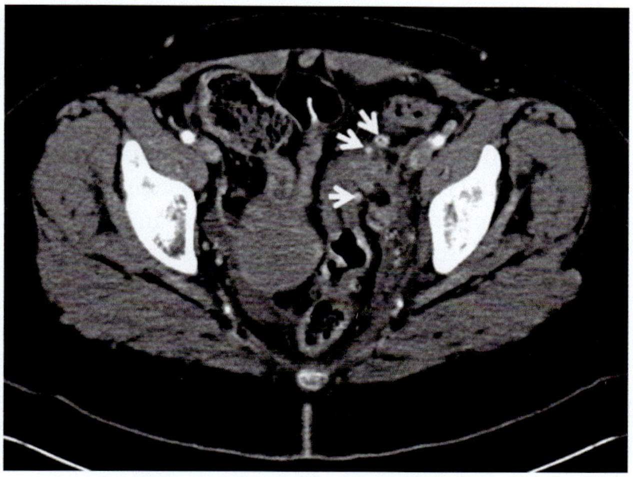

Fig. 26.2 Axial CT of the pelvis demonstrating sigmoid diverticula with significant wall thickening of the sigmoid colon, consistent with acute sigmoid diverticulitis. *White arrows: diverticula*

What Two Diagnostic Studies Are Contraindicated in the Acute Setting of Suspected Diverticulitis, and Why?

A barium enema introduces fluid under pressure, which may unseal a contained perforation. Barium would then leak into the peritoneum, causing barium peritonitis (CT scans with oral contrast are safe as they use water-soluble contrast). Colonoscopy may similarly worsen diverticulitis, as it increases pressure due to air insufflation.

Management

What Is the First Step in the Management of Suspected Acute Diverticulitis?

Determine if the patient needs admission to the hospital. If the episode of diverticulitis is uncomplicated and without evidence of a systemic response, the patient can be discharged home with oral antibiotics and clear liquids. Patients with acute diverticulitis who have significant pain or have a systemic response (fever, tachycardia, and leukocytosis) should be admitted to the hospital, placed NPO, and given IV antibiotics, fluids, and analgesia.

What Is the Subsequent Management for Uncomplicated Diverticulitis?

The majority will resolve with the approach described above, without the need for surgery, and will not have another episode. The patient should be counseled on dietary modification (decrease fats and increase fibers). If the patient fails to improve while hospitalized (persistent abdominal pain and tenderness, worsening leukocytosis), the options are to broaden the antibiotics, to repeat the CT scan to look for an abscess that might require drainage, or to take the patient to the operating room for a colon resection.

What Operation Is Performed in the Elective Setting for Sigmoid Diverticulitis? How Is This Operation Different Than Surgery in the Urgent or Emergent Setting?

In cases of recurrent uncomplicated diverticulitis, preventive surgery may be performed, and patients may undergo a one-step procedure wherein the diseased colon is resected and the proximal and distal segments are connected to one another. This is known as primary anastomosis. In the emergent or urgent situationssetting, resection of the diseased colon with an anastomosis (with or without a proximal diverting ostomy) or resection without an anastomosis (resulting in an ostomy) is often performed. At a later time, the proximal and distal ends of the remaining colon can be anastomosed if diversion was performed.

> **Watch Out**
> The ureters are retroperitoneal structures and are at risk of damage or complete transection during colonic resection if not identified.

Complicated Diverticulitis

What Is the Management of Complicated Diverticulitis?

Depending on the specific complication, the recommendation is either urgent surgery, CT-guided drainage, or delayed surgery.

What Are the Indications for Urgent Surgery? What Operation Is Recommended in the Urgent Setting?

Patients with evidence of diffuse peritonitis as a result of free colonic perforation should undergo urgent surgery. In this setting, the diseased colon is removed, and an end colostomy is performed with the distal rectum closed and left in the abdomen (known as a Hartmann procedure). After the inflammation of acute diverticulitis resolves, the end colostomy may be reversed and reattached to the rectum (usually 6 months later).

How Does One Determine the Proximal and Distal Extent of Colon Resection? What if There Are Diverticula Throughout the Colon?

The proximal margin of resection should be proximal to the diseased colon (as evidenced by soft and non-inflamed bowel), but it is *not necessary* to resect all diverticula-containing colon if it is not inflamed. The distal extent of resection should remove all sigmoid colon so as to prevent recurrent diverticulitis. The start of the rectum can be identified by the absence of distinct taenia coli.

What Is the Recommended Treatment for Diverticulitis Complicated by a Localized Abscess?

Patients with a pericolic abscess with a diameter less than 4 cm and without peritoneal signs can be treated with bowel rest and broad-spectrum antibiotics. If the abscess is larger than 4 cm and they only have localized tenderness, antibiotics plus CT-guided percutaneous drainage is indicated, as this will facilitate resolution of acute inflammation, which may allow for a one-stage surgical resection of the affected bowel at a later date. It is important to note that the presence of an abscess (Hinchey stage II or higher) indicates complicated diverticulitis.

What Is the Recommended Treatment for Diverticulitis with a Colovesical Fistula?

The affected segment of the colon should be resected electively to eliminate the fistula and prevent recurrence. Because the bladder defect is often very small, direct bladder repair is not always necessary. Postoperatively, temporary Foley catheter drainage is recommended to allow the bladder to heal. In patients who are poor surgical candidates, medical management alone with antibiotic therapy may be considered.

Is Free Air on CT an Absolute Indication for Emergency Surgery?

Not necessarily. The presence of free intraperitoneal air on CT imaging indicates a perforation; it does not automatically require immediate surgical intervention. Patients without signs of diffuse peritonitis on physical examination may be managed nonoperatively with intravenous antibiotics, bowel rest, and close monitoring. If a drainable fluid collection (abscess) is present, percutaneous drainage may be performed (◘ Table 26.3). However, patients with diffuse peritonitis require emergent operative intervention, typically with sigmoid colectomy and end colostomy.

◘ **Table 26.3** Management of complicated diverticulitis

Complication	Management
Free perforation without peritonitis	IV antibiotics, supportive care, and elective sigmoid colectomy
Free perforation with diffuse peritonitis	Emergent colectomy with end colostomy (Hartmann procedure)
Large bowel obstruction	Urgent colectomy with or without end colostomy
Large (>4 cm) localized abscess	CT-guided drainage followed by elective colon resection
Small (<4 cm) localized abscess	IV antibiotics
Colovesical fistula	Elective colon resection, close fistula, and bladder drainage with Foley

Following an Episode of Acute Diverticulitis, What Study Is Recommended 6–8 Weeks Later?

A colonoscopy should be performed 6–8 weeks after recovering from the acute episode in patients with complicated diverticulitis as there is an association between diverticulitis and colonic cancer/polyps.

Areas Where You Can Get in Trouble

Elderly Patient with Chronic Constipation and NSAID Use, with Sudden Abdominal Pain

This is concerning for a stercoral ulceration complicated by perforation, a rare condition that typically affects elderly patients with chronic constipation. The hard stool travels through the rectosigmoid colon and develops into a fecaloma, which can result in local ischemia, ulceration, and subsequent perforation leading to a sudden onset of abdominal pain. In some patients, chronic laxative use may be the only indication of underlying constipation. Additionally, NSAIDs use has been found to be a risk factor for stercoral ulceration.

Areas of Controversy

How Many Episodes of Uncomplicated Diverticulitis Are Acceptable Before Elective Surgery Is Recommended?

Most studies show that the rate of recurrence after diverticulitis is 10–30%. There is no strict threshold for the number of episodes that necessitates elective surgery. Therefore, even patients with repeated episodes of uncomplicated diverticulitis may be managed medically as long as symptoms remain controlled. The decision is individually based and depends on medical comorbidities and the patient's preference.

Is There a Role for Aspirin in the Prevention or Management of Diverticulitis?

Recent studies suggest that acute uncomplicated diverticulitis is primarily an inflammatory, rather than infectious, process. Because of this, there is growing interest in the potential role of anti-inflammatory agents such as low-dose aspirin. Some observational studies have suggested that aspirin may reduce the incidence or severity of diverticulitis by limiting mucosal inflammation. However, aspirin use also carries a risk of gastrointestinal bleeding, particularly in patients with diverticulosis. At this time, the use of aspirin specifically to treat or prevent diverticulitis remains investigational and is not part of standard clinical practice. Decisions regarding aspirin use should be individualized based on a patient's overall cardiovascular and gastrointestinal risk profiles.

One Stage Colon Resection and Immediate Reanastomosis for Perforated Diverticulitis

Rather than performing a two-stage procedure for perforated diverticulitis (Hartmann's procedure followed 6 months later by colostomy takedown), recent data suggest that a single-stage operation—sigmoid resection with primary anastomosis, with or without a proximal diverting ostomy—may be appropriate. The decision should be individualized based on patient-specific factors such as hemodynamic stability and comorbid conditions.

Should Patients with Prior Episodes of Diverticulitis Avoid Eating Nuts, Popcorn, or Corn?

At one time there was concern that these foods might get caught in the diverticulum and trigger diverticulitis, but this has been disproven.

Complications of Diverticulitis (◘ Fig. 26.3)

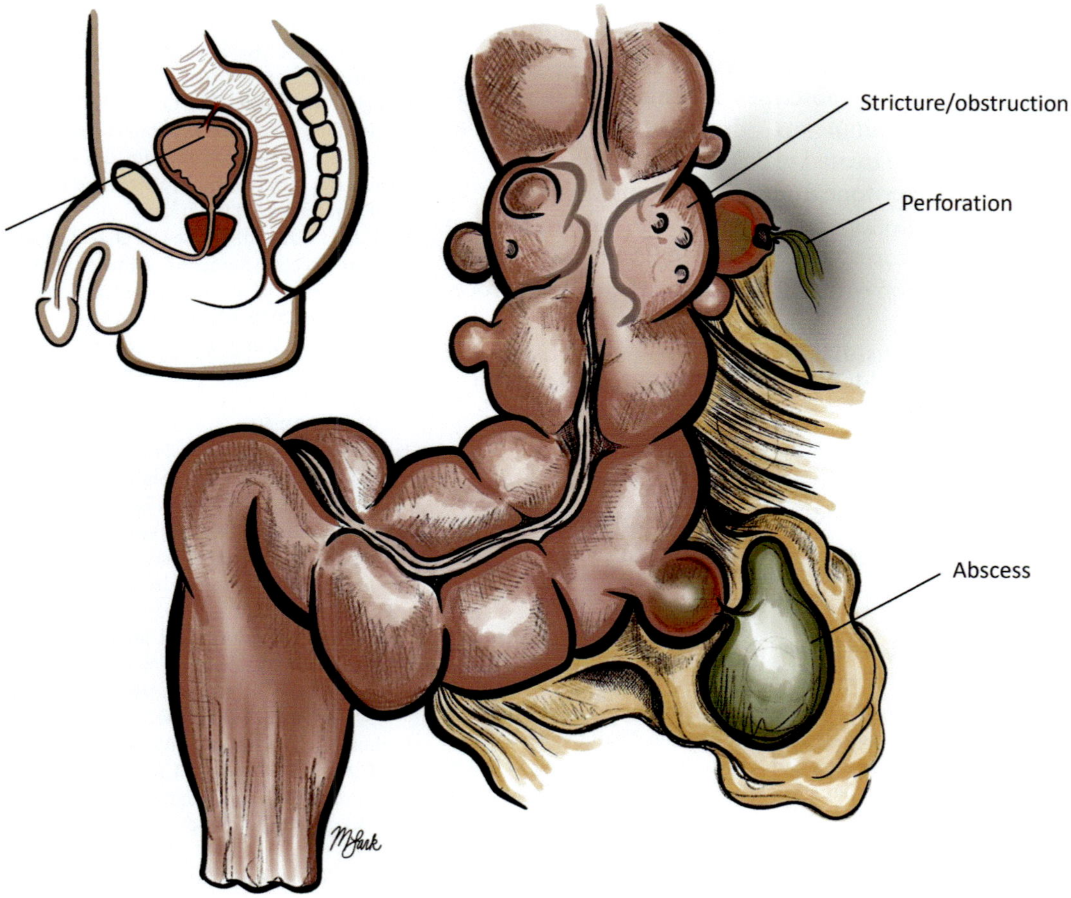

Fig. 26.3 Diverticulitis complications: Local inflammation from diverticulitis can lead to numerous complications, including the formation of an abscess, perforation, stricture causing obstruction, or a colovesicular fistula

Summary of Essentials

History and Physical

- Diverticulitis typically presents with left lower quadrant pain and tenderness, fever, leukocytosis, and bowel habit changes.
- Major risk factors are obesity, advanced age, and a diet low in fiber, high in fat, high in red meat, and opiate abuse.
- Approximately 5–15% of patients with diverticulosis develop diverticulitis.

Pathophysiology

- Diverticula occur most commonly in the sigmoid colon, where intraluminal pressures are greatest.
- Left-sided diverticula are more prone to infection (diverticulitis), while right-sided diverticula are more likely to bleed.
- Complicated diverticulitis: abscess, free perforation, fistula, stricture, and obstruction.

Diagnosis

- CT scan is the first-line imaging modality.
- Avoid barium enemas and colonoscopies in acute presentations because of increased risk of perforation.
- Determine if complicated or uncomplicated.
- Presence or absence of systemic markers (fever, tachycardia, leukocytosis).

Management

- Uncomplicated diverticulitis without systemic signs (fever, tachycardia, leukocytosis) can be treated as an outpatient with oral antibiotics and a clear liquid diet.

- Follow-up colonoscopy is recommended 6–8 weeks after recovery to rule out underlying malignancy or polyps in complicated diverticulitis.
- Large (>4 cm) abscesses are managed with CT-guided percutaneous drainage, while smaller abscesses are treated with IV antibiotics.
- Free intraperitoneal air without peritonitis may be managed nonoperatively with IV antibiotics and close monitoring; diffuse peritonitis requires emergent resection with end colostomy (Hartmann procedure).
- Colovesical fistulas typically require elective colon resection and bladder drainage with a Foley catheter.

Acknowledgement The editors would like to acknowledge and thank Paul N. Frank for his valuable contributions to the previous edition of this chapter.

Suggested Reading

Costi R, Le Cauchy F, Bian A, et al. Challenging a classic myth: pneumoperitoneum associated with acute diverticulitis is not an indication for open or laparoscopic emergency surgery in hemodynamically stable patients. A 10-year experience with a nonoperative treatment. Surg Endosc. 2012;26(7):2061–71.

Desai M, Fathallah J, Nutalapati V, Saligram S. Antibiotics Versus No Antibiotics for Acute Uncomplicated Diverticulitis: A Systematic Review and Meta-analysis. *Dis Colon Rectum.* 2019;62(8):1005–1012.

Feingold D, Steele SR, Lee S, Kaiser A, Boushey R, Buie WD, Rafferty JF. Practice parameters for treatment of sigmoid diverticulitis. Dis Colon Rectum. 2014;57(3):284–94.

Glemo BT. Elective surgical treatment of diverticulitis. Clin Colon Rectal Surg. 2004;17(3):183–6.

Hall, J., Hardiman, K., Lee S., et al. The American Society of Colon and Rectal Surgeons Clinical Practice Guidelines for the Treatment of of Left-Sided Colonic Diverticulitis. Dis Colon Rectum. 2020; 63(6): 728–747.

Huang WS, Wang CS, Hsieh CC, Lin PY, Chin CC, Wang JY. Management of patients with stercoral perforation of the sigmoid colon: report of five cases. World J Gastroenterol WJG. 2006;12(3):500.

Jacobs DO. Diverticulitis. N Engl J Med. 2007;357:2057–66.

Kumar AS, Kelleher DC, Sigle GQ. Bowel preparation before elective surgery. Clin Colon Rectal Surg. 2013;26(03):146–52.

Lau KC, Spilsbury K, Farooque Y, et al. Is colonoscopy still mandatory after a CT diagnosis of left-sided diverticulitis: can colorectal cancer be confidently excluded?. Dis Colon Rectum. 2011;54(10):1265–1270.

Tian BWCA, Vigutto G, et al. WSES consensus guidelines on sigmoid volvulus management. World J Emerg Surg. 2023 May 15;18(1):34. https://doi.org/10.1186/s13017-023-00502-x. PMID: 37189134; PMCID: PMC10186802.

Richter, S., Lindemann, W., Kollmar, O., Pistorius, G.A., Maurer, C.A. and Schilling, M.K., 2006. One-stage sigmoid colon resection for perforated sigmoid diverticulitis (Hinchey stages III and IV). World journal of surgery, 30(6), pp.1027–1032.

Fatigue and Bloody Diarrhea

James McDermott, Areg Grigorian, and Christian de Virgilio

Contents

C. de Virgilio, A. Grigorian (eds.), *Surgery*, https://doi.org/10.1007/978-3-032-09799-6_27

Case Study

A 19-year-old female presents with fatigue for the past 3 months. She is of Ashkenazi Jewish origin. She reports a 2-year history of diarrhea accompanied by abdominal pain and cramping. Her stool is sometimes tinged with blood as well as mucus. She also has intermittent aches and malaise. Her stature is short relative to her parents. She smokes ½ a pack of cigarettes per day. On physical examination, the patient appears pale and thin. She has several, small painful sores inside her mouth. Her abdominal exam is unremarkable. Her legs demonstrate several red nodules that are tender to palpation. Anal exam reveals perianal skin tags. Her laboratory studies show a hemoglobin of 7.5 g/dL (normal 12–15.5 g/dL).

Diagnosis

What Is the Differential Diagnosis of Chronic Diarrhea with Mucus and/or Blood? (Table 27.1)

Table 27.1 Differential diagnosis of chronic diarrhea

Diagnosis	Comments
Irritable bowel syndrome (IBS)	Chronically altered bowel habits (constipation and/or diarrhea, and stool form), bloating, crampy abdominal pain, mucus in stool, but *without* blood
Infectious colitis (Shigella, Salmonellae, Campylobacter, Yersinia)	Fever, watery diarrhea, nausea, vomiting, abdominal cramping; acute onset; may present with bloody stools and mucus
Inflammatory bowel disease (Ulcerative colitis and Crohn's)	Abdominal pain, fatigue, anemia, weight loss, intermittent diarrhea
Celiac disease	Flatulence, weight loss, malabsorption, steatorrhea
Pseudomembranous colitis	*Clostridium difficile* infection; abdominal pain/cramping, diarrhea; recent antibiotic use (e.g., clindamycin); yellow plaques found on colonoscopy

What Are the Key Differences Between Ulcerative Colitis and Crohn's? (Table 27.2)

Table 27.2 Distinguishing features of Crohn's and ulcerative colitis

	Crohn's	Ulcerative colitis
Location	Anywhere from the mouth to anus, "Gum to bum," terminal ileum is the most common site	Starts in the rectum and extends proximally to colon; does not involve small bowel
Distribution	Discontinuous (skip lesions)	Continuous
Symptoms	Varies but may include abdominal pain, weight loss, bloating, diarrhea, and mucus in stool	Abdominal pain with bloody diarrhea and mucus
Gross appearance	Cobblestone mucosa, creeping fat, fistulas, and strictures	Pseudopolyps, barium enema may show "lead pipe" colon devoid of haustra; no fistulas present
Depth of inflammation	Transmural (entire bowel wall affected)	Shallow, mucosal
Histology	Lymphoid aggregates with noncaseating granulomas in only 15% of endoscopic biopsy	Crypt abscesses with neutrophils
Complications	Malabsorption and nutritional deficiency, oral ulcers, fistula formation, calcium oxalate nephrolithiasis, gallstones, colorectal cancer	Primary sclerosing cholangitis, toxic megacolon, colorectal cancer with increasing risk after 10 years with the disease
Cancer risk	Increased 8–10 years after diagnosis	Increased 8–10 years after diagnosis
Labs	cANCA frequently positive, pANCA rarely positive	cANCA rarely positive, pANCA frequently positive
Granulomas	Yes	No

Watch Out

Use "*G*reen *CHRISTMAS*" to help remember the key features of Crohn's: *g*ranuloma, *c*obblestones, *h*yperthermia, *r*educed lumen, *i*ntestinal fistula, *s*kip lesions, *t*ransmural, *m*alabsorption, *a*bdominal pain, *s*ubmucosal fibrosis.

What Is the Diagnosis for This Patient?

In a young patient presenting with short stature, an insidious history of diarrhea with blood or mucus, perianal disease (skin tags), and extracolonic manifestations such as joint ache, aphthous ulcer, and erythema nodosum, the most likely diagnosis is Crohn's disease. In addition, inflammatory bowel disease (IBD) is more common in patients of Ashkenazi Jewish origin.

History and Physical

What Is the Age Distribution of IBD?

IBD typically demonstrates a bimodal distribution with initial (and greater) incidence of the disease occurring between ages 20 and 30. In this younger age group, Crohn's occurs more commonly than ulcerative colitis (UC). The second (and lower) peak in incidence of IBD occurs between ages 60 and 80 with a greater propensity for UC over Crohn's. While the exact etiology of this bimodal distribution remains unknown, potential hypotheses include changes in the immune system during aging and increased exposure to environmental stimulants.

What Are the Risk Factors for IBD?

Risk factors for IBD are multifactorial, including genetics, environmental exposures, and host microbiome. Particular ethnic groups predisposed to higher rates of IBD include certain Jewish populations. The hygiene hypothesis has been postulated as a risk factor as well. Children raised in urban settings with presumably more hygienic upbringings have higher rates of IBD. A reduction in enteric antigen exposure during childhood may lead to altered immunological function. Crohn's has been demonstrated to occur at higher rates in families with fewer siblings. Reduction in the biodiversity of the gut flora has been associated with a higher incidence of IBD.

Is Smoking a Risk Factor for Both Crohn's and UC?

Smoking is a risk factor for Crohn's, with higher rates in patients who are active smokers as well as ex-smokers. Smoking is the only modifiable risk factor for the severity and progression of Crohn's. In comparison, smoking correlates with a decreased incidence of UC. UC patients who are active smokers tend to experience less severe symptoms of UC. Nicotine appears to induce a complex effect on mucosal epithelial cells and T-cell function resulting in modulation of cytokine levels and immune function.

How Do Patients with IBD Typically Present Clinically?

The classic presentation differs between UC and Crohn's. Since UC begins in the rectum, it typically presents with crampy abdominal pain and bloody diarrhea. Since Crohn's can affect any part of the GI tract, the presentation is much more variable. Classically it presents with intermittent or insidious onset of abdominal pain, weight loss/growth failure, and diarrhea. Bloody diarrhea is less common with Crohn's. Secondary effects include volume depletion, anemia, electrolyte disturbances, and hypoalbuminemia. Due to the effect of Crohn's on the small bowel, nutritional deficiencies and malabsorption are more common in comparison to UC. Acute episodes of Crohn's can be associated with intra-abdominal abscesses. Crohn's can lead to intestinal strictures (leading to bowel obstructive symptoms) and fistulas to the skin. In addition, Crohn's is associated with perianal disease including skin tags, perianal abscesses, and anal fistulas; UC does not present with fistulas or perianal disease.

What Are the Extraintestinal Manifestations of IBD?

Musculoskeletal conditions (peripheral and axial arthropathy) are the most common extraintestinal manifestations of IBD. Cutaneous disorders include erythema nodosa or pyoderma gangrenosum. Oral manifestations including aphthous ulcers and mucosal/gingival lesions are more common with Crohn's. Similarly, Crohn's has a stronger association with ophthalmologic manifestations such as uveitis and episcleritis. Primary sclerosing cholangitis (PSC), an inflammatory fibrotic process affecting the intrahepatic and extrahepatic biliary ducts, has been strongly associated with IBD, more commonly with UC. The clinical presentation of PSC includes progressive jaundice and pruritus, with periodic acute episodes of hepatitis and jaundice. Progressive dysfunction associated with PSC culminates in cirrhosis, ascites, and hepatic encephalopathy. PSC is a strong risk factor for the development of cholangiocarcinoma. Gallstones are more common with Crohn's.

What Is the Significance of Short Stature and Delayed Onset of Puberty?

IBD has been associated with impaired oral intake, vitamin and mineral deficiencies, and abnormal intestinal absorption, all of which contribute to a detrimental effect on growth and delayed puberty or start of menses. The pro-inflammatory state and elevated levels of cytokines such as TNF-α contribute to anorexia. This has been shown to affect up to 80% of children diagnosed with Crohn's.

What Is Tenesmus?

Tenesmus is the sensation of incomplete defecation, even when the rectum is empty. It is characterized by a continual or recurrent inclination to evacuate the bowels. It may be associated with rectal pain, abdominal cramps, and fecal urgency. It is associated with irritable bowel syndrome and with conditions that cause inflammation of the colonic or rectal mucosa.

Pathophysiology

What Is the Final Common Pathway for the Pathogenesis of IBD?

Inflammation: This is important because most therapeutic interventions directly or indirectly downregulate the immune system.

Are Patients with IBD at Increased Risk for Cancer?

Yes, patients with IBD are at increased risk for certain cancers due to chronic intestinal inflammation. These cancers include colorectal cancer, cholangiocarcinoma (commonly associated with PSC and UC), small bowel adenocarcinoma (more frequently linked to Crohn's, particularly in the ileum), and intestinal lymphoma (more common with Crohn's). The risk of cancer correlates with both the duration of the disease and the extent of intestinal involvement. Unlike sporadic colon cancers, which typically arise from a localized dysplastic polyp, IBD-related dysplasia is often multifocal and diffuse. For patients with UC, the cancer risk remains low during the first 10 years of disease (2–3%) but increases by approximately 1–2% annually thereafter.

What Is the Screening Recommendation for Colon Cancer in IBD?

Current screening guidelines recommend the first screening colonoscopy 8 years after initial diagnosis of UC. The same guideline is recommended for patients with Crohn's who have colonic involvement. Colonoscopy is recommended immediately in patients with newly diagnosed PSC (much higher risk of colon cancer). Because cancer can develop in the absence of polyps, random biopsies are recommended. Subsequent endoscopic surveillance is performed every 1–3 years depending on prior endoscopic findings and risk stratification.

What Portion of the GI Tract Is Most Commonly Affected in Crohn's?

Crohn's can affect any part of the gastrointestinal tract, but involvement of the terminal ileum is most common and occurs in up to 2/3 of patients.

What Complications Affect IBD Patients?

Patients with Crohn's tend to form fistulas to other organs since the inflammation is full thickness. These include enterovesical (small bowel to bladder) and colovesical (colon to bladder) fistulas. The latter can present with pneumaturia, fecaluria, or recurrent multi-organism urinary tract infections. Crohn's commonly features perianal disease including skin tags, perirectal abscesses, and anal fissures. The transmural inflammation associated with Crohn's can also lead to stricture formation. Strictures and intra-abdominal adhesions can both contribute to intestinal obstruction. Malabsorption and impaired bile salt reabsorption can lead to protein loss, vitamin deficiencies, and gallstone formation. With UC, patients may develop intractable bloody diarrhea. The severe mucosal inflammation, with interruption of the protective mucosal barriers, may lead to secondary bacterial infection and a life-threatening toxic megacolon.

How Does Crohn's Lead to Gallstones or Kidney Stones?

Patients with Crohn's disease are at increased risk of developing gallstones and kidney stones due to malabsorption of bile salts and fat, respectively. Malabsorption of bile salts may result from inflammation in the ileum (terminal ileitis) or from surgical resection (ileocecectomy) of the ileum since this is the primary location where bile salts are reabsorbed. Decreased absorption and enterohepatic circulation of bile acids reduce the amount of bile in the gallbladder, allowing cholesterol to precipitate and form gallstones. Calcium-oxalate kidney stones are a sequelae of decreased fat absorption. In healthy patients, calcium binds oxalate in the bowel which can then be excreted. In the setting of malabsorption, increased fat in the bowel lumen will bind calcium, leaving free oxalate to be absorbed. The subsequent increase in oxalate delivery to the kidneys predisposes patients to calcium-oxalate kidney stones.

Watch Out
A Crohn's patient presenting with flank pain and hematuria should raise suspicion for nephrolithiasis secondary to hyperoxaluria.

What Types of Anemia Are Seen with IBD?

Both UC and Crohn's patients frequently have iron deficiency anemia. This is related to chronic loss of blood in the GI tract, effects of chronic inflammation, and decreased duodenal iron absorption (more often in Crohn's). Less commonly, B12 deficiency anemia may occur in Crohn's patients since vitamin B12 is absorbed in the terminal ileum. These patients may present with the pernicious anemia triad:

1. Megaloblastic anemia due to inhibition of DNA synthesis
2. GI symptoms: bowel motility changes
3. Neurological symptoms: absent reflexes, diminished vibration or soft touch sensation, subacute combined degeneration of spinal cord, seizures, and dementia

What Nutritional Deficiencies May IBD Patients Have?

Approximately 20–85% of IBD patients have varying degrees of nutritional deficiencies (◘ Table 27.3). Protein malnutrition has been characterized as the most common feature.

◘ **Table 27.3** Nutritional deficiencies in IBD

Risk factor	Comment
Vitamin B9 (folate)	Present in 30% of Crohn's patients and 10% of ulcerative colitis. This can contribute to megaloblastic anemia
Vitamin B12	Ileal inflammation or prior resection of the terminal ileum can reduce intrinsic factor absorption. This can contribute to pernicious anemia
Vitamin A	Low serum retinol levels detected in up to 30% of Crohn's disease patients
Vitamin D	Associated with low serum calcium levels in IBD patients
Vitamin E	Acts as a free scavenger radical, supplementation may sometimes be necessary for IBD patients
Vitamin K	Plays a role in coagulation factor production as well as development of bone mineral density

What Conditions Will Prevent Fistulas from Resolving Spontaneously?

Conditions that prevent fistulas from spontaneously closing can be remembered by the acronym "HIS FRIEND": high fistula output (>500 cm^3/day), IBD, short fistula (<2.5 cm), foreign body, radiation, infection, epithelialization, neoplasm, and distal obstruction.

Workup

What Laboratory Studies Are Recommended? What Serology Is Recommended?

Patients should have a complete blood count and vitamin B12 level checked. Other studies that may help in evaluating for IBD include ESR, CRP, and albumin. pANCA is more frequently positive in UC, while cANCA positivity is more common in Crohn's.

What Is the Primary Modality for Diagnosing IBD?

Colonoscopy serves as the preferred diagnostic modality and to determine the extent of disease. Ideally, this should not be performed during an acute or initial presentation of IBD as it increases the risk of iatrogenic perforation. Once inflammation has resolved, a colonoscopy can be performed after a bowel preparation. With Crohn's, the colonoscope should include inspection of the terminal ileum (ileoscopy). Since Crohn's does not always involve the colon (or even the ileum), other imaging may be necessary.

What Are the Classic Findings on a CT Scan?

CT imaging is the primary imaging modality for evaluating an acute presentation of IBD and its complications. IBD patients will have a thickened bowel wall, increased mural enhancement with hyper-enhancing mucosa, and fibrofatty proliferation of the mesenteric fat (creeping fat sign).

Watch Out

Creeping fat refers to the encroachment of mesenteric fat toward the antimesenteric border of the bowel. It is classically associated with Crohn's and can be seen grossly in the operating room. This is considered a pathognomonic finding.

Management

What Are the Medical Therapies Available?

Treatment for IBD is tailored to the degree of inflammation and disease extent. Mild UC is defined by fewer than four bowel movements per day, intermittent hematochezia, normal inflammatory markers, and no anemia. First-line treatment for mild UC involves 5-aminosalicylic acid (5-ASA) agents, such as mesalamine. Rectosigmoid-limited UC is typically treated with mesalamine suppositories or enemas, while oral therapy is preferred for more extensive disease. For moderate to severe cases of IBD, medical therapies include corticosteroids, immunosuppressants (e.g., azathioprine), and biologics (e.g., infliximab). While 5-ASA agents are effective in UC, they are generally less useful in Crohn's. Most clinicians now practice a "top-down" approach where there is an early initiation of more aggressive medications such as biologics, which is eventually tailored to more benign medications, such as a steroid taper.

Watch Out

5-ASA appears to have a protective effect for colorectal cancer in patients with UC.

Will Most IBD Patients Eventually Require Surgery?

About ¾ of Crohn's patients will eventually need surgery, whereas only about ¼ of UC patients will. Unfortunately, for Crohn's patients, surgery is not curative. In contrast, surgery for UC can be curative but usually requires complete removal of the colon and rectum (total proctocolectomy). A pouch or reservoir for stool (much like a new rectum) is created from the ileum (termed a J-pouch) and is anastomosed to the anus. Though it is possible to leave a rectal cuff, this would create the need for lifelong surveillance for malignant transformation of the remaining rectal mucosa.

Watch Out

The newly created ileal J-pouch can develop recurrent inflammation or infection (termed "pouchitis"). This is treated with metronidazole or ciprofloxacin. However, occasionally pouchitis represents Crohn's disease that was incorrectly diagnosed as UC.

What Are the Surgical Indications for Crohn's? Ulcerative Colitis?

Since Crohn's has a tendency to create strictures, the most common indication for surgery is small bowel obstruction. Other indications include fistulas and abscesses. Since UC only affects the colorectal mucosa, the most common indication for surgery is intractability (failure of medical management to control bloody diarrhea). Another indication is toxic megacolon. Surgery may be required for both Crohn's and UC patients with fulminant acute disease unresponsive to steroid therapy. In addition, patients with high-risk dysplasia or colon cancer require surgical resection.

Watch Out

Patients with IBD are at much higher risk of postoperative venous thromboembolic events such as pulmonary embolism and deep vein thrombosis.

Why Is it Recommended to Avoid Small Bowel Resection with Crohn's Disease if Possible?

Since the entire GI tract of Crohn's patients is susceptible to inflammation and thus stricturing, there is a high risk of requiring multiple areas of resection over the lifespan of the patient, predisposing patients to short bowel syndrome. For this reason, it is recommended to only resect small bowel when it is absolutely necessary. Alternative options to bowel resection are to perform a stricturoplasty or to bypass the segment of bowel.

Watch Out

Crohn's patients undergoing small bowel resection with primary anastomosis have the highest risk of recurrence of inflammation at the anastomosis.

In a UC Patient, What Would Be the Concern if They Presented with Sepsis, Diffuse Abdominal Pain, and a Markedly Distended Colon?

This presentation is concerning for toxic megacolon, a potentially lethal complication of IBD that is characterized by an acute dilation of the colon, typically larger than 6 cm in diameter with a high risk for perforation. The etiology has not been fully elucidated. It is much more common with UC than with Crohn's. These patients are at high risk for septic shock and present with fever, chills, leukocytosis, tachycardia, lactic acidosis, and eventually hypotension and organ failure. In the case of perforation, patients may have free air on x-ray or develop a rigid abdomen with guarding (peritonitis). These patients should be started on IV fluid resuscitation and broad-spectrum IV antibiotics and taken to the operating room for total abdominal colectomy.

Areas Where You Can Get in Trouble

Bloating and Watery Diarrhea After Terminal Ileum Resection in Crohn's

Small intestinal bacterial overgrowth (SIBO) is an excess of bacteria in the small intestine, resulting in bloating, flatulence, watery diarrhea, and malabsorption. Patients with Crohn's disease are particularly at risk of SIBO after ileocecal resection, as the removal of the ileocecal valve may permit reflux of colonic bacteria into the ileum. In addition to anatomic abnormalities of the bowel, other risk factors include motility disorders, immunodeficiency, chronic pancreatitis, decreased gastric acid production (i.e., use of proton-pump inhibitors), and antibiotic use. The gold standard of diagnosis is an endoscopy with a small bowel aspirate and culture. However, diagnosis is usually based on a hydrogen breath test given that it is reliable and non-invasive. The quantity of exhaled hydrogen is measured after the patient consumes sugar (lactose or glucose). A rapid increase in exhaled hydrogen suggests that bacteria, particularly anaerobic bacteria, are fermenting the carbohydrate and have colonized the small bowel. Treatment is antibiotics, typically rifaximin, ciprofloxacin, or doxycycline.

Watch Out

The symptoms of SIBO may resemble those of celiac disease. Patients with celiac disease will have tissue transglutaminase antibodies (tTG-IgA).

Cecal or Terminal Ileum Inflammation in Association with Suspected Appendicitis

Crohn's can mimic acute appendicitis. If during surgery the appendix appears normal and without inflammation, but the terminal ileum and cecum are red and inflamed, the presumptive diagnosis is Crohn's (in this setting the term "regional enteritis" is used). These patients may have creeping fat around the ileum. If the cecum is red and inflamed, do not perform an appendectomy, as there is a risk that the stump of the appendix will blow out and form a fistula. These patients should have a postoperative colonoscopy performed. Biopsy of an inflamed cecum should also be avoided as this increases the risk for enterocutaneous fistula. If only the terminal ileum is inflamed (and not the cecum), the risk of a fistula is low. It is then reasonable to still proceed with appendectomy so as to avoid future confusion in the event of future recurrent right lower quadrant pain.

Inflammatory Bowel Disease (Fig. 27.1)

Some of the differences in IBD include:

1. Depth of mucosal involvement: Crohn's disease involves transmural inflammation, whereas ulcerative colitis is limited to the mucosa and submucosa.
2. Lesion distribution: Crohn's disease demonstrates skip lesions, in which patches of diseased tissue are interspersed between normal areas of bowel, often affecting the terminal ileum, as well as other segments of small and large intestine. Ulcerative colitis presents with continuous lesions, usually starting at the rectum and progressing proximally through the colon.
3. Mucosal appearance: Mucosa in Crohn's disease exhibits signs of cobblestoning from the deep nature of mucosal involvement, whereas ulcerative colitis shows pseudopolyps.
4. Complications: Crohn's disease is more likely to cause strictures and fistulas, whereas ulcerative colitis may lead to toxic megacolon and severe bleeding.

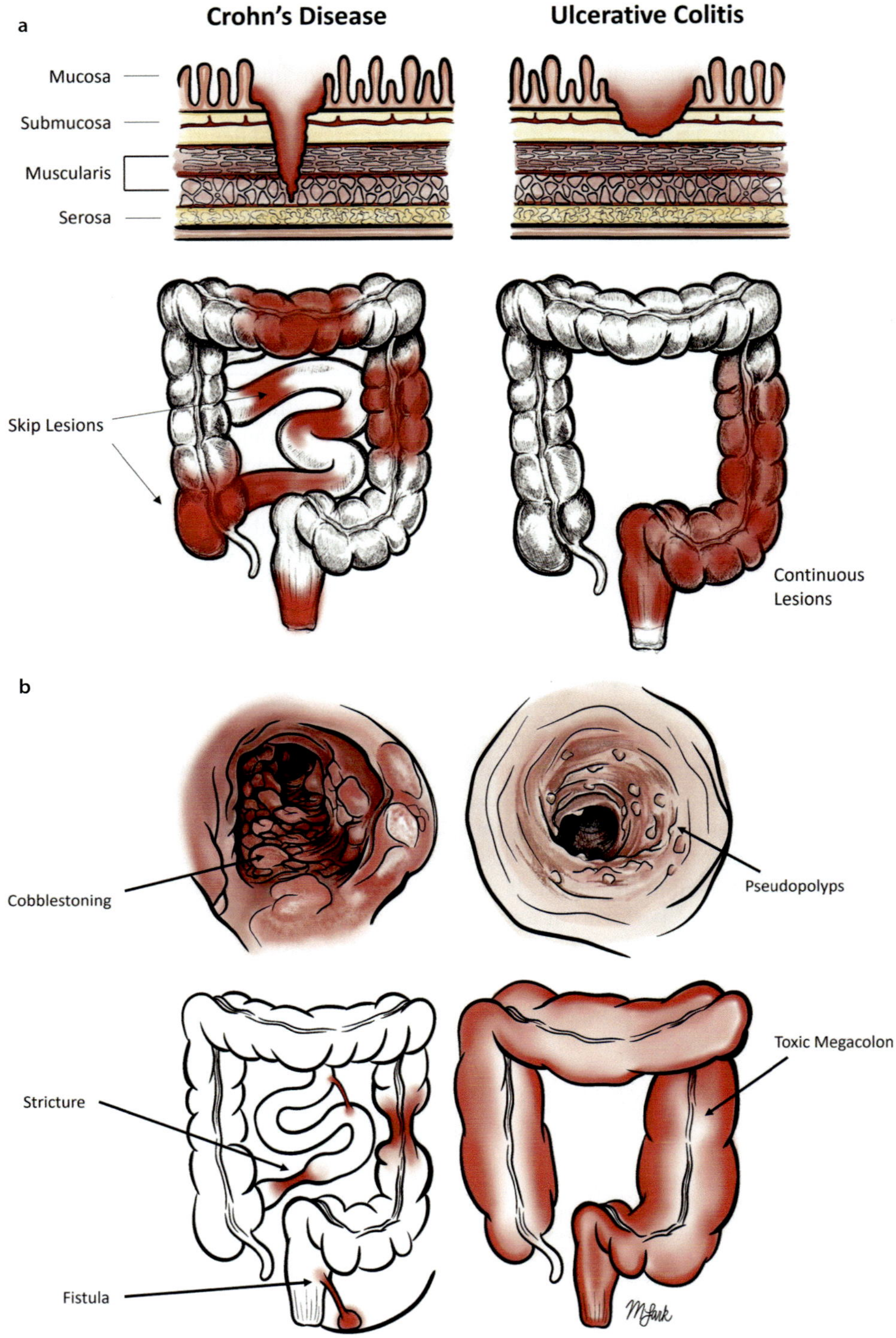

Fig. 27.1 **a** and **b**, Differences between Crohn's disease (*left*) and ulcerative colitis (*right*), specifically related to depth of mucosal involvement, gross lesion distribution, mucosal appearance on colonoscopy, and complications

Summary of Essentials

History and Physical

- IBD is multifactorial: genetic components, environmental exposures, and host microbiome.
- Bimodal distribution: age 20–30 and 60–80.
- Smoking is a risk factor for Crohn's but protects against UC.

Pathophysiology

- Crohn's occurs "gum to bum" but most commonly terminal ileum, characterized by skip lesions.
- UC starts in rectum and only extends to colon continuously.
- Iron, vitamin B12, and fat-soluble vitamin deficiencies can occur.
- Cancer risk increased 8–10 years after diagnosis and need to be screened with a colonoscopy 8 years after diagnosis.

Diagnosis

- Colonoscopy is the primary modality for diagnosis.
- Creeping fat is a pathognomonic finding for IBD in the operating room, most commonly Crohn's.

Management

- Top-down approach with biologics, immunosuppressant agents, 5-ASA agents, and steroids.
- Most Crohn's patients ultimately require surgery, most commonly for obstruction.

Acknowledgments The editors would like to acknowledge and thank the following authors for their contributions to the previous edition of the chapter: Sarath Sujatha-Bhaskar.

Suggested Reading

Brant SR, Nguyen GC. Is there a gender difference in the prevalence of Crohn's disease or ulcerative colitis? Inflamm Bowel Dis. 2008;14(Suppl 2):S2–3.

Cushing K, Higgins PDR. Management of Crohn Disease: A Review. JAMA. 2021;325(1):69–80. doi:https://doi.org/10.1001/jama.2020.18936

Santos MPC, Gomes C, Torres J. Familial and ethnic risk in inflammatory bowel disease. Ann Gastroenterol. 2018;31(1):14–23.

Soares-Mota M, Silva TA, Gomes LM, et al. High prevalence of vitamin A deficiency in Crohn's disease patients according to serum retinol levels and the relative dose-response test. World J Gastroenterol. 2015;21(5):1614–20.

Sonnenberg A. Age distribution of IBD hospitalization. Inflamm Bowel Dis. 2010;16(3):452–7.

Pimentel M, Saad RJ, Long MD, Rao SSC. ACG Clinical Guideline: Small Intestinal Bacterial Overgrowth. *Am J Gastroenterol*. 2020;115(2):165–178. https://doi.org/10.14309/ajg.0000000000000501

Yamamoto-Furusho JK. Genetic factors associated with the development of inflammatory bowel disease. World J Gastroenterol. 2007;13(42):5594–7.

Lower Gastrointestinal

Question Set: Lower Gastrointestinal

Questions

1. A 68-year-old man with a history of prostate cancer treated with external beam radiation therapy 6 months ago presents with intermittent rectal bleeding and a sensation of incomplete evacuation. He reports no abdominal pain, fever, or weight loss. He denies any history of inflammatory bowel disease. On physical exam, his abdomen is soft and non-tender. Rectal examination reveals no masses. Colonoscopy reveals telangiectasias and pallor of the rectal mucosa without ulcerations, polyps, or signs of active infection. Which of the following is the most appropriate next step in management?
   (A) Oral mesalamine
   (B) Metronidazole and ciprofloxacin
   (C) Endoscopic thermal coagulation
   (D) Loperamide and butyrate enemas
   (E) Total proctocolectomy

2. A 50-year-old woman undergoes screening colonoscopy. She is asymptomatic. During the procedure, she is found to have a dark discoloration of the entire colon with lymph follicles shining through as pale patches. What is the most likely underlying etiology?
   (A) Drinking lots of prune juice
   (B) Colon cancer
   (C) Laxative abuse
   (D) Normal anatomic variation
   (E) Inflammatory bowel disease (IBD)

3. An 88-year-old man with Parkinson's disease and chronic obstructive pulmonary disease (COPD) is brought to the emergency department from a skilled nursing facility because his nurse noticed bright red blood in his stool. His medications include hydrochlorothiazide, metformin, levodopa, salmeterol, and docusate. On admission, he is afebrile with normal blood pressure and pulse. Colonoscopy shows bright red blood within the colon, multiple diverticula, and no blood proximal to the ileocecal valve. Although he has a large amount of stool and blood clots, no active bleeding sources are able to be seen. He continues to have blood per rectum over the next hour. Blood pressure is 120/70 mmHg and heart rate is 90/min. Which of the following is the most appropriate next step in management?
   (A) Exploratory laparotomy
   (B) Transfuse two units of packed red blood cells (RBCs)
   (C) 99mTc red blood cell (RBC) scintigraphy
   (D) Esophagogastroduodenoscopy (EGD)
   (E) Omeprazole and antibiotics

4. A 62-year-old female arrives to the emergency department with acute abdominal pain. She has a past medical history significant for diverticulitis. She is diagnosed with uncomplicated diverticulitis and managed with bowel rest and antibiotics. A year later, she has another episode of diverticulitis that was again successfully managed on an outpatient basis. Which of the following is this patient at higher risk of developing?
(A) Crohn's disease
(B) Ulcerative colitis
(C) Pancreatic cancer
(D) Anal cancer
(E) Stricture formation

5. A 55-year-old male has been receiving serial ultrasound examinations to follow his abdominal aortic aneurysm (AAA). Over the past year, the aneurysm has rapidly enlarged to 5.8 cm, and he undergoes endovascular abdominal aortic aneurysm repair (EVAR). The operation itself is uneventful. However, on postoperative day 1, the patient develops a low-grade fever, left lower quadrant pain, and diarrhea that appears to be blood tinged. On physical examination, he has mild-to-moderate tenderness in the left lower quadrant without rebound or guarding. What is the next step in the workup?
(A) CT scan of the abdomen and pelvis with oral and intravenous (IV) contrast
(B) Exploratory laparotomy
(C) Formal mesenteric arteriography
(D) Flexible sigmoidoscopy
(E) Abdominal ultrasound

6. A 30-year-old man with colon cancer secondary to familial adenomatous polyposis (FAP) arrives for follow-up after receiving a total proctocolectomy with end ileostomy. He was found to have colon cancer after presenting at the age of 27 with unexplained rectal bleeding, diarrhea, and abdominal pain. Subsequent colonoscopy found multiple adenomatous polyps in his colon. He has a 5-year-old son, who is screened and is positive for the adenomatous polyposis coli (APC) gene. What is the recommended screening for his son?
(A) Colonoscopy starting at age 20
(B) Flexible sigmoidoscopy starting at age 10
(C) Flexible sigmoidoscopy starting at age 17
(D) Annual fecal occult blood test (FOBT)
(E) Annual barium enema

7. A 75-year-old man arrives to the emergency department with abdominal pain. He has never experienced this before but reports having left-sided abdominal pain over the last 2 days that is relieved temporarily after defecation. He has a temperature of 38.5 °C with a blood pressure of 142/88 mmHg and pulse of 88/min. His laboratory examination is significant for a white blood cell (WBC) of $14 \times 10^3/\mu L$ (normal $4.1–10.9 \times 10^3/\mu L$) with 10% bands. Hematocrit is 30%. CT imaging reveals focal sigmoidal wall thickening with significant paracolic inflammation. He was treated in the hospital for 3 days and discharged home without complications. Which of the following is the most appropriate follow-up option?
(A) High-fiber diet alone
(B) CT scan 2 weeks after resolution
(C) Elective sigmoid colectomy
(D) Barium enema
(E) Colonoscopy

8. A 28-year-old woman presents to the emergency department because of abdominal pain that started 2 h ago. She has nausea and vomited twice in the last hour. She reports that the pain is predominantly in the right lower quadrant (RLQ). On physical exam, her blood pressure is 120/60 mmHg, heart rate is 100/min, and she is afebrile. She is very tender at McBurney's point and has pain on passive extension of the right hip. Her WBC is 14 × $10^3/\mu L$ (normal 4.1–10.9 × $10^3/\mu L$), hemoglobin is 12 g/dL (12–15.2 g/dL), hematocrit is 36% (37–46%), and platelet count is 250,000 μ/L (140–450,000 μ/L). Her urinalysis shows 1+ white blood cells. Which of the following is the best next step in management?
   - (A) Admit for observation
   - (B) CT scan of the abdomen
   - (C) Laparoscopic appendectomy
   - (D) Beta-human chorionic gonadotropin (B-hCG)
   - (E) Oral antibiotics covering gram-negative flora

9. A 38-year-old male presents with a history and exam suggestive of acute appendicitis and undergoes laparoscopic appendectomy. At surgery, the terminal ileum and cecum appear to be red and inflamed. The appendix is removed uneventfully. Final pathology of the appendix demonstrates no evidence of acute appendicitis. Two weeks later, he presents back to the emergency department with feces draining from his right lower quadrant wound. Which of the following is the most likely explanation for why the drainage may not spontaneously stop?
   - (A) A distal colonic obstruction
   - (B) Chronic inflammation
   - (C) An occult intra-abdominal abscess
   - (D) A retained sponge in the abdomen
   - (E) A missed malignancy

10. Which of the following is most likely to require *urgent* colectomy?
   - (A) Cecal volvulus
   - (B) Sigmoid volvulus
   - (C) Acute diverticulitis
   - (D) Cecal adenocarcinoma
   - (E) Pseudomembranous colitis

11. A 55-year-old man is about to start a new security job that requires a physical exam by a doctor. He has no past medical history, and everyone in his family is healthy. He has a well-balanced diet and exercises every day. He is evaluated during a routine examination which includes a discussion of health maintenance issues. He is surprised to hear that it is recommended for a man of his age to get a colonoscopy. He asks if there are any other options available. Which of the following is an appropriate recommendation with respect to this health maintenance screening strategy?
   - (A) Fecal occult blood test (FOBT) every 5 years
   - (B) Annual rectal examination
   - (C) Flexible sigmoidoscopy every 5 years + FOBT every 3 years
   - (D) Annual CT colonography
   - (E) Annual carcinoembryonic antigen (CEA) levels

of the appendix or for tumors of any size located at the base of the appendix (thus, involving the margins), a right colectomy is indicated. Otherwise, no further treatment is needed. The other answer choices are not appropriate for a carcinoid tumor (A–D).

14. Answer B
Carcinoembryonic antigen (CEA) is a glycoprotein, which is present in normal mucosal cells, but increased amounts are associated with adenocarcinoma, especially colorectal cancer. The major role of CEA in colon cancer patients is to allow clinicians to monitor for recurrence after intended curative treatment. Typically, patients achieve normal levels about 4–6 weeks after surgical intervention. Smoking up to 4 h prior to checking serum CEA can falsely elevate levels. CEA levels are also elevated with other cancers (e.g., medullary carcinoma of the thyroid, pancreatic, gastric cancer) as well as benign conditions (inflammatory bowel disease, pancreatitis and cirrhosis), but not with the other choices provided (A, C–E). It is recommended to counsel all patients to quit smoking as it can affect postoperative monitoring and improves overall health.

15. Answer C
Sigmoid volvulus occurs in debilitated and/or psychiatric patients. The twist in the colon leads to a closed loop obstruction which, if left untreated, leads to colonic ischemia, sepsis, and eventual colonic gangrene and perforation. Patients present with abdominal distention, pain, constipation, and vomiting. X-ray films may show an air filled closed loop of massively distended colon, referred to as a "bent inner tube" or "coffee bean" sign. Most patients can be managed by decompression with colonoscopy. However, this patient demonstrates evidence that the colon is already ischemic/gangrenous (fever, tachycardia, hypotension, peritonitis, leukocytosis). Thus, colonic decompression is contraindicated (A). Following fluid resuscitation and antibiotics, the patient requires urgent exploratory laparotomy with sigmoid colon resection and proximal colostomy. Similarly, with peritonitis and the classic plain X-ray finding, CT scan is unnecessary and in fact may cause renal injury given his pre-renal azotemia (B). Placing a rectal tube and admitting to the hospital without surgery would not be appropriate (D–E).

16. Answer A
Ogilvie's syndrome is a pseudo-obstruction of the colon that is associated with bedridden, neurologically impaired or older patients, opiate use, recent surgery, trauma, or infection. The mechanism for this colon dysfunction is unknown. X-ray films will predominantly show a markedly dilated colon without evidence of a bowel obstruction. Management consists of removing any drugs that may interfere with gut motility (e.g., opiates) and replacement of electrolytes (especially potassium). A colon larger than 10 cm is at risk for perforation and requires decompression with neostigmine and/or colonoscopy. Due to the law of Laplace (tension = [pressure × radius]/wall thickness), the cecum, being the part of the colon with the largest diameter and thinnest wall, is the most common site for perforation (B–E).

17. Answer B
The first step in the workup for GI bleeding is to determine if the source is the upper or lower GI tract. If the patient is vomiting blood or has coffee ground emesis, then the source is clearly an UGI one. Since a massive UGI bleeding can cause bleeding per rectum, it is imperative that an UGI source is ruled out first when working up a patient with a massive lower GI bleeding. This is achieved by performing an EGD. Previously, these patients received a nasogastric tube to examine the aspirate for blood. However, EGD is more sensitive to detect an UGI bleeding and can serve as a therapeutic modality. CT scan with IV contrast is sometimes utilized for GI bleeding, but is not the first line study

(A). Colonoscopy is not yet indicated nor is surgery (C–D). A central venous line should be considered if ongoing massive fluids/blood are needed (E).

18. Answer B

Patients with inflammatory bowel disease are at increased risk of colon cancer. The risk is much greater for ulcerative colitis (UC) than with Crohn's disease and is related to the duration of illness and the extent of disease. For UC, the risk is low in the first 10 years of the disease (2–3%) but grows to 1–2% per year afterwards. UC patients should begin getting screened 8 years after disease onset and continue getting screened every 1–2 years after. *Random biopsies* are necessary in patients with UC undergoing screening with colonoscopy because in these patients, cancers do not follow the typical progression from polyp to cancer (A, C–E). A proctocolectomy removes the entire rectum and colon, which prevents patients with UC from developing cancer, and no further surveillance is required.

19. Answer C

Streptococcus bovis and *Clostridium septicum* are both associated with colon cancer. The clinical context *S. bovis* comes up in most often is in that of patients suffering from endocarditis. *C. septicum* can spread hematogenously to muscle tissue and is also associated with the concomitant presence of hematologic malignancy. All patients found to be infected with these organisms should be scheduled for a colonoscopy to rule out colorectal malignancy. *Diphyllobothrium latum* (fish tapeworm) and *Cryptococcus neoformans* have not been linked to an increased risk of developing colon cancer (D–E).

20. Answer A

Acute appendicitis is triggered by an obstruction of the appendiceal lumen. In adults, the obstruction is most commonly caused by a fecalith (B). However, in children the obstruction is most often due to lymphoid hyperplasia within the appendix that may be triggered by an antecedent viral infection. Thus, patients may have a history of a recent viral infection prior to the acute appendicitis. Parasites, such as pinworm, and foreign body ingestion can rarely obstruct the appendiceal lumen and cause appendicitis (C, E). Acute mesenteric adenitis can mimic acute appendicitis (D). However, this is less common, and the vast majority present with mild diffuse abdominal pain as opposed to localized pain and tenderness at McBurney's point.

Neurosurgery

Richard G. Everson

Contents

Neck Pain and Extremity Weakness Following Trauma

Richard G. Everson, Jose Manuel Sarmiento, and Isaac Yang

Contents

C. de Virgilio, A. Grigorian (eds.), *Surgery*, https://doi.org/10.1007/978-3-032-09799-6_28

28

Case Study

A 25-year-old man was snowboarding down a slope and attempted to perform a trick off a ramp. He miscalculated the jump and landed directly on his head, without a helmet. He denied any loss of consciousness but immediately had difficulty moving his arms and legs. The ambulance crew placed him supine on a board with a hard cervical collar and blocks. In the emergency department, he is alert and oriented to person, place, and time, but he complains of severe neck pain. His heart rate is 80 beats/min, blood pressure is 130/85 mmHg, respiratory rate is 13/min, and temperature is 37.4 °C. He has 2/5 strength in his upper and lower extremities. He reports decreased sensation to pinpricks and cold packs in all extremities but has preserved sensation to deep touch and pressure throughout the body. He has nonsustained clonus and brisk reflexes in his biceps, brachioradialis, triceps, patellar tendons, and Achilles tendons. His big toe points upward with all other toes fanning out when the sole of his foot is stimulated with a blunt instrument. Rectal examination reveals preserved anal tone. His imaging is shown below (◘ Fig. 28.1).

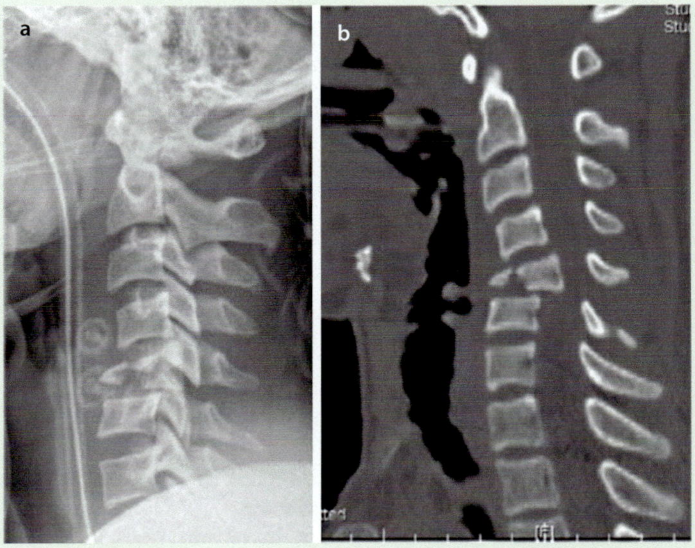

◘ **Fig. 28.1** **a** Lateral radiograph and **b** computed tomographic scan. (Reprinted from Vollmer et al. (2011). Copyright 2011, with permission from Elsevier)

Diagnosis

What Spinal Cord Syndromes Are Associated with Cervical Spine Injury? (Table 28.1)

Table 28.1 Spinal cord syndromes associated with cervical spine injury

Diagnosis	History and physical
Complete spinal cord injury	Complete loss of motor and sensory function (>3 segments) below the level of injury, including absence of voluntary anal contraction and perineal sensation (no sacral sparing), in the absence of spinal shock
Brown-Sequard syndrome	Ipsilateral motor weakness with associated upper motor neuron signs (spasticity, hyperreflexia, clonus, and positive Babinski's sign) and loss of proprioception and light touch below the level of injury; contralateral loss of pain and temperature sensation starting one to two levels below the lesion
Central cord syndrome	Weakness and loss of sensory function that is disproportionately worse in the upper extremities than in the lower extremities; distal lower extremities are typically spared; typically occurs after hyperextension injury in patients with preexisting cervical spondylosis
Anterior spinal artery syndrome	Paraplegia (quadriplegia if higher than C7) with loss of pain and temperature sensation below the level of injury; the posterior columns are unaffected, leading to preserved two-point discrimination, deep touch/pressure, vibration, and proprioception

Clinically, What Is the Difference Between a Complete and Incomplete Spinal Cord Injury?

Patients with complete spinal cord injuries have no motor or sensory function below the level of injury, whereas those with incomplete spinal cord injuries have some residual function below the injury level.

What Is the Most Likely Diagnosis?

Anterior spinal artery syndrome due to burst fracture dislocation at C5. This is an *incomplete* spinal cord injury because the patient has some motor and sensory function in his extremities, as well as preserved anal tone. The patient's pertinent neurological examination findings (e.g., bilateral loss of motor, pain, and temperature with preserved deep touch and pressure throughout the body) are consistent with an anterior cord syndrome with associated myelopathic signs. Radiographic studies show evidence of a burst fracture at the C5 level. Additionally, he has signs of upper motor neuron dysfunction (Babinski's sign). The patient does not show evidence of spinal shock (no flaccid paralysis in extremities and reflexes are present) or neurogenic shock (no hypotension or bradycardia).

History and Physical

What Are the Most Common Cervical Spinal Levels Involved After Trauma?

The most common level of cervical vertebral fracture is C2 (approximately one-third of all C2 fractures are odontoid fractures), followed by C6 and C7. The most common level of subluxation injury is the C5–C6 interspace, which is the area of greatest flexion and extension in the cervical spine.

What Dermatome Level Supplies the Shoulders? What Must You Remember About the Dermatome Map When Testing Sensation on the Chest?

The shoulders are supplied by C4 (Table 28.2). When testing sensation on the chest, remember that there is a skip from C4 to T2, with C5 through T1 represented in the upper extremities.

> **Watch Out**
> A dermatome is a sensory region of the skin innervated by a nerve root.

Why Is it Important to Check Deep Tendon Reflexes?

Patients with injured nerve roots can have abnormal deep tendon reflexes (Table 28.3). Some patients with acute spinal cord injuries may initially have completely blunted reflexes during the acute stage of spinal shock but later develop hyperactive and brisk reflexes as the inhibitory forces from upper motor neurons are lifted.

28

Table 28.2 Common dermatomal levels

Anatomical site	Dermatomal level
Shoulders	C4
Nipples	T4
Umbilicus	T10
Knees	L4
Perianal region	S4–S5

Table 28.3 Deep tendon reflexes

Reflex	Involved nerve root(s)
Biceps	C5/C6
Brachioradialis	C6
Triceps	C7
Patellar tendon (knee jerk)	L4
Achilles tendon (ankle jerk)	S1

How Are Deep Tendon Reflexes Graded?

These are graded as 0 to 4+ with *2+ being normal*. 0 is no response, while 1+ is a sluggish one. A reflex that is more brisk than usual is 3+, and those with a clonus present are 4+.

What Are the Devastating Clinical Examination Findings in Patients with Complete Spinal Cord Injury in the High Cervical Cord (at or Above C3)?

Inability to breathe due to diaphragmatic paralysis, as well as paralysis of all four limbs. The phrenic nerve originates from the C3 to C5 spinal nerves.

Watch Out
Remember: C3, C4, and C5 keep the diaphragm alive!

What Is the Term for Sensory or Motor Dysfunction Caused by Pathology of a *Nerve Root*? What Are the Clinical Signs and Symptoms Associated with This Disorder?

Radiculopathy. The main symptom associated with radiculopathy is a burning, tingling pain that radiates down the limb. Clinical signs of radiculopathy include lower motor neuron signs such as loss of reflexes, weakness, and diminished sensation along dermatomal distributions.

What Is the Term for Sensory or Motor Dysfunction Caused by Pathology of the *Spinal Cord*? What Are the Clinical Signs and Symptoms Associated with This Disorder?

Myelopathy. Patients experience intermittent neck pain that radiates into the shoulders or occiput. Clinical findings of myelopathy result from a spinal cord injury and include bilateral upper motor neuron signs (Table 28.4) such as diffuse hyperreflexia, weakness, and numbness in the extremities, and upward-going toes (Babinski's sign).

Watch Out
Babinski's sign can be a normal finding in infants as old as 2 years.

What Does the Presence of Lower Motor Neuron Signs in the Upper Extremities and Upper Motor Neuron Signs in the Lower Extremities Suggest?

This pattern suggests cervical spinal cord compression. Associated findings may include a positive Lhermitte sign, described as an electric shock-like sensation radiating down the spine with neck flexion, which is highly suggestive of cervical myelopathy.

Table 28.4 Upper motor neuron (UMN) and lower motor neuron (LMN) signs

Sign	UMN lesion	LMN lesion
Weakness	Yes	Yes
Fasciculations	No	Yes
Atrophy	No	Yes
Tone	Increased	Decreased
Reflexes	Increased	Decreased
Babinski's sign (plantar reflex)	Yes	No
Hoffmann's sign	Yes	No
Clonus	Yes	No

Pathophysiology

What Is the Difference Between Spinal Shock and Neurogenic Shock?

Spinal shock is not a true form of shock. It is a term used for a temporary (one day to a few weeks) loss of spinal cord function. It manifests with flaccid paralysis below the level of injury and loss of all reflexes, including urinary and rectal tone (loss of *bulbocavernosus reflex*). With time (months), the deep tendon reflexes return and may become hyperreflexive, and a Babinski sign may appear. Return of motor and sensory function depends on the type and severity of the spinal cord injury. Neurogenic shock is a true shock wherein sympathetic outflow through the spinal cord has been disrupted. The loss of sympathetic tone results in vasodilation, bradycardia, and dangerous hypotension. Neurogenic shock is typically associated with more severe spinal cord injuries (typically above T6). A patient may have both neurogenic and spinal shock present simultaneously.

Watch Out

In a paralyzed trauma patient, hypotension should be presumed to be due to bleeding (hypovolemic shock) until proven otherwise, especially if they are *tachycardic*. Also, keep in mind that the abdominal exam is unreliable.

What Is Sacral Sparing? What Is Its Significance in the Setting of Spinal Shock?

Sacral sparing refers to the sparing of function at the sacral nerve level, such as an intact anal sphincter or perianal sensation. When there is sacral sparing in a patient with spinal shock, the chance of functional neurological recovery is better compared to a situation where the sacral roots are affected.

What Are the Common Mechanisms for Neck Injuries?

Flexion, extension, axial loading (vertical compression), and rotational injuries.

What Is Atlanto-Occipital Dislocation?

Atlanto-occipital dislocation is the most unstable and dangerous injury of the cervical spine. This occurs when the superior facets of the atlas vertebra lose their articulation with the occipital condyles at the base of the skull, resulting from ligamentous disruption between the occiput and the cervical spine. Severe neurological morbidity and mortality are due to high cervical cord injury that can lead to quadriparesis, diaphragm paralysis, and cardiac arrest.

Watch Out

Patients with *trisomy-21* (Down's syndrome) are at particularly high risk for atlantoaxial and atlanto-occipital instability and should always be screened before participating in contact sports or undergoing anesthesia.

28

What Is the Pathophysiology of the Three Most Common Incomplete Spinal Cord Injuries? (Table 28.5)

Table 28.5 Pathophysiology of incomplete spinal cord injuries

Syndrome	Comments
Brown-Sequard syndrome	Hemisection of the spinal cord, usually from penetrating trauma such as a gunshot or a stabbing, causing injury to the corticospinal tract (motor), posterior columns (proprioception, deep touch/pressure), and spinothalamic tracts (contralateral pain and temperature)
Anterior cord syndrome	Damage to the anterior two-thirds of the spinal cord is classically due to severe flexion injury; this area receives its blood supply from the anterior spinal artery; the corticospinal and lateral spinothalamic tracts are affected bilaterally
Central cord syndrome	Damage to the central portion of the spinal cord is classically associated with severe hyperextension injury; patients who present with central cord syndrome are often elderly and have preexisting cervical stenosis

Why Are the Distal Lower Extremities Typically Spared in Central Cord Syndrome?

This reflects the unique topographical organization of the spinal cord in which upper extremity motor function is represented at the medial aspects of the cord, while lower extremity motor function is represented at the lateral aspects of the cord. The central portion of the spinal cord is a vascular watershed zone that is more susceptible to injury and ischemia from edema. Thus, motor function and sensation in the distal lower extremities are spared.

Which Incomplete Cord Syndrome Carries the *Best* Prognosis for Recovery of Neurological Function, Bowel and Bladder Function, and Ambulatory Capacity?

Brown-Sequard syndrome

Which Incomplete Cord Syndrome Carries the *Worst* Prognosis for Functional Recovery?

Anterior cord syndrome (about 10% recover to ambulation)

What Spinal Cord Injury Can Occur After Surgery on the Thoracic Aorta?

Anterior spinal cord infarction (due to interruption of the artery of Adamkiewicz, a branch of the anterior spinal artery). They may develop bilateral flaccid paralysis with loss of pain/temperature below the lowest level of infarction shortly after surgery.

Workup

How Do You Diagnose Spinal Cord Injuries and Cervical Vertebral Fractures?

Spinal cord injuries may be diagnosed with a thorough history and neurological examination. The diagnosis may be confirmed with the help of radiographic imaging modalities such as X-ray, CT scan, and MRI. The American Spinal Injury Association (ASIA) scale should be used for functional assessment.

What Are the NEXUS Criteria?

This is a validated tool to determine which adult trauma patients may have their C-spine cleared (cervical collar removed) without first obtaining imaging. Attempting such clearance is *contraindicated* if they have any of the following criteria (remembered as the *NSAID* mnemonic):

- *N*eurologic deficit
- *S*pinal tenderness
- *A*ltered mental status
- *I*ntoxicated
- *D*istracting injury

What Type of Imaging Should Be Obtained?

A high-quality cervical spine CT scan is the imaging modality of choice in adults following trauma. If CT is not available, or in pediatric patients under 9 years of age where radiation exposure is a concern, plain radiographs can be obtained. To adequately evaluate the cervical spine on plain films, the craniocervical junction through the C7-T1 junction must be visualized. The initial views should include anteroposterior (AP), lateral, and open-mouth (odontoid) projections. If these views are normal but symptoms persist, oblique views and a swimmer's view (with one arm elevated) may be obtained to better visualize the cervicothoracic junction. Finding a single vertebral fracture on imaging in a trauma patient mandates imaging of the entire spine, as noncontiguous spine injuries are common. A CT scan of the thoracic and lumbar spine should be obtained.

What Is the Indication for Ordering an MRI Scan of the Cervical Spine?

An MRI of the cervical spine is indicated in patients with neurologic deficits suggestive of spinal cord injury or when there is concern for instability despite a negative CT scan. MRI provides additional information by detecting spinal cord edema, contusion, hematoma, and ligamentous injury. In patients with persistent neck pain but no neurologic deficits and a normal CT scan, MRI is not routinely required. Instead, these patients can be placed in a soft cervical collar and monitored clinically with outpatient follow-up. If symptoms do not improve after two weeks, further evaluation with an MRI may be considered.

Can a Spinal Epidural Abscess Occur After Trauma?

Yes. Trauma can predispose to spinal epidural abscess, especially in immunocompromised patients such as those with diabetes or alcohol use disorder. Clinical features include progressively worsening neck or back pain, neurologic deficits, and systemic signs of infection (e.g., fever, leukocytosis). MRI of the spine with contrast is the diagnostic modality of choice. Prompt diagnosis and treatment are critical to prevent permanent neurologic injury.

What Is SCIWORA and SCIWOCTET?

SCIWORA is a term to describe "spinal cord injury without radiographic abnormalities" and is not typically used anymore. SCIWOCTET is a term to describe "spinal cord injury without computed tomography evidence of trauma." Since the advent of high-quality CT and MRI imaging over the past 10 years, most of these injuries are now identified.

> **Watch Out**
> C2 is the most common level injured in the spinal cord.

Management

What Are the General Treatment Principles for Patients with Cervical Spine Injury?

- Transport the patient with a rigid cervical collar on a spine board for immobilization.
- Early closed reduction with tongs or halo traction devices is recommended for awake patients with obvious subluxation on imaging, causing spinal cord compression.
- Avoid hypotension (SBP <90 mmHg) and maintain mean arterial pressure between 85 and 90 mmHg for 7 days after spinal cord injury. Maintain minimum blood pressure goals with intravenous fluids and vasopressors (phenylephrine or dopamine) to reduce secondary injury.
- Insert a Foley catheter to monitor urinary output and prevent bladder distention. In patients with spi-

nal cord injury, acute bladder paralysis from neurogenic shock should be suspected if a suprapubic or lower abdominal mass is palpated.

- Order venous thromboembolism prophylaxis (i.e., low-molecular-weight heparin, heparin) within 48 h and maintain for 3 months.
- Restore spinal stability by external orthoses (cervical collars, cervicothoracic devices, and halo orthosis) or surgical reduction, decompression, and/or fusion.

Watch Out

Among trauma patients, those with spinal cord injury have the highest rate of venous thromboembolic events.

How Is Neurogenic Shock Treated?

Hypotension is treated with rapid infusion of crystalloid normal saline (0.9% NaCl). If intravenous fluids are inadequate to maintain organ perfusion, phenylephrine (an alpha agent) is often used (but may cause reflex bradycardia). Norepinephrine (with both alpha and beta effects) may be better at addressing both bradycardia and hypotension. Bradycardia can also be treated with atropine or dopamine.

What Are the Goals of Management for Patients with Complete Spinal Cord Injuries or High Cervical Cord Injuries?

Spinal stabilization to facilitate nursing and rehabilitation. Surgical decompression aims to maintain and regain function in the uppermost section of the injured cord where an incomplete injury may exist. Nonsurgical care focuses on functional rehabilitation, prevention of decubitus ulcers, bowel and bladder management, and avoidance of pneumonia and deep vein thrombosis.

Watch Out

Complete high cervical spinal cord injuries (above C3) can mimic brain death due to apnea and quadriplegia. Brainstem reflexes must be carefully assessed before making a diagnosis of brain death in trauma patients.

Why Is There a Lower Threshold for Surgical Intervention in Patients with Incomplete Spinal Cord Injury Versus Patients with Complete Spinal Cord Injury?

Expedient open or closed reduction and cord decompression in patients with incomplete spinal cord injury have a higher likelihood of maintaining or regaining neurological function.

What Are the General Indications for Emergent Surgery with Spinal Cord Injury?

- Unstable vertebral fracture
- Non-reducible spinal cord compression with deficit
- Ligamentous injury with facet instability
- Progressive neurologic deficit

Watch Out

Restoration of spinal stability is important to minimize the risk for secondary injury and to allow early mobilization.

Areas Where You Can Get in Trouble

Complications with the Exposure of the Anterior Cervical Spine

The most common complication of exposing the anterior cervical spine for decompressive surgery is recurrent laryngeal nerve injury. Injury to this nerve can paralyze the vocal cord on one side and lead to a hoarse voice (unilateral nerve injury) and can cause airway obstruction (if bilateral nerve injury). Patients may also have transient dysphagia and, rarely, perforation of the esophagus—a life-threatening condition due to the high risk of infection. Injuries of the carotid artery, jugular vein, and superior and inferior thyroid arteries are uncommon. Injury of the vertebral artery is a rare complication.

Impaired Upper Extremity Strength After Whiplash

Patients who experience whiplash may not have any acute symptoms, but <5% are at risk for post-traumatic syringomyelia, which can develop within the following year. This occurs as a result of cerebrospinal fluid retention, enlarging the central spinal cord canal. Post-traumatic syringomyelia can result in weakness of the upper extremities along with decreased pain/temperature sensation bilaterally.

Area of Controversy

Steroid Therapy for Acute Spinal Cord Injury

The administration of methylprednisolone is not recommended for the treatment of acute spinal cord injury. Current guidelines advise against its use due to the lack of high-quality evidence demonstrating clinical benefit and the potential for significant complications, such as infections and gastrointestinal bleeding. Methylprednisolone is not FDA-approved for this indication, and despite several randomized controlled trials, no Class I or II evidence supports its routine use.

Timing of Decompressive Surgery with Acute Spinal Cord Injury

The timing of decompressive surgery for acute spinal cord injury is controversial and is divided into ultra-early (within 12 h), early (within 24 h), and late (>24 h). Recent studies suggest that ultra-early surgery may be associated with improved outcomes, particularly in those with cervical injuries and those with incomplete injuries. However, this is not as yet the standard of care.

MRI for Obtunded Patients

In obtunded trauma patients or patients with traumatic brain injury, some guidelines allow cervical spine clearance with a negative high-quality CT scan alone, without the need for MRI. However, other institutions advocate obtaining an MRI to rule out occult ligamentous injury. The decision often depends on hospital protocol and the patient's clinical status.

Spinal Cord Injury (Fig. 28.2)

1. **Brown-Sequard syndrome** (A)—injury resulting from hemisection of the spinal cord, typically due to penetrating trauma. Injury pattern usually manifests as ipsilateral motor loss and proprioceptive deficits below the level of injury (due to damage to the corticospinal tract and dorsal columns) and contralateral pain and temperature loss (due to disruption of the spinothalamic tract), starting a few levels below the injury.
2. **Anterior cord syndrome** (B)—injury resulting from damage to the anterior portion of the spinal cord, usually due to ischemia or compression. Injury pattern usually manifests as loss of motor function and pain/temperature sensation below the level of injury (damaged corticospinal and spinothalamic tracts) and preserved proprioception and vibration sense (spared dorsal columns).
3. **Central cord syndrome** (C)—injury resulting most commonly from hyperextension injuries. Injury pattern manifests as motor weakness of the upper extremities with loss of pain and temperature sensation.

28

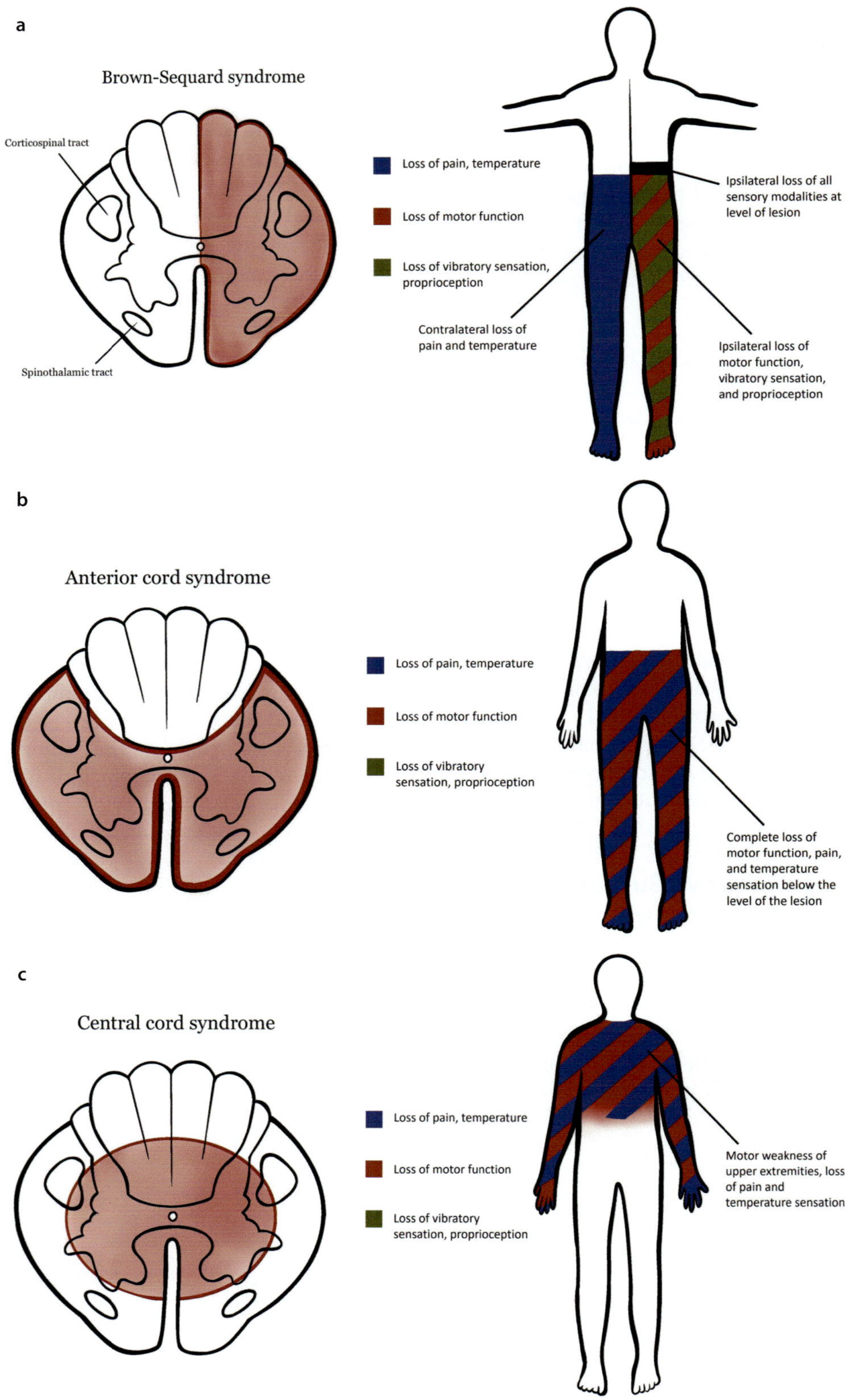

Fig. 28.2 These illustrations demonstrate three common patterns of spinal cord injury

Summary of Essentials

History and Physical

- A thorough neurological examination is necessary for the localization of spinal cord injuries
- Complete spinal cord injury: no motor and sensory function below the level of injury
- Incomplete spinal cord injury: some residual function below the level of injury
- Recognize spinal cord syndromes: Brown-Sequard syndrome, Central cord syndrome, Anterior cord syndrome

Pathophysiology

- Spinal shock: temporary flaccid paralysis below the level of injury with loss of all reflexes, as well as urinary and rectal tone
- Neurogenic shock: a hemodynamic state wherein sympathetic outflow through the spinal cord has been disrupted, resulting in vasodilation, bradycardia, and dangerous hypotension
- Atlanto-occipital dislocation is the most dangerous cervical spine injury

Workup

- CT C-spine is useful for detecting vertebral fractures and identifying hematomas or disk fragments within the spinal canal
- If CT cannot be obtained, and in pediatric traumas, X-rays are appropriate: anteroposterior (AP), lateral, and open-mouth (odontoid)
- MRI C-spine is indicated for neurologic deficits or suspected ligamentous injury despite normal CT
- Trauma patients with a single vertebral fracture must undergo imaging of the entire spine

Management

- Rigid cervical collar on a spine board
- Early closed reduction with tongs or halo traction devices for awake patients with obvious subluxation on imaging, causing spinal cord compression
- IV fluids to avoid hypotension
- Vasopressors (phenylephrine or norepinephrine) if neurogenic shock
- Insert a Foley catheter to monitor for a neurogenic bladder
- Stool softeners
- Venous thromboembolism prophylaxis

Suggested Reading

Badhiwala JH, Ahuja CS, Fehlings MG. Time is spine: a review of translational advances in spinal cord injury. J Neurosurg Spine. 2018 Dec 20;30(1):1–18. https://doi.org/10.3171/2018.9.SPINE18682. PMID: 30611186.

Greenberg MS. Head trauma. In: Greenberg MS, editor. Handbook of neurosurgery. 8th ed. New York: Theime Medical Publishers; 2016. p. 930–60.

Hadley MC, Walters BC. Introduction to the guidelines for the management of acute cervical spine and spinal cord injuries. Neurosurgery. 2013;72:5–16.

Hurlbert RJ, Hadley MN, Walters BC, Aarabi B, Dhall SS, Gelb DE, et al. Pharmacological therapy for acute spinal cord injury. Neurosurgery. 2013;72:93–105.

Kokoska ER, Keller MS, Rallo MC, Weber TR. Characteristics of paediatric cervical spine injuries. J Pediatr Surg. 2011;36(1):100–5.

Rozzelle CJ, Aarabi B, Dhall SS, Gelb DE, et al. Management of pediatric cervical spine and spinal cord injuries. Neurosurgery. 2013;72(suppl_3):205–26.

Sonntag V, Hadley M. Management of nonodontoid upper cervical spine injuries. In: Cooper P, editor. Management of posttraumatic spinal instability: neurosurgical topics. Rolling Meadows: AANS Publications; 1990. p. 99–109.

Sonntag V, Hadley M. Management of upper cervical spinal instability. In: Wilkins R, editor. Neurosurgery update. New York: McGraw-Hill; 1991. p. 222–3.

Vollmer DG, Eichler ME, Jenkins AL III. Chapter 312: Assessment of the cervical spine after trauma. In: Youmans neurological surgery. Philadelphia: Elsevier; 2011. p. 3166–79.

Loss of Consciousness Following Head Trauma

James McDermott, Isaac Yang, and Richard G. Everson

Contents

C. de Virgilio, A. Grigorian (eds.), *Surgery*, https://doi.org/10.1007/978-3-032-09799-6_29

Case Study

A 40-year-old male motorcyclist is brought to the emergency department by paramedics after rear-ending a car at highway speeds. He was wearing a helmet but was thrown from his motorcycle. He was initially awake in the field but then quickly became unconscious. His airway is patent, and his respirations are shallow and irregular. His blood pressure is 190/90 mmHg, heart rate is 60/min, and respiratory rate is 20/min and irregular. In response to a sternal rub, the patient moans and withdraws his right upper and lower extremities, but he does not move the left upper or lower extremities, and he does not open his eyes. His Glasgow Coma Scale (GCS) is 7. His right pupil is 6 mm and nonreactive, while his left is 3 mm and reactive to light. There is no obvious head injury or laceration. There is no discharge from the nose or ears; however, there is a right hemotympanum. The oropharynx is clear. The remainder of the physical examination is normal.

Diagnosis

What Is the Differential Diagnosis for a Severe (GCS ≤8) Traumatic Brain Injury? (Table 29.1)

Table 29.1 Differential diagnosis for severe TBI

Diagnosis	Pathophysiology	Comments
Epidural hematoma (EDH)	Laceration of the middle meningeal artery by temporal bone fracture; blood accumulates between the dura and skull	Classic presentation: Brief loss of consciousness, followed by a lucid interval, then a rapid decline in level of consciousness; better prognosis than subdural hematoma
Subdural hematoma (SDH)	Tearing of bridging veins resulting in the accumulation of blood between the dura mater and the arachnoid membrane	More likely to have associated brain parenchymal injury than epidural hematoma; acute and chronic forms; worse prognosis than epidural hematoma
Intraparenchymal hematoma	Hemorrhage occurs in the area of the contused brain parenchyma	More likely to occur in association with hypertensive hemorrhage or arteriovenous malformation than with trauma; bleeding may be delayed
Diffuse axonal injury (DAI)	Rotational acceleration and deceleration result in shearing of axons between the gray and white matter	DAI is typically the underlying injury in shaken baby syndrome
Subarachnoid hemorrhage (SAH)	Accumulation of blood in CSF-filled subarachnoid spaces; trauma is the most common cause, but it also can occur spontaneously when caused by aneurysm rupture or AVM	Patient complains of "worst headache of my life," sudden onset, thunderclap headache when associated with spontaneous forms (aneurysm and AVM)

CSF cerebrospinal fluid, *AVM* arteriovenous malformation

What Is the Most Likely Diagnosis?

This patient has sustained a severe traumatic brain injury (TBI) as evidenced by a GCS of 7 (eyes-1, verbal-2, motor-4). He likely has a right-sided EDH, which is supported by evidence of a right temporal bone fracture (hemotympanum). He also displays the classic sequence for EDH: loss of consciousness, a brief lucid interval, and then progression to coma. The patient has objective signs of intracranial hypertension (Cushing's triad: hypertension, bradycardia, and irregular respiration) and uncal herniation, with a dilated nonresponsive right pupil and left-sided hemiplegia.

History and Physical

What Is the Definition of a TBI?

TBI results in a disruption of brain function. To meet the definition of TBI, at least one of the following criteria must be met: a period of loss of consciousness, loss of memory for events immediately before or after the accident, alteration in mental state at the time of the accident, or evidence of intracranial hemorrhage due to trauma, with or without a focal neurologic deficit. While not all patients with TBI exhibit intracranial hemorrhage, every patient with traumatic intracranial hemorrhage meets the definition of TBI.

How Do You Calculate the GCS?

The GCS (Table 29.2) is composed of three components: eye opening, verbal response, and motor response.

Table 29.2 Glasgow Coma Scale (GCS)

Eye opening	Best verbal response	Best motor response	Points
		Follows commands	6
	Oriented	Localizes pain	5
Spontaneous	Confused	Withdraws from pain	4
To voice	Inappropriate words	Decorticate posturing	3
To pain	Incomprehensible	Decerebrate posturing	2
None	None	None	1

By definition, a neurologically intact person has a GCS score of 15. A GCS score of 3–8 indicates severe TBI, 9–12 indicates moderate injury, and 13–15 indicates mild injury. There is a 30% probability of mortality associated with scores of 7 or 8.

Watch Out

A patient with a GCS of 8 or less is considered to be in a coma and mandates immediate establishment of an airway. Remember, "if GCS is 8 or less, intubate". It is essential to document a neurologic exam prior to paralysis and intubation, as this baseline information will be unobtainable once the patient is sedated/paralyzed.

Watch Out

The GCS score should be frequently reassessed to determine if the patient's TBI is worsening.

What Non-head Trauma Factors Affect GCS?

The GCS can be temporarily lowered by alcohol and drug intoxication, seizures, sedatives, severe hypoxia, shock, and severe hypothermia.

What Are Raccoon Eyes? What Is Battle's Sign?

Raccoon eyes are bilateral periorbital ecchymosis. Battle's sign is retroauricular ecchymosis. These signs should raise the suspicion of a *basilar* skull fracture.

How Does the Physical Exam Help to Localize the Site of Intracranial Bleeding?

Hemiparesis, or weakness on one side of the body, typically occurs on the side opposite the brain lesion due to decussation of motor pathways in the brainstem. Abnormal pupillary findings, such as a "blown pupil," are ipsilateral to the lesion because they result from compression of the oculomotor nerve (cranial nerve III) by brain structures such as the uncus of the temporal lobe. The above patient has a left hemiparesis and a blown pupil on the right, localizing the lesion to the right.

What Is the Implication of Abnormal Arm Flexion/Leg Extension with Pain Stimulation? Arm/Leg Extension?

Abnormal flexion in the upper extremity and extension in the lower extremity in response to painful stimuli is called *decorticate posturing*. Abnormal extension in upper and lower extremities in response to painful stimuli is called *decerebrate posturing*. These are primitive reflexes mediated by the brain stem when higher brain function is absent. While both are grave signs, decorticate posturing carries a better prognosis than decerebrate posturing.

How Does the Presentation of Chronic SDH Differ from Acute SDH?

Acute SDH typically presents within 72 h of head injury. Chronic SDH can have a delayed onset, even months later. Chronic SDH typically affects the elderly, as they have brain atrophy, allowing more room for a slow bleed to accumulate without elevating the intracranial pressure (ICP). The presentation is often insidious: gait abnormalities, decreased levels of consciousness, aphasia, cognitive dysfunction, memory loss, and/or personality changes.

What Is the Implication of Clear Fluid Leaking from the Ear?

This is highly suggestive of a basilar skull fracture with leaking cerebrospinal fluid (CSF).

How Would a Cerebellar Hemorrhage Present?

Cerebellar hemorrhage typically results from longstanding hypertension but can also be associated with antithrombotic therapy, cerebral amyloid angiopathy, and, rarely, trauma. It presents vertigo, dysarthria, nystagmus, and ipsilateral truncal ataxia (vermis involvement) or limb ataxia (hemisphere involvement), along with general intracerebral hemorrhage symptoms such as headache, nausea, vomiting, and meningismus. Unlike other forms of intracerebral hemorrhage, a cerebellar hemorrhage does not cause hemiparesis or sensory loss. Surgical decompression is indicated for a hematoma larger than 3 cm, neurologic deterioration, brainstem compression, or obstructive hydrocephalus.

Pathophysiology

What Is a Concussion?

This term refers to a mild TBI that presents without identifiable abnormalities on imaging. A concussion temporarily alters brain function by causing problems with memory, balance, coordination, and/or concentration. It may be associated with symptoms such as headaches, dizziness, confusion, personality changes, and irritability. Loss of consciousness (LOC) is not required to establish the diagnosis of a concussion.

What Is Uncal Herniation?

Uncal herniation occurs when a space-occupying lesion above the tentorium displaces the uncus of the temporal lobe medially and inferiorly over the tentorial incisure, compressing the ipsilateral oculomotor nerve (cranial nerve III) and the ipsilateral cerebral peduncle, which contains the corticospinal tract. This results in an ipsilateral blown pupil and contralateral paralysis.

What Is Subfalcine Herniation?

Subfalcine herniation (also called cingulate herniation) is the most common form of intracranial herniation and occurs when the cingulate gyrus (part of the medial cerebral cortex) herniates under the falx cerebri. This typically results from a unilateral frontal, parietal, or temporal lobe lesion, such as a bleed or mass. Unlike uncal herniation, subfalcine herniation does not involve the brainstem or cranial nerves and, therefore, does not cause symptoms like a blown pupil, respiratory center compression, or coma. The hallmark clinical feature is contralateral leg weakness, caused by compression of the ipsilateral anterior cerebral artery. Elevated intracranial pressure may also result in papilledema.

What Is the Pathophysiology of an Epidural Hematoma?

An epidural hematoma is the accumulation of blood between the dura mater and skull. The most common cause is a temporal bone fracture from a head injury that results in bleeding from a laceration of the middle meningeal artery. EDHs have a biconvex appearance on

CT that *does not cross* suture lines. Because the hematoma is from an arterial source, it may expand rapidly, leading to mass effect, which requires urgent surgical evacuation.

What Is the Implication of a "Lucid" Interval Seen in Patients with an EDH?

Initial loss of consciousness results from disruption of the reticular activating system located in the brainstem, while the subsequent loss of consciousness results from the expanding hematoma and mass effect. The interval between the first and second LOC is called the lucid interval, which may last minutes to hours.

What Is the Pathophysiology of an Acute Subdural Hematoma?

Acute subdural hematoma is an accumulation of blood between the dura and arachnoid membrane. It results from tearing of bridging veins, which run from the cortex to the dural venous sinuses. SDHs have a crescent-shaped appearance on CT that can cross suture lines. The elderly, patients with alcohol use disorder, and patients on anticoagulation therapy are particularly susceptible. The force required to tear these veins is typically greater than for an epidural. As such, SDH is more often associated with parenchymal injury and therefore carries a worse prognosis (despite it being a venous bleed).

Watch Out

The relatively atrophic brain parenchyma in the elderly increases tension on bridging veins, making them more susceptible to injury after head trauma.

What Is Cerebral Perfusion Pressure (CPP)?

CPP is the difference between mean arterial pressure (MAP) and intracranial pressure (ICP). Three components contribute to the ICP: brain tissue, cerebrospinal fluid (CSF), and cerebral blood. According to the Monro-Kellie doctrine, in order to maintain constant ICP, an increase in one must result in a decrease in the volume of the other two components. As such, bleeding and edema may result in increased ICP, leading to complications such as reduced cerebral blood flow and brain ischemia.

What Is the Most Powerful Intracranial Vasodilator?

The most powerful intracranial vasodilator is associated with an elevated serum CO_2 level.

Watch Out

A closed head injury does not cause hypovolemic shock. If a patient with TBI is hypotensive, search for sources of hypovolemic shock in the abdomen, chest, pelvis or extremities. Hypotension in the presence of TBI significantly increases mortality, as does hypoxia. A goal SBP >90 mmHg and PaO_2 >60 mmHg should be maintained.

What Is the Pathophysiology of Cushing's Triad?

Cushing's triad (hypertension, bradycardia, and irregular respirations) or Cushing's reflex is the physiologic response to increased ICP. In the presence of elevated ICP, systemic blood pressure increases in order to maintain CPP. The increased pressure results in negative feedback at the carotid sinus, leading to bradycardia. The respiratory center is located in the medulla and will become impaired as a result of elevated ICP.

What Is a Coup vs. Contrecoup Injury?

Coup refers to injury to brain tissue directly below the skull at the point of impact. However, the force of impact may thrust the brain tissue against the skull on the opposite side and cause injury. This is referred to as a contrecoup injury. Thus, contusion may occur on opposite sides of the brain.

What Is Paroxysmal Sympathetic Hyperactivity?

TBI patients may experience paroxysmal sympathetic hyperactivity (PSH), a clinical diagnosis characterized by excessive sympathetic activity, resulting in episodes of hypertension, tachycardia, diaphoresis, and hyperthermia. Typically, these episodes occur after stimuli such as postural changes, pain, movement, or suctioning. Treatment is with supportive care, minimizing stimuli, and use of medications to prevent and/or abort PSH episodes, including morphine, alpha-2 agonists, beta-blockers, and gabapentin.

Initial Management

What Initial Management Is Recommended for the Above Patient?

Initial management of this patient should follow the ABCDE model of primary assessment. A GCS of ≤8 (as in the present patient) is an indication for intubation to protect the airway and assure optimal oxygenation and ventilation. Moreover, intubation and paralysis can help facilitate ICP management. Next, he should receive a non-contrast head CT with anticipation that expedient evacuation of a likely epidural hematoma will follow.

What Are the Indications for Head CT with TBI?

All patients with moderate (GCS 9–12) and severe (3–8) TBI should get a non-contrast CT scan. Patients with mild brain injury who have certain risk factors (anticoagulation, alcohol abuse, or being elderly) should also undergo a CT scan.

> **Watch Out**
> Ketamine can increase ICP and is relatively contraindicated in the setting of TBI. Etomidate would be a better option during rapid sequence intubation.

Describe the Findings on CT Head for Various Intracranial TBIs (Table 29.3)

Table 29.3 CT findings for TBI

Diagnosis	Findings
Acute epidural hematoma	Hyperdense lens-shaped (Fig. 29.1) density adjacent to the skull *does not cross* suture lines and is usually associated with a skull fracture
Acute subdural hematoma	Hyperdense crescent-shaped (Fig. 29.2) density adjacent to brain parenchyma but not within sulci, crosses suture lines but not the falx
Chronic subdural hematoma	*Isodense or hypodense* crescent-shaped density adjacent to brain parenchyma but not within sulci, crosses suture lines but not the falx, and often presents with mass effect out of proportion to clinical findings
Traumatic subarachnoid hemorrhage	Hyperdense material adjacent to brain parenchyma, tracing along gyri and sulci
Intraparenchymal contusion	Hyperdense irregular lesions within the brain parenchyma
Diffuse axonal injury	Multifocal punctate hemorrhages are typically located at the gray-white matter junction; MRI is the modality of choice for assessing diffuse axonal injury (demonstrating blurring of the gray-white junction), as CT may appear normal

> **Watch Out**
> Patients with severe TBI are at risk of developing disseminated intravascular coagulation because of the exposed underlying tissue factor of the injured brain parenchyma; be sure to follow coagulation labs and platelet count.

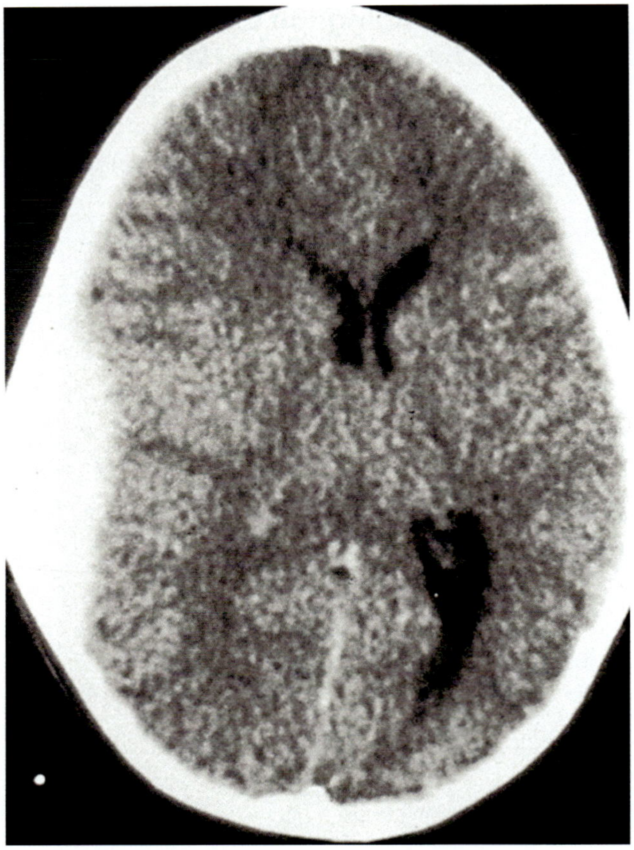

Fig. 29.1 Non-contrast head CT demonstrating an acute epidural hematoma. (From Hanley DF, et al. Coma and intensive care neurology. In: Rosenberg RN, editor. *Atlas of clinical neurology*. London: Current Medicine Group; 2003. Reprinted with permission from Springer Nature)

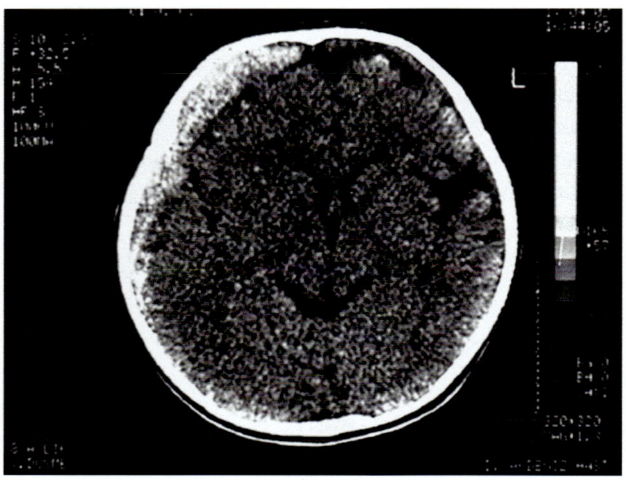

Fig. 29.2 Non-contrast head CT demonstrating an acute subdural hematoma. (From Erdogan B, et al. Hemispheric cerebrovascular venous thrombosis due to closed head injury. *Childs Nerv Syst*. 2004;20:239. ► https://doi.org/10.1007/s00381-003-0845-7. Reprinted with permission from Springer Nature)

What Medical Treatment Options Are There for Intracranial Hypertension?

The head of the bed should be elevated to 30–45° to facilitate venous outflow. The cervical collar should be removed as soon as it is safe to do so. Hyperthermia should be treated if present. Osmotic therapy is another cornerstone of treatment. Mannitol can be used for its osmotic diuretic effect, though it may cause hypotension and is generally avoided in acutely undifferentiated trauma patients. Hypertonic saline (3% or higher) is a better alternative that effectively reduces ICP without the same risk of hypotension. Neuromuscular blockade may be employed to prevent ICP spikes caused by agitation or coughing, and some clinicians advocate for therapeutic hypothermia, although this approach remains controversial. If ICP cannot be controlled with these measures, more aggressive interventions such as a barbiturate coma or decompressive craniectomy may be required.

What Is the Role of Hyperventilation in TBI?

Mild hyperventilation serves as a temporizing measure in patients with radiographic (CT) or clinical signs of elevated ICP prior to the initiation of more definitive interventions. Hyperventilation is used to achieve a $PaCO_2$ of 30–35 mmHg, which induces cerebral vasoconstriction and temporarily reduces ICP by lowering blood CO_2 levels. However, $PaCO_2$ should not be reduced below 30 mmHg to avoid decreasing cerebral blood flow. Importantly, hyperventilation is only a short-term strategy and should be discontinued once more definitive ICP control methods are in place.

Watch Out

Avoid Lactated Ringers (LR) in TBI. LR is slightly hypotonic (sodium content of only 130 meq/L) so it can worsen cerebral edema. Normal Saline is the ideal maintenance fluid for TBI patients.

How Does Mannitol Work?

Mannitol is an osmotic diuretic. Mannitol increases the tonicity of the extracellular space, which causes a shift of water from the intracellular space (brain parenchyma) to the extracellular space, reducing ICP.

Initially, it expands the plasma volume and reduces blood viscosity, which increases cerebral blood flow (and O_2 delivery).

> **Watch Out**
> Mannitol should be avoided in patients with hypotension or hypovolemia due to its volume-depleting effects.

Is There a Role for Corticosteroids in the Treatment of TBI? What Is the Difference Between Vasogenic and Cytotoxic Edema?

There is no role for corticosteroids in the setting of TBI. Corticosteroids such as dexamethasone are routinely used in the treatment of cerebral edema caused by brain tumors and other inflammatory CNS processes. The mechanisms of edema in tumors and in trauma are fundamentally different. Tumors produce edema by causing inflammation and blood-brain barrier breakdown (vasogenic edema) and will respond to corticosteroids. Trauma, in contrast, causes cerebral edema (cytotoxic edema) as a result of impaired cellular metabolism, causing failure of the sodium and potassium pump at the cell membrane, leading to accumulation of intracellular sodium. Cytotoxic edema is not responsive to corticosteroids.

What Are the Criteria for Brain Death? What Conditions Must Be Ruled Out?

Brain death refers to the irreversible cessation of the entire brain function, including the brain stem. To perform the exam, the patient must have a GCS of 3. The patient must be euthermic (>36 °C), the PaO_2 must be greater than 90 mmHg, the SBP must be greater than 100 mmHg, and the patient cannot be sedated or paralyzed (a serum or urine drug screen may be needed). Declaration of brain death requires the absence of brainstem reflexes (corneal, gag, oculocephalic, and oculovestibular), no response to deep central pain, and the agreement of two physicians. If the above criteria are met, an apnea test is performed. The patient is preoxygenated for 10 min with 100% O_2 with confirmation of a PaO_2 of at least 200 mm Hg. They are then disconnected from the ventilator and observed for respiratory effort. If after 10 min, there is no evidence of spontaneous respirations with a $PaCO_2$ >60 mmHg, and the other criteria are met, the patient is declared brain dead. Although not typically necessary, an adjunctive test is a cerebral blood flow study. It is used in cases where the apnea test would be contraindicated (i.e., cervical spinal cord injury).

Area You Can Get in Trouble

Guidelines for Head CT in Children

Children have a higher sensitivity to ionizing radiation than adults, increasing their long-term risk of malignancy. As a result, stricter criteria are applied when deciding whether to perform a head CT in pediatric patients. The Pediatric Emergency Care Applied Research Network (PECARN) scoring tool is widely used to identify children at risk for clinically significant TBI who may require head CT imaging. PECARN provides specific, evidence-based criteria for stratifying patients based on age (younger or older than 2 years) and clinical presentation. For children younger than 2 years, PECARN recommends head CT imaging if they exhibit signs such as a GCS of ≤ 14 or less, a palpable skull fracture, or altered mental status. For children 2 years and older, indications include GCS of ≤14, signs of basilar skull fracture, or altered mental status. Additional factors evaluated using PECARN include LOC lasting more than 5 s, a severe mechanism of injury, occipital, parietal, or temporal scalp hematomas (in children under 2), a history of vomiting, severe headache, worsening symptoms, or parental concern about the child not acting normally.

Patient with No Obvious Trauma Presenting with "Worst Headache of My Life"

Subarachnoid hemorrhage (SAH) should be suspected in a patient with a sudden-onset severe headache with lethargy and nuchal rigidity. SAH may be traumatic or a result of a ruptured saccular aneurysm. Risk factors for aneurysmal SAH include cigarette smoking, hypertension, and genetic factors including autosomal dominant polycystic kidney disease and Ehlers-Danlos syndrome. A non-contrast CT head should be obtained, which will often show blood in the basal cisterns. If CT is negative, but clinical suspicion is high, a lumbar puncture should be performed. Lumbar puncture will typically reveal an elevated opening pressure, red blood cells, and xanthochromia (a yellow hue resulting from the breakdown of red blood cells into bilirubin).

Persistent Headaches and Papilledema in a Chronic SDH Patient

Idiopathic intracranial hypertension (IIH) (also called pseudotumor cerebri) most commonly affects females of childbearing age with obesity. It typically presents as a daily, throbbing headache and may be associated with papilledema, transient visual obscuration, and tinnitus. Although the cause of IIH is not known, symptoms occur from excessive CSF in the brain, either via increased production or decreased removal of CSF. An urgent MRI or CT should be performed to rule out other causes of elevated ICP, such as an intracranial mass or vascular lesion. A subsequent lumbar puncture will only be remarkable for an elevated opening pressure. The principal management of IIH is weight loss. If there is a concern for vision loss, patients may require surgery to shunt CSF.

Summary of Essentials

History and Physical

- TBI may present with confusion, loss of consciousness, decreased level of consciousness, and amnesia
- GCS, cranial nerve exam, and sensory and motor exam
  - GCS of 8 or less = severe TBI
- Signs of basilar skull fracture
  - Raccoon eyes (periorbital ecchymoses) and Battle's sign (postauricular ecchymoses)
- Intracranial hypertension.
  - Hypertension, bradycardia, and respiratory irregularity (Cushing's triad)
  - Signs of uncal herniation: blown pupil and contralateral hemiparesis

Pathophysiology

- Primary injury: occurs at the time of trauma from deformative and concussive forces and includes laceration, hemorrhage, and fracture
- Secondary injury: brain's response to injury and includes cellular ischemic injury, edema, inflammation, and disruption of blood flow
- Types of brain injury:
  - Epidural hematoma: laceration of the middle meningeal artery (most common source)
  - Subdural hematoma: tearing of the bridging veins
  - Diffuse axonal injury: stretching of axons between gray and white matter
  - Concussion: disruption of inflow and outflow tracts from the reticular activating system
  - Contusion: hemorrhage within the brain parenchyma
  - Subarachnoid hemorrhage: accumulation of blood in subarachnoid space

Initial Management

- Start with ABCs
- Intubate if severe TBI (GCS ≤8)
  - Protects the patient's airway
  - Facilitates ICP management
- STAT non-contrast head CT
- Coagulopathy should be sought and corrected
- ICP monitoring for select patients with moderate to severe TBI
- An ICP >20 mmHg should be treated aggressively
  - Elevate the head of a bed
  - Intubate and paralyze
  - Mannitol
  - Hypertonic saline
  - Mild hyperventilation (avoid prolonged hyperventilation)
  - Control pyrexia/therapeutic hypothermia
  - Barbiturate coma
- Craniotomy with hematoma evacuation.
  - Epidural hematomas >30 ml in volume or causing >5 mm of midline shift
  - Acute subdural hematomas >10 mm in thickness or causing >5 mm of shift
  - Decompressive craniectomy
  - Persistent severe intracranial hypertension despite medical management
- Criteria for brain death.
  - GCS of 3, while not hypoxic, normotensive, and euthermic, not on sedatives or paralytics
  - No cranial nerve reflexes
  - No respiratory effort observed during an apnea test

Suggested Reading

Bernat JL, Culver CM, Gert B. On the definition and criterion of death. Ann Intern Med. 1981;94(3):389–94.

Bullock MR, Chesnut R, Ghajar J, Gordon D, Hartl R, Newell DW, et al. Guidelines for the surgical management of traumatic brain injury. Neurosurgery. 2006;58(Supplement):S2–1–3. https://doi.org/https://doi.org/10.1227/01.NEU.0000210361.83548.D0.

Carney N, Totten AM, O'Reilly C, Ullman JS, Hawryluk GW, Bell MJ, et al. Guidelines for the management of severe traumatic brain injury, Fourth Edition. Neurosurgery. 2017;80(1):6–15.
Greenberg MS. Head Trauma. In: Greenberg MS, editor. Handbook of neurosurgery. 8th ed. New York: Theime Medical Publishers; 2016. p. 824–929.
Hawryluk GWJ, Lulla A, Bell R, et al. Guidelines for Prehospital Management of Traumatic Brain Injury 3rd Edition: Executive Summary. Neurosurgery. 2023;93(6):e159–e169. doi:https://doi.org/10.1227/neu.0000000000002672
Mollan SP, Davies B, Silver NC, et al. Idiopathic intracranial hypertension: consensus guidelines on management. *J Neurol Neurosurg Psychiatry*. 2018;89(10):1088–1100. doi:https://doi.org/10.1136/jnnp-2017-317440

Neurosurgery

Question Set: Neurosurgery

Questions

1. A 34-year-old woman with a history of breast cancer presents to the emergency department with progressive headache, nausea, and visual blurring over the last 2 days. On examination, she is alert but has bilateral papilledema. MRI of the brain demonstrates a 2.5-cm enhancing mass in the right cerebellar hemisphere with surrounding vasogenic edema and mild compression of the fourth ventricle. What is the most appropriate next step in management?
   (A) Intravenous (IV) mannitol
   (B) Surgical resection of the mass
   (C) Whole brain radiation therapy
   (D) IV dexamethasone
   (E) Lumbar puncture

2. A 29-year-old male with no past medical history presents to the emergency department with the worst headache of his life. He was watching television when the headache started and is unlike any headache he has experienced before. It is located near the back of his head. He reports that his father had a kidney transplant at a young age. He is managed appropriately for his acute condition. His recovery is complicated by progressive lethargy, agitation, and eventual coma. Which of the following would most likely explain this complication?
   (A) Nephrogenic diabetes insipidus
   (B) Central (neurogenic) diabetes insipidus
   (C) Poor oral intake
   (D) Cerebral salt-wasting syndrome
   (E) Thyroid dysfunction

3. A 31-year-old male with human immunodeficiency virus (HIV) presents with headaches and night sweats. He is poorly compliant with his medications. His headaches are severe in the morning but subside throughout the day. He has no other complaints. His last CD-4 count was 95/mm^3. His temperature is 37.7 °C, blood pressure is 110/76 mmHg, and pulse is 88/min. His physical exam is normal. CT scan of the head shows a ring-enhancing lesion near the right primary motor cortex. What is the best next step in management?
   (A) Radiation
   (B) Chemotherapy and radiation
   (C) Pyrimethamine and sulfadiazine
   (D) Stereotactic brain biopsy
   (E) Restart highly active antiretroviral therapy (HAART)

4. A 61-year-old man with a past medical history of opioid dependence and diabetes presents with focal back pain and right leg weakness. He does not recall any recent trauma. He reports having "back surgery" nearly 20 years ago but does not remember why. He also reports helping his friend move furniture last week. His temperature is 38.8 °C, blood pressure is 104/76 mmHg, and pulse is 102/min. Physical examination is significant for focal pain on palpation of his lower lumbar spine. Laboratory examination is significant for elevated erythrocyte sedimentation rate (ESR). Imaging is obtained. Which of the following is the most likely best management approach for this condition?
   (A) Nonsteroidal anti-inflammatory drug (NSAID)
   (B) High-dose IV corticosteroids
   (C) Long-term antibiotics alone
   (D) Physical therapy and education
   (E) Long-term antibiotics with surgical drainage

5. Which of the following findings would be expected in a patient presenting with a transtentorial (uncal) herniation?
   (A) Loss of gag reflex
   (B) Diplopia on attempted lateral gaze
   (C) Medial rectus palsy on attempted lateral gaze
   (D) Ptosis and a "down-and-out" eye
   (E) Paralysis of the sternocleidomastoid muscle

6. A 40-year-old female presents to her family physician with progressive weakness in both her arms for the past year. She is healthy and does not take any medications but reports being hospitalized 5 years ago for 2 days following a motor vehicle accident in which she sustained severe and sudden whiplash injury. On physical examination, she has atrophy of the intrinsic muscles of both hands and an inability to differentiate between hot and cold in bilateral upper extremities. All other sensations are intact. What is the most likely underlying etiology?
   (A) Spinal spondylosis
   (B) Brachial plexus injury
   (C) Syringomyelia
   (D) Autoimmune condition
   (E) Herniated disk

7. In a patient with an isolated head injury and concerns for increased intracranial pressure (ICP), which of the following would have the most potential to benefit the patient?
   (A) Hypertonic (3%) saline solution
   (B) Ventilation with permissive hypercapnia
   (C) Trendelenburg position of bed
   (D) Intermittent D-5 (dextrose) boluses
   (E) Nitroprusside drip

8. A 20-year-old female arrives to the emergency department after slipping and hitting her head on ice and briefly losing consciousness. In the emergency room, she vomits twice. She denies amnesia. Her temperature is 37.6 °C, blood pressure is 110/80 mmHg, and pulse is 80/min. Her Glasgow Coma Scale (GCS) score is 15. Her physical exam is normal with no papilledema. What is the most appropriate next step in management?
   (A) Admit for observation and order CT scan of the head only if she develops a neurologic deficit
   (B) Admit for observation and start corticosteroids
   (C) Order CT scan of the head without contrast
   (D) Discharge home
   (E) Order CT scan of the head with contrast

9. A 48-year-old woman arrives for her 6-month follow-up after undergoing breast-conserving therapy to treat stage-IIA breast cancer. Her only postoperative complication has been red patches of skin on her chest following radiation therapy. She does not complain of any pain or pruritus but does report having intense headaches in the mornings when she wakes up. Her temperature is 37.7 °C, blood pressure is 110/80 mmHg, and pulse is 90/min. Her physical examination is normal. She is worried that the red patches on her chest are suggestive of something more serious. Which of the following studies would be the most appropriate next step in management?
   (A) Excisional skin biopsy
   (B) Cerebral angiogram
   (C) Skin punch biopsy
   (D) Carotid duplex
   (E) CT scan of the head

10. A 29-year-old woman arrives to the emergency department following a Jet Ski accident. She has multiple bruises on her head, torso, and legs. She did not lose consciousness. Her temperature is 37.8 °C, blood pressure is 108/78 mmHg, and pulse is 102/min. She only opens her eyes when you speak loudly to her. She is confused and screams in pain and withdraws when you palpate her left lower leg. Her imaging is pending. What is her Glasgow Coma Scale (GCS) score?
   (A) 6
   (B) 8
   (C) 10
   (D) 11
   (E) 14

11. A 22-year-old patient arrives to the emergency department after falling off his bicycle and hitting his head. He is clearly intoxicated and his speech is slurred. He denies any neck pain but is not cooperative during the exam. He is placed in a cervical spine collar. What is the optimal method for clearance of the cervical spine in this patient?
   (A) CT scan of the cervical spine alone, regardless of exam findings
   (B) MRI of the cervical spine as the initial imaging modality
   (C) Physical exam alone is sufficient to clear the cervical spine
   (D) CT scan of the cervical spine, with MRI considered if concern persists
   (E) Lateral cervical spine X-ray followed by flexion-extension views

12. A 32-year-old man presents with progressive frontal headaches. His symptoms started 2 months ago and often wake him up from his sleep. His vital signs are stable, and neurologic examination reveals no focal deficits. MRI brain imaging reveals a mass, and subsequent biopsy is consistent with a type IV astrocytoma. Which of the following is true regarding this patient's illness?
   (A) It is considered the most common primary malignant brain tumor.
   (B) Prognosis is good since the tumor is slow growing.
   (C) The biopsy should demonstrate psammoma bodies.
   (D) This tumor does not cross the corpus callosum.
   (E) Interferon beta and glatiramer acetate are used in the management of this tumor.

13. Which of the following is true regarding diffuse axonal injury (DAI)?
   (A) It is often associated with a lucid interval.
   (B) Blurring of gray–white junctions can be found on imaging.
   (C) It occurs following a tensile force.
   (D) Persistent vegetative state is rare.
   (E) Patients often have hyperdense fluid in the ventricles, sulci, and cisterns.

14. A 55-year-old female restrained driver arrives to the emergency department following a motor vehicle accident. She sustained hyperextension of the cervical spine and hit her chest on the steering wheel. Neurologic examination shows spastic paraplegia and loss of pain sensation in both upper extremities. She is able to move both her legs and can differentiate vibratory sensation and light touch in both feet. What is the most likely etiology for her acute condition?
   (A) Central cord syndrome
   (B) Anterior spinal artery syndrome
   (C) Brown-Séquard syndrome
   (D) Cauda equina syndrome
   (E) Subacute combined degeneration of the spinal cord

15. Which of the following is the most common brain cancer?
   (A) Lung metastasis
   (B) Glioblastoma multiforme
   (C) Colon metastasis
   (D) Breast metastasis
   (E) Astrocytoma

16. A 64-year-old man is brought to the emergency department by paramedics after being found confused on the street. He has bruises on his head and arms with a few that appear to be new. He has alcohol on his breath. He is awake in the emergency department but unable to follow commands or answer questions. CT scan of the head without contrast demonstrates a crescent-shaped lesion. Which of the following is most associated with this patient's condition?
   (A) Family member with polycystic kidney disease
   (B) Congenital malformation
   (C) Torn bridging veins
   (D) Injured middle meningeal artery
   (E) Temporal bone fracture

17. A 50-year-old woman arrives to the emergency department after she was witnessed having two generalized tonic–clonic seizures over 15 min without recovering consciousness between episodes. Her seizures are resolved by the time she gets to the hospital. She had a toe removed for a skin tumor 10 years ago but does not remember any details. Review of systems reveals a loss of nearly 15 lb over the last 2 months. She has no other complaints. CT scan of the head reveals a solitary mass in the gray–white junction of the left temporal lobe with some surrounding edema but no calcifications. After further imaging and workup are done, no other lesions are identified. Which of the following most likely represents the mass?
   (A) Type IV astrocytoma
   (B) Metastasis
   (C) Oligodendroglioma
   (D) Meningioma
   (E) Ependymoma

Answers

1. Answer D
   This patient presents with signs of increased intracranial pressure (ICP), including headache, nausea, and papilledema, in the setting of known malignancy and imaging showing a cerebellar metastasis with surrounding edema. The most appropriate immediate intervention is administration of intravenous corticosteroids, classically dexametha-

sone. Dexamethasone is used to reduce vasogenic edema surrounding brain tumors and can rapidly improve neurologic symptoms by decreasing mass effect and ICP. It is indicated in patients with brain metastases or spinal cord compression causing neurologic compromise. IV mannitol is used for emergent reduction in ICP in cases such as acute herniation or traumatic brain injury, but it is not first-line in patients with tumor-related edema and no acute deterioration (A). Surgical resection may eventually be indicated depending on tumor characteristics and symptom progression, but steroids are given first to stabilize the patient and limit inflammation (B). Whole brain radiation therapy is often part of definitive management for brain metastases, but not the immediate next step when a patient is symptomatic from mass effect (C). Lumbar puncture is contraindicated in patients with elevated ICP due to mass lesion, as it risks precipitating brain herniation (E). In patients with spinal cord compression from tumors (e.g., spinal meningioma), corticosteroids are similarly used acutely to reduce edema and preserve neurologic function prior to surgical or radiation-based treatment. Spinal meningiomas typically present as homogeneously enhancing extramedullary lesions on MRI and cause upper motor neuron signs due to cord compression.

2. Answer D
Patients with subarachnoid hemorrhage (SAH) can have multiple complications after their initial presentation including rebleeding, hyperglycemia, acute hypoxia, and electrolyte abnormalities. Patients are at risk for symptomatic hyponatremia secondary to *cerebral salt-wasting syndrome*. This is characterized by excessive renal sodium excretion and volume depletion, often triggered by brain injury such as SAH. It is thought to result from elevated levels of natriuretic peptides (e.g., atrial and brain natriuretic peptide), which promote sodium loss and diuresis, leading to hypovolemia and hyponatremia. This distinguishes CSWS from the syndrome of inappropriate antidiuretic hormone secretion (SIADH), in which patients are typically euvolemic or mildly hypervolemic. Patients with hyponatremia may present with seizures, lethargy, agitation, confusion, and nausea, and if untreated, patients can eventually fall into a coma. Nephrogenic diabetes insipidus is a renal dysfunction in which the collecting ducts are unresponsive to ADH, while central diabetes insipidus is associated with decreased levels of ADH released from the posterior pituitary (A–B). Both of these conditions are associated with hypernatremia. Thyroid dysfunction can rarely lead to loss of sodium (E). However, there is no evidence to believe the presented patient has any thyroid problems.

3. Answer C
HIV-positive patients that present with CD-4 counts between 50 and 100 per mm^3, and ring-enhancing lesions found on CT scan of the head should be suspected of having either *toxoplasmosis* or *central nervous system (CNS) lymphoma*. These are clinically indistinguishable and occur in similar frequencies. Patients should always be started first on an empiric therapeutic trial of pyrimethamine and sulfadiazine to treat a presumed toxoplasmosis infection. If this does not resolve the patient's symptoms and/or findings (e.g., ring-enhancing lesions on CT), the next best step is to perform a stereotactic brain biopsy to confirm CNS lymphoma (D). On imaging, toxoplasmosis typically presents as multiple ring-enhancing lesions in the basal ganglia or corticomedullary junction, whereas CNS lymphoma often presents as a solitary lesion that is subependymal or periventricular. Additionally, HIV-positive patients with CNS lymphoma almost always exhibit evidence of Epstein–Barr virus (EBV) in their cerebrospinal fluid (CSF). Although no consensus exists on treatment for HIV-related CNS lymphoma, few studies have looked at treatment with radiation therapy or chemotherapy and have reported only modest gains (A–B). Restarting HAART in a patient suspected of having toxoplasmosis or CNS lymphoma increases the risk of developing immune reconstitution inflammatory syndrome (IRIS) (E).

4. Answer E

This patient is most likely presenting with an *epidural abscess*. Patients with previous spinal surgeries (even if remote) or a history of IV drug abuse are at higher risk. The clinical triad of epidural abscesses includes focal back pain (or headache, if abscess is located intracranial), abnormal inflammatory parameters (fever, leukocytosis, elevated ESR), and neurologic deficits (e.g., right leg weakness). MRI is the imaging modality of choice to confirm the diagnosis. Patients should be started on long-term IV antibiotics and undergo surgical drainage of the abscess. NSAIDs, physical therapy, and education would be appropriate recommendations for patients with lumbar strain (A, C–D). These patients would not be expected to have fevers or focal neurologic deficits. Current guidelines do not recommend corticosteroids after acute spinal cord injury (B).

5. Answer D

The uncus is a part of the medial temporal lobe and can herniate through the tentorium and compress the midbrain and brainstem during significant brain swelling. This will present with features that can be explained by local compression of nearby structures by the herniated uncus (e.g., mydriasis or "blown pupil," ipsilateral ptosis, and "down-and-out" eye). These occur due to the compression of the parasympathetic fibers of the oculomotor nerve (cranial nerve III) by the uncus. Loss of gag reflex would be expected in patients with an injured glossopharyngeal nerve (cranial nerve IX) (A). This can occur in a patient with a posterior fossa tumor. Diplopia on attempted lateral gaze is expected in patients with injury to the abducens nerve (cranial nerve VI), as in those patients with cavernous sinus malignancy (B). Medial rectus palsy on attempted lateral gaze is commonly seen in patients with multiple sclerosis that have medial longitudinal fasciculus (MLF) syndrome (C). Paralysis of the sternocleidomastoid muscle would be expected in patients with a spinal accessory nerve (cranial nerve XI) injury.

6. Answer C

This patient's arm weakness and inability to differentiate between hot and cold in the bilateral upper extremities are most likely due to *syringomyelia*, which is the presence of a cystic structure in the central cervical spinal cord. This most commonly occurs from congenital conditions (e.g., Arnold Chiari malformations) but may also occur months or years after a cervical spinal injury, such as whiplash (e.g., sudden distortion of the neck associated with extension). Trauma-induced syringomyelia typically involves the cervical spinal cord and results from impaired CSF drainage in the central canal of the spinal cord which may lead to a fluid-filled cavity that compresses the surrounding spinal cord. Patients will present with weakness and decreased pain and temperature sensation in bilateral upper extremities with no other sensory deficits. Spinal spondylosis occurs as a result of degenerative joint disease (e.g., osteoarthritis) and presents with radiculopathy secondary to affected nerve roots. Trauma-induced brachial plexus injuries are more likely to occur immediately following the traumatic incident and will not present with an inability to differentiate between hot and cold in the upper extremities (B). An autoimmune condition, such as multiple sclerosis, will more than likely have two lesions and present in a relapsing-remitting course (D). A herniated disk is likely but will present with radiculopathy in the affected nerve roots (E). Decreased sensation to hot and cold would not be expected.

7. Answer A

Patients with increased ICP will benefit with therapy aimed at decreasing ICP. Hypertonic (3%) saline solution will decrease cerebral edema by acting as an osmotic force, drawing fluid out of the tissues and into the blood and thus decrease ICP. Fluids that contain hypotonic saline (such as dextrose 5% water) would have a deleterious effect (D). Mild hyperventilation to create *hypocapnia* is also beneficial as it induces mild vasoconstriction (CO_2 is the most potent cerebral vasodilator). Excessive hyperventilation can be deleterious as it will decrease overall perfusion. Ventilation with permissive hypercapnia is a technique used in acute respiratory distress syndrome (ARDS) that helps prevent barotrauma (B). However, hypercapnia (high CO_2) would lead to cerebral vasodilation and worsen ICP. Patients with head injury should be placed with the head 30° elevated. Trendelenburg position will increase ICP by using gravity to increase cerebral blood flow (C). Hyperglycemia (injured brain metabolizes glucose, leading to an increase in cerebral lactate with subsequent acidosis) and nitroprusside drip (vasodilation) have also been associated with increased ICP (E).

8. Answer C

Numerous guidelines exist for when to perform a non-contrast CT in the setting of head trauma. The Canadian guidelines state that a head CT is indicated following minor head trauma and more than one episode of emesis, GCS <15 at 2 h after injury, evidence of basilar skull fracture (Battle's sign, raccoon eyes), focal neurologic deficit, age >65, dangerous mechanism of injury (e.g., ejected out of car), and suspected open or depressed skull fracture. Although she has a normal GCS, since she has vomited twice, a CT scan is indicated (A). Discharging the patient would be inappropriate because she meets the criteria for getting a head CT without contrast (D–E). A patient with a minor, isolated head injury and a negative CT could be safely discharged with instructions given to the patient and/or family/caregiver to look for signs of increased intracranial pressure (e.g., lethargy, vomiting, intense headaches, deficits in short-term memory, seizures, or focal neurologic deficits). Patients with these signs should return to the hospital immediately. Administration of corticosteroids is not indicated in patients with head injury (B).

9. Answer E

Any postoperative breast cancer patient with a severe headache should be evaluated for metastasis to the brain with a CT scan of the head. Postoperative radiation therapy is offered in conjunction with breast-conserving therapy (e.g., lumpectomy) to appropriate patients. Complications of radiation therapy include pneumonitis, ulceration, sarcoma, contralateral breast cancer, and red patches of skin or "radiation burns." Skin biopsy is not needed to confirm this (A, C). These can be severe and very painful or, in this patient's case, can only be a cosmetic burden. Cerebral angiogram does not typically help in the evaluation for brain metastasis (B). Carotid disease does not typically present with headaches, so duplex scan would not be indicated (D).

10. Answer D

Once the ABCs have been addressed in a patient presenting with traumatic brain injury, one can assess a patient's level of consciousness by using the GCS as part of the primary neurologic survey. GCS is composed of three components: eye opening, verbal response, and motor response. The sum total of the three components is the GCS score, which ranges from 3 to 15. This patient has an eye score of 3 (open eyes to voice), verbal score of 4 (confused speech), and a motor score of 4 (withdraws to pain). Thus, her GCS is 11 and classified as a moderate head injury (A–C, E).

11. Answer D

In trauma patients with altered mental status or intoxication, clinical examination cannot be relied upon to clear the cervical spine. These patients require imaging. The preferred first-line modality is a high-resolution CT scan of the cervical spine due to its speed, accessibility, and high sensitivity for bony injury. If the CT is negative and the patient has no neurologic deficits, many institutions now permit cervical spine clearance without further imaging, even in the setting of impaired mentation. However, some centers may choose to obtain an MRI to evaluate for occult ligamentous injury

depending on institutional protocol or clinical concern. MRI is particularly useful if neurologic symptoms are present, or if the patient cannot participate in a reliable exam even after sobering. CT alone may be sufficient in many institutions, but it does not account for those that still require MRI in select cases (A). MRI alone is not the appropriate first-line imaging for trauma due to its lower sensitivity for bony injury and longer acquisition time (B). Physical examination alone is inappropriate in this patient due to intoxication and lack of cooperation, which precludes a reliable exam (C). Lateral cervical spine X-ray and flexion–extension views are outdated and insufficient in the acute trauma setting (E).
Thus, the most appropriate and widely accepted approach is to begin with a CT scan and consider an MRI only if clinical suspicion for instability persists despite a negative CT.

12. Answer A
Glioblastoma multiforme is a type IV astrocytoma and considered to be the most common primary malignant brain tumor in the United States. This tumor has a grave prognosis with life expectancy estimated to be less than 1 year from the time of diagnosis (B). On gross appearance, it can cross the corpus callosum (butterfly glioma) (D). On histologic appearance, it will stain with GFAP. Psammoma bodies are spindle cells concentrically arranged in a whorled pattern and are characteristic of a meningioma (C). Interferon beta and glatiramer acetate have been shown to decrease the frequency of future attacks in patients with multiple sclerosis (E).

13. Answer B
Patients with DAI following rapid deceleration trauma typically suffer instantaneous loss of consciousness followed by a persistent vegetative state if the DAI is severe (D). Prognosis is very poor, although some may regain some level of function. It occurs as a result of shearing forces (C). A CT scan of the head will show numerous minute punctate hemorrhages with blurring of gray–white junctions. A lucid interval is often associated with an epidural hematoma (A). Hyperdense fluid in the ventricles, sulci, and cisterns would be suggestive of a subarachnoid hemorrhage (E).

14. Answer A
This patient has central cord syndrome which classically occurs following hyperextension of the cervical spine but may also result from hyperflexion. The lateral corticospinal fasciculus is home to the motor tracts of the lower extremities and is often spared in central cord syndrome. The medial aspect hosts the motor tracts for the upper extremities and is disproportionately affected, often with profound hand weakness. Most patients regain functional recovery in a predictable fashion starting first with the lower extremities (if affected), then bladder/bowel function, and finally the upper extremities. Elderly patients with preexisting cervical spondylosis are most at risk. Anterior spinal artery syndrome results from a compressed anterior spinal artery (B). This presents with bilateral loss of motor, pain, and temperature below the lesion with partial sensory sparing (e.g., proprioception, vibration) since the posterior dorsal columns remain viable. Brown-Séquard syndrome presents with ipsilateral motor weakness with associated upper motor neuron signs (spasticity, hyperreflexia, clonus, and positive Babinski sign) and touch/proprioception loss below the level of the injury, also contralateral loss of pain and temperature sensation beginning one or two dermatome levels below the level of the injury (C). Cauda equina syndrome may occur in a traumatic setting following compression of the lumbar nerve roots by a spinal fracture (D). Patients will present with perineal sensory deficit (saddle anesthesia), bowel/bladder incontinence, and pain/weakness in the lower extremities. Subacute combined degeneration of the spinal cord is the term used to describe the neurologic deficits (e.g., peripheral sensory deficits, loss of deep tendon reflexes) seen in patients with vitamin B_{12} deficiency (E).

15. Answer A

Malignant brain tumors are more commonly metastatic than primary (B, E). An estimated 24–45% of all patients with cancer have metastatic lesions to the CNS. Nearly half of all brain metastasis are attributed to lung cancer. The second most common cancer to metastasize to the brain is breast (15%), followed by genitourinary (11%), melanoma (9%), and head and neck cancers (6%) (D). Prostate and colon cancers do not commonly metastasize to the brain (C).

16. Answer C

This patient's history and CT findings are most consistent with a subdural hematoma which is caused by torn bridging veins. Patients will experience progressive neurologic deficits which if left untreated can be fatal. CT scan of the head will demonstrate a crescent-shaped lesion that may extend across the entire hemisphere. This typically occurs in older or alcoholic patients with recent head trauma, often due to a fall. Elderly patients are at increased risk due to age-related cerebral atrophy which can exert tension on the bridging veins. A family member with polycystic kidney disease is often seen in patients with subarachnoid hemorrhage due to the disease's association with berry aneurysms in the circle of Willis that are prone to rupture (A). Cerebral arteriovenous malformations can spontaneously bleed and result in a sudden intense headache and/or loss of consciousness (B). A temporal bone fracture and subsequent injury to the middle meningeal artery can result in an epidural hematoma (D–E). This classically presents with a loss of consciousness in patients with head trauma, followed by a lucid interval and then a loss of consciousness again. The hematoma is lenticular (lens shaped) or convex in shape.

17. Answer B

A solitary brain mass in the gray–white junction with surrounding edema is most consistent with a metastatic tumor. Although the most common source would be lung cancer, the history of a toe amputation highly suggests a subungual melanoma. This may occur even in patients with a remote history of melanoma. Type IV astrocytoma (glioblastoma multiforme) is considered to be the most common *primary* malignant brain tumor in the United States (A). It can cross the corpus callosum, giving it a "butterfly" appearance. However, the most common *overall* brain tumor is from metastasis. Meningioma is the second most common primary tumor in adults. Meningioma is a benign tumor that presents as an extra-axial well-circumscribed dural-based mass that may have scattered calcifications (D). Primary tumors can also present with mass effect (seizures, headaches, focal neurologic deficits). Oligodendroglioma is a rare, slow-growing tumor often found in the frontal lobes (C). It arises from arachnoid cells and is characterized by psammoma bodies on histologic examination. Ependymoma primarily affects children and commonly occurs in the fourth ventricle leading to hydrocephalus (E). Patients have a poor prognosis.

Multiple Extremity Injuries After Motor Vehicle Collision

Areg Grigorian and Kevin W. Rolfe

Contents

C. de Virgilio, A. Grigorian (eds.), *Surgery*, https://doi.org/10.1007/978-3-032-09799-6_30

30

Case Study

A 35-year-old male is involved in a motor vehicle collision and is brought in by paramedics, complaining of severe pain in his right leg and arm. In the emergency department, the patient is awake and alert. He has an obvious deformity of his right mid-humerus. There are no open wounds on the arm. He has a noticeable wrist-drop on the right and is unable to dorsiflex the wrist or extend the metacarpophalangeal joints. The radial pulse on the right is 2+. There is a 2 cm laceration over his mid-shin, with visible bone exposed. Distal motor and sensory function in his right leg is intact, and pedal pulses are 2+. There is no tenderness or deformity in his left thigh or left lower leg. He also has tenderness to palpation of his right clavicle, and on auscultation, a faint bruit is heard underneath the right clavicle. X-ray imaging confirms a right clavicle fracture, a right mid-shaft humerus fracture (Fig. 30.1), a right femur fracture, and a right tibia and fibula fracture. X-rays of the left knee are negative.

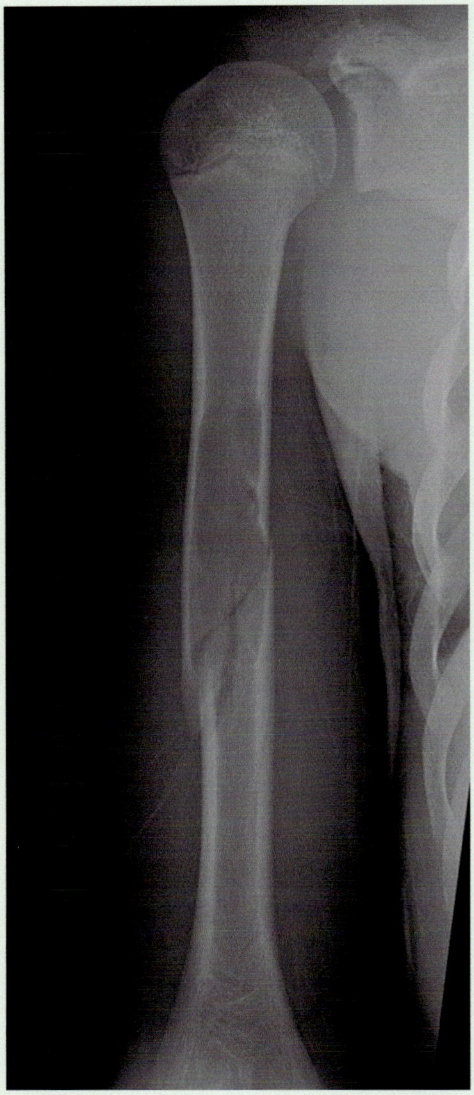

Fig. 30.1 Right mid-shaft humerus fracture. (From Jordanov MI. The "rising bubble" sign: a new aid in the diagnosis of unicameral bone cysts. *Skeletal Radiol*. 2009;38:597. ► https://doi.org/10.1007/s00256-009-0685-y. Reprinted with permission from Springer Nature)

Diagnosis

What Is the Most Likely Diagnosis?

Given the vignette and radiographic findings, the diagnosis is straightforward. This is a polytrauma patient with multiple extremity fractures, including a right clavicle fracture, a closed right humerus fracture with a nerve deficit, a closed right femur fracture, an open right tibia fracture, and possibly a left knee injury.

History and Physical

What Should Be Assessed During Extremity Evaluation of a Trauma Patient?

After the primary survey is completed and all life-threatening injuries are addressed, the extremities should be evaluated to assess the four functional components (nerves, blood vessels, bones, and soft tissues). Injury to three of these four elements constitutes a "mangled extremity."

What Is an Open Fracture?

Open fractures are those in which the fracture communicates with the outer environment due to disruption of the intervening soft tissue and skin. Because of the open communication, there exists a higher risk for osteomyelitis and infection of any hardware placed for fixing the fracture. Bone healing is also slowed in open fractures and more often results in nonhealing, known as a nonunion. Antibiotics should ideally be administered within one hour of presentation for open fractures.

What Is the Likely Etiology of the Neurologic Deficit in His Right Arm?

The most likely etiology of the patient's neurologic deficit is radial nerve injury. The radial nerve travels along the medial aspect of the humerus before coursing posteriorly into the spiral groove, where it lies in close contact with the bone. As a result, fractures of the middle or distal third of the humerus place the nerve at particular risk for injury due to either mechanical stretching from fracture displacement or entrapment between the fracture fragments. Because the branches to the triceps muscle originate proximal to the spiral groove, triceps function is usually preserved. However, patients typically present with wrist-drop due to impaired wrist extension, loss of metacarpophalangeal joint extension, and sensory deficits over the dorsal aspect of the hand.

> **Watch Out**
> Finger extension at the interphalangeal (IP) joints can still be accomplished by the intrinsic muscles controlled by the ulnar nerve (interossei and ulnar two lumbricals) and median nerve (radial two lumbricals).

What Is the Significance of Hearing a Bruit on Auscultation of the Right Clavicle?

This is concerning for an underlying vascular injury, particularly of the subclavian artery. Trauma to the clavicle can lead to pseudoaneurysm, arteriovenous fistula, and dissection of the subclavian artery. This needs to be further evaluated with a CT angiogram.

How Does Fat Embolism Syndrome Present?

Fat embolism syndrome occurs in up to 15% of polytrauma patients, particularly in association with fractures of marrow-containing bone (e.g., femur, pelvis). It typically presents between 24 and 72 h following the trauma. The classic triad consists of respiratory symptoms, neurological changes, and a reddish-brown petechial rash. Respiratory findings such as hypoxemia, dyspnea, and tachypnea are the earliest manifestations, followed by neurologic abnormalities such as confusion, drowsiness, or altered level of consciousness, and, in severe cases, seizure or paralysis. Lastly, the classic petechial rash develops, but in only 50–60% of cases. The petechial rash results from extravasation of erythrocytes secondary to the occlusion of dermal capillaries by fat emboli. The rash, in the proper clinical context, is pathognomonic for fat embolism syndrome.

What Is a Dangerous Sequela for a Tibia Fracture (or Forearm Fracture)?

Compartment syndrome. Don't forget the Ps: pain out of proportion to injury, pain with gentle passive stretch of the involved muscles, pressure (swollen and tense compartments), paresthesia, pallor, poikilothermia, paralysis, and pulselessness (rare, very late sign). This is a surgical emergency and requires emergent fasciotomy.

What Concomitant Fracture Is Important to Consider in All Femur Fractures?

A concomitant femoral neck fracture. A missed femoral neck fracture may lead to avascular necrosis (AVN) if not treated. AVN is largely irreversible and leads to end-stage dysfunction of the hip joint.

Watch Out

Femoral neck fracture is common in elderly, debilitated patients after a fall. Although this is best treated with urgent surgical intervention to prevent avascular necrosis, repair can be delayed for up to 3 days if the patient requires medical stabilization and more urgent issues need to be addressed.

How Do Distal Forearm Fractures Typically Present in Children, and What Is Their Management?

Distal forearm fractures in children, including greenstick fractures, are common following a fall onto an outstretched hand. Patients present with pain, swelling, and decreased range of motion at the wrist. Greenstick fractures occur due to the relatively strong and pliable periosteum, resulting in an incomplete fracture. Management typically involves immobilization with casting to prevent refracture. Prognosis is excellent, and long-term complications are rare.

Pathophysiology

What Are Seddon's Three Basic Categories of Nerve Injury? (◘ Table 30.1)

◘ **Table 30.1** Seddon's classification of nerve injury

Type	Features
Neuropraxia	Minimal injury (myelin), but not axon or nerve sheath. Temporary nerve conduction block, loss of motor and sensory function, but not autonomic. Full recovery expected, hours to months
Axonotmesis	Myelin plus axon disrupted, nerve sheath intact. Wallerian degeneration with motor, sensory, and autonomic paralysis. Recovery is often incomplete, taking weeks to months, and axon sprouts within the nerve sheath
Neurotmesis	Myelin, axon, and nerve sheath are also damaged. Recovery variable and incomplete at best, usually requires surgery or results in permanent paralysis

How Fast Does an Injured Axon Regenerate?

Approximately 1 mm per day, though factors like age and nutritional status may affect the rate.

Does Wallerian Degeneration Occur with Neurapraxia?

Not with neuropraxia. It does for axonotmesis and neurotmesis.

What Are the Three Layers of the Nerve Sheath?

Endoneurium, perineurium, and epineurium.

What Are the Classic Nerve Injuries Associated with Fractures? (Table 30.2)

Table 30.2 Common nerve injuries associated with fractures

	Fracture	Classic nerve injury	Symptoms
Upper extremity	Humeral head/proximal humerus	Axillary	Impaired shoulder abduction, sensory loss over the deltoid
	Mid-shaft of the humerus	Radial	Wrist-drop, impaired extension of wrist and fingers, sensory loss over the dorsal hand
	Supracondylar (humerus)	Median (anterior interosseous branch)	Weakness in thumb and index finger flexion (impaired pinch), preserved sensation
	Distal radius	Median	Impaired thumb opposition, thenar atrophy, and sensory loss over the lateral palm
Lower extremity	Hip fracture dislocation	Sciatic (tibial and peroneal branches)	Impaired knee flexion, foot drop, and sensory loss over the posterior leg and foot
	Fibular head	Common peroneal nerve	Foot drop, impaired eversion/dorsiflexion, and sensory loss over the lateral leg and dorsum of foot

What Is the Presumed Pathophysiology of Fat Embolism Syndrome?

Embolization of fat and marrow from the fracture (or from surgical intramedullary rodding) into the bloodstream. There are both mechanical and metabolic theories as to how this embolization occurs after injury.

What Artery Is Most at Risk with a Supracondylar Humerus Fracture?

The brachial artery can be injured with this type of fracture (more common in children). Make sure to assess distal radial and ulnar pulses. In rare cases, compartment syndrome can develop, and, if left untreated, can result in *Volkmann's contracture*.

> **Watch Out**
> Growth plate (physis) fractures can lead to premature physeal closure, resulting in leg length discrepancies or angular deformities.

Workup

What Is the Extent of Imaging Recommended with All Long Bone Fractures?

The joint above and below any long bone fracture must always be evaluated radiographically.

What Is a Floating Knee?

This is a term for the knee when ipsilateral femur and tibia fractures are present. A floating knee tends to flail or float between bony disconnections above and below the injury.

Management

How Are Open Fractures Graded?

The Gustilo-Anderson grading system (Table 30.3) is used to grade open fractures. An increased grade correlates with a higher risk of *infection*, nonunion, and amputation. All open fractures should receive antibiotics.

Table 30.3 Gustilo-Anderson grading system

Grade	Characteristics	Antibiotic coverage/ duration
I	Wound <1 cm, minimal contamination or soft tissue injury	Gram-positive with first-generation cephalosporin (e.g., cefazolin) for 24 h
II	Wound 1–10 cm, moderate soft tissue injury, no flaps or avulsions	Gram-positive with first-generation cephalosporin (e.g., cefazolin) for 24 h
IIIA	Wound >10 cm or high-energy, but with adequate soft tissue coverage	Gram-positive and Gram-negative (e.g., cefazolin and gentamicin) for 72 h
IIIB	IIIA with significant soft tissue injury requiring a flap or free tissue transfer	Gram-positive and Gram-negative (e.g., cefazolin and gentamicin) for 72 h
IIIC	IIIA with vascular injury that requires a vascular repair	Gram-positive and Gram-negative (e.g., cefazolin and gentamicin) for 72 h

What Is the Most Important Determinant of Severity for Fractures?

The energy imparted to the limb is the most important consideration. The greater the force, the higher the likelihood of a large associated soft tissue injury. For open fractures, any segmental or severely comminuted fracture should be at least a grade IIIA, even if the wound is small. In some cases, a limb may have no open wounds but may be at significant risk for amputation due to significant crush or high-energy injury.

What Antibiotics Are Indicated for Open Fractures in Farm Accidents or Soil-Contaminated Wounds?

Penicillin or its equivalent is *added* to cover anaerobes, especially *Clostridium perfringens*. Gas gangrene has led to many amputations in the past.

What Else Should Be Considered for Wounds Contaminated with Dirt and Soil?

Tetanus immune globulin (TIG) or tetanus toxoid (TT) administration depending on vaccine history and level

Table 30.4 *Clostridium tetani* infection

History of TT vaccination	Clean wounds	Dirty wounds
<3 doses	All should receive TT	All should receive both TT and TIG
≥3 doses	Should receive TT only if the last dose was more than 10 years ago	Should receive TT only if the last dose was more than 5 years ago

of contamination (Table 30.4). Wounds at the highest risk for *Clostridium tetani* infection include those containing foreign bodies and/or necrotic tissue.

What Are the Principles of Surgical Management of an Open Fracture? What Is the Optimal Timing?

Open fractures should be taken to the operating room as soon as the patient is medically stable for surgical irrigation and debridement (Grade IIIC injuries are a surgical emergency), ideally within six hours, but starting antibiotics within one hour is the most important step in management. All devitalized skin, tissue, and bone should be excised.

How Are Skin Wounds Closed?

Grade I, II, and IIIA injuries typically receive primary closure, though some IIIA injuries may require multiple debridements before secondary closure due to significant contamination or inability to ascertain tissue viability at first look.

Why Is It Important to Have Early Stabilization of Open Fractures?

Restoring length, alignment, and rotation helps protect the soft tissues around the injury and prevent further damage secondary to mobile fracture fragments. Restoration of length also helps reduce dead space, which decreases rates of infection. Patients who receive earlier stabilization also have quicker recovery.

Which Should Be Repaired First in a Patient with Concurrent Bone Fracture and Associated Vascular Injury with a Hard Sign (e.g., No Distal Pulse)?

These patients require a coordinated effort between the trauma, orthopedic, and vascular surgery services. The accepted sequence of events should be (1) temporary vascular shunting, (2) orthopedic stabilization, and (3) definitive vascular repair. This establishes early blood flow to the extremity.

What Is the Difference Between Open and Closed Reduction?

Reduction is the process of putting displaced bones back to their normal anatomic positions. This can either be done by direct manipulation of the bone through a surgical incision (open reduction) or indirectly by external manipulation of the limb manually or with a fracture table (closed reduction). Isolated diaphyseal fractures without neurovascular compromise, limb shortening, or significant displacement are generally managed with closed reduction and immobilization. Open reduction is reserved for cases involving open fractures, neurovascular injury, polytrauma, or pathologic fractures.

What Is the Difference Between Internal and External Fixation? What Are the Advantages/Disadvantages?

Fixation refers to the stabilization of a fracture using orthopedic hardware. Internal fixation involves placing hardware such as plates, screws, or rods entirely beneath the skin. These implants are usually permanent and offer rigid stabilization. In contrast, external fixation involves inserting pins or wires into bone that are connected to a stabilizing frame outside the body. External fixators are temporary and carry a higher risk of pin site infection, necessitating eventual removal. The choice between internal and external fixation depends on fracture pattern, soft tissue condition, and overall patient status.

What Are the Main Management Concerns for a Femur Fracture?

Patients with long bone fractures (e.g., femur, humerus) are at risk for fat embolism syndrome (discussed above). Femur fractures can also present with considerable blood loss since bone is highly vascular, and the thigh compartment can accommodate a large volume of blood. Patients should also be monitored for signs of hemorrhagic shock.

What Single Type of Orthopedic Fracture Is at the Greatest Risk for Hemorrhagic Shock?

Pelvic fractures. Some are benign and cause minimal blood loss, while some are highly unstable and may require a massive blood transfusion protocol due to the high pelvic volume into which blood may accumulate.

What Is the Optimal Timing of Femur Fracture Repair? What Is the Main Risk if Repair Is Delayed? What Are the Main Options in Repair?

The American College of Surgeons recommends definitive surgical management of femur fractures within 2–12 h of injury, provided that they are hemodynamically and medically stable. Patients who undergo surgical repair within 24 hours have decreased rates of mortality and morbidity. Definitive management is most often accomplished with *intramedullary nailing* in the adult, though external fixation is sometimes used temporarily in unstable patients, as this can be performed more quickly and easily and does not involve reaming the canal, which can increase the risk of developing fat embolism syndrome (◘ Fig. 30.2).

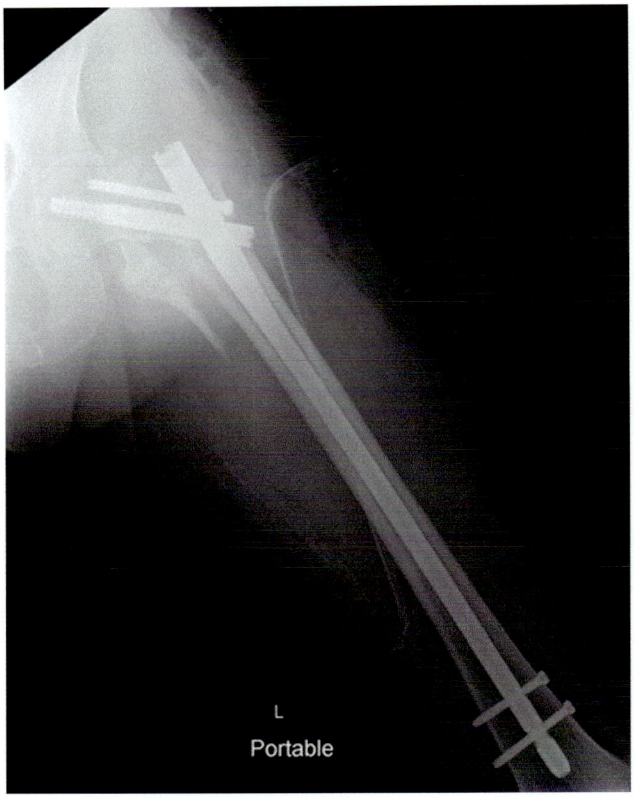

◘ **Fig. 30.2** Intramedullary nail for femoral fracture (From Li X, et al. Pseudoaneurysm of the profunda femoris artery following a long anterograde intramedullary nail for an unstable intertrochanteric hip fracture: a case report and review of the literature. *Eur J Orthop Surg Traumatol*. 2011;21:293. ► https://doi.org/10.1007/s00590-010-0700-y. Reprinted with permission from Springer Nature)

Do All Femur Fractures Require Fixation? Do All Radius Fractures Require Fixation?

No, children less than 3–5 years old are usually managed with spica casting and do not carry the same risk of morbidity and mortality associated with femur fractures as in adults. In young children who fall onto an outstretched hand, buckle fractures of the distal radius are common. These incomplete fractures result from cortical compression without disruption of the bone cortex, appearing as a bulge on radiographs. They heal rapidly with immobilization. Unlike pathologies such as rickets or osteosarcoma, buckle fractures occur following trauma and have no associated systemic symptoms.

What Should Be Considered in a Child Who Is Not Yet Walking and Presents with a Femur Fracture?

Child abuse. In some cases, these children are found to have fragile bones, as in osteogenesis imperfecta.

What Is the Management for Fat Embolism Syndrome?

Management of fat embolism syndrome consists of supportive care with oxygenation and ventilatory support.

What Is the Most Important Factor to Prevent Fat Embolism Syndrome Before It Occurs in a Polytrauma Patient?

Early stabilization of long bone fractures within the first 24 h.

What Is the Management for a Clavicle Fracture?

Most clavicle fractures involve the middle and proximal third, which can be managed with a sling/brace, rest, and ice. Significantly displaced fractures that cause tenting of the skin can lead to pressure necrosis and may require open reduction with internal fixation.

What Are the Complications Associated with Colles Fracture?

A Colles fracture, characterized by dorsal displacement of the distal radius, is commonly associated with median nerve compression and potential injury to the radial artery. Neurovascular assessment is important. Closed reduction and immobilization are typically the initial management.

Why Is CT Angiography Recommended After Posterior Knee Dislocation?

Posterior dislocation of the knee carries a significant risk of popliteal artery injury. Even if reduction restores distal motor function and palpable pulses, CT angiography is recommended to evaluate for occult vascular injuries that may threaten limb viability.

Postoperative

What Are the Important Risks Associated with Fracture Treatment?

Infection, iatrogenic nerve or vessel injury, nonunion (failure to heal), malunion (healing in an improper position or alignment), or instrumentation failure.

Area of Controversy

Limb Salvage or Amputation

In cases of severe lower extremity trauma (mangled extremity), determining whether to pursue limb salvage or primary amputation can be challenging. Factors favoring amputation include hemodynamic instability, prolonged ischemia, and high-energy mechanisms resulting in combined vascular, nerve, soft tissue, and osseous injury. Although scoring systems such as the Mangled Extremity Severity Score exist, they play a limited role in decision-making and should not replace clinical judgment. More important considerations include the patient's overall stability, associated complications such as compartment syndrome or rhabdomyolysis, and anticipated deterioration of the affected limb. Patient preference is also an important factor, as most individuals strongly favor limb preservation despite the potential for prolonged recovery. Limb salvage often requires multiple operations and extended hospitalization and can have a significant psychological impact. Amputation, while allowing for faster initial mobilization, may carry comparable or greater long-term costs due to the need for prosthetic care. Importantly, the outdated notion that plantar insensitivity alone warrants amputation is no longer accepted as a definitive indication.

Areas Where You Can Get in Trouble

Missing Other Fractures

A joint above and below any fracture must always be assessed radiographically. This is one of the greatest sources of missed injury, aside from incomplete clinical secondary surveys, for additional injury. In some cases, a missed foot injury that was not treated properly at the outset will plague the patient more than the dangerous femur fracture, which has subsequently healed without sequelae. The most commonly missed fractures in trauma patients are of the hand and foot.

Failure to Recognize a Neurologic Deficit

A radial nerve deficit is important to determine, as it may need separate treatment or dictate treatment options. Also, if a preoperative nerve deficit was missed and not documented, then a postoperative nerve deficit may be attributed by the patient to an operative complication and/or lead to medicolegal issues.

Summary of Essentials

30

History and Physical

- Inquire about the mechanism of injury and perform a complete secondary survey to avoid missing fractures or soft tissue injuries.
- Fat embolism syndrome (24–72 h after injury): respiratory symptoms, neurological changes, and reddish-brown petechial rash.
- Examine the four functional components of the extremity: nerves, vessels, bones, and soft tissues.

Pathophysiology

- Fat embolism syndrome results from fat and marrow embolization, primarily affecting the lungs and brain.
- Three nerve injuries: neuropraxia, axonotmesis, and neurotmesis.
- Humeral shaft fractures associated with radial nerve injury and wrist-drop.
- Open fracture communicates with the environment due to disruption of soft tissue and skin and requires special treatment due to infection risk.

Diagnosis

- Diagnosis is usually straightforward with fractures after acute trauma.
- Radiographs must include the joint above and below all fractures seen on X-ray.
- Any soft tissue wounds in conjunction with a fracture constitute an open fracture.
- In patients with femoral fractures, always evaluate for a femoral neck fracture.

Management

Open Fracture

- All open fractures should receive antibiotic coverage: first-generation cephalosporin +/−aminoglycoside.
- Irrigation and surgical debridement.
- External fixation for immediate and temporary control of an unstable patient.
- Definitive management with internal fixation.

Closed Femur Fracture

- Managed within 2–12 h with intramedullary nailing.
- Reduces the risk of fat embolism syndrome.

Postoperative

- Main surgical risks include infection, nonunion, malunion, nerve or vessel injury, and amputation in some cases.

Acknowledgements The editors would like to acknowledge and thank the following authors for their contributions to the previous edition of the chapter: C. Max Hoshino, Spencer Albertson.

Suggested Reading

American College of Surgeons Committee on Trauma. *ATLS: Advanced Trauma Life Support Student Course Manual*. 10th ed. Chicago, IL: American College of Surgeons; 2018.

Ashford RU, Mehta JA, Cripps R. Delayed presentation is no barrier to satisfactory outcome in the management of open tibial fractures. Injury. 2004;35:411–6.

Lieurance R, Benjamin JB, Rappaport WD. Blood loss and transfusion in patients with isolated femur fractures. J Orthop Trauma. 1992;6(2):175–9.

Müller EJ, Siebenrock K, Ekkernkamp A, et al. Ipsilateral fractures of the pelvis and the femur–floating hip? A retrospective analysis of 42 cases. Arch Orthop Trauma Surg. 1999;119:179.

Pollak AN. Timing of debridement of open fractures. J Am Acad Orthop Surg. 2006;14:S48–51.

Immediate Swelling After Trauma to the Knee

D'Ann E. Arthur and Kevin W. Rolfe

Contents

C. de Virgilio, A. Grigorian (eds.), *Surgery*, https://doi.org/10.1007/978-3-032-09799-6_31

Case Study

A 26-year-old otherwise healthy female presents to the clinic with right knee pain after a skiing accident 3 days ago. The patient landed awkwardly after attempting a jump and experienced the immediate onset of right knee pain necessitating ski patrol to bring her down the mountain. The patient reports hearing a "popping" noise when landing. Shortly after, she noticed swelling around her knee. She was still able to bear weight on her leg. Today, in clinic, the patient can ambulate with a single crutch on a slightly flexed knee without the knee buckling. On physical exam, a large effusion is present over her anterior knee. There is mild warmth and tenderness to palpation around the medial joint line. Muscle compartments in the leg are soft and pulses are 2+. Neurologic exam reveals normal motor and sensory function distal to the knee. The patient is able but hesitant to perform active and passive knee range of motion. There is increased knee laxity of 1 cm when an anterior force is applied to the tibia at 30° and 90°. There is no laxity with varus or valgus stress applied to the knee. Compression and axial rotation across the knee joint while extending it from a fully flexed position produces neither pain nor a palpable or audible snap.

Diagnosis

What Is the Differential Diagnosis for Acute Knee Pain? (Table 31.1)

Table 31.1 Differential diagnosis of acute knee pain

Diagnosis	Comments
Hemarthrosis, bone infarct	History of hemophilia or sickle cell disease
Septic arthritis	Fever, erythema and warmth of knee; unwillingness to bear weight or range the knee and instead hold it constantly around 30° of flexion; *Neisseria gonorrhoeae* common in sexually active young individuals
Prepatellar bursitis	Occurs in patients that are repetitively kneeling (e.g., gardener); normal passive motion but very painful active range of motion
Acute osteomyelitis	Fever and constitutional symptoms especially in association with immunocompromise (HIV, sickle cell, diabetes, alcohol use disorder, chronic corticosteroid use), or intravenous drug use
Neoplastic	Constitutional symptoms, typically more insidious onset (except pathologic fracture through tumoral bone); acute fracture across a benign preexisting bone lesion or cyst would not be distinguishable from ordinary fracture without imaging studies
Inflammatory	History of rheumatoid arthritis (flare up) or crystalline arthropathy; focal tenderness over the affected area (bursitis, tendinitis)
Traumatic	Onset of pain at time of acute sporting or vehicular injury; fractures associated with *unwillingness to bear weight* more than ligamentous or soft-tissue injuries but may occur together; acute patellar or quadriceps tendon rupture prevents ability to actively extend knee despite adequate passive motion
Iatrogenic/drugs	History of recent knee injection (postinjection inflammation and/or infection)

HIV human immunodeficiency virus

Watch Out
Ligamentous injuries classically present with immediate swelling, while meniscal tears develop swelling the next day.

What Is the Most Likely Diagnosis?

In a young healthy female with sudden knee pain immediately following a skiing accident, a traumatic etiology is most likely. Since the patient can bear weight, fracture is less likely, though not entirely ruled out. Anterior knee laxity on physical exam suggests anterior cruciate ligament (ACL) disruption. Varus and valgus stability make associated medial collateral ligament (MCL) and/or lateral collateral ligament (LCL) disruptions less likely. As the patient's knee does not buckle despite a flexed knee gait during weight bearing in conjunction with no palpable tendon defects, quadriceps or patellar tendon rupture is less likely. Though commonly associated with ACL tears, a meniscal tear is less likely in the presence of a negative McMurray sign (no pain, no palpable or audible snap with a compression and axial rotation maneuver of the knee while extending it from a fully flexed position).

History and Physical Exam

What Is the Classic History for the Various Ligamentous Injuries in the Knee? (◘ Table 31.2)

◘ **Table 31.2** Classic history for ligamentous injuries

Ligament	Classic history
Anterior cruciate ligament (ACL)	Posterior blow to the lateral knee
Posterior cruciate ligament (PCL)	Direct blow to the anterior tibia (e.g., dashboard injury)
Medial collateral ligament (MCL)	Lateral blow to the knee (valgus stress)
Lateral collateral ligament (LCL)	Medial blow to the knee (varus stress)

What Are the Classical Physical Exam Signs for Knee Injuries and How Are They Performed?

◘ Table 31.3 describes the clinical tests used to evaluate knee pain. All are performed supine, and side-to-side comparison is most important to determine the presence of laxity.

What Does a History of Locking or Catching Signify?

Intermittent locking or catching with range of motion of the knee most commonly signifies a mechanical blockage to motion. This is most often associated with meniscal tears, especially tears with mobile flaps. Patients often have medial joint tenderness. Loose osteochondral bodies in the joint space can also present with locking/catching.

◘ **Table 31.3** Knee maneuvers

Structure	Clinical test	Description
Anterior cruciate ligament (ACL)	Anterior drawer or Lachman's test	Knee flexed at 90°, forward traction on the lower leg causes the tibial plateau to move forward relative to the knee suggesting a torn ACL
Posterior cruciate ligament (PCL)	Posterior drawer test or "tibial sag" on 90° flexion	Knee flexed at 90°, posterior force on the lower leg causes the tibial plateau to move posteriorly relative to the knee suggesting a torn PCL
Meniscal cartilage	McMurray's test	Involves extending the knee from full flexion while applying compression and axial rotation across the joint
Lateral collateral ligament (LCL)	Varus instability	Thigh pushed on medial side in lateral direction while foot pushed on lateral side in medial direction, significant laxity suggests LCL tear
Medial collateral ligament (MCL)	Valgus instability	Thigh pushed on lateral side in medial direction while foot pushed on medial side in lateral direction, significant laxity suggests MCL tear

Why Is It Important to Perform a Careful Vascular Exam?

Injuries such as posterior knee dislocation or proximal tibia fracture can damage the popliteal artery leading to acute limb ischemia which may lead to amputation if not recognized and treated promptly. Pulses should always be assessed, and ankle-brachial indices (ABIs) must be performed if there is any uncertainty. An ABI < 0.9 indicates a high likelihood of vascular injury and warrants further workup with a CT angiogram.

Why Is It Important to Perform a Careful Neurologic Exam?

Global instability after knee dislocation, significant ligamentous disruption, or fracture can damage the major nerves or branches traversing the region. The common peroneal nerve (as it passes around the fibular neck at knee) is the most common nerve injured in the lower leg and results in a foot drop (with "slapping" gait) and numbness of dorsum of foot. Immediate stabilization of an unstable knee may be indicated to protect these structures and thus prevent further damage. Surgical exploration and nerve repair are sometimes needed.

What Is the Significance of Having Soft Muscular Compartments in the Lower Leg?

This helps rule out compartment syndrome, which is a true surgical emergency with a limited window of time for intervention (fasciotomy) before irreversible tissue death. The most sensitive clinical finding for compartment syndrome is pain with passive stretch. This can be performed by performing a passive range of motion of the great toe. Don't forget the six Ps of compartment syndrome: pain (out of proportion to injury, and to passive motion), pallor, paresthesia, poikilothermia (cold limb compared to unaffected side), paralysis, and pulselessness (rare and very late finding).

What Is the Importance of Asking About Previous Knee Surgery?

Patients with previous knee surgery may have hardware/prosthesis used in the repair. This can serve as a nidus for subsequent infection.

Watch Out

Patients presenting with knee infection within the first 3 months after knee surgery with hardware/prosthesis implants likely are to be infected with a highly virulent organism such as *Staphylococcus aureus*. Those who have a delayed onset (>6 months) with chronic pain are more likely to be infected with a less-virulent organism such as a coagulase-negative *Staphylococcus epidermidis*.

What Should Be Considered in Patients with Recurrent Fractures?

Although a patient with a recurrent fracture may report minor trauma as the inciting event, recurrent fractures should raise the suspicion for infection (osteomyelitis) or neoplasms within the bone resulting in pathologic fracture. Osteosarcomas are malignancies that lay down bony osteoid material that can mimic healing fracture callus on radiographs.

What Is the Significance of Being Able to Bear Weight?

When the patient can bear substantial weight on the limb, fractures and septic arthritis are less likely.

Why Is It Important to Look for Lacerations or Wounds?

Wounds or lacerations after a trauma may signify an *open fracture* which is a surgical emergency. Ideally, antibiotics should be administered within one hour of presentation.

Pathophysiology

What Two Basic Mechanisms Lead to ACL Injury?

Contact and noncontact pivoting injuries. Contact injuries involve a direct blow to the knee, often a lateral or hyperextension blow to the knee (e.g., with a helmet as may be seen in football). Noncontact ACL injuries are far more common. These typically occur during pivoting sports including football, basketball, and soccer, and are commonly associated with awkward landings.

Is ACL Injury More Common in Males or Females?

Among active sports participants, the incidence of ACL injury is four to five times more common in females. This difference in rate is likely multifactorial. Anatomically, females tend to have a smaller ACL and a narrower intercondylar notch. Biomechanically, they often land with greater knee valgus and extension, which increases stress on the ACL. Muscular imbalances also contribute, as females generally exhibit a lower hamstring-to-quadriceps strength ratio. Hormonal fluctuations associated with the menstrual cycle further influence injury rates, with the preovulatory phase posing the highest risk for ACL rupture.

What Is the Terrible (Aka "Unhappy") Triad of the Knee?

A combination of MCL, ACL, and medial meniscus injuries. Medial meniscus injuries commonly result from twisting the knee while the foot is fixed.

> **Watch Out**
> Don't confuse the terrible triad of the knee with that of the elbow (elbow dislocation with coronoid and radial head fractures).

What Is the Distribution of Blood Supply to the Meniscus and Why Is It Important?

The menisci receive blood peripherally from outside-in to cover only the outer 25–30% of their diameter. Tears occurring in the outer "red" zone have the potential to heal and are often repaired. Inner tears in the "white zone" without a direct blood supply have little healing potential. As such, tears in the "white zone" are not repaired but surgically debrided if needed.

What Is the Significance of a "Popping" Noise on Traumatic Injury?

Although a "popping" noise can occur with meniscal injuries, it is most commonly associated with ACL rupture. High tension on the ligament immediately before the tear may cause the audible noise. Some believe that the noise occurs due to a sudden collision between the bone ends of the femur and tibia.

What Injury Would You Expect from a Dashboard Knee Injury?

A dashboard knee injury occurs in a motor vehicle accident when a flexed knee hits the dashboard subjecting it to an anterior force. This mechanism is associated with PCL injury and a positive posterior drawer test.

What Is the Normal Range of Motion of the Knee?

The range of motion of the knee is tested with the patient lying supine and the hip partially flexed. The normal range is 0–5° extension to 130–140° flexion.

What Is the Significance of Being Unable to Actively or Fully Extend the Knee While the Examiner Can Do So Passively?

Inability to actively extend the knee with normal passive extension suggests disruption of the extensor mechanism, such as quadriceps or patellar tendon rupture, or fracture of the patella or tibial tubercle. These injuries are common in middle-aged "weekend warrior" athletes. Severe pain with active motion but minimal to no pain with passive motion is highly suggestive of prepatellar bursitis, an inflammation of the bursa anterior to the patella. It often occurs in individuals who frequently kneel, earning the nickname "housemaid's knee." NSAIDs are the primary treatment for bursitis.

What About Pain Inferior to the Patella with an Intact Extensor Mechanism of the Knee?

Pain along the patellar tendon near its attachment to the patella suggests patellar tendinitis ("jumper's knee"), common in sports involving frequent jumping (e.g., basketball) or repetitive knee extension (e.g., soccer). Pes anserine pain syndrome causes pain on the medial tibial condyle, 2–3 inches below the joint line. It results from quadriceps overuse and weakness, leading to inflammation of the pes anserine bursa and tendons of the sartorius, gracilis, and semitendinosus muscles. It tends to occur in obese, diabetic patients with abnormal gait. NSAIDs are the primary treatment for this.

Workup

What Is the Next Step in the Workup of This Patient?

Radiographs of the knee are taken to evaluate for fracture, alignment or deformity, infection, and tumor.

What Is the Meaning of Patella Alta and Baja on an X-Ray?

The patella may ride high (alta) due to unopposed pull from the quadriceps in the setting of a patellar tendon rupture. Conversely, it may ride low (baja) with quadriceps rupture.

What Are the Characteristic Radiographic Features of Osteoarthritis of the Knee, and Why Is It Important to Consider After ACL Injury?

Radiographic changes consistent with degenerative arthritis in the knee include joint space narrowing, osteophytes (bone spurs), subchondral sclerosis, and subchondral cysts (◘ Fig. 31.1). These changes are critical to recognize as ACL surgery is not appropriate in the setting of significant arthritis of the knee as it does not prevent or reverse the preexisting degenerative process.

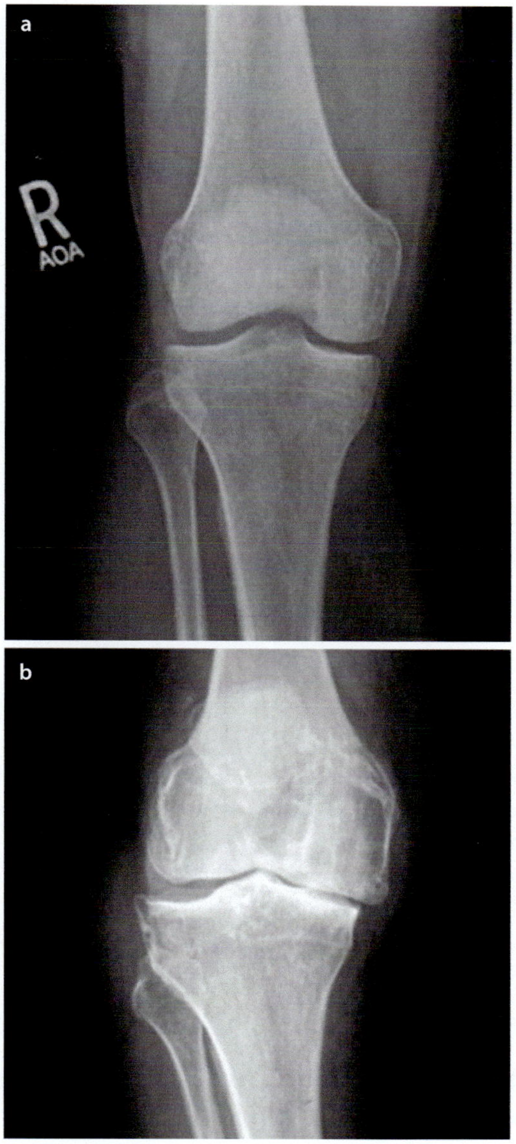

◘ **Fig. 31.1** (**a**) Normal radiograph of the knee. (From Abdul-Jabar HB, et al. Primary meningococcal oligoarthritis of the knee—case report and review of the literature. *Eur Orthop Traumatol*. 2011;2:149. ► https://doi.org/10.1007/s12570-011-0078-2. Reprinted with permission Springer Nature). (**b**) Arthritic knee. (From Leonard M, Murphy PG. End-stage osteoarthritis of the knee presenting with foot drop. *Eur J Orthop Surg Traumatol*. 2007;17:399. ► https://doi.org/10.1007/s00590-007-0200-x. Reprinted with permission from Springer Nature)

How Should Suspected Septic Arthritis or Crystalline Arthropathy Be Worked Up?

A hot, swollen knee without a preceding trauma should prompt knee *arthrocentesis* (needle aspiration to obtain *synovial fluid* for culture and pathology including cell counts and crystal analysis). Unwillingness to bear weight or range the knee, especially with fever, suggests a serious joint infection that requires emergent intervention. Gross purulence on aspiration is infectious until proven otherwise (although pseudogout can give this appearance as well). Pseudogout crystals are formed of calcium pyrophosphate and are rhomboid in shape and positively birefringent (purple) on crystal analysis. Gout crystals are formed of monosodium urate and are needle-shaped and negatively birefringent (yellow) on crystal analysis. White blood cell (WBC) counts in synovial fluid of less than 200/μL are normal. Inflammatory conditions range from 200 to 50,000/μL, and above 50,000/μL is infectious. There may be diagnostic ambiguity near the overlapping ranges between disease processes. ◘ Table 31.4 describes arthrocentesis findings of various joint pathologies.

Table 31.4 Arthrocentesis findings

Type	Color/Clarity	WBC count	Culture	Crystals
Normal	Clear, translucent	<200/μL	Negative	Negative
Non-inflammatory (osteoarthritis)	Straw colored/ yellow, translucent	200–2000/μL	Negative	Negative
Inflammatory (rheumatoid arthritis, psoriatic arthritis, gout, pseudogout)	Yellow, cloudy	2000–50,000/ μL	Negative	Positive in gout (needle shaped, negatively birefringent) and pseudogout (rhomboid, positively birefringent)
Septic	Yellow/green, opaque	>50,000/μL	Positive	Negative
Hemarthrosis	Red, bloody	200–2000/μL	Negative	Negative

Watch Out

When performing an arthrocentesis or injection, skin flora may be introduced into the joint. If a patient presents with worsening pain around the joint, erythema, and fever several days after an arthrocentesis or injection, consider iatrogenic septic bursitis. When infection is suspected, an image-guided (e.g., ultrasound) aspiration of the bursa and/or joint is necessary.

What Imaging Would You Use to Confirm a Suspected ACL Injury?

MRI is the *best* technique to evaluate the integrity of the ACL and the menisci.

Management

Is There a Role for Nonoperative Management of ACL Tears?

Nonoperative management of ACL tears can be considered with (1) partial tears and no instability symptoms; (2) those with complete tears with no symptoms of knee instability during low-demand sports who are willing to give up high-demand sports; (3) those who do light manual work or live sedentary lifestyles; (4) those with advanced osteoarthritis; and (5) those with significant comorbidities precluding surgery. These may be managed nonoperatively with activity modification, bracing, and physical therapy focused on strengthening the muscles which serve to dynamically stabilize the knee, especially the hamstrings. Note that acute symptomatic treatment includes the RICE formula: rest, ice, compress, and elevate.

What Is the Management for the Patient in This Case?

A young, healthy, athletic patient without preexisting arthritis involved in a high-energy injury who, most likely, wishes to return to a high level of athletic function is an excellent surgical candidate. Surgery entails arthroscopic *reconstruction* of the ACL, not repair. Reconstruction involves the use of a tendon graft placed into bone tunnels across the knee in the femur and the tibia approximating the normal position of the ACL. Attempts at repair of the native ligament do not heal due to the intra-articular location and presence of synovial fluid which inhibits local healing.

What Is the Management of a Meniscal Tear?

Most tears that are small or causing infrequent symptoms can be managed successfully with the RICE (rest, ice, compression, elevation) approach followed by physical therapy. Surgery is considered for patients with persistent and/or disabling symptoms and those involving large, complex tears in contact with the articular cartilage.

Areas Where You Can Get in Trouble

Failure to Recognize a Knee Dislocation or Vascular Injury

The knee should be examined fully after significant trauma. Significant instability needs to be assessed and recognized on exam as it will change the acute management. Static radiographs may not reveal a globally unstable knee after dislocation due to spontaneous reduction or positioning of the knee during the x-ray. The vascular status of the limb must be evaluated with a pulse exam and ABIs.

Failure to Recognize a Septic (Infected) Knee Joint

If a septic knee is missed, the intra-articular cartilage can be completely destroyed by the bacteria. Cartilage has little to no capacity to heal, so the patient will be left with an end-stage arthritic knee joint that is painful and functions poorly.

Summary of Essentials

Diagnosis

- Acute trauma to knee with anterior knee laxity suggests ACL injury
- If the patient can bear weight, fracture is less likely

History and Physical Exam

- Components of knee exam: gait, observation, palpation, range of motion, joint line tenderness, neurovascular, and knee maneuvers
- Knee maneuvers: anterior drawer/Lachman's, posterior drawer, McMurray's test, and varus/valgus instability
- Knee dislocations can damage vasculature, creating a dysvascular limb risking amputation
- Ligament injury presents with immediate swelling; meniscal injury has delayed swelling

Etiology/Pathophysiology

- ACL injury:
  - Contact versus noncontact (more common) pivoting injuries
  - Audible pop during an acute sports-related injury involving an awkward landing or twisting mechanism
- Unhappy triad:
  - MCL
  - ACL
  - Medial meniscus

Workup

- Start with radiographs to look for fractures, alignment or deformity, infection, and tumors
- If there is concern for infection, perform an arthrocentesis
- MRI for confirmation

Management

- Treatment made on individualized basis
- Treatment for all patients begins with:
  - Rest
  - Ice
  - Compress
  - Elevate
- Patients begin physical therapy as soon as they are able to tolerate treatment to restore the range of motion prior to surgical intervention
- Consider nonoperative management for elderly and low-demand patients
- Surgery for reconstruction, not repair

Acknowledgements The editors would like to acknowledge and thank the following authors for their contributions to the previous edition of the chapter: Spencer Albertson.

Suggested Reading

Beynnon BD, Johnson RJ, et al. Treatment of anterior cruciate ligament injuries, part I. Am J Sports Med. 2005;33(10):1579–602.

Jackson JL, O'Malley PG, Kroenke K. Evaluation of acute knee pain in primary care. Ann Intern Med. 2003;139:575.

LaBella CR, Hennrikus W, Hewett TE. Anterior cruciate ligament injuries: diagnosis, treatment and prevention. Pediatrics. 2014;133(5):1437–50.

Prodromos CC, Han Y, Rogowski J, et al. A meta-analysis of the incidence of anterior cruciate ligament tears as a function of gender, sport, and a knee injury-reduction regimen. Arthroscopy. 2007;23:1320.

Spindler KP, Wright RW. Clinical practice. Anterior cruciate ligament tear. N Engl J Med. 2008;359:2135.

Sutton KM, Mntgomery Bullock J. Anterior cruciate ligament rupture: differences between males and females. J Am Acad Orthop Surg. 2013;21(1):41–50.

Adolescent Male with Right Groin Pain and Limp

Cameron Gerhold, John F. Fleming III, and Kevin W. Rolfe

Contents

C. de Virgilio, A. Grigorian (eds.), *Surgery*, https://doi.org/10.1007/978-3-032-09799-6_32

Case Study

A 12-year-old moderately obese boy presents with right groin pain and a limp. He states that the pain is worse with walking and relieved by rest. The pain begins in his right groin and radiates to his right knee. The pain began about 1 month ago without antecedent trauma and has progressively worsened. He has no pain in any other joints or extremities. He has no recent infections and reports no associated fevers, chills, or malaise. He participates in physical education at school but is otherwise not involved in sports. He has no recent travel or camping trips and lives in an urban area. He takes no medications. There is no family history of joint problems. On physical examination, he is afebrile. The right lower extremity rests in a slightly externally rotated position compared to the contralateral extremity, and he resists internal rotation. There is no leg length discrepancy (LLD). The neurologic and vascular exams are normal. Erythrocyte sedimentation rate (ESR) and C-reactive protein (CRP) are within normal limits.

Diagnosis

What Is the Differential Diagnosis for Groin Pain with a Limp or Refusal to Bear Weight? (▫ Table 32.1)

▫ **Table 32.1** Differential diagnosis for groin pain

Infectious	History and physical
Septic arthritis	Triad of fever, pain, and impaired range of motion; a surgical emergency
Lyme disease	*Ixodes* tick bite (*Borrelia burgdorferi* bacteria); early signs include chills, fatigue, erythema chronicum migrans (bull's-eye rash); late signs include chronic synovitis, monoarthritis or oligoarthritis, aseptic meningitis
Psoas abscess	Fever, patient holds thigh in slight hip flexion and internal rotation, passive hip extension which stretches the psoas muscle is met with significant pain; can be associated with osteomyelitis of the spine, appendicitis, or other intraabdominal infections
Inflammatory	
Juvenile idiopathic arthritis	Nonmigratory arthropathy affecting one or more joints for >3 months, morning stiffness, fevers
Transient synovitis	History of a recent upper respiratory tract or other viral infections in the presence of hip pain; average age 2–5 years; most common cause of hip pain during childhood; pain is usually worse upon awakening and improves as the day progresses; often self-limiting
Mechanical	
Developmental dysplasia of the hip	In infants, it is seen with positive Barlow's and Ortolani's tests (provocation of hip dislocation or reduction, respectively), Galeazzi's sign (knees at unequal heights when hips/knees flexed); in toddlers, positive Trendelenburg sign; untreated will have delayed walking or abnormal gait
Legg-Calve-Perthes disease	Idiopathic osteonecrosis of femoral head; most common ages 4–8 years; gradual progressive limp, slow onset of pain, decreased range of motion
Stress fracture	Insidious onset of pain with activity or repeated loading; typically, the patient has no history of recent trauma; pain subsides at rest; local tenderness and swelling
Slipped capital femoral epiphysis	Obese, adolescent male aged 10–16 years old presenting with groin pain, painful limp, externally rotated hip, and pain with forced internal rotation
Osteogenesis imperfecta	Should be considered in patients with a history of multiple fractures, blue sclerae, or dentinogenesis imperfecta; although uncommon, mechanical pain or limping may arise due to pathologic fractures in the lower extremities
Neoplastic	
Benign	
Osteoid osteoma	Continuous, deep, aching bone pain in a young patient; typically, affects the neck or back; unexplained, rigid, painful scoliosis
Malignant	
Osteosarcoma	Most common primary malignant bone tumor; age range 10–30 years but more common in adolescent males; deep bony pain that progresses to palpable bony mass; typically affects distal femur
Ewing's sarcoma	Affects children 5–15 years old; bony pain, fever, fatigue, weight loss, pathologic fractures, palpable mass

What Is the Most Likely Diagnosis?

The most likely diagnosis is slipped capital femoral epiphysis (SCFE). There are a number of factors from the patient's history and physical exam that support this diagnosis (discussed below).

History and Physical

What Important Demographic Factor Limits the Differential Diagnosis for This Patient?

The patient's age limits the differential. Primary tumors or metastasis in the proximal femur typically affect older patients (multiple myeloma, bone metastasis) or younger (<5 years) children (acute lymphoblastic leukemia or neuroblastoma). Among the mechanical processes, transient synovitis peaks at 2–5 years (max around 12), and Legg-Calve-Perthes at 4–8 years. Also, it would be highly unusual for developmental dysplasia of the hip (DDH) to have its first presentation at age 12 years (screening for these begins at birth using Ortolani and Barlow maneuvers). Coupled with the absence of fever and other constitutional symptoms, only a few diagnoses remain for groin pain with a painful limp in a 12-year-old.

What Is an Antalgic Gait?

An antalgic gait refers to a limping pattern that arises due to pain, typically localized to one lower extremity. It is characterized by a shortened stance phase on the affected limb, as the patient minimizes the duration of weight-bearing to reduce discomfort. This compensatory gait allows continued ambulation while limiting stress on the painful area.

What Risk Factors Are Shared by Patients That Develop SCFE?

SCFE commonly presents at age 10–16 years old; males are more commonly affected than females (2:1), and the condition is more common among Black, Hispanic, and Polynesian children. Obesity is one of the strongest risk factors, presumably due to an increased load across the physis. 50% of SCFE patients are >90th percentile for weight; 70% of patients are >80th percentile. Patients undergoing puberty-related hormonal changes are also at higher risk due to the temporary and unstable widening of the epiphyseal growth plate of the proximal femur.

What Is the Most Common Presentation of SCFE and Physical Exam Findings?

Children commonly present with an antalgic gait (painful limp) and occasionally an inability to bear weight because of pain. The pain is most commonly in the groin but can also radiate and localize to the thigh or knee. On physical exam, patients have decreased internal rotation, and the thigh is held most comfortably resting in external rotation. Internal rotation maneuvers recreate the pain. Though a painful limp can be a sign of a tumor or infection, the absence of fever, malaise, and other constitutional symptoms makes these less likely.

What Is the Significance of External Rotation of His Leg and Resisting Internal Rotation?

External rotation of the leg is the most common resting position of children with SCFE because of the direction in which the metaphysis slips in relation to the epiphysis. Often, this external rotation can be exaggerated when the hip is brought into flexion and the leg involuntarily externally rotates. This is called obligatory external rotation.

What If the Patient Holds the Thigh in Slight Hip Flexion and Internal Rotation?

This position is classic for a psoas abscess with reflexive contracture of the psoas muscle due to spasm, especially in conjunction with fever and other signs of infection. Attempts at passive hip extension that stretches the psoas muscle are usually met with significant pain and resistance. Psoas abscess is often a sign of another underlying etiology, such as osteomyelitis of the spine, appendicitis, or Crohn's. Thus, once the diagnosis of a psoas abscess is determined, it is important to search for the primary source of the abscess.

Watch Out

A hip held in flexion and internal rotation after trauma, without signs of infection, should be presumed to be a dislocation and treated as a surgical emergency. Delays significantly increase the risk of avascular necrosis.

Why Is It Important to Examine the Hip in the Setting of Knee Pain?

Hip pathology may cause referred pain to the knee. Legg-Calve-Perthes disease and SCFE can both initially present as knee pain, with no complaint of hip discomfort. Therefore, it is important to perform a complete physical exam to determine if knee pain is native to the knee or referred from the hip.

Watch Out

In older adults, a shortened and externally rotated leg after trauma raises suspicion for hip fracture. Intracapsular fractures (femoral head and neck) carry a higher risk of avascular necrosis, while extracapsular fractures (intertrochanteric and subtrochanteric) are more likely to show bruising and displacement.

Why Is It Important to Consider Delayed Growth, Puberty, or Endocrinological Signs or Symptoms If SCFE Is Suspected?

SCFE typically presents in overweight patients older than 10 years. Patients who are younger (<10 years old) or thin (<50th percentile for weight) should be worked up for underlying endocrine disorders that are associated with SCFE. These include hypothyroidism, growth hormone abnormalities, renal osteodystrophy, hypopituitarism, and hyper- or hypoparathyroidism. These conditions physiologically weaken the physis, increasing the likelihood of slippage.

Watch Out

Hernias, testicular disease, and kidney stones are important entities that cause pain that radiates to the groin.

Why Is It Important to Clarify the Meaning of Hip Pain in History?

Clarifying the meaning of "hip pain" during the history is important because patients often misidentify the location. Many describe pain in the lateral thigh near the greater trochanter or in the buttock, which is anatomically distinct from true hip joint pain. The hip joint, formed by the articulation of the femoral head with the acetabulum, typically causes pain localized to the groin due to its medial position. When patients report lateral or posterior pain, alternative diagnoses such as trochanteric bursitis, sciatica, neurogenic claudication (leg pain with walking due to nerve compression), or sacroiliac joint pathology should be considered, as these conditions affect structures outside the joint itself. Posterior pain that worsens with lumbar extension or prolonged walking may suggest neurogenic claudication, while buttock pain could reflect referred symptoms from sacroiliac inflammation or lumbosacral radiculopathy.

What Would Be the Significance of a History of a Recent Upper Respiratory Tract or Other Viral Infections?

A recent history of upper respiratory tract infection or viral infection in the presence of hip pain would suggest a post-infectious inflammatory etiology, such as *transient synovitis*. Transient synovitis is the most common cause of hip pain during childhood, and though most common under 5 years of age, it can be seen into late adolescence. The pain is usually worse upon awakening and improves as the day progresses. As opposed to septic arthritis, transient synovitis presents with a mild or absent fever. The treatment for transient synovitis is usually observation, as this condition is self-limiting. Note that this is a diagnosis of exclusion, and a full workup for septic arthritis, including aspiration if needed, should be done if there is any doubt. Unlike SCFE, children with transient synovitis typically maintain the ability to bear weight, and hip range of motion is only mildly restricted. Inflammatory markers are usually normal or only mildly elevated, and constitutional symptoms are absent.

Why Is It Important to Ask About Travel or Exposure to Wildlife?

Recent travel or exposure to wildlife can raise the concern for special cases of septic arthritis. Travel outside the United States can risk exposure to tuberculosis (TB). Children with TB are more likely than adults to present with extrapulmonary involvement. The most common site of musculoskeletal involvement is the spine, followed by large joints (hip, knee). Domestically, exposure to wildlife in the upper Midwest and New England can raise the concern for Lyme disease. Children with Lyme arthritis are usually able to bear weight, and the pain is typically less severe than with typical bacterial arthritis. A target-shaped rash, erythema migrans, presents in the early stages of Lyme disease and is very helpful for early detection if seen. Although the hip may be involved, the knee is the most commonly affected joint in Lyme arthritis. These patients are typically afebrile and may present weeks after the initial tick bite, often without any recollection of a rash. Unlike septic arthritis, their symptoms are less acute, and aspiration often reveals high white counts but less dramatic clinical findings.

Why Is a Family History of Joint Disease Important?

A family history of joint pain is an important clue for some disease processes. DDH is thought to be largely multifactorial; however, family history is a strong risk factor. There is a 10% risk of DDH when at least one parent has a history of DDH and a 40% risk if both do. Additionally, juvenile idiopathic arthritis often has a genetic component.

Watch Out

A *nonpainful* limp while walking is common in early DDH and many neurological disorders.

Why Would a History of Corticosteroid Use Be Important?

A history of steroid use can predispose the pediatric population to *avascular necrosis* of the femoral head, also known as *osteonecrosis*. An adequate history is important because this diagnosis is clinically similar to Legg-Calve-Perthes disease, which has an entirely different treatment algorithm.

What Are Other Important Risk Factors for Secondary Osteonecrosis of the Hip?

In pediatric patients, sickle cell disease and marrow-replacing processes such as Gaucher's disease are important risk factors. In children with sickle cell disease, avascular necrosis is a common cause of atraumatic hip pain and should always be considered in the differential. MRI is the preferred modality for early detection. In adults, alcohol use disorder, dysbarism (decompression sickness, "the bends," or caisson disease), antiretroviral medications, previous history of hip trauma, systemic lupus erythematosus, and corticosteroid use are important etiologies to consider in the differential.

What Is the Significance of a Leg Length Discrepancy with This Clinical Presentation?

LLD points toward a mechanical pathology. Disruptions in the structural integrity of the long bones of the lower limb can lead to LLD. This is common in DDH and Legg-Calve-Perthes disease. Infections, tumors, or trauma can lead to disruption of the physis or bone, ultimately leading to an LLD, but not in the acute phase. SCFE may have a mild or apparent LLD due to the posture of the hip and thigh. A child with a long-standing LLD can develop a compensatory scoliosis.

What Is the Importance of the Ability to Bear Weight or Range the Hip?

The inability to bear weight or move through a range of motion for the hip indicates a potentially serious condition. Septic arthritis presents as the refusal to walk or bear weight in the setting of high fever. Fever combined with inability to bear weight should always raise concern for septic arthritis, which is a surgical emergency and must be presumed until ruled out. SCFE can present with or without the ability to bear weight. The inability to bear weight is what differentiates an *unstable* SCFE from a stable one. An unstable SCFE has a significantly higher rate of osteonecrosis of the femoral head. Both types of patients require surgical intervention on an urgent basis.

What Are the Component Steps in the Orthopedic Examination of a Painful Hip?

Gait, observation/inspection, palpation, range of motion (active, passive), neurologic (motor, sensory), vascular (pulses), and special physical exam tests.

What Are Some Common Physical Exam Tests Utilized in the Examination of the Hip? (Table 32.2)

Table 32.2 Physical exam tests for the hip

Test	Comments
Thomas test for flexion contracture	Patient lies supine and brings one knee to chest; if the opposite leg is unable to remain completely extended, then this is indicative of a flexion contracture of the hip
Trendelen-burg test	Patient in standing position and asked to lift one leg; the pelvis should remain level but if falls or dips inferiorly on the side of the raised leg, this is indicative of abductor muscle weakness on side of standing leg
FABER	*F*lexion, *ab*duction, *e*xternal *r*otation maneuver of the hip while patient is supine; if this position results in pain, it suggests sacroiliac joint pathology

Pathophysiology

What Is the Pathophysiology for the Orthopedic Mechanical Diagnoses? (Table 32.3)

Table 32.3 Pathophysiology for orthopedic mechanical diagnoses

Diagnosis	Pathophysiology and features
Develop-mental dysplasia of the hip	Abnormal hip development resulting in laxity, subluxation, or dislocation of the hip; initial instability/laxity of the hip results in malpositioning of the femoral head in the developing acetabulum and incomplete formation of the hip socket; dysplasia can lead to gradual dislocation, difficulty with ambulation, degenerative arthritis, and pain
Legg-Calve-Perthes disease	Unknown pathophysiology; idiopathic osteonecrosis of femoral head; typically presents at age 4–8 years
Stress fracture	Repetitive overloading causing a fatigue fracture, which overwhelms the body's remodeling and repair capacity, typically minimally or non-displaced
Slipped capital femoral epiphysis	Displacement of the metaphysis of the femoral neck relative to the epiphysis of the femoral head through the growth plate is likely due to obesity and mechanical overloading, and less commonly due to a weakened physis from an underlying endocrine disorder; the femoral neck displaces anteriorly and superiorly relative to the femoral epiphysis; typically, presents at age 10–16 years during puberty

Are "Shin Splints" the Same as Tibial Stress Fractures?

No. Medial tibial stress syndrome (shin splints) presents with *diffuse* tenderness along the tibia of overweight individuals that are on their feet for a prolonged period of time (e.g., security guard). In contrast, a tibial stress fracture presents with *focal* tenderness along the anterior tibia worsened with exercise and occurs in individuals with a sudden increase in activity (e.g., new gym membership, athletes). Radiographs are often normal.

Watch Out

Stress fractures of the metatarsals can also occur after sudden increases in activity. The second metatarsal is the most commonly injured, and most patients only require rest and analgesia. The fifth metatarsal is the only one that has increased risk for nonunion and so may require surgical intervention.

Workup

What Laboratory Tests Would Be Useful and Why?

Laboratory values are important to determine the etiology of musculoskeletal pathology. In this case, one must rule out infection via laboratory testing. Complete blood count, complete chemistry panel, ESR, and CRP should be drawn to check for signs of infection. Septic arthritis in the pediatric population can be diagnosed using the Kocher criteria (◘ Table 32.4). The predicted probability of septic arthritis is 5% with one predictor, 40% with two predictors, 95% with three predictors, and 99% with all four predictors. Additionally, a CRP >2.0 mg/dl coupled with refusal to bear weight carries a 75% probability of septic arthritis. Blood cultures and joint aspirations should be drawn if there is a suspicion of infection.

◘ Table 32.4 Kocher criteria to diagnose septic arthritis in pediatric population

Fever >38.5 °C
Inability to bear weight
ESR >20 mm/h
WBC >12,000/μl

These criteria are especially useful in the early diagnostic phase, and their predictive value increases with the number of positive findings. A child with all four criteria should be taken for surgical evaluation without delay.

What Analysis Should Be Done if Joint Aspiration (Arthrocentesis) Is Done for Suspected Infection?

Samples of joint fluid should be sent for cultures, including aerobic and anaerobic bacteria, fungi, and mycobacteria. Gram stain, fungal prep, and acid-fast stains must be done in addition to culture. It is also important to perform cell counts and crystal analysis.

What Is the First Imaging That Would Be Recommended?

Plain film radiographs (x-rays) should be ordered first. AP and frog-leg lateral views of the pelvis should be ordered for any suspected hip pathology. If knee pathology is in question, additional plain radiographs of the knee are ordered (AP, lateral, and sunrise views). In pediatric populations, a complaint of hip or knee pain should both prompt hip radiographs.

What Are the Classic X-ray Findings of Pediatric Orthopedic Mechanical Hip Disease? (◘ Table 32.5)

◘ Table 32.5 X-ray findings of pediatric orthopedic mechanical hip diseases

Disease	X-ray finding
Developmental dysplasia of the hip	Subluxation or dislocation of the femoral head from the acetabulum; difficult to assess on x-ray in infants, for which ultrasound is typically used (◘ Fig. 32.1)
Legg-Calve-Perthes disease	Subchondral (under the cartilage) collapse of the bone of the femoral head
Slipped capital femoral epiphysis	Asymmetry of the femoral head on the neck. The appearance is commonly described as "ice cream sliding off the cone" (◘ Figs. 32.2 and 32.3)

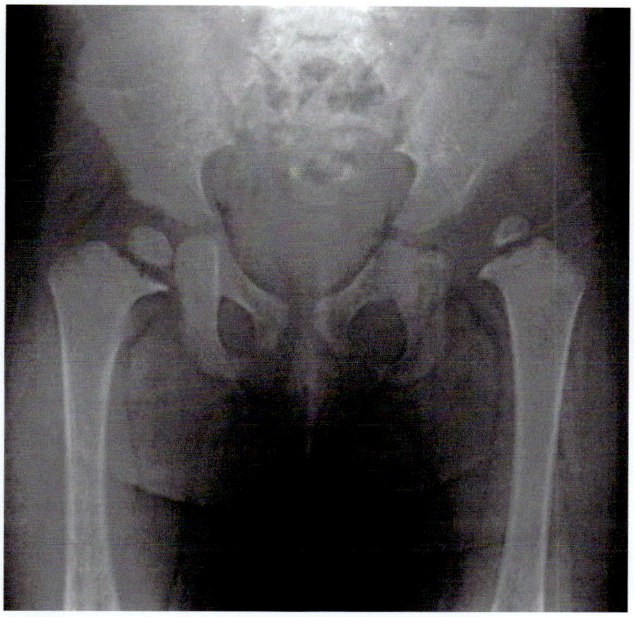

Fig. 32.1 Developmental dysplasia of the hip radiograph showing normal right and subluxated left hip

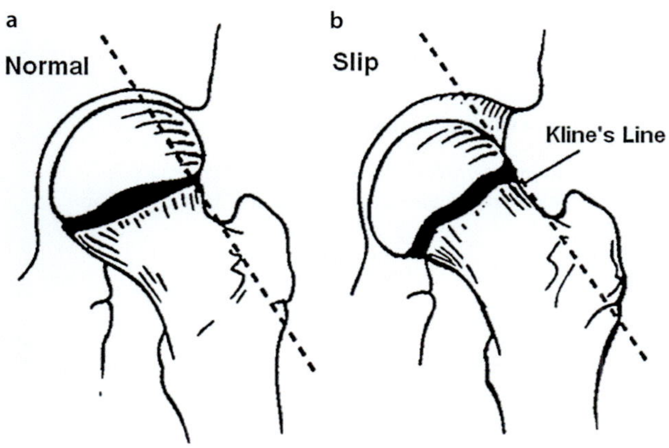

Fig. 32.2 SCFE schematic

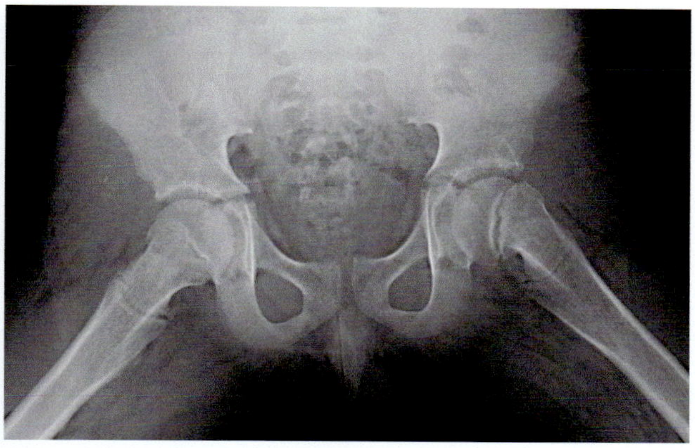

Fig. 32.3 SCFE radiograph (frog lateral) showing SCFE on the left and normal on the right

What Other Imaging Is Useful if the Diagnosis Is Unclear?

MRI is excellent at visualizing non-displaced stress fractures, early avascular necrosis, or Legg-Calve-Perthes disease, as well as soft-tissue abnormalities of the ligaments, tendons, and labrum. MRI also adds to the workup for local tumors and osteomyelitis about the hip. CT is excellent for fine evaluation of bone but is used sparingly in children to avoid unnecessary radiation exposure. CT of the chest, abdomen, and/or pelvis is used in the workup of malignant tumors to assess for metastases. Bone scans evaluate the metabolic activity of the bone by recording uptake of venous-injected radioactive material (i.e., technetium-99 m). They can be used to highlight an active area of infection or tumor when the lesion is not otherwise evident (e.g., an osteoid osteoma: a small, but painful, benign bone tumor).

Management

What Is the Management for the Following Diagnoses on the Differential? (Table 32.6)

32

Table 32.6 Management of diagnoses for the differential

Infectious	**Management**
Septic arthritis	Joint aspiration and blood cultures will dictate antibiotic selection, but start with broad-spectrum IV antibiotics; emergent incision and drainage
Lyme disease	Antibiotics (doxycycline, amoxicillin, or cefuroxime)
Psoas abscess	Antibiotics +/– surgical drainage
Inflammatory	
Juvenile idiopathic arthritis	DMARDs, NSAIDs, +/– steroid injections, frequent ophthalmologic exams; watch for C1–2 instability and myelopathy; as disease progresses, surgery for diseased joints is often necessary
Transient synovitis	Observation and NSAIDs; rule out septic arthritis
Mechanical	
Developmental dysplasia of the hip	0–6 months: Pavlik harness 6–18 months: Surgical closed vs. open reduction with spica casting >18 months: Surgical open reduction with pelvic osteotomies
Legg-Calve-Perthes disease	Most patients do not require treatment (symptomatic and supportive measures); treatment of advanced disease aims at *containment* (casting/bracing, femoral/pelvic osteotomies)
Stress fracture	Period of non- or protected weight bearing +/– casting/bracing
Slipped capital femoral epiphysis	In situ screw fixation across the capital physis
Snapping hip syndrome	Rest, ice, physical therapy; surgical intervention may be indicated in persistent case
Neoplastic	
Benign	
Osteoid osteoma	Percutaneous RFA if symptoms are not controlled with NSAIDs
Other benign bone lesions	Observation vs. intralesional curettage and grafting
Malignant	
Osteosarcoma	Neoadjuvant chemotherapy plus wide surgical resection
Ewing's sarcoma	Neoadjuvant chemotherapy plus wide surgical resection, possible radiation

DMARD disease-modifying antirheumatic drugs, *NSAID* nonsteroidal anti-inflammatory drugs, *RFA* radiofrequency ablation

Complications

What Are the Important Potential Complications of Surgery for SCFE?

Most patients with SCFE undergo in situ (directly through the growth plate) percutaneous screw fixation of the femoral head. The area for the screw placement is very small, and it is sometimes difficult to obtain purchase across the capital physis into the epiphysis from the femoral neck. If the screw is too long, it may penetrate the hip joint and destroy the cartilage and lead to chondrolysis. If the screw is too short, further slippage may occur, often necessitating additional, more involved surgeries to correct the alignment of the hip. Avascular necrosis of the femoral head due to disruption of the blood supply is also a dreaded complication. This complication may lead to the development of early-onset hip osteoarthritis and a need for hip replacement at a young age.

Area of Controversy

Do Both Hips Require In Situ Screw Fixation in Patients with SCFE?

At the time of presentation, most patients present with unilateral SCFE (80%). Ultimately, bilateral involvement ensues in 10–60% of cases. When a patient presents with unilateral SCFE requiring surgical fixation, some surgeons support prophylactic fixation of the contralateral, unaffected hip. It has been suggested that contralateral fixation should be considered in high-risk patients. Patients with a high risk for slippage of the contralateral hip include those <10 years old, those with endocrinopathies, renal osteodystrophy, or a history of radiation therapy.

Area Where You Can Get in Trouble

Never Miss Septic Arthritis

Most of the conditions in the differential for this case do not require immediate intervention, though symptomatic SCFEs are typically admitted and surgically pinned on an urgent basis. The only exception to this rule is septic arthritis due to bacterial pathogens like *Staphylococcus* or *Streptococcus*, which is a surgical emergency. Irreversible cartilage damage leading to dysfunction of the joint can occur in a matter of hours, so every minute counts. Thus, it is important to investigate and attempt to rule out this diagnosis early in the workup. The patient's history and laboratory values are primarily used to make the diagnosis of septic arthritis. Fever with refusal to move or bear weight on the joint is septic arthritis until proven otherwise. Laboratory values can be used along with the Kocher criteria to confirm the diagnosis. It is also important to note that a negative gram stain does not definitely rule out this diagnosis. Once septic arthritis is suspected, the patient should be taken to the OR for emergent debridement.

Summary of Essentials

History and Physical

- SCFE: Obese, adolescent male aged 10–16 years old presenting with groin pain, painful limp, externally rotated hip, and not irritable with gentle flexion or extension
- Family history of SCFE
- Knee pain is referred from hip pathology in young children until proven otherwise
- Acute or chronic onset

Pathophysiology

- Excess loading across the physis causes slippage of the epiphysis on the metaphysis of the proximal femur in SCFE
- Predisposing factors for weak physis in SCFE: endocrine disorders, prior trauma, osteodystrophy, hypothyroid/hypopituitarism, and hormonal changes during puberty

Workup

- SCFE confirmed by displacement of proximal femoral epiphysis from metaphysis, seen on AP and/or frog lateral view of the hip
- Obtain bilateral hip x-rays. If x-rays are nondiagnostic, order an MRI
- Imaging will reveal a femoral head that is not located in the correct anatomic position and widening of the epiphyseal growth plate
- Rule out septic arthritis (an emergency)

Management

- Ensure the patient is nonweight-bearing
- Admit for urgent in situ surgical pinning of the hip
- In patients that are not great candidates for in-situ pinning of the epiphysis, open reduction is an appropriate alternative
- Prophylactic fixation of the contralateral epiphysis may be indicated if the patient is at high risk of contralateral SCFE
- Short period of protected weight bearing with crutches

Complications

32

- Screw too short or long, inadequate fixation, additional slippage, avascular necrosis, early osteoarthritis of the hip, deformity due to premature epiphyseal plate closure

Acknowledgements The editors would like to acknowledge and thank the following authors for their contributions to the previous edition of the chapter: Tracy Kim Kovach.

Suggested Reading

Katz DA. Slipped capital femoral epiphysis: the importance of early diagnosis. Pediatr Ann. 2006;35(2):102–11.

Kehl DK. Slipped capital femoral epiphysis. In: Lovell WW, Winter RB, Morrissy RT, Weinstein SL, editors. Lovell and Winter's pediatric orthopaedics. 4th ed. Philadelphia: Lippincott, Williams & Wilkins; 1996.

Kocher MS, Zurakowski D, Kasser JR. Differentiating between septic arthritis and transient synovitis of the hip in children: an evidence-based clinical prediction algorithm. J Bone Joint Surg Am. 1999;81(12):1662–70.

Shultz WR, Weinstein JN, Weinstein SL, Smith BG. Prophylactic pinning of the contralateral hip in slipped capital femoral epiphysis: evaluation of long-term outcome for the contralateral hip with use of decision analysis. J Bone Joint Surg Am. 2002;84-A(8):1305–14.

Uglow MG, Clarke NM. The management of slipped capital femoral epiphysis. J Bone Joint Surg Br. 2004;86(5):631–5.

Weinstein SL, Mibarak SJ, Wegner DR. Developmental hip dysplasia and dislocation. J Bone Joint Surg Am. 2003;85:1824–32.

Chronic Right-Hand Pain

Cameron Gerhold, Arezou Yaghoubian, and Kevin W. Rolfe

Contents

C. de Virgilio, A. Grigorian (eds.), *Surgery*, https://doi.org/10.1007/978-3-032-09799-6_33

Case Study

A 45-year-old seamstress presents to the clinic with a 4-year history of paresthesias of the volar right thumb, index, and middle finger with associated pain. She reports that the symptoms are worse at night. She has no past medical history and no history of cancer. On examination, she has decreased sensation on the volar thumb, index, and middle finger as well as the dorsal fingertips and a positive Tinel's sign and Phalen's test at the wrist. Strength in her abductor pollicis brevis is abnormal at 3/5 compared to the contralateral side. She has moderate thenar atrophy but no hypothenar or intrinsic muscle atrophy. The hand is well perfused. There are no surgical or traumatic scars on the hand or wrist. Bilateral radial and ulnar pulses are normal.

Diagnosis

What Is the Differential Diagnosis? (Table 33.1)

Table 33.1 Differential diagnosis of clinical presentation

Etiology	Differential diagnosis
Vascular	Thoracic outlet syndrome, compression of the brachial plexus by ribs or muscle
Infectious	Medical neuropathy (e.g., leprosy, Lyme disease, HIV, hepatitis, post-herpetic neuralgia)
Neoplastic	Pancoast tumor invading the brachial plexus, intracranial neoplasm, peripheral nerve tumor (e.g., schwannoma)
Inflammatory or degenerative	Cervical root pathology (radiculopathy), cervical cord pathology (myelopathy), carpal tunnel syndrome, pronator syndrome, cubital tunnel syndrome, ulnar tunnel (Guyon's canal) syndrome, radial neuropathy
Traumatic	Injury (median nerve, brachial plexus, spinal nerve, or cord), post-traumatic syrinx, CRPS/RSD
Iatrogenic/drugs	Local radiation-induced or systemic chemotherapy-induced plexopathy or neuropathy, injury from prior surgery
Metabolic/endocrine	Diabetic or other medical peripheral neuropathy, including hypothyroidism, vitamin deficiency, heavy metal, or other toxicity
Autoimmune	Multiple sclerosis, Guillain-Barré syndrome, sarcoidosis

HIV human immunodeficiency syndrome, *CRPS* complex regional pain syndrome, *RSD* reflex sympathetic dystrophy

What Clues on History and Physical Examination Might Direct You Toward Specific Diagnoses? (Table 33.2)

Table 33.2 History and physical exam findings

Diagnosis	History and physical
Thoracic outlet syndrome	Positive Adson's or Wright's test, ulnar nerve symptoms most likely
Medical neuropathy (infectious, metabolic, iatrogenic)	Often diffuse and bilateral; history of cancer treatment, HIV, diabetes, nutritional deficiency, or toxic exposure
Traumatic	Acute injury with new onset of symptoms; usually obvious; CRPS/RSD occurs later to a previously injured area that never fully recovered
Autoimmune	Generalized symptoms including diffuse weakness (multiple sclerosis, Guillain-Barré syndrome) or other systemic findings involving lung (sarcoid) or eye (MS)
Cervical root	Dermatomal distribution (vs. peripheral nerve), positive Spurling's test
Cervical myelopathy	Hyperreflexia, hand clumsiness, and gait unsteadiness on exam
Carpal tunnel	Positive Tinel's, Phalen's, or Durkan's test; median distribution of sensory symptoms
Pronator syndrome	Overlaps carpal tunnel, palmar cutaneous branch over thenar eminence also affected
Other compressive neuropathies	Radial or ulnar syndromes affect their respective peripheral nerve distributions or muscles; key is remembering the anatomy and innervation

HIV human immunodeficiency syndrome, *CRPS* complex regional pain syndrome, *RSD* reflex sympathetic dystrophy

What Is the Most Likely Diagnosis?

Carpal tunnel syndrome (CTS). Nighttime dysesthesias in the median nerve distribution without prior injury or congenital defect, particularly in association with isolated thenar muscle wasting, are most likely due to CTS and are highly specific for this clinical entity. However, the differential diagnosis remains very broad, as CTS rarely presents exactly in the median nerve distribution, is often bilateral, and often occurs in association with other overlapping aches, pains, and medical conditions such as diabetes.

History and Physical

What Is the Most Common Nerve Entrapment Syndrome in the Upper Extremity?

CTS. The condition affects approximately 1% of the general population and 5% of the working population engaged in repetitive motion and grasping activities. Reports of prevalence of up to 25% or more have been made for full-time computer operators.

What Are the Major Risk Factors for CTS?

Women are affected 2–3 times more often than men with the most common age range of 40–60 years. Other risk factors include obesity, pregnancy, smoking, activities involving repetitive movements or sustained wrist flexion or extension, rheumatoid arthritis, diabetes, hypothyroidism, and alcohol use disorder.

What Are the Best-Known Classic Signs of CTS?

Tinel's sign and Phalen's test. *Tinel's sign* is elicited by gently percussing over the median nerve at the carpal tunnel. A positive sign is present if the patient describes an electrical shock sensation in the median nerve distribution. *Phalen's test* is performed by having the patient place the dorsal sides of each hand against each other in a position of maximal wrist flexion for 30–60 seconds. The test is considered positive if the patient reports new or worsening paresthesias in the median nerve distribution of the affected hand(s).

Are There Any Other Overlapping Median Nerve Diagnoses to Consider?

Proximal median nerve compression at the elbow is often referred to as pronator teres syndrome, acute CTS, traumatic median nerve injury, or median nerve tumor (e.g., schwannoma).

What Is Acute CTS?

Acute CTS may be seen after a fracture or dislocation of the distal radius or wrist with acute compression of the median nerve. It is an emergency and requires immediate reduction of the fracture or dislocation and often surgical release of the carpal tunnel.

What Physical Exam Finding Helps Distinguish Proximal Median Nerve Compression at the Elbow (Pronator Teres Syndrome) from Compression at the Carpal Tunnel?

The palmar cutaneous branch of the median nerve branches prior to the carpal tunnel and travels above the transverse carpal ligament. It innervates the skin over the thenar eminence. Thus, typical CTS will not show sensory dysesthesias in this area, whereas pronator teres syndrome will.

What Findings Help Distinguish CTS from Cervical Spine Root Pathology?

Much like the straight leg raise for sciatica of the lumbar spine, Spurling's test may be used to elicit cervical root pathology (radiculopathy). The patient is asked to extend the neck and tilt and turn the head laterally to the affected side to determine if the hand dysesthesias occur or worsen with the maneuver. Radiculopathy, often mimicking CTS symptoms, is a clinical diagnosis based on dermatomal patterns of pain or sensory changes. Neuroimaging is typically unnecessary unless conservative management fails. Initial treatment of radiculopathy includes NSAIDs and avoiding provocative maneuvers, with glucocorticoids or epidural corticosteroid injections as second-line options. Other causes of back pain relevant to peripheral neuropathies include ankylosing spondylitis, disc herniation, lumbosacral strain, and spondylolysis. These should be considered in the broader context of axial and radicular pain evaluation.

Watch Out

C-6 and C-7 nerve roots overlap the median nerve distribution to the hand. A key sensory distinction is that CTS does not affect the dorsal hand except for the fingertips. C-6 and C-7 nerve root compression also affects the dorsum of the hand in the radial nerve distribution in addition to the median distribution.

What Is Thoracic Outlet Syndrome and What Physical Exam Tests Distinguish It from Spinal Root Pathology?

Thoracic outlet syndrome (TOS) involves compression of the lower brachial plexus (ulnar symptoms predominate) or compression of the subclavian vessels (vein or artery) between the anterior and middle scalene muscles. This is sometimes associated with a *cervical rib* (obtain chest x-ray to look for this). Two classic tests are used, Adson's and Wright's, both of which are frequently confused with the Spurling's test. *Adson's test* involves extension of the shoulder with the neck turned *toward* the affected side and may reproduce TOS symptoms or a reduction or loss of the radial pulse. *Wright's test* involves abduction and external rotation of the shoulder with the neck rotated *away* from the affected side and may similarly reproduce TOS symptoms or cause reduction or loss of the pulse at the wrist.

Watch Out

Look for a Pancoast tumor of the lung on x-ray if the presentation suggests thoracic outlet syndrome symptoms or brachial plexopathy.

Watch Out

Adhesive capsulitis, also known as frozen shoulder, presents with significant stiffness and pain in the shoulder, often limiting range of motion. Risk factors include diabetes, thyroid disease, and prolonged immobilization.

What About Myelopathy?

Myelopathy, which results from compression of the spinal cord (as opposed to radiculopathy, which compresses nerve roots), is a dangerous and irreversible entity that often presents with hand pain or dysesthesias. It should always be considered, especially when the hand pain does not follow an exact pattern of CTS. Myelopathy typically involves symptoms in both arms or in arms and legs, whereas radiculopathy is usually unilateral. Hyperreflexia (and pathologic reflexes like Hoffmann's or suprapatellars) and heel-toe tandem gait should be checked. The patient may likewise complain of dropping things but also incoordination of the hands for fine motor skills and decreased balance during ambulation. Many patients are referred to hand surgeons for alleged CTS, which is really myelopathy.

What Are Ganglion Cysts?

Ganglion cysts are commonly found at the wrist but can also occur in the lower extremities. They present as firm masses on the dorsal aspect of the wrist joint that transilluminate (indicating fluid). They are smooth and somewhat mobile. They should be distinguished from epidermoid cysts, which have a central punctum, and rheumatoid nodules, which are firm and non-mobile.

Pathophysiology

What Nerve Is Compressed in CTS?

The median nerve is compressed in CTS.

What Is the Motor Distribution of the Median Nerve in the Hand?

Median nerve innervates the thenar muscles (abductor pollicis brevis, flexor pollicis brevis, superficial head; and opponens pollicis) and the two radial lumbricals.

What Is the Sensory Distribution of the Median Nerve in the Hand?

Sensory distribution provides sensation to the radial volar 3½ fingers and dorsal tips (thumb, index, middle, and half of the ring).

> **Watch Out**
> Finger numbering is not used by hand surgeons, as it is unclear. Always label the digits as thumb, index, middle, ring, and small fingers.

What Is the Origin of the Median Nerve from the Cervical Spine Roots?

The origin of the median nerve from the cervical spine roots is C5-T1.

Where Is the Median Nerve Located in the Wrist?

The median nerve is located in the carpal tunnel.

What Are the Boundaries of the Carpal Tunnel?

Carpus dorsally (floor) and transverse carpal ligament volarly (roof). The scaphoid, trapezium, and sheath of flexor carpi radialis form its radial margin. The ulnar boundary consists of the triquetrum, hook of the hamate, and the pisiform.

How Many Structures Course Through the Carpal Tunnel? What Are the Contents of the Carpal Tunnel?

Ten structures (nine tendons and one nerve). Flexor digitorum superficialis (four tendons), flexor digitorum profundus (four tendons), flexor pollicis longus (one tendon), and the median nerve.

> **Watch Out**
> The median nerve is the most *superficial* structure in the carpal tunnel.

What Is the Pathophysiology of CTS and Potential Causes?

The primary cause is compression of the median nerve, typically as a result of an increase in the interstitial pressure in the carpal tunnel. This increased pressure may be due to numerous factors, including hormonal (pregnancy, hypothyroidism), repetitive movements causing trauma/inflammation, and obesity. Women tend to have smaller carpal tunnel sizes.

What Is the Significance of Thenar Wasting?

Since the recurrent motor branch of the median nerve innervates the thenar muscle mass, long-standing or severe CTS can result in denervation of the thenar muscles. The profile of the thenar eminence of both hands as well as the strength of abductor pollicis brevis (palmar abduction) should always be checked.

What Systemic Conditions Are Often Associated with CTS?

Hypothyroidism and Diabetes. One proposed mechanism involves the associated myxedema, which leads to excess deposition of glycosaminoglycans and hyaluronic acid in subcutaneous tissue and the median nerve sheath. Diabetes causes neuropathy, making nerves more susceptible to injury, and tendons in the carpal tunnel to become glycosylated, making them thickened, leaving less space for the median nerve.

Workup

How Is Carpal Tunnel Diagnosed?

Semmes-Weinstein filament testing (as for diabetic or neuropathic feet) is the most sensitive sensory modality to diagnose CTS. Electromyography/nerve conduction studies (EMG/NCS) are useful in equivocal cases, typically due to an uncertain distribution of the symptoms. Classic findings on NCS are increased latencies and decreased conduction velocities across the wrist. EMG is most useful to rule out other pathologies. EMG may show slowing of median sensory or motor nerve conduction velocity at the wrist, prolonged distal motor or sensory latency, or denervation of the abductor pollicis brevis muscle.

Do Any Medical Neuropathies Need to Be Ruled Out?

Several medical causes of neuropathy must be considered and ruled out, including vitamin deficiencies, heavy metal toxicity, infections, and thyroid disease. Recommended studies include vitamin B12 levels (to evaluate for subacute combined degeneration of the spinal cord), rapid plasma reagin for syphilis (tabes dorsalis), HIV testing, thiamine levels (particularly in those with alcohol use), thyroid-stimulating hormone for thyroid dysfunction, antinuclear antibody for autoimmune disease, HbA1c for diabetes, and C-reactive protein for inflammatory conditions. Electromyography and nerve conduction studies should also be obtained. In select cases, a lumbar puncture or nerve biopsy may be indicated. It is important to remember that the diagnosis of CTS may not be straightforward, especially when symptoms present bilaterally, in an atypical nerve distribution, or in elderly patients with multiple comorbidities. Before initiating treatment with gabapentin for presumed medical neuropathy, reversible and treatable causes should first be excluded.

How Is Suspected Cervical Spine Disease Worked Up?

MRI and x-rays of the cervical spine would evaluate root or cord pathology.

Watch Out

If the patient cannot have an MRI due to an incompatible stent, pacemaker, etc., then the test of choice for spinal pathology is a CT *myelogram*. This involves a dural puncture and injection of contrast into the thecal sac to outline the spinal cord and nerve roots. It is not the same as a CT with intravenous contrast injected peripherally.

Management

What Is the Initial Treatment for CTS?

Splinting of the wrist (not hand) in a neutral position. This position affords the lowest pressure in the carpal tunnel. NSAIDs and activity modifications are also first-line treatment modalities.

What Is the Second Line of Treatment?

Carpal tunnel injection with local anesthetic and corticosteroid medication. Response to steroid injection is a good prognostic indicator for improvement with surgery, if required later. Similarly, failure to respond to injection (at least temporarily) suggests surgery is unlikely to improve symptoms.

What Are Indications for Surgical Intervention for CTS?

Failure to respond adequately to conservative nonoperative management or thenar motor involvement is an indication for surgical intervention for CTS.

Watch Out

Thenar atrophy or denervation of the abductor pollicis brevis muscle on EMG should prompt early surgical treatment, as these are late-stage findings and largely irreversible. At this point, surgery should be performed primarily to prevent progression.

What Is the Gold Standard Treatment for CTS?

Carpal tunnel release. This involves surgical cutting of the transverse carpal ligament, the roof of the carpal tunnel. This is performed through a small open incision or endoscopically. Neurolysis or manipulation of the median nerve and its tissue coverings *does not* improve outcomes and is not typically performed.

How Is CTS Associated with Hypothyroidism Managed?

This is initially treated conservatively with splinting of the wrist in a neutral position and NSAIDs while the hypothyroidism is treated. Typically, once the hypothyroidism is resolved, the CTS will improve.

Areas Where You Can Get in Trouble

What Is the "Million-Dollar Nerve"?

The recurrent motor branch of the median nerve can be injured if the transverse carpal tunnel ligament is transected too radially. This nerve has a variable anatomic course and sometimes runs through the ligament without recurring, thereby increasing the risk of its transection. It has been called the million-dollar nerve, as iatrogenic injury to it has led to many million-dollar lawsuits. The thumb will show greatly impaired function if the nerve is injured.

Summary of Essentials

History

- Sensory dysesthesias in the median nerve distribution ($3^1/_2$ radial digits volar and dorsal tips), dropping things, symptoms worse at nighttime, job or activity involving repetitive movements of the hand/wrist

Physical Exam

- Tinel's and Phalen's
- Check for thenar atrophy

Pathophysiology

- Majority of cases are idiopathic involving synovial inflammation and increased pressure within the carpal tunnel

Diagnosis

- Diagnosis is clinically based on history and exam
- Equivocal cases should prompt EMG/NCS
- Rule out spinal disease with MRI and medical neuropathies with laboratory testing as indicated based on history and exam

Management

- NSAIDs, wrist splinting, carpal tunnel injection
- Surgical release (open or endoscopic) for cases that fail conservative treatment or if muscle involvement (thenar wasting) is present

Additional Important Facts

- Beware of overlooking myelopathy or Pancoast tumor
- Beware of overlooking a treatable peripheral neuropathy (e.g., syphilis, HIV, vitamin deficiency, heavy metal toxicity, cancer, rheumatologic condition, diabetes, thyroid disease)
- Beware of acute carpal tunnel syndrome, an emergency occurring after acute fracture or dislocation

Suggested Reading

Bland JD. Carpal tunnel syndrome. BMJ. 2007;335:43.

MacDermid JC, Wessel J. Clinical diagnosis of carpal tunnel syndrome: a systematic review. J Hand Ther. 2004;17:309.

Wipperman J, Goerl K. Carpal Tunnel Syndrome: Diagnosis and Management. Am Fam Physician. 2016;94(12):993–999.

Orthopedic

Question Set: Orthopedic Surgery

Questions

1. A 22-year-old man presents to the clinic with right thigh pain that has worsened over the last two weeks. He was involved in a motor vehicle accident six weeks ago and sustained a femoral shaft fracture treated with intramedullary nailing. He completed an inpatient rehabilitation program and has been ambulating with assistance. On physical exam, there is a firm, mobile, and tender mass over the lateral thigh with overlying skin induration. Passive range of motion at the hip is limited due to pain. Laboratory studies show an elevated alkaline phosphatase level and mildly increased erythrocyte sedimentation rate (ESR). X-ray of the thigh shows a well-circumscribed, calcified, soft tissue mass adjacent to the femur. Which of the following is the most likely diagnosis?
   (A) Soft tissue sarcoma
   (B) Osteomyelitis
   (C) Myositis ossificans
   (D) Hematoma
   (E) Desmoid tumor

2. An 18-year-old soccer player presents to her doctor two days after getting kicked in the knee during her championship game. She reports hearing a snap immediately after the injury, but her knee looked normal. The next day, she had a swollen kneecap with progressive pain. On physical exam, she has medial joint line tenderness and effusion. Her doctor notices an audible snap occurring when extending the knee from a fully flexed position while applying tibial torsion. What is the most likely diagnosis?
   (A) Collateral ligament tear
   (B) Anterior cruciate ligament (ACL) tear
   (C) Stress fracture
   (D) Tendon displacement
   (E) Meniscus tear

3. A 32-year-old housekeeper comes to the physician for hip pain localized to the lateral aspect of the hip. The hip pain is interrupting her sleep. She denies any muscle weakness or numbness and tingling. The pain is not worse with physical activity. On physical exam, there is tenderness to palpation on the lateral aspect of her hip while in the lateral decubitus position. Which of the following is the most likely etiology of the hip pain?
   (A) Hip osteoarthritis
   (B) Meralgia paresthetica
   (C) Trochanteric bursitis
   (D) Osteonecrosis
   (E) Hip fracture

4. A 17-year-old male comes to the emergency department for the third time over the last month due to pain in his right thigh above his knee that is particularly bothersome at night. He was previously diagnosed with growing pains. Now he has developed swelling above his right knee and states his pain is worse. On physical exam, there is a soft tissue mass that is tender to palpation. The skin overlying the mass is erythematous. An X-ray is obtained and shows a "sunburst" pattern in the distal femur. What is the most likely diagnosis?
   (A) Ewing's sarcoma
   (B) Osteosarcoma
   (C) Osteomyelitis

(D) Osteochondroma
(E) Osteoid osteoma

5. A 35-year-old female telemarketer presents with complaints of pain in her right wrist for the past 6 months. She also reports having numbness in her right hand that occurs with wrist flexion or extension. For the past month, she has been receiving corticosteroid injections after her doctor diagnosed her with carpal tunnel syndrome (CTS). However, her pain has dramatically increased over the past week and has started to affect her job performance. Her mother has rheumatoid arthritis. Her hand appears to be swollen and is tender to palpation. She is scheduled for a synovial fluid aspiration. Which of the following findings in the aspirate would indicate surgical intervention?
(A) Glucose of 90 mg/dL
(B) White blood cell (WBC) of 200 cells/μL
(C) High abundance of rheumatoid factor
(D) Negatively birefringent crystals
(E) Thick yellow-green fluid

6. An 11-year-old boy presents to his pediatrician because his mother is concerned that he has been limping for the past three days. He states that he is limping because of a dull, aching pain in the right groin and thigh that extends down to his right knee. He has no history of preceding trauma. The pain is increased by physical activity. On physical exam, there is a shift of the torso over the affected hip with standing. Which of the following explains this physical exam finding?
(A) Weakness in hip abduction
(B) Weakness in hip flexion
(C) Weakness in hip extension
(D) Weakness in knee extension
(E) Weakness in knee flexion

7. A 45-year-old male with alcohol use disorder presents with fevers and right-hand pain. He cannot recall what happened but thinks he may have punched someone in the face during a bar fight two days earlier. He has tried over-the-counter anti-inflammatory agents, but they have not helped decrease the pain. His temperature is 37.7 °C, blood pressure is 132/88 mmHg, and pulse is 78/min. On physical exam, he has a skin break over his second phalanx–metacarpal region. He is holding his second finger in slight flexion. He has a sausage-shaped swelling of the finger, as well as flexor tendon sheath tenderness that extends the entire length of the tendon. His pain increases with passive motion of the finger. What is the most likely diagnosis?
(A) Suppurative tenosynovitis due to *Eikenella corrodens*
(B) Gout
(C) Dupuytren's contracture
(D) Suppurative tenosynovitis due to *Pasteurella multocida*
(E) Felon

8. A five-year-old boy is brought to the pediatrician because of left knee pain that is causing him to limp. His history is significant for severe asthma. He was recently hospitalized for a severe exacerbation requiring a prolonged steroid taper. On physical exam, his temperature is 37.6 °C, blood pressure is 88/56 mmHg, pulse is 76/min, and respirations are 16/min. He has a normal knee exam. Labs are drawn and show WBC of $7.4 \times 10^3/\mu L$ (normal $4.1–10.9 \times 10^3/\mu L$) and hemoglobin of 12.7 g/dL (12–15 g/dL). ESR and C-reactive protein (CRP) are within normal limits. Which of the following is the most likely diagnosis?
(A) Septic arthritis
(B) Osteomyelitis
(C) Slipped capital femoral epiphysis (SCFE)
(D) Torn anterior cruciate ligament (ACL)
(E) Osteonecrosis of the hip

9. A college athlete presents with shoulder pain. He reports that he was injured during basketball practice two days ago when his teammate ran into his shoulder. On physical examination, he has an edematous left shoulder. The clinician passively abducts the patient's shoulders to 90° and flexes to 30° while asking the patient to point his thumbs down. The patient is unable to smoothly lower the arm. What muscle is the clinician trying to evaluate?
   (A) Supraspinatus
   (B) Infraspinatus
   (C) Teres minor
   (D) Teres major
   (E) Subscapularis

10. A 45-year-old Internet insurance salesman presents to his doctor with progressive pain in his left hand for one year. His pain is primarily limited to the left thumb and index finger. After finishing the physical examination, his doctor believes he has carpal tunnel syndrome (CTS). Which of the following did the doctor most likely find on physical examination to support this diagnosis?
   (A) Percussing the wrist elicits pain in all five fingers and the palmar surface
   (B) Pain felt along the left thumb, index, and middle finger when placing the elbow on a table and flexing the wrist for 60 seconds
   (C) Pain felt along the left thumb, index, middle finger, and palmar surface when placing the elbow on a table and flexing the wrist for 60 seconds
   (D) Radial deviation of the wrist upon wrist flexion
   (E) Posterior and lateral forearm sensory deficit

11. A two-week-old female born at 39 weeks gestation to a 36-year-old G2P1 female via normal spontaneous vaginal delivery comes to her pediatrician for her two-week well-baby exam. The birth was unremarkable, and the baby went home with her mother after two days. She received prenatal care starting at 10 weeks gestation and had a normal, healthy pregnancy with no issues. On physical exam, as the hip is gently adducted and posterior pressure is applied, there is a palpable clunk. Which of the following is the next step in management?
   (A) Reexamine at one-month exam
   (B) CT scan of the hips
   (C) X-ray of the hips
   (D) Reassurance
   (E) Ultrasound of the hips

12. A 45-year-old woman presents with pain in her right hand for two days. She reports falling down and attempting to break her fall with an outstretched hand. Physical examination is significant only for pain in the anatomic snuffbox of her right hand. She has no motor weakness or sensory deficits. What is the most appropriate next step in management?
   (A) Radiograph of hand and if normal, recommend supportive care with follow-up
   (B) Radiograph of hand and if even if normal, recommend thumb spica cast with follow-up
   (C) Thumb spica cast without radiograph
   (D) Supportive care without radiograph
   (E) CT scan of hand

13. An 88-year-old woman is brought in by ambulance after falling in her house. She complains of right hip pain. On physical exam, her temperature is 37.6 °C, blood pressure is 110/75 mmHg, pulse is 110/min, and respirations are 20/min. The leg appears externally rotated and shortened. X-ray shows femoral neck fracture. Which of the following is a complication of femoral neck fracture?
   (A) Avascular necrosis (AVN)
   (B) Lumbar radiculopathy
   (C) Long-term loss of hip abduction

motor vehicle accident. This should be considered if the patient presents with chest pain and/or hemodynamic instability. Given his age, the bruit heard in his chest is unlikely to be related to underlying cardiovascular disease. For these reasons, an echocardiogram is not indicated (E).

22. Answer A

Pregnant patients with preeclampsia or eclampsia that present with an inability to move the arm following a seizure are most likely suffering from a posterior shoulder dislocation. These are rare and occur most often in patients that have had generalized seizures or have been electrocuted. Pregnant patients suffering from eclampsia are also at risk because of its association with seizures. Regular anteroposterior radiographs will often miss the diagnosis, and so patients suspected of having a posterior dislocation should receive *axillary and lateral view* radiographs. The axillary view is essential for diagnosis as it can help estimate the size of the defect in the humeral head. If radiographs are equivocal, a CT scan can be ordered next (C). MRI is considered for older patients with shoulder dislocation as they are more likely to have concurrent rotator cuff injury (B). Reassurance is not appropriate for shoulder dislocation (E). Most patients are able to manage a shoulder dislocation with nonoperative therapy (D).

23. Answer D

The patient is most likely exhibiting slipped capital femoral epiphysis (SCFE), which affects obese adolescent males. In SCFE, the femoral head separates from the neck and slips posteriorly, resulting in a limp and impaired internal rotation. Patients often present with knee pain, so a high index of suspicion is necessary to diagnose SCFE. The physical exam finding includes altered gait such that the patient takes a short step on the affected side to minimize weight-bearing due to pain and tenderness to palpation at the anterior hip. The diagnosis of SCFE is made with X-rays, which show the classic "ice cream slipping off the cone" suggesting posterior displacement of the femoral head. Obesity seems to be the strongest risk factor for SCFE, likely due to excessive mechanical stress on the physis (growth plate). Weight loss can be beneficial to the overall health of the child and will decrease the risk of SCFE in the contralateral hip but is not considered a definitive management intervention for SCFE (C). Treatment involves operative stabilization using pinning of the hip joint. Supportive therapy with rest and ibuprofen would be the appropriate treatment for transient synovitis (A). Aspiration of the synovial fluid along with appropriate antibiotic therapy would be the treatment for septic arthritis (B). Pavlik harness is used in the management of developmental dysplasia of the hip to keep the hip in a flexed and abducted position (E).

Pediatric

Steven L. Lee

Contents

Full-Term Male Infant with Respiratory Distress

Veronica F. Sullins and Steven L. Lee

Contents

C. de Virgilio, A. Grigorian (eds.), *Surgery*, https://doi.org/10.1007/978-3-032-09799-6_34

Case Study

A full-term male infant becomes cyanotic immediately after birth. His mother states she had no access to prenatal care. Her pregnancy was otherwise uncomplicated. On examination, the newborn is tachypneic and tachycardic, and his oxygen saturation is 75%. He is grunting and has supracostal retractions. He has a barrel-shaped chest with decreased breath sounds on the left side. His abdomen is scaphoid, and his heartbeat is displaced to the right. The amniotic fluid is clear.

Diagnosis

What Is the Differential Diagnosis of Surgical Causes of Neonatal Respiratory Distress? (Table 34.1)

Table 34.1 Differential diagnosis of surgical causes of neonatal respiratory distress

Diagnosis	Comments
Choanal atresia	Neonates are obligate nasal breathers; inability to pass a nasogastric tube suggests diagnosis
Congenital diaphragmatic hernia	Bowel loops visible in the thoracic cavity on chest radiograph; scaphoid abdomen and mediastinal shift are common
Pulmonary cystic lesions	Cystic lesion may represent congenital cystic adenomatoid malformation (CCAM), bronchopulmonary sequestration, or congenital lobar emphysema (CLE); each may cause mass effect and respiratory distress
Esophageal atresia +/− tracheo-esophageal fistula (TEF)	Associated with excessive salivation, choking with feeds, and inability to pass an orogastric tube; abdominal gas pattern may suggest distal fistula
Mediastinal lesions	Diagnosed incidentally or patient develops infected cyst, secondary mass effects if large enough; includes bronchogenic cysts and mediastinal masses
Pneumothorax	Decreased breath sounds on affected side with collapsed lung on CXR

CXR chest X-ray

What Is the Most Likely Diagnosis?

Congenital diaphragmatic hernia (CDH). The constellation of severe respiratory distress in a full-term neonate with decreased breath sounds on the left and a scaphoid abdomen should be highly suspicious for this condition, and a chest radiograph will confirm the diagnosis (Fig. 34.1). A scaphoid abdomen describes a sunken abdominal wall with a concave, rather than normal convex shape. It implies a smaller volume of abdominal contents than normal and may also be seen in cases of proximal bowel obstruction and malnutrition. In CDH, the abdomen is scaphoid because the intra-abdominal contents have herniated into the chest.

What Cardiac Lesion Can Mimic Respiratory Distress in a Neonate?

A ventricular septal defect (VSD) can present with respiratory distress in a neonate due to left-to-right intracardiac shunting. This leads to right ventricular volume overload, increased left atrial preload, and enlargement of the left-sided chambers. A holosystolic murmur at the left lower sternal border is characteristic, and chest radiograph may show an enlarged cardiac silhouette.

What Are the Most Common Causes of Neonatal Respiratory Distress?

It is important to note that the most common causes of neonatal respiratory distress are not surgical. Transient tachypnea of the newborn, a benign condition,

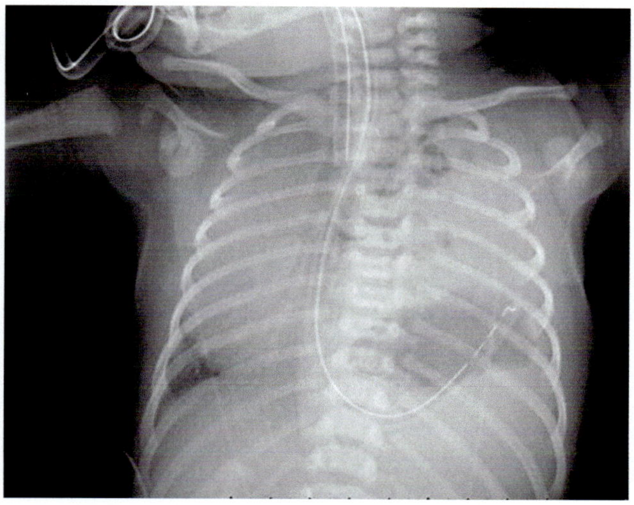

Fig. 34.1 Chest radiograph of an infant with CDH

accounts for more than 40% of cases. It results from delayed clearance of fetal lung fluid and typically presents with diffuse parenchymal infiltrates and a "wet silhouette" around the heart on chest radiograph. Symptoms usually resolve within a few hours to several days. In premature infants, the most common cause of respiratory distress is respiratory distress syndrome (hyaline membrane disease) due to insufficient surfactant production by type II alveolar cells. Chest radiograph typically demonstrates homogenous ground-glass opacities with air bronchograms. In term or post-term infants, meconium aspiration syndrome is a frequent cause, often associated with meconium-stained amniotic fluid. Other, less common, causes include persistent pulmonary hypertension, neonatal pneumonia, and nonpulmonary conditions such as congenital cardiac or renal anomalies.

History and Physical

What Is the Significance of the Supracostal Retractions and Grunting?

Grunting and costal retractions (subcostal, intercostal, or supracostal) indicate ongoing or impending severe respiratory distress and should alert the clinician to impending cardiorespiratory collapse. Patients of all ages who exhibit signs of severe respiratory compromise should be intubated and placed on mechanical ventilation.

What Information Does the Pulmonary Examination Provide?

Decreased or absent breath sounds in a newborn may be due to abnormal lung development as seen with pulmonary agenesis or bronchial atresia. Alternately, there may be a pneumothorax or a space-occupying lesion as in CDH, teratoma, bronchopulmonary sequestration, and bronchogenic cyst.

Why Is the Heartbeat Displaced?

A displaced heartbeat occurs when a space-occupying lesion has enough volume to shift the mediastinum toward the contralateral side. Frequently a barrel-shaped chest will accompany this finding.

Why Is the Absence of Prenatal Care Important?

The majority of CDH is diagnosed prenatally by maternal ultrasound or, less commonly, fetal MRI. CDH can be successfully diagnosed as early as 15 weeks gestation; however, most are diagnosed by 24 weeks. Ultrasound findings such as bowel loops within the thoracic cavity or a mediastinal shift toward the contralateral side are diagnostic. Therefore, the absence of prenatal care should alert the physician of the possibility of a malformation that is typically diagnosed in utero.

What Is a Common Benign Cause of Stridor in Newborns?

Laryngomalacia is the most common cause of chronic stridor in infants. It presents with inspiratory stridor that worsens in the supine position and improves when prone. Laryngoscopy shows collapse of the supraglottic structures during inspiration. Although most cases resolve by 18 months, concurrent gastroesophageal reflux should be treated if present.

Pathophysiology

What Is Thought to Be the Etiology of CDH?

CDH results from failure of the septum transversum to completely divide the pleural and coelomic (later becomes the peritoneal) cavities during fetal development. Fusion of this diaphragmatic precursor is usually completed posteriorly by the twelfth week of gestation. Herniation of intra-abdominal contents occurs during a critical period of lung development when the pulmonary arteries and bronchi are branching. Pulmonary hypoplasia results from decreased pulmonary mass and bronchiolar branching as well as dysfunctional surfactant production.

Watch Out
In CDH, pulmonary hypoplasia occurs in *both* lungs.

Are There Different Type of CDHs?

Approximately 85% of CDH occurs on the left side, 10% on the right side, and <5% bilaterally. The most common variant is a posterolateral defect, known as a Bochdalek hernia. Anteromedial defects, or Morgagni hernias, are much rarer and occur in a parasternal or retrosternal location. Most Morgagni hernias are asymptomatic and less severe and do not therefore present with neonatal respiratory compromise. They are more likely to present later in childhood or early adulthood with gastrointestinal symptoms or obstruction.

How Is Fetal Blood Shunted Away from Pulmonary Circulation in Utero?

In utero, high pressure in the fetal pulmonary vasculature causes blood to flow away from pulmonary circulation and into systemic circulation. This is achieved through two fetal shunts. Most blood entering the right atrium is shunted through the foramen ovale into the left atrium, away from the right ventricle and lungs. Blood pumped into the pulmonary arteries from the right ventricle is shunted away from the pulmonary arterial tree and the lungs into systemic circulation through the ductus arteriosus, which connects the main pulmonary artery to the aortic arch and is just distal to the left subclavian artery.

What Are the Changes That Occur During Childbirth That Allow the Neonate to Transition to Breathing Air?

When a newborn takes the first breath of air, the pulmonary vascular bed transitions from a high resistance to a low resistance system leading to more oxygenated blood reaching the left atrium, which increases left atrial pressure relative to the right atrium. Blood flow then reverses across the foramen ovale, which subsequently closes. The increase in oxygen concentration in the blood causes a local decrease in prostaglandins and subsequent closure of the ductus arteriosus. Thus, both shunts close leading to the standard adult circulation.

How Is This Transition Affected By CDH?

Herniation of the abdominal contents into the thoracic cavity causes pulmonary hypoplasia on the ipsilateral side and to the contralateral side. The mediastinum is shifted, thereby compressing the contralateral lung. Pulmonary hypoplasia combined with the muscular hyperplasia of the pulmonary arterial tree causes high resistance in the pulmonary arterial bed that does not reverse with the infant's first breath. The resultant hypoxemia, acidosis, and hypotension cause pulmonary vasoconstriction, worsening the patient's pulmonary hypertension. In summary, pulmonary hypertension results in decreased pulmonary blood flow and hypoxia, and pulmonary hypoplasia results in decreased gas exchange and carbon dioxide retention.

Are There Associated Anomalies?

Approximately 50–60% of affected infants have isolated CDH. CDH is considered complex when it exists in conjunction with other associated anomalies including structural malformations, chromosomal abnormalities, and single-gene mutations (▫ Table 34.2).

▫ **Table 34.2** Most common anomalies associated with CDH

Associated anomalies	Incidence
Malrotation or nonrotation	60–100%
Cardiovascular	63%
VSD/ASD	
Hypoplastic left heart	
Genitourinary	18–23%
Undescended or ectopic testes	
Ectopic or horse shoe kidney	
Limb	10–16%
Polydactyly	
Syndactyly	
Central nervous system	10–14%
Neural tube defects	
Hydrocephalus	
Chromosomal abnormality	10%
Trisomy 13, 18, or 21	
Single-gene/chromosome defect	

VSD ventricular septal defect, *ASD* atrial septal defect

Workup

What Is the Best Initial Diagnostic Test?

A chest X-ray. In meconium aspiration syndrome or pneumonia, chest X-ray may show patchy atelectasis or consolidation. By placing an orogastric (OG) tube prior to the X-ray, many surgical causes for newborn respiratory distress can be identified or ruled out. If the OG tube curls up in the upper esophagus, this is highly suggestive of esophageal atresia with or without a TEF. In CDH, the tip of the tube may be seen in the thoracic cavity. If the hernia is on the left side, air- or fluid-filled bowel loops may be seen above the diaphragm. If the lesion is on the right side, the liver may be seen as a soft tissue mass in the thoracic cavity with absence of the normally seen intra-abdominal liver shadow. The heart and other mediastinal structures are shifted to the contralateral side, compressing the lung. Similarly, there will be abnormal lung fields in primary pulmonary lesions, such as CCAM, CLE, pulmonary atresia, bronchogenic cysts, and pulmonary agenesis. Choanal atresia can be diagnosed by inability to pass a nasogastric (NG) tube. A diagnostic algorithm for surgical causes of newborn respiratory distress is shown in ◘ Fig. 34.2.

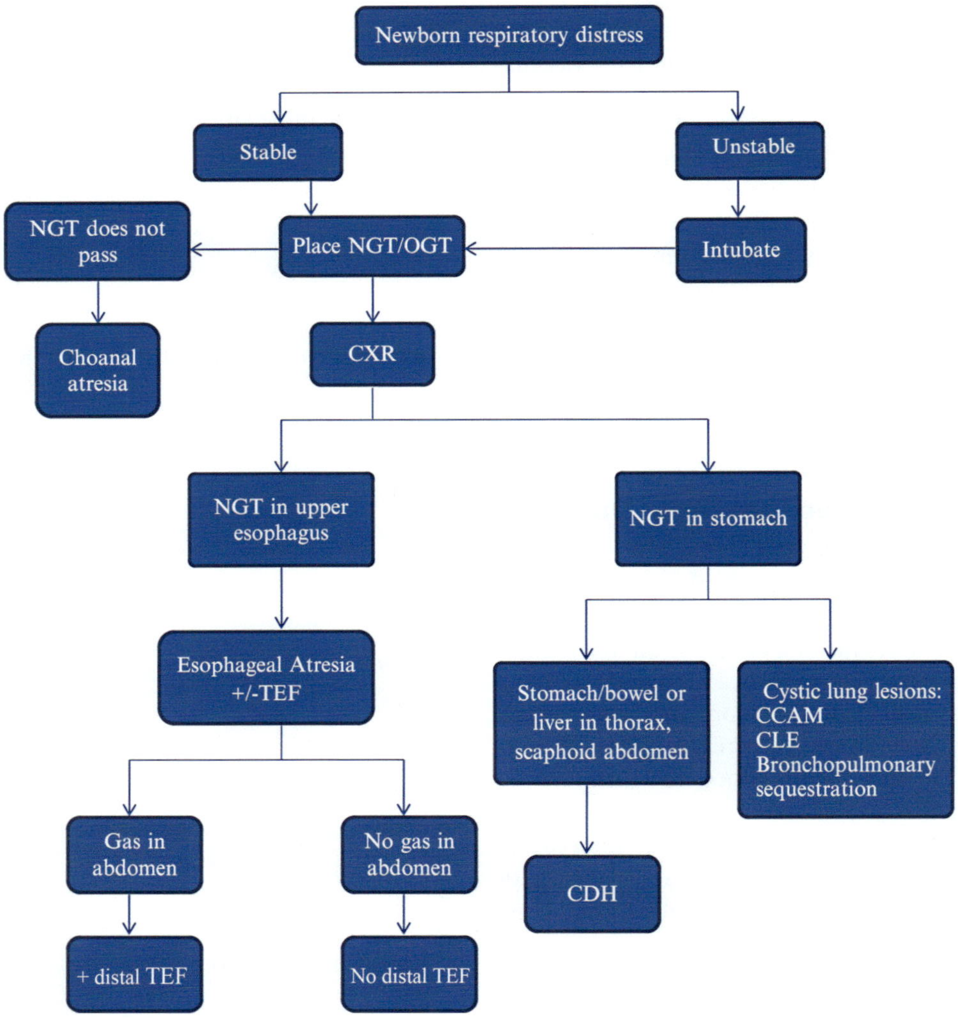

◘ **Fig. 34.2** Diagnostic algorithm for surgical causes of neonatal respiratory distress

Management

What Is the Most Important Step in Clinical Management?

Newborns with respiratory distress should be immediately intubated. An OG tube should be placed to low continuous suction to decompress the stomach and proximal small bowel and to help available lung tissue expand further. To minimize injury to remaining lung tissue, low-pressure ventilation settings should be used. Neonatal ICU admission and blood pressure support should be initiated as necessary.

What Type of Ventilation Is Recommended? What if the Patient Cannot Be Adequately Oxygenated and/or Ventilated?

If standard mechanical ventilation is inadequate, high-frequency oscillatory ventilation is often utilized as it permits lower airway pressures and less lung damage. If this is unsuccessful, the patient is placed on extracorporeal membrane oxygenation (ECMO). With standard ECMO, a cannula is placed into the jugular vein and another into the carotid artery.

What Is the Timing of Surgical Repair?

In the early era of surgical management of patients with CDH, surgery was performed immediately to repair the diaphragmatic defect. However, overall survival did not improve beyond 50%. The goal in management of CDH is supporting lung function because survival is directly related to the degree of pulmonary hypoplasia and pulmonary hypertension. Repairing the diaphragm will not improve pulmonary function. Patients with mild symptoms requiring minimal support likely have little or no pulmonary hypertension and may undergo surgical repair after just 48–72 hours. However, in most patients, the timing of surgery is *generally delayed*. It is important to provide cardiopulmonary support and avoid lung injury while awaiting lung maturation and reversal of pulmonary hypertension. In most cases, time will improve lung function.

> **Watch Out**
> Associated anomalies are common, and therefore an appropriate family history, examination, and workup with *echocardiogram*, limb radiographs, and renal and cranial ultrasounds are required prior to definitive surgical repair of the diaphragmatic defect.

Area Where You Can Get in Trouble

Initial Intubation

The infant should be intubated as quickly as possible. Every effort should be made to avoid blow-by oxygen or bag-mask ventilation prior to endotracheal intubation as these can worsen lung compression and mediastinal shift by filling the herniated stomach/intestines with additional air. In addition, any delay in securing an airway may worsen hypoxia and acidosis, thereby increasing the risk of persistent pulmonary hypertension.

Area of Controversy

Type of Repair: Open Versus Minimally Invasive Surgery (MIS)

Recently, with improvements in minimally invasive surgery (MIS) techniques and technology, CDH repairs have been successfully performed thoracoscopically with encouraging reports of less pain, earlier recovery, and shorter length of hospitalization. However, there remain some concerns over hernia recurrence with the MIS technique. To date, most evidence is based on retrospective review, and selection bias limits comparative data. Although no consensus currently exists, it has been suggested that the MIS approach be reserved for stable patients with isolated CDH (no additional anomalies), delayed presentation, and small diaphragmatic defects (not requiring patch repair).

Prognosis

What Is the Prognosis for CDH? What Are the Factors Affecting Prognosis?

Overall mortality has improved since the development of extracorporeal membrane oxygenation (ECMO) and surgical repair with current survival rates between 60% and 80%. Mortality is directly related to the degree of pulmonary hypoplasia and pulmonary hypertension as well as the presence of congenital anomalies.

Summary of Essentials

History, Physical Examination, and Diagnosis

- The most common causes of newborn respiratory distress are not surgical
- Grunting and costal retractions and abnormal vital signs indicate severe respiratory compromise
- Severe respiratory distress with absent breath sounds and a scaphoid abdomen suggests CDH; this is typically diagnosed in utero by prenatal ultrasound

Etiology/Pathophysiology

- The majority occur on the left side and the most common defect is posterolateral or Bochdalek hernia
- Herniation of abdominal contents results in bilateral pulmonary hypoplasia
- Pulmonary hypertension → decreased pulmonary blood flow and hypoxia; pulmonary hypoplasia → decreased gas exchange and carbon dioxide retention
- Common associated anomalies: chromosomal defects, rotational, cardiac (VSD/ASD), central nervous system, limb, and genitourinary defects
- Mortality directly related to degree of pulmonary hypoplasia and pulmonary hypertension and presence of congenital anomalies

Management

- Immediate intubation with ventilator support is necessary to avoid worsening lung compression
- Survival directly related to the degree of pulmonary hypoplasia and pulmonary hypertension
- Delay surgery to allow lungs to mature and for pulmonary hypertension to improve or reverse
- Evaluate for other anomalies prior to surgery

Acknowledgements The editors would like to acknowledge and thank the following author for their contributions to the previous edition of the chapter: Rivfka Shenoy.

Suggested Reading

Dingemann C, Ure B, Dingemann J. Thoracoscopic procedures in pediatric surgery: what's the evidence? Eur J Pediatr Surg. 2014;24(1):14–9.

Fauza DO, Wilson JM. Congenital diaphragmatic hernia and associated anomalies: incidence, identification, and impact on prognosis. J Pediatr Surg. 1994;29(8):1113–7.

Haroon J, Chamberlain RS. An evidence-based review of the current treatment of congenital diaphragmatic hernia. Clin Pediatr. 2013;52(2):115–24.

Infant with Bilious Emesis

James McDermott, Veronica F. Sullins, and Steven L. Lee

Contents

C. de Virgilio, A. Grigorian (eds.), *Surgery*, https://doi.org/10.1007/978-3-032-09799-6_35

> **Case Study**
>
> A 7-month-old male infant presents with two episodes of green emesis, lethargy, oliguria, and decreased stool output. The mother states he was a full-term baby with no prior illnesses or surgery. He fed normally for months until the day prior to presentation. His last normal bowel movement was 24 hours ago. His heart rate is slightly elevated. He is normotensive and afebrile. He is lethargic but otherwise has a normal physical examination. His abdomen is soft, nontender, and nondistended.

Diagnosis

What Is the Differential Diagnosis for Bilious Emesis in an Infant? (◘ Table 35.1)

◘ **Table 35.1** Differential diagnosis for bilious emesis in an infant

Diagnosis	Specific findings
Adhesions	Prior abdominal surgery, dilated loops of bowel with a transition point to decompressed bowel on contrast study
Enteric duplication cyst	Fluid-filled structure not contiguous with stomach or small bowel on MRI/US
Gastroenteritis	History of fever, diarrhea, initial nonbilious emesis, diagnosis of exclusion
Hirschsprung's disease	Transition zone (caliber change) on contrast enema, absence of ganglion cells with hypertrophied nerve trunks on rectal biopsy
Ileus secondary to other medical diseases	Metabolic derangements, electrolyte abnormalities, sepsis, multiple etiologies
Incarcerated inguinal hernia	Inguinal hernia with evidence of incarceration on physical exam
Intussusception	Target sign on US, possible preceding viral upper respiratory illness, "currant-jelly" stool
Malrotation with midgut volvulus	"Corkscrew" appearance of duodenum on contrast UGI, misplaced ligament of Treitz
Duodenal atresia	Double bubble sign on ultrasound or radiograph, vomiting within hours of birth, epigastric distension, associated with Down syndrome

MRI magnetic resonance imaging, *US* ultrasound, *UGI* upper gastrointestinal study

How Does Age Affect the Differential Diagnosis of Bilious Emesis? (◘ Table 35.2)

◘ **Table 35.2** Differential diagnosis of bilious emesis by age

All ages[a]	Adhesions
	Hirschsprung's disease
	Incarcerated inguinal hernia
	Malrotation with midgut volvulus
Neonate (0–1 month)	Annular pancreas
	Duodenal atresia
	Imperforate anus
	Jejunoileal/colonic atresia
	Meconium ileus/plug
	Necrotizing enterocolitis
Infant (1–24 months)	Intussusception
Child (2–12 years)	Ileus secondary to appendicitis
	Intussusception

[a]In all ages, underlying sepsis or metabolic derangements may lead to ileus and bilious vomiting

What Is the Diagnosis?

Malrotation with midgut volvulus (◘ Fig. 35.1) should always be suspected in any infant or child presenting with bilious vomiting. While over half of children with malrotation present with volvulus (the twisting of the small bowel around its mesentery leading to intestinal ischemia) before the first month of age, one-third can present between 1 and 12 months.

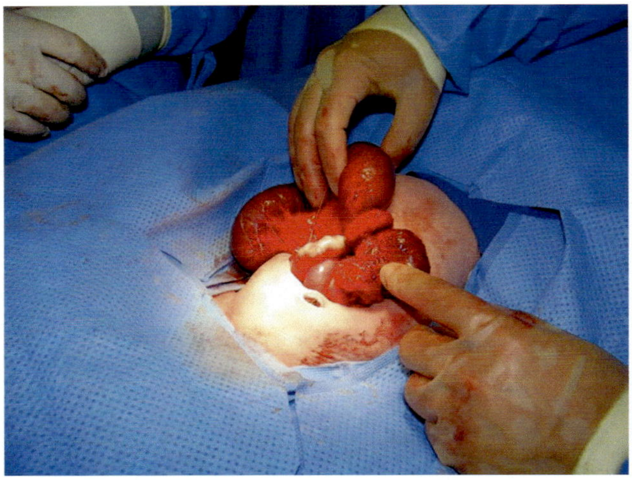

Fig. 35.1 Photograph of malrotation with midgut volvulus

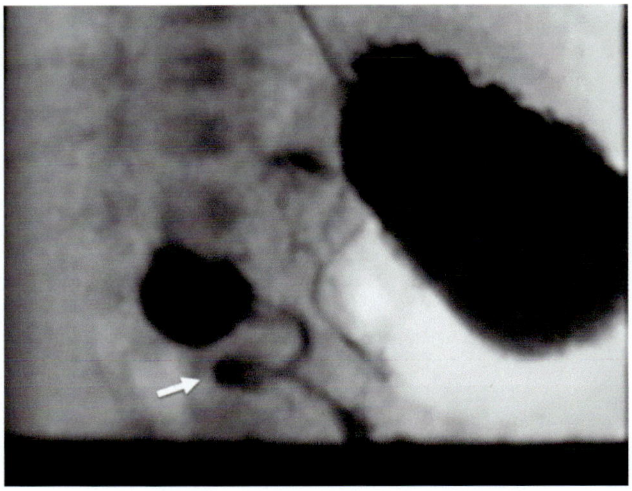

Fig. 35.2 UGI contrast study with small bowel follow-through

35

History and Physical

Why Is It Important to Distinguish Between Bilious and Nonbilious Vomiting in an Infant?

Bilious emesis, defined as green or yellow vomitus, should always be considered a sign of a surgically correctable lesion until proven otherwise. Nonbilious emesis suggests an obstruction proximal to the ampulla of Vater, such as pyloric stenosis, whereas bilious emesis indicates that the obstruction lies distal to this point. Differentiating between proximal and distal causes helps guide the appropriate diagnostic evaluation.

Workup

What Is the First Imaging Study to Obtain?

Given that the patient is hemodynamically stable, the first study to obtain is a plain abdominal radiograph. While plain radiographs are rarely diagnostic in midgut volvulus, they may reveal free air under the diaphragm, consistent with bowel perforation. If there is evidence of perforation, no additional studies are needed, and the patient should be taken to the operating room for urgent laparotomy. The film may demonstrate other diagnoses, such as bowel obstruction; in that case, the pattern of distended bowel loops and the distribution of gas can help determine whether the patient has a proximal (duodenum or proximal jejunum) or distal (ileum or colon) obstruction, which will then guide further workup based on the differential diagnosis.

What Is the Next Step in Diagnosis?

If no free perforation is seen, an upper gastrointestinal (UGI) contrast series (Fig. 35.2) should be obtained to visualize the duodenum and proximal small intestine. In cases of malrotation with volvulus, the UGI will typically show all of the small bowel positioned to the right of the midline. If the volvulus has spontaneously untwisted, the UGI will still be abnormal and indicate malrotation if the duodenojejunal junction is to the right of the spine (it is usually on the left).

Pathophysiology

What Defines the Midgut?

The midgut is the portion of the gut receiving blood supply from the superior mesenteric artery (SMA). In a fully developed fetus, it extends from the second part of the duodenum to two-thirds of the way across the transverse colon. The foregut structures are supplied by the celiac axis, and the hindgut structures are supplied by the inferior mesenteric artery.

What Is the Normal Developmental Sequence of Events of the Human Midgut?

During the sixth week of gestation, the midgut elongates rapidly and temporarily herniates into the umbilical cord. At this stage, it rotates 90° counterclockwise around the SMA, positioning the proximal limb (small bowel) on the right and the distal limb (colon) on the left side of the artery. Between the 10th and 12th week of gestation, the midgut returns into the abdominal cavity. The proximal limb passes behind the SMA and anchors to the left as the duodenojejunal flexure (ligament of Treitz), while the distal limb rotates an additional 180° counterclockwise, positioning the cecum in the right lower quadrant and the transverse colon anterior to the SMA. The duodenum and ascending colon then fix in retroperitoneal positions. Proper midgut rotation establishes a broad mesenteric base from the ligament of Treitz to the ileocecal junction, securing attachment to the posterior abdominal wall.

What Is the Etiology of Malrotation?

Malrotation results from failure of the midgut to rotate and fix properly, typically during its return into the abdominal cavity. Although there are various degrees of malrotation, classically the ligament of Treitz is situated to the right of midline, and the cecum fails to rotate the final 180° counterclockwise down to the right lower quadrant, placing it in the epigastrium.

Does Malrotation Always Result in Midgut Volvulus? Is It Always Acute?

No. The diagnosis of malrotation is not itself a surgical emergency. However, it predisposes the infant to midgut volvulus. It is also not always acute, and acute presentations vary from intermittent to complete obstruction. If the acute volvulus is incomplete or intermittent, the infant may appear well between episodes of vomiting. If the volvulus is chronic, the patient may present in childhood with chronic vomiting and recurrent abdominal pain or failure to thrive.

Workup

Are Plain Radiographs Always Necessary?

No. If an infant has symptoms of acute gastrointestinal obstruction, has peritonitis, or is hemodynamically unstable, no additional evaluation is necessary. Rapid fluid resuscitation and immediate surgical intervention will provide the best chance at saving ischemic bowel.

> **Watch Out**
> In a patient with midgut volvulus, the most common bowel gas pattern seen on plain radiograph is normal. Suspicion should actually be heightened when a "normal" abdominal gas pattern is observed in an infant with bilious vomiting.

How Do You Distinguish Midgut Volvulus from Duodenal Atresia?

Duodenal atresia presents with neonatal bilious emesis and is characterized by the classic "double-bubble" sign on abdominal X-ray, which reflects a dilated stomach (first bubble) and proximal duodenum (second bubble) with no distal gas. This condition results from failure of gut recanalization and is associated with epigastric distension that typically resolves with nasogastric decompression. Unlike midgut volvulus, duodenal atresia is rarely a surgical emergency. Initial management includes fluid resuscitation and correction of electrolyte abnormalities to prevent complications during anesthesia. Echocardiography is recommended due to the high incidence of associated congenital heart defects, and approximately 25% of cases occur in infants with Down syndrome.

How Do You Distinguish Midgut Volvulus from Jejunoileal Atresia?

Jejunoileal atresia also presents with neonatal bilious emesis but results from an in utero vascular insult leading to ischemia, resorption, and absence of a segment of small bowel. Abdominal X-rays typically show dilated loops of small bowel with air-fluid levels and absence of gas in the colon and rectum. A contrast enema reveals a microcolon, reflecting a lack of meconium filling due to disuse of the distal bowel in utero.

How Do You Distinguish Midgut Volvulus from Necrotizing Enterocolitis (NEC)?

NEC primarily affects preterm infants due to immature mucosal barriers and immune responses. It involves bacterial translocation into the bowel wall, triggering inflammation, ischemia, and necrosis. Early signs include feeding intolerance, increasing gastric residuals, and abdominal distention, which may progress to bilious vomiting, bloody stools, and lethargy. Diagnosis is made with abdominal radiographs showing dilated bowel loops and pneumatosis intestinalis. Ultrasound can detect bowel wall gas earlier in some cases. Management includes bowel rest and intravenous antibiotics for 10 to 14 days. Neonates with evidence of bowel necrosis or perforation should undergo exploratory laparotomy with resection of necrotic intestine.

Management

What Is the Most Important Immediate Management Issue?

Acute midgut volvulus is a surgical emergency. Any delay in operating may result in gangrene of the entire midgut. The patient should be rapidly fluid resuscitated, started on broad-spectrum IV antibiotics, and taken to the operating room for exploratory laparotomy. An orogastric or nasogastric tube should be placed to decompress the stomach while preparing for the operating room.

What Operation Is Required?

The Ladd's procedure. The goals of surgery are to relieve any intestinal obstruction and prevent recurrent volvulus. First, because volvulus typically occurs in a clockwise direction, the volvulus must be reduced by gently rotating the gut counterclockwise. Next, Ladd's bands, or the peritoneal attachments from the right upper quadrant to the ascending colon, must be divided. The duodenum is then straightened and examined for intrinsic obstruction. The base of the mesentery must be widened by dividing peritoneal adhesions. Finally, the small bowel is positioned on the right side of the abdomen and the large bowel on the left, in complete nonrotation. These positions ensure the maximum distance between the duodenum and the ileocecal junction. Because the cecum and appendix are relocated to the left upper quadrant, most surgeons perform an appendectomy to avoid misdiagnosis if the patient later develops appendicitis.

Area Where You Can Get in Trouble

Delays in Diagnosis

Delays in diagnosis may lead to extensive necrosis of the small bowel, which is highly lethal. If the infant survives, they may develop short bowel syndrome, which may require lifelong intravenous parenteral nutrition and eventual small bowel transplantation.

Diagnosis in Older Children

In older children and even adults with malrotation, the small bowel may intermittently twist and untwist chronically. Symptoms may be milder, making the diagnosis more challenging.

Malrotation (◻ Fig. 35.3)

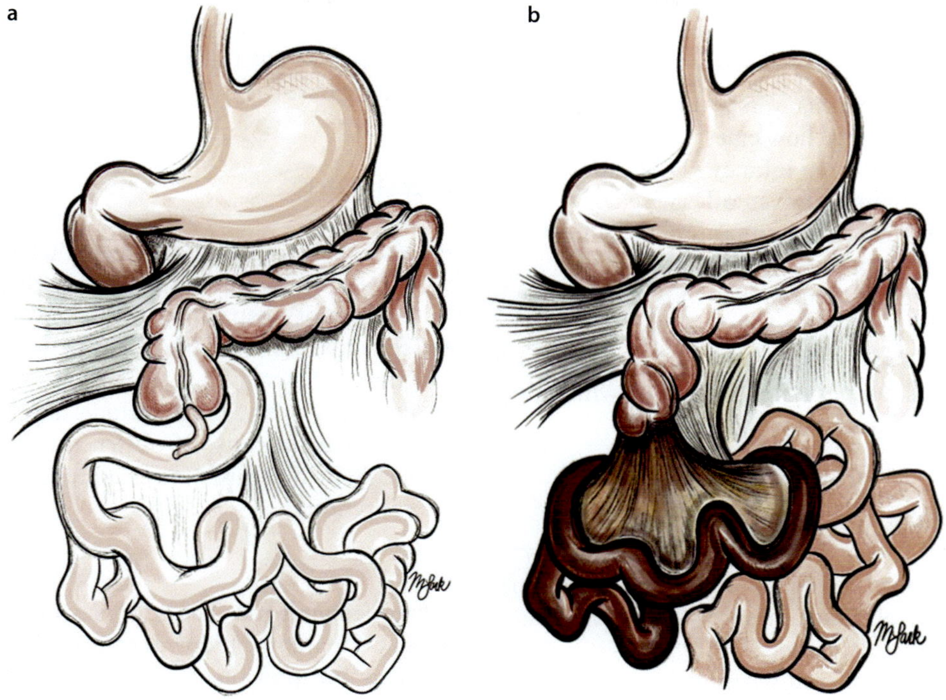

◻ **Fig. 35.3** Abnormal positioning of the bowel (**a**) due to malrotation and Ladd's bands, which can progress to midgut volvulus (**b**)

Summary of Essentials

History, Physical Examination, and Diagnosis

- Must determine bilious versus nonbilious emesis. Remember: green or yellow emesis = bilious emesis
- Bilious vomiting during infancy (1–24 months) is a surgical problem until proven otherwise
- Stable patient: plain abdominal radiographs first to exclude gross perforation
- If initial radiograph is negative: UGI contrast study to evaluate the proximal small intestine
- Always suspect malrotation with midgut volvulus in infants with bilious vomiting or children with bilious vomiting and abdominal pain

Etiology/Pathophysiology

- Midgut is supplied by the superior mesenteric artery: second portion of duodenum → two-thirds of transverse colon
- Malrotation due to developmental failure of normal 270° counterclockwise midgut rotation
- Classic malrotation = narrow mesenteric base, ligament of Treitz located right of midline, cecum in the epigastrium, Ladd's bands from cecum to right upper quadrant, crossing duodenum
- Volvulus = midgut rotates around superior mesenteric artery axis → duodenal obstruction, vascular compromise of bowel
- Classic UGI radiograph: "corkscrew" appearance of contrast in bowel lumen

Management

- Place nasogastric tube to decompress stomach; give antibiotics and IVF while preparing for laparotomy
- Hemodynamically unstable infant with acute gastrointestinal obstruction → rapid fluid resuscitation, immediate surgical intervention without additional studies
- Ladd's procedure: relieve obstruction by untwisting bowel; prevent future episodes by broadening mesenteric base

Watch Out

- Malrotation with midgut volvulus may present with bilious or nonbilious vomiting depending on the location of obstruction
- The most common bowel gas pattern on plain radiograph is normal
- During surgery, must exclude duodenal stenosis or atresia as the cause of obstruction
- Delay in diagnosis may result in complete midgut infarction

Acknowledgements The editors would like to acknowledge and thank the following authors for their contributions to the previous edition of the chapter: Rivfka Shenoy.

Suggested Reading

Lampl B, Levin TL, Berdon WE, Cowles RA. Malrotation and midgut volvulus: a historical review and current controversies in diagnosis and management. Pediatr Radiol. 2009;39(4):359–66.

Millar AJ, Rode H, Cywes S. Malrotation and volvulus in infancy and childhood. Semin Pediatr Surg. 2003;12(4):229–36.

O'Neill J. Chapter 47: Rotational anomalies and volvulus. In: Principles of pediatric surgery. 7th ed. Mosby; New York, NY; 2003. p. 477–58.

Strouse PJ. Disorders of intestinal rotation and fixation ("malrotation"). Pediatr Radiol. 2004;34(11):837–51.

Infant with Nonbilious Emesis

Veronica F. Sullins and Steven L. Lee

Contents

C. de Virgilio, A. Grigorian (eds.), *Surgery*, https://doi.org/10.1007/978-3-032-09799-6_36

Case Study

A 6-week-old full-term male is brought into the emergency room for nonbilious emesis. The mother reports that he began regurgitating breast milk 1 week ago. Although intermittent at first, nonbilious emesis now occurs after every feeding and has become progressively more forceful with increased volume. His appetite remains vigorous, even immediately after vomiting. He is the mother's first child and his delivery was uneventful. His blood pressure is normal and he is afebrile but tachycardic. On physical examination, he is irritable and has a sunken fontanelle. A small, firm mass is palpated in the right upper quadrant.

Diagnosis

What Is the Differential Diagnosis? (Table 36.1)

Table 36.1 Differential diagnosis of nonbilious emesis in neonate

Diseases managed medically	Diseases managed surgically
Acute gastroenteritis	Antral web
Gastroesophageal reflux disease	Enteric duplication cyst
Metabolic disorders (congenital adrenal hyperplasia, electrolyte imbalance, glycogen storage disease)	Gastroesophageal reflux disease
Pylorospasm	Pyloric atresia
	Pyloric stenosis

36

What Is the Most Likely Diagnosis?

Infantile hypertrophic pyloric stenosis (HPS). The incidence is approximately 1.5–4 in 1000 live births. HPS affects predominantly males over females, with reported ratios of 2:1 to 5:1 and is found more frequently in *first-born males*. There is occasionally a positive family history.

History and Physical

Why Is It Important to Distinguish Between Bilious and Nonbilious Vomiting in an Infant?

The presence or absence of bile in the emesis is useful diagnostic information and is indicative of the anatomical location of the lesion. If the obstruction is proximal to the pylorus, the emesis will always be nonbilious. Bile-stained emesis implies that the obstruction is distal to the ampulla of Vater. Children with *bilious emesis* are presumed to have a surgical problem (usually urgent/emergent) unless proven otherwise.

What Is the Classic History for HPS?

Projectile, nonbilious vomiting in an otherwise healthy infant is classic for HPS. The infant may have been vomiting for 1–2 weeks, but the emesis will become progressively more forceful and voluminous (consistent with progressively worsening pyloric stenosis). Infants will typically be brought to medical attention between 4 and 8 weeks of age, although the diagnosis can be made outside of this window.

What Are the Classic Physical Examination Findings?

The classic findings are a volume-depleted infant, as evidenced by a sunken fontanelle, and a palpable mass in the right upper quadrant, described as an "olive," which represents the thickened and elongated pyloric muscle. However, the mass is often difficult to palpate, especially if the infant is crying or tense. Reverse peristaltic waves may be visible across the upper abdomen. Because examination can be challenging, it is important to keep the infant warm and comfortable, using techniques such as bending the legs and offering a pacifier dipped in sugar water. If the classic history and a palpable "olive" are present, no additional studies are needed. If a mass cannot be appreciated, further diagnostic evaluation is warranted.

Pathophysiology

What Is the Pathophysiology of This Condition?

There is universal consensus that HPS is characterized by hypertrophy and hyperplasia of the circular muscle layer of the pylorus. Muscle thickening causes the pyloric channel to become increasingly narrowed and elongated, eventually leading to gastric outlet obstruction. The smooth muscle of the stomach hypertrophies and dilates in response to vigorous peristalsis against an obstructed pylorus. As the stomach dilates and peristaltic contractions become stronger, the classic projectile vomiting of a large volume of gastric content occurs.

Watch Out
There is a reported association with use of oral erythromycin and HPS in infants.

Workup

What Is the First Imaging Study to Obtain?

If the diagnosis of hypertrophic pyloric stenosis is suspected but the mass is not palpable, an abdominal ultrasound is the diagnostic study of choice and typically reveals a thickened and elongated pyloric muscle (◘ Fig. 36.1). Ultrasound diagnostic criteria include

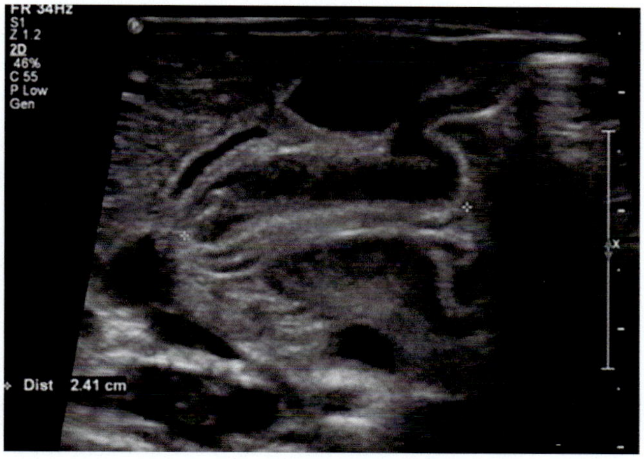

◘ **Fig. 36.1** Ultrasound image of pyloric stenosis (pyloric length is 24 mm)

pyloric muscle thickness greater than 3 mm and length greater than 15 mm. If ultrasound results are equivocal or the pylorus cannot be adequately visualized, an upper gastrointestinal (UGI) series may be performed. This study would demonstrate a "string sign," representing a narrowed pyloric channel, or delayed gastric emptying. However, imaging beyond ultrasound is rarely needed.

Watch Out
Contrast UGI studies have a risk of causing aspiration in infants, especially those with HPS (since they have gastric outlet obstruction), and should therefore be reserved for cases where the diagnosis is uncertain or malrotation with midgut volvulus cannot be ruled out.

What Electrolyte Abnormalities Would You Expect?

Protracted, nonbilious vomiting results in a *hypochloremic, hypokalemic metabolic alkalosis*. Chloride ions are lost in gastric secretions, and alkalosis is initially caused by loss of gastric HCl. Hypokalemia is primarily the result of kidney excretion of K^+, and to a lesser extent, the loss of potassium ions with vomiting. Volume depletion and subsequent hypovolemia increase aldosterone secretion, which in turn leads to activation of the Na+/K+ pump in the renal tubules. In an attempt to increase water reabsorption, Na^+ is conserved at the expense of K^+ excretion (this is the main driver of K+ loss). As K^+ levels in the blood decrease, the kidney preferentially uses Na^+/H^+ pump to maintain Na^+ and water reabsorption and prevent profound hypokalemia. This change leads to H^+ secretion and worsens the metabolic alkalosis. Accordingly, urinalysis often reveals paradoxical aciduria.

Management

What Is the Most Important Immediate Management Issue?

The first step in management is to secure intravenous access and begin fluid resuscitation. Volume depletion in patients with HPS is common due to prolonged, high-volume emesis. An initial isotonic fluid (normal saline) bolus of 20 ml/kg should be given to children with severe volume deficits. A nasogastric tube is not routinely necessary. Any electrolyte abnormalities should be corrected prior to taking the patient to the operating room.

> **Watch Out**
> Children have a higher body surface area-to-volume ratio than adults and are therefore more sensitive to volume loss. Any child with physical exam findings indicating volume depletion (decreased skin turgor and sunken fontanelle) or vital sign derangements should be considered to have moderate to severe hypovolemia.

What Is the Treatment?

Surgery provides definitive treatment for pyloric stenosis. The procedure of choice is a pyloromyotomy. The abdomen is entered either laparoscopically or through a small transverse right upper quadrant incision. The pylorus is identified, and an incision is made through the overlying serosa and the thickened pyloric muscularis. The pylorus muscle is then spread apart until the intact submucosa and mucosa are seen. Air or methylene blue is instilled through a nasogastric tube into the stomach to confirm there is no leak.

> **Watch Out**
> Remember that HPS is a medical emergency, not a surgical one. Restoration of fluids and electrolytes is paramount.

What Is the Timing of Surgery?

Surgery is delayed until effective fluid resuscitation and electrolyte replacement have been performed. While not an emergency, surgery should be performed during the same admission. Most patients require 24 hours for adequate resuscitation. Patients with severe volume depletion may require a longer period of repletion prior to surgery. In general, patients are optimized for surgery when there is adequate urine output, the serum bicarbonate is less than 30 mmol/L, and the serum potassium is normal.

When Can the Patient Resume Eating?

Following surgery, many children may begin oral feeding within a few hours. There continues to be wide variation in structured feeding regimens. It is very common, however, for patients to vomit after surgery. This is most often due to either postoperative edema around the pylorus or, less commonly, an incomplete pyloromyotomy. Edema will resolve over a few days and the vomiting will subside. An incomplete pyloromyotomy will not likely resolve, and the patient may require a repeat operation. Persistent vomiting beyond 3–4 days postoperatively is often indicative of this complication. Patients are typically discharged home 1 day after surgery.

Areas Where You Can Get in Trouble

Inadequate Resuscitation Prior to Surgery

Operating prior to adequate resuscitation is perilous for children with HPS. Anesthesia induction in hypovolemic children with electrolyte disturbances may precipitate catastrophic outcomes, including cardiovascular collapse and death. Children with severe electrolyte derangements or kidney disease may experience rapid fluid and electrolyte shifts, and potassium repletion in the setting of hypovolemia could lead to iatrogenic hyperkalemia or seizures.

Area of Controversy

Nonsurgical Management

In North America, surgical management remains the standard of care; pyloromyotomy is regarded as the definitive treatment. Some European centers have explored dietary modification and prolonged supportive care in hopes of spontaneous resolution of pyloric hypertrophy. In some Asian countries, atropine has been used to medically manage HPS with variable success.

Summary of Essentials

History, Physical Examination, and Diagnosis

- Always determine if vomiting is bilious (green or yellow) or nonbilious
- The most common surgical cause of nonbilious vomiting in an infant is HPS
- Classic history: projectile, nonbilious vomiting in healthy 4–8-week-old male
- Classic physical examination: palpable right upper quadrant "olive" mass (ensure patient is calm during exam), visible peristalsis over the epigastrium
- Ultrasound if diagnosis is unclear; pyloric muscle thickness greater than 3 mm and length greater than 15 mm
- Laboratory abnormalities common: hypochloremic, hypokalemic metabolic alkalosis, and paradoxical aciduria

Pathophysiology

- Etiology not known
- Hyperplasia and hypertrophy of pylorus → gastric outlet obstruction

Management

- Medical management first: fluid resuscitation, correct electrolyte imbalances
- Pyloromyotomy is the gold standard: incise and split the muscular layers, leaving the mucosa and submucosa intact
- Delay surgery until infant is resuscitated and electrolyte levels are normal (may take 24–48 hours)
- Feeding starts hours after surgery; vomiting is common but should resolve

Acknowledgements The editors would like to acknowledge and thank the following author for their contributions to the previous edition of the chapter: Rivfka Shenoy.

Suggested Reading

Iqbal CW, Rivard DC, Mortellary VE, Sharp SW, St Peter SD. Evaluation of ultrasonographic parameters in the diagnosis of pyloric stenosis relative to patient age and size. J Pediatr Surg. 2012;47(8):1542–7.

Pandya S, Heiss K. Pyloric stenosis in pediatric surgery: an evidence-based review. Surg Clin N Am. 2012;92(3):527–39. vii–viii.

St Peter SD, Holcomb GW, Calkins CM, Murphy JP, Andrews WS, Sharp RJ, Snyder CL, Ostlie DJ. Open versus laparoscopic pyloromyotomy for pyloric stenosis: a prospective, randomized trial. Ann Surg. 2006;244(3):363–70.

Infant Born with Abdominal Wall Defect

Justin P. Wagner and Steven L. Lee

Contents

C. de Virgilio, A. Grigorian (eds.), *Surgery*, https://doi.org/10.1007/978-3-032-09799-6_37

Case Study

An infant at 39-week gestation is born to a thin 19-year-old Caucasian grava-1, para-0 woman with no prior medical history. Her body mass index (BMI) is 20. She quit smoking when she discovered she was pregnant. The pregnancy was uncomplicated. Prenatal maternal laboratory studies were significant for an elevated serum alpha-fetoprotein (AFP) level. Prenatal ultrasound examinations showed a fetus with free loops of intestine present in the amniotic cavity extruding through a small abdominal defect lateral to the base of the umbilical cord. The infant's APGAR scores are 8 and 9 at birth and 5 min later, respectively. Vital signs are within normal limits. The abdomen is scaphoid with loops of matted and inflamed small bowel protruding from a defect to the right of the umbilicus, and the umbilicus appears to be intact.

Diagnosis

What Is the Differential Diagnosis for a Newborn with an Abdominal Wall Defect? What Are the Common and Distinguishing Features? (Table 37.1)

Table 37.1 Differential diagnosis and distinguishing features for a newborn with an abdominal wall defects

Diagnosis	Common features	Distinguishing features
Gastroschisis	Medial abdominal wall defect with evisceration of abdominal contents	No membrane over abdominal contents
		Evisceration usually to the *right* of umbilical stalk
		Higher risk to intestinal viability
		Diagnosis impossible before 12 weeks of gestation
Omphalocele	Midline abdominal wall defect with herniation of abdominal contents	Amnioperitoneal membrane covers abdominal contents
		Umbilical cord inserts into membrane
		Associated with other birth defects
		Diagnosis possible before 12 weeks gestation only if liver herniation is present
Urachal abnormality	Communication of bladder and anterior abdominal wall; may be associated with cyst or sinus	Communication between the bladder and a cystic mass pathognomonic for patent urachus
		Often associated with omphalocele and neural tube defects
Umbilical hernia	Umbilical ring fails to close after separation of the umbilical cord, leading to a bulge in the area of umbilicus	May be more prominent during coughing, crying, or bearing down; often reducible and painless

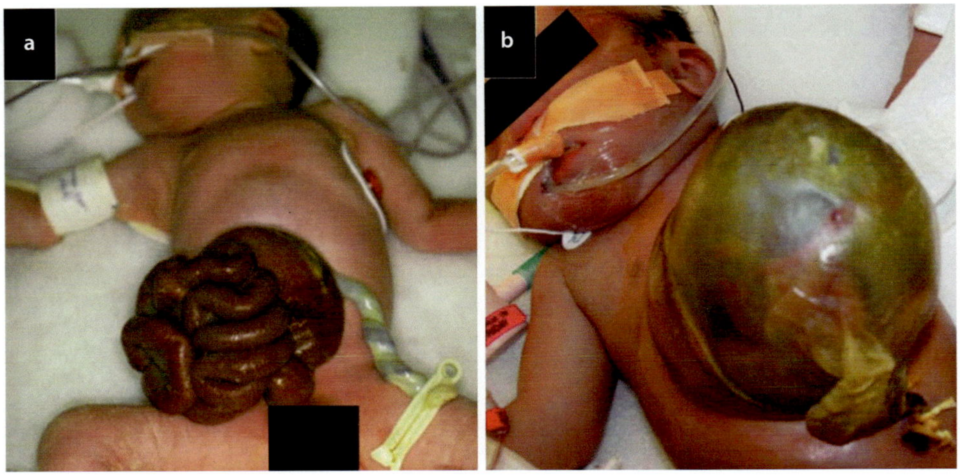

Fig. 37.1 Gastroschisis (**a**) and omphalocele (**b**)

What Is the Most Likely Diagnosis in This Case?

Gastroschisis is the most likely diagnosis. The infant's mother has several risk factors associated with gastroschisis, including young age, Caucasian race, low BMI, singleton pregnancy, and recent tobacco use. Prenatal ultrasound detects gastroschisis in about 70% of cases. Ultrasound is effective in distinguishing gastroschisis from omphalocele and is useful to evaluate visceral blood flow. In this case, the patient is born with eviscerated bowel, no sac, a defect to the right of the umbilicus, and an intact umbilicus, strongly suggesting a diagnosis of gastroschisis (Fig. 37.1a).

> **Watch Out**
> The absence of a sac does not automatically make the diagnosis gastroschisis, as on occasion, the omphalocele sac ruptures before delivery.

History and Physical Examination

Which of the Above Diagnoses Are the Most Common?

Up to 20% of newborns present with umbilical hernias. Gastroschisis occurs in 2–4 in 10,000 live births, while omphalocele occurs in 1 in 4000–5000 live births.

What Are the Specific Differences Between Gastroschisis and Omphalocele? (Table 37.2)

Table 37.2 Differences between gastroschisis and omphalocele

Factor	Gastroschisis (Fig. 37.1a)	Omphalocele (Fig. 37.1b)
Location	Paraumbilical (usually *right* side)	Umbilical
Defect size	Often small (<5 cm)	Variable, often large
Cord insertion	Normal in umbilicus	Inserts in membrane
Membrane	Absent	Present (10–20% rupture)
Contents	Bowel (gonads, liver, stomach)	Bowel, liver
Bowel	Matted, dilated, or thickened	Normal
Malrotation	Often present	Present
Abdominal cavity	Small	Small
Maternal AFP level	Elevated (greater than omphalocele)	Elevated
Intrauterine growth restriction (IUGR)	Present	Absent
GI function	Ileus	Normal
Associated GI anomalies	Intestinal atresia (10–25%)	Nonspecific, but higher overall risk
Other associated anomalies	Rare	Common (30–70%)
		Beckwith-Wiedemann, trisomies 13 and 18, pentalogy of Cantrell
		Chromosomal in 50–70% without liver herniation

AFP alpha-fetoprotein

Pathophysiology

What Is the Etiology of Gastroschisis?

While the etiology of gastroschisis is relatively unclear, it is thought to result from a *vascular accident* within the umbilical ring, leading to a local defect in the developing body wall and evisceration.

What Is the Etiology of Omphalocele?

Omphalocele is thought to develop from an arrest of lateral-body fold migration and body wall closure. This process takes place during the organogenesis phase. At embryonic week 5 of normal development, the midgut extrudes through the base of the umbilical cord and undergoes proliferation and rotation. The viscera return to the peritoneal cavity at week 11 of gestation. Omphalocele is a result of persistent herniation of viscera contained within a sac that never returned to the abdomen during development. The failure of cell migration may be a manifestation of an underlying disease process that affects several other migrating cell types during development. Frequently, omphalocele is part of an association of birth defects with a common congenital cause.

Which Condition Is More Urgent? Which Is Associated with Greater Long-Term Problems?

Gastroschisis generally creates more urgent problems at delivery that require immediate pediatric surgical intervention. This derives from two problems: the fact that the bowel is not covered by a protective membrane and the associated intestinal abnormalities. The longstanding exposure of the bowel in utero to amniotic fluid often leads to markedly inflamed bowel. Concurrent malrotation with volvulus or intrauterine vascular compromise may result in intestinal atresia, obstruction, stenosis, necrosis, or perforation. Furthermore, the exposed bowel creates significant risk of insensible fluid and heat losses that can be substantial if the bowel remains unprotected. With omphalocele, the membrane covering the bowel protects against these urgent problems. Of greater long-term concern for patients with omphalocele, however, are the associated conditions such as Pentalogy of Cantrell, trisomy 13, and trisomy 18, all of which carry poor prognoses.

Management and Work Up

What Is the Next Step in the Management of Gastroschisis?

Neonatal management of gastroschisis prioritizes airway protection, thermal support, protection of herniated viscera, and fluid resuscitation. Intravenous antibiotics are administered due to the exposed bowel. The bowel should be covered with a plastic wrap and a sterile plastic bag should be applied immediately around the torso to minimize heat and fluid loss from exposed viscera. Gastroschisis often leads to prolonged ileus due to intestinal inflammation, necessitating parenteral nutrition.

After the Initial Management, What Is the Next Step?

Small defects may then undergo primary surgical repair, while larger defects require temporary placement of herniated contents in a Dacron-coated silastic silo to allow gradual reduction and resolution of inflammation. Omphaloceles rupture in up to 20% of cases, requiring the same management as gastroschisis if rupture occurs.

How Does the Initial Management of Omphalocele Differ?

Since the bowel is covered by a membrane, there is not the same concern for bowel injury and fluid losses, and therefore no need for emergency surgery to close the defect or cover the bowel with a silastic wrap. The membrane covering is covered with a nonadherent dressing. If surgery is delayed, the membrane can be covered with topical antibiotics and the torso wrapped with an elastic wrap (termed "paint and wait"). Since the bowel is intact and protected by a membrane, the infant can be fed enterally. Stabilized infants with omphalocele undergo echocardiography to evaluate for associated congenital cardiac defects.

What Is the Timing of the Closure of the Abdominal Wall Defect?

The defect is surgically repaired when the herniated contents have reduced significantly and there is sufficient abdominal wall laxity to accommodate a low-tension repair. Small gastroschisis and omphalocele defects may undergo primary operative repair if the contents reduce easily. For large defects, a silo is used for temporary coverage, and the herniated contents are gradually reduced each day into the abdominal cavity, and once there is no tension, the defect can be closed (■ Fig. 37.2).

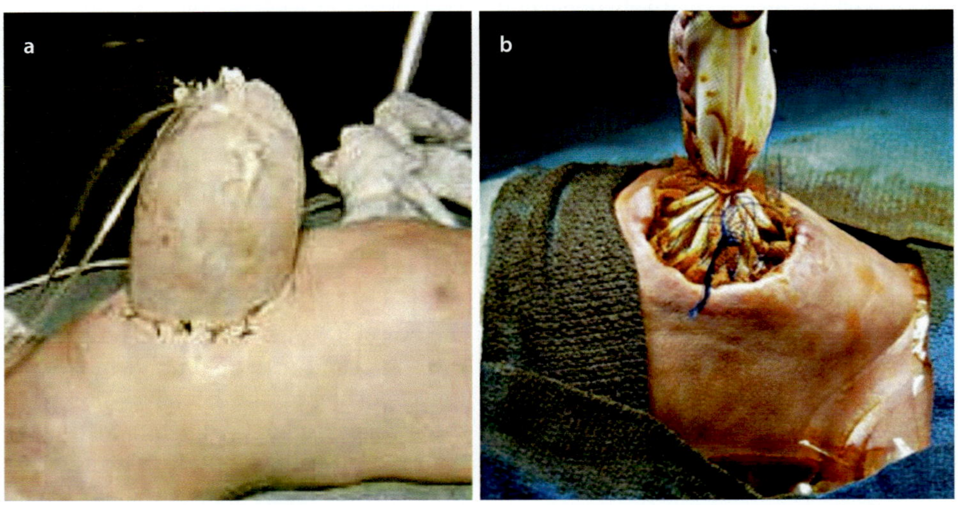

■ **Fig. 37.2** Initial silo placement for gastroschisis (**a**) and complete reduction (**b**)

What Is the Management of Pediatric Umbilical Hernias?

Pediatric umbilical hernias are often reducible, painless, and will resolve with observation alone. Therefore, expectant management is acceptable for asymptomatic umbilical hernias until the child is 5 years old. Surgical repair is indicated if the hernia does not resolve by age 5 or becomes incarcerated or strangulated.

Areas Where You Can Get in Trouble

Not Properly Protecting the Bowel

Upon securing the airway, thermal support is usually provided by a heating lamp. The viscera are wrapped with a sterile plastic covering. Plastic wrap is a reasonable temporizing option if there is a delay in acquiring a silo. Moist gauze dressings alone should be avoided because the infant can lose significant fluid and heat without a watertight plastic dressing.

Not Addressing Nutritional Needs

The appearance of the bowel will dictate the nutritional support the child receives. Matted, inflamed intestines will likely be slow to function, and ileus is likely. In cases where gastrointestinal dysmotility is suspected, the infant should be supported with total parenteral nutrition (TPN) until the bowel is functional.

Not Recognizing Abdominal Compartment Syndrome After Repair

After the defect is surgically repaired, the infant must be monitored closely for signs of increased intra-abdominal pressure. Low urine output, insufficient ventilation, tense abdominal distension, and positive fluid balance signify development of abdominal compartment syndrome. Prolonged mechanical ventilation may be necessary after reduction and abdominal closure.

Summary of Essentials

Diagnosis

- Gastroschisis and omphalocele can be diagnosed on prenatal ultrasound in most cases
- Gastroschisis is paraumbilical (typically to the right of the umbilicus) and has exposed bowel
- Omphalocele has a sac (the umbilicus inserts into the sac) and is associated with more congenital defects

Omphalocele-Associated Conditions

- Beckwith-Wiedemann Syndrome
- Trisomy 13
- Trisomy 18
- Pentalogy of Cantrell

Etiology

- Gastroschisis: in utero vascular insult, abdominal wall defect
- Omphalocele: arrest of cell migration, incomplete return of midgut to the peritoneal cavity

Neonatal Management

- Ventilation
- Normothermia and fluid management:
  - Radiant heater
  - Orogastric suction
  - Protect exposed viscera with plastic wrap
  - IV fluids and broad-spectrum antibiotics
  - Gastroschisis: surgical evaluation for atresia, ischemia, or volvulus; low threshold to start TPN
  - Primary surgical repair (small defects)
  - Silo (large defects) silo, serial reduction, then closure

Postoperative Care

- Ventilator requirement after reduction may persist
- Administer TPN if necessary
- Monitor for abdominal compartment syndrome

Acknowledgements The editors would like to acknowledge and thank the following authors for their contributions to the previous edition of the chapter: Rivfka Shenoy.

Suggested Reading

Henrich K, Huemmer HP, Reingruber B, Weber PG. Gastroschisis and omphalocele: treatments and long-term outcomes. Pediatr Surg Int. 2008;24(2):167–73.

Mac Bird T, Robbins JM, Druschel C, Cleves MA, Yang S, Hobbs CA. Demographic and environmental risk factors for gastroschisis and omphalocele in the National Birth Defects Prevention Study. J Pediatr Surg. 2009;44(8):1546–51.

Sadler TW. The embryologic origin of ventral body wall defects. Semin Pediatr Surg. 2010;19(3):209–14.

Zens T, Nichol PF, Cartmill R, Kohler JE. Management of asymptomatic pediatric umbilical hernias: a systematic review. J Pediatr Surg. 2017;52(11):1723–1731. https://doi.org/10.1016/j.jpedsurg.2017.07.016.

Excessive Drooling in a Newborn

Veronica F. Sullins and Steven L. Lee

Contents

C. de Virgilio, A. Grigorian (eds.), *Surgery*, https://doi.org/10.1007/978-3-032-09799-6_38

Case Study

A full-term female newborn presents with excessive drooling. She is noted to have white, frothy mucus building up in her mouth and nose, which recurs despite suctioning. She is also unable to tolerate any feedings. During her first feeding, she gagged and immediately spit up. There were no complications during birth. On examination, the newborn is normotensive and has a normal heart rate. Her oxygen saturation is 98% but decreases to 80% during feeding. She has bilateral rales and rhonchi on lung auscultation. Her abdomen is distended and nontender. The patient receives anteroposterior and lateral chest radiographs after orogastric tube placement (Fig. 38.1).

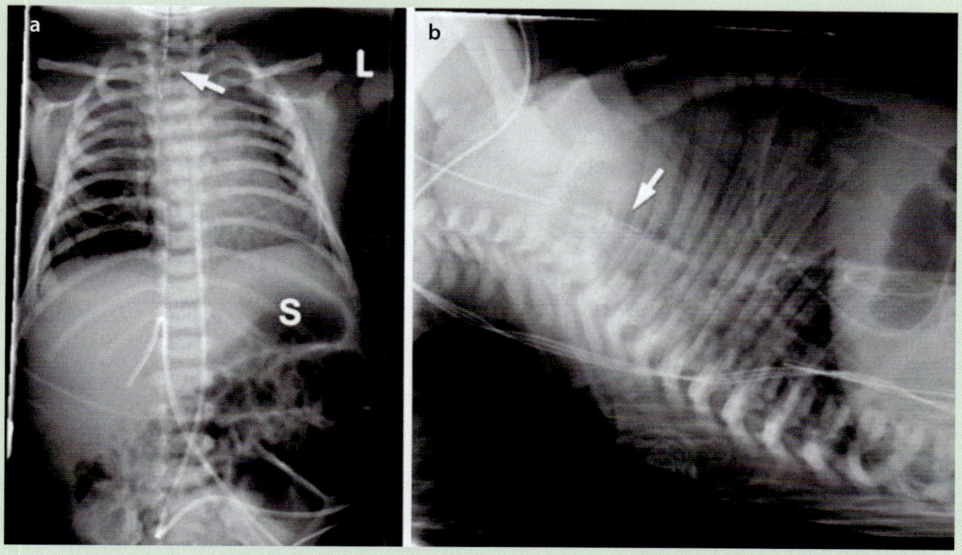

Fig. 38.1 (**a**, **b**) Anteroposterior and lateral chest radiographs after orogastric tube placement *(arrows)*. The stomach (S) is shown in the anteroposterior radiograph

Table 38.1 Differential diagnosis of excessive drooling/feeding intolerance in a newborn

Diagnosis	Distinguishing features
Choanal atresia	Neonates are obligate nasal breathers; inability to pass NG tube; may present with cyanosis that improves with crying
Cleft palate	Defect seen on physical examination of the oral cavity
Esophageal atresia with or without tracheo-esophageal fistula	OG/NG tube seen curled in upper esophageal pouch on AP and lateral radiographs
Esophageal web or ring	Usually asymptomatic until later in life, vomiting if symptomatic, circumferential partial obstruction on contrast esophagram
Food sensitivity	Normal anatomy, accompanying rash or diarrhea, specific food intolerance
Gastroesophageal reflux	Normal anatomy, frequent regurgitation, or vomiting
Laryngotracheoesophageal cleft	Midline defect between posterior wall of larynx/trachea and anterior esophagus
Mediastinal or tracheal compression	Extrinsic compression of esophagus, lesion (tumor, vascular ring, foregut duplication, etc.) on chest XR, ultrasound, or CT scan
Neurologic disorder	Patent esophagus on contrast esophagram, uncoordinated peristalsis on swallow study

NG nasogastric, *OG* orogastric, *AP* anteroposterior, *XR* radiograph, *CT* computed tomography

Diagnosis

What Is the Differential Diagnosis of Excessive Drooling/Feeding Intolerance in a Newborn? (Table 38.1)

38

What Is the Most Likely Diagnosis?

Esophageal atresia (EA) with distal tracheoesophageal fistula (TEF) is the most likely diagnosis. Chest radiographs show the orogastric tube curled in the upper esophageal pouch, confirming the diagnosis of EA. The presence of air in the gastrointestinal tract suggests a connection from the trachea to the distal esophagus or a distal TEF. Absence of a gastric bubble is diagnostic of either EA without a TEF or EA with a proximal TEF. Focal infiltrates may indicate pneumonia secondary to aspiration of gastric contents or feedings.

History and Physical

What Are Other Possible Presentations of TEF?

In addition to excessive drooling or choking with feeds, newborns may also present with respiratory distress or pneumonia. The presentation of TEF is determined by the presence or absence of EA as well as the presence and severity of associated anomalies. Patients with small fistulas with a normal esophagus (H-type) may be asymptomatic at birth and present later in infancy or childhood with recurrent pneumonia, chronic cough, or feeding difficulties.

Pathophysiology

What Is the Significance of Oxygen Desaturation that Only Occurs While Feeding?

Normal oxygen saturation at rest implies intact tracheobronchial anatomy. When a newborn has desaturations while feeding, it implies that there is a significant anatomic or functional problem with the proximal alimentary tract (nasopharynx, oropharynx, esophagus, or stomach).

What Is Thought to Be the Etiology of EA?

Although the pathogenesis remains unknown, EA with or without TEF is thought to be caused by a defect in the development of the longitudinal tracheoesophageal fold that separates the most caudal part of the primitive foregut into the trachea and esophagus. It is believed that the fistula tract is derived from defective epithelial-

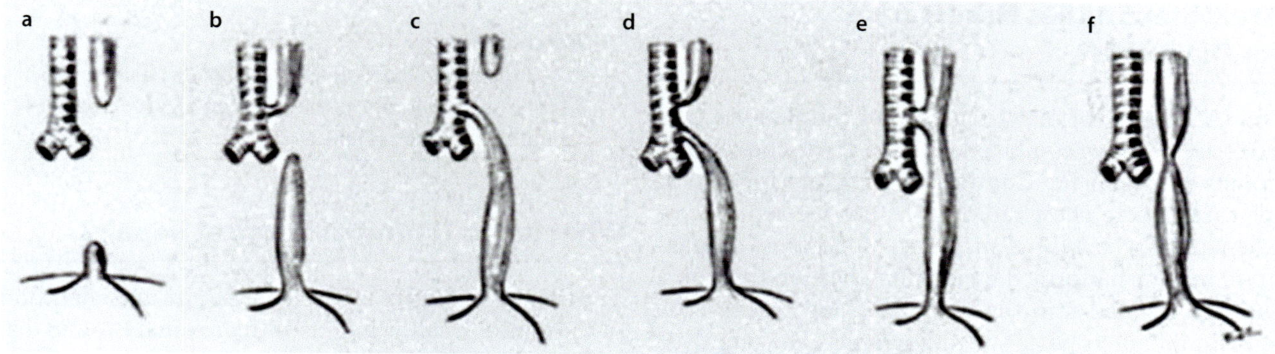

■ **Fig. 38.2** (a–f) Gross classification of esophageal atresia and tracheoesophageal fistula. (From Harmon CM, Coran AG. Congenital anomalies of the esophagus. In: Coran AG, et al. *Pediatric Surgery*, 7th edition. Copyright Elsevier (2012). Reprinted with permission)

■ **Table 38.2** Anomalies found in VACTERL

Category of anomaly	Specific anomalies
*V*ertebral	Hypoplastic or hemivertebrae
*A*norectal	Anal atresia or imperforate anus
*C*ardiovascular	ASD, VSD, tetralogy of Fallot, truncus arteriosus, transposition of the great arteries
*T*racheo-esophageal	Tracheoesophageal fistula
*E*sophageal	Esophageal atresia
*R*enal	Renal agenesis, hypoplastic or dysplastic kidney, horseshoe kidney, renal ectopia, ureteral obstruction, vesicoureteral reflux
*L*imb	Displaced or hypoplastic thumb, polydactyly, syndactyly, radial aplasia

ASD atrial septal defect, *VSD* ventricular septal defect

mesenchymal interactions in a branch of the embryonic lung bud that fails to develop. An alternate theory is that the primitive foregut occludes, and then there is a failure of recanalization.

How Are the Different Types Classified?

EA and TEF are classified by their anatomic configuration, specifically the location of the TEF (■ Fig. 38.2). The *most common is type C*, a proximal esophageal pouch with a distal TEF, accounting for approximately 85% of cases. The next most common is pure EA without TEF, also known as type A (8%).

What Are the Associated Anomalies?

Approximately 50% of children with TEFs have associated anomalies including cardiac (most common), urogenital, skeletal, vertebral, anorectal, gastrointestinal, and palatal or laryngeal anomalies. Associations and syndromes known as VACTERL (■ Table 38.2) are frequently diagnosed. In addition, there are reports of associations with trisomies 18, 21, and 13 as well as single-gene deletions.

Work-up

What Is the Best Initial Diagnostic Test?

If the newborn is stable, the best initial study is a chest radiograph (anteroposterior *and* lateral) after placement of a nasogastric or orogastric tube. Abnormal lung fields may demonstrate a pneumonia, primary lung lesion, or congenital diaphragmatic hernia. EA is diagnosed by visualization of the nasogastric or orogastric tube coiled in the upper mediastinum, posterior to the larynx or trachea.

Watch Out

An anteroposterior chest radiograph alone may be misleading if the nasogastric or orogastric tube is inadvertently placed in the trachea. A lateral chest radiograph is essential to confirm that the tube is coiled in the proximal esophageal pouch.

Are Other Studies Necessary for Diagnosis?

No. A history of newborn feeding intolerance and excessive drooling combined with the above chest radiographs is diagnostic. Contrast esophagram is reserved for cases where chest radiographs are inconclusive or when an H-type TEF is suspected. A contrast esophagram may be performed by instilling barium through a catheter inserted into the esophagus and taking both lateral and anteroposterior radiographs. The improved quality of CT scans has made three-dimensional imaging popular; however, it exposes the newborn to a much larger radiation dose and is not usually necessary to make the diagnosis.

Watch Out

Contrast esophagrams have a risk of causing aspiration pneumonitis and should therefore be reserved for cases where the location of the fistula cannot be ascertained or the diagnosis is uncertain.

Can the Diagnosis of TEF Be Made Prenatally?

EA may be manifested by polyhydramnios on prenatal ultrasound. However, the presence of an accompanying TEF may be difficult to determine prenatally, as air will not have entered into the alimentary tract through the fistula until after birth.

Management

What Is the First Step in Clinical Management?

If the patient is exhibiting signs of respiratory compromise, endotracheal intubation and mechanical ventilation are required. Preoperative management is aimed at minimizing the risk of aspiration. This may be achieved by continuous suction of the blind upper esophageal pouch and elevation of the infant's head. For patients who have developed pneumonia, broad-spectrum antibiotics should be given, and a gastrostomy tube may be placed to prevent further reflux into the trachea. Patients without a pulmonary infection should be started on prophylactic antibiotics.

Watch Out

Avoid the use of bag valve masks, as this will further distend the gastrointestinal tract and cause further aspiration and lung injury.

What Is the Timing of Surgical Repair?

The timing of surgery is based on the size and condition of the infant. Healthy infants with proximal EA and distal TEF (Type C) may undergo surgical repair within the first few days of life. Infants who are premature with low birth weight, unstable, or have severe pneumonia may initially undergo ligation of the TEF and placement of a gastrostomy tube for feeding, with delayed esophageal repair after clinical stabilization. Definitive treatment consists of surgical division of the fistula tract with repair of the trachea and primary anastomosis of the esophagus.

Are Any Other Studies Needed Prior to Surgery?

Even stable infants who are fit for early repair must have a complete work-up, including a thorough physical exam, cardiac and renal ultrasounds, and plain radiographs to evaluate for associated anomalies (▫ ▫ Table 38.2) prior to operation. In addition, *echocardiography* provides essential anatomic information required for surgical repair.

What Are the Complications After Surgical Repair?

Approximately 15% of patients have a leak at the esophageal anastomosis. Typically, leaks heal spontaneously, resulting in a stricture. If a leak occurs within the first few days postoperatively, surgical revision is usually required. Anastomotic strictures are common and typically managed with serial esophageal dilations under endoscopic guidance. Typical management includes esophagoscopy and balloon dilation of the stricture. Gastroesophageal reflux disease is very common after TEF repair, and such reflux is associated with an increased risk of Barrett's esophagus and esophageal cancer. Long-term, approximately 30% will need a surgical anti-reflux procedure. Recurrence of the TEF has also been described and requires surgical repair.

What Is the Prognosis?

In infants without severe associated anomalies, survival rates are near 100%. However, patients may have significant morbidity, including anastomotic leak, tracheomalacia, gastroesophageal reflux disease, dysphagia, esophageal dysmotility, and pulmonary problems due to recurrent aspiration. In infants with significant comorbid conditions or who are not candidates for early repair, the survival rate is 80–95%. Those with low birth weight and major cardiac anomalies have the lowest survival rates. Pulmonary complications, such as recurrent aspiration and tracheomalacia (which can present with a characteristic "barking cough"), are also common.

Area Where You Can Get in Trouble

Intubation and TEF

In the presence of a TEF, intubation and mechanical ventilation should be avoided if possible, as positive pressure can distend the gastrointestinal tract through the fistula, leading to severe respiratory compromise. Positive pressure ventilation causes air to preferentially enter the stomach and intestines instead of the lungs, resulting in progressive gastric and abdominal distension. Increasing abdominal pressure decreases lung expansion and worsens respiratory function. In addition, excessive gastrointestinal distension complicates intraoperative ventilation, increases the risk of visceral perforation, and may necessitate emergent surgical intervention.

Summary of Essentials

Diagnosis

- Differential diagnosis of feeding intolerance and excessive drooling in a newborn includes anatomic malformations of the nasopharynx, oropharynx, trachea, and esophagus; gastroesophageal reflux; extrinsic esophageal compression; food sensitivity; and neurologic disorders
- Best initial diagnostic test is anteroposterior and lateral chest radiography after nasogastric or orogastric tube placement

History and Physical Examination

- Desaturations only while feeding imply anatomic or functional problem within proximal aerodigestive tract
- In esophageal atresia with or without tracheoesophageal fistula, patients typically present with excessive drooling, feeding intolerance, and respiratory distress

Pathophysiology

- EA ± TEF caused by defect in the development of longitudinal tracheoesophageal fold separating foregut into trachea and esophagus
- >50% have associated anomalies: cardiovascular most common, frequent VACTERL association
- Excellent prognosis in absence of significant anomalies, but patients may have significant clinical sequelae resulting from surgical repair

Management

- Preoperative management aims to minimize aspiration risk with continuous suction of the upper esophageal pouch, head elevation, and administration of prophylactic antibiotics
- Mechanical ventilation is avoided if possible; if required, care must be taken to prevent gastric distension.
- All need evaluation for associated anomalies: echocardiogram, renal ultrasound, radiographs
- Timing of surgery depends on patient's clinical condition, size, and associated anomalies; healthy infants typically undergo repair within the first few days of life

Acknowledgements The editors would like to acknowledge and thank the following authors for their contributions to the previous edition of the chapter: Rivfka Shenoy.

Suggested Reading

Alberti D, Boroni G, Corasaniti L, Torri F. Esophageal atresia: pre and post-operative management. J Matern Fetal Neonatal Med. 2011;24(Suppl 1):4–6.

Kunisaki SM, Foker JE. Surgical advances in the fetus and neonate: esophageal atresia. Clin Perinatol. 2012;39(2):349–61.

Lal DR, Gadepalli SK, Downard CD; Midwest Pediatric Surgery Consortium. Perioperative management and outcomes of esophageal atresia and tracheoesophageal fistula. J Pediatr Surg. 2017 Aug;52(8):1245–1251. https://doi.org/10.1016/j.jpedsurg.2016.11.046. Epub 2016 Dec 5. PMID: 27993359.

Pinheiro P, Silva A, Pereira R. Current knowledge on esophageal atresia. World J Gastroenterol. 2012;18(28):3662–72.

Sulkowski JP, Cooper JN, et al. Morbidity and mortality in patients with esophageal atresia. Surgery. 2014 Aug;156(2):483–91. https://doi.org/10.1016/j.surg.2014.03.016. Epub 2014 Mar 14. PMID: 24947650; PMCID: PMC4099299.

Pediatric

Question Set: Pediatric Surgery

Questions

1. A three-year-old boy is brought to the pediatrician due to fatigue and pallor. His mother reports that he has been increasingly tired and less active over the past month. He has no history of fever, vomiting, or abdominal pain. Physical examination reveals conjunctival pallor but is otherwise unremarkable. Laboratory studies show a hemoglobin of 8.9 g/dL and mean corpuscular volume (MCV) of 68 fL. Fecal occult blood testing is positive. Which of the following is the most appropriate next step in diagnosis?
   (A) Colonoscopy
   (B) Upper endoscopy
   (C) Technetium-99m pertechnetate scan
   (D) Abdominal ultrasound
   (E) Upper gastrointestinal (GI) series with small bowel follow-through

2. A four-week-old boy presents with a three-day history of forceful vomiting. The mother states that the vomitus only contains partially digested milk. She notes that the infant seems very hungry between feedings and drinks vigorously. Past history is significant for a skin infection for which the infant received oral erythromycin. On examination, the infant appears to be healthy appearing and in no acute distress. The physician feels there may be a small palpable mass in the right upper quadrant but is not certain. Electrolytes are normal. What is the best way to establish the most likely diagnosis?
   (A) Plain abdominal X-rays
   (B) Laparoscopy
   (C) CT of the abdomen
   (D) Upper GI study with contrast
   (E) Ultrasound

3. A two-hour-old male born at 39 weeks' gestation with difficulty breathing is diagnosed with esophageal atresia with a tracheoesophageal fistula and undergoes surgical repair, which was uncomplicated. Ten years later, the patient develops difficulty swallowing and often vomits undigested food shortly after eating. Which of the following is the most likely explanation for this?
   (A) Scleroderma
   (B) Gastroesophageal reflux
   (C) Esophageal cancer
   (D) Esophageal leak
   (E) Esophageal stricture

4. A two-week-old male infant born at 26 weeks' gestation is in the neonatal ICU when he becomes hypotensive and begins passing bloody stools. Which of the following is the most likely finding?
   (A) Palpable olive-shaped mass in the epigastric region
   (B) Double-bubble sign on abdominal X-ray
   (C) Loops of intestine in the left hemithorax on chest X-ray
   (D) Gas in the walls of the intestine
   (E) Donut sign on abdominal ultrasound

5. A one-week-old male presents with intolerance of breastfeedings as well as several episodes of bilious vomiting. On physical exam, the patient's blood pressure and temperature are normal. The infant appears to be in pain. However, the abdomen does not appear to be distended, and there is no tenderness to palpation. Plain abdominal X-ray shows an absence of gas within the bowel but is otherwise unremarkable. A complete blood count and electrolytes are normal. What is the next step in the management?
   (A) Admit for observation
   (B) Discharge patient and offer parents reassurance
   (C) Exploratory laparotomy
   (D) Upper GI study with oral contrast
   (E) Abdominal ultrasound

6. A male infant is born via normal spontaneous vaginal delivery at 39 weeks' gestation to a 32-year-old G1P1. She had good prenatal care. The infant is heard grunting while trying to breathe, and he shows bilateral subcostal and intercostal retractions. The patient is observed closely for several hours following delivery, and his respiratory status improves over that time. Which of the following is the most likely explanation of this patient's course?
   (A) Spontaneous reduction in congenital diaphragmatic hernia
   (B) Closure of the ductus arteriosus
   (C) Resorption of excess pulmonary fluid
   (D) Paramyxovirus infection
   (E) Closure of the foramen ovale

7. A five-week-old boy presents with a six-day history of vomiting. The parents report that his vomiting is more forceful than his usual spit ups and contain significantly more volume. The mother describes the vomit as partially digested milk. Between episodes of vomiting, the baby feeds vigorously. The parents report that he has made only one wet diaper today. On physical exam, the baby appears lethargic. Mucous membranes are dry, and the anterior fontanelle is open and sunken. Capillary refill is 2 s. The growth chart reveals a 0.5-lb weight loss since his clinic visit seven days ago. What is the next step in management?
   (A) Surgical intervention
   (B) CT of the abdomen
   (C) Upper GI contrast study
   (D) Fluid resuscitation
   (E) Ultrasound

8. A two-week-old infant delivered at 35 weeks' gestation is brought to the pediatrician by his mother who reports that he has had a harsh, barking cough and makes a high-pitched whistling sound when he inhales. He has been feeding poorly but has not had a fever. The mother also says that the patient has bouts of blue discoloration around his lips, more frequently when he is lying on his back than on his stomach. Chest X-ray is normal. What is the most likely diagnosis?
   (A) Foreign body aspiration
   (B) Asthma
   (C) Transient tachypnea of the newborn
   (D) Tracheomalacia
   (E) Congenital diaphragmatic hernia

9. A two-hour-old male infant born at 39 weeks' gestation is noted to be drooling. Prenatal ultrasound demonstrated polyhydramnios. Attempts at placement of an orogastric (OG) tube are unsuccessful as the tube only passes about 10 cm from the lips. What is the most important immediate concern for an infant with this condition?
   (A) Prevention of aspiration
   (B) Nutrition

(C) Urgent surgical exploration
(D) Establishing positive pressure ventilation
(E) Confirmatory contrast esophagram

10. Which of the following is the next best step in the management of a one-week-old infant born at full term with bilious emesis?
(A) Abdominal ultrasound
(B) Broad-spectrum antibiotics and blood cultures
(C) Immediate operative repair
(D) Contrast enema
(E) Intravenous (IV) fluids and nasogastric (NG) tube placement

11. A six-week-old boy presents with a six-day history of non-bilious, forceful vomiting. Between episodes of vomiting, the baby feeds vigorously. On physical exam, the baby has dry mucous membranes with a sunken anterior fontanelle. Capillary refill is 2 s. He is otherwise asymptomatic without findings on physical exam. Ultrasound is obtained and demonstrates a thickened pyloric channel. What electrolyte abnormality would you expect?
(A) Hypochloremic metabolic alkalosis
(B) Hyperkalemic metabolic acidosis
(C) Hyponatremic metabolism acidosis
(D) Hyperkalemic metabolic alkalosis
(E) Hyponatremic metabolic alkalosis

12. A two-hour-old male born at 39 weeks' gestation is noted to have difficulty breathing. Which of the following would most strongly suggest a diagnosis of esophageal atresia with a tracheoesophageal fistula?
(A) Worsening respiratory status with feeding
(B) Olive-shaped mass palpable in the epigastric region
(C) Improvement of respiratory status over 24-hour after birth
(D) Chest X-ray showing dilated loops of small bowel in the left hemithorax
(E) Scaphoid abdomen

13. A newborn male infant was diagnosed prenatally with trisomy 21. Delivery was uneventful, but pregnancy was complicated by polyhydramnios. The infant has had several episodes of bilious vomiting after breastfeeding but is otherwise stable. Which of the following would be the most likely finding on further workup?
(A) Dilated loops of small bowel with air–fluid levels on abdominal X-ray
(B) Inability to pass a nasogastric tube
(C) Abdominal distention with erythema of the overlying skin
(D) Two large air bubbles on abdominal X-ray
(E) Narrowing of the distal rectum on GI contrast study

14. A 12-day-old male born at 33 weeks becomes lethargic and hypothermic over the course of 24-h. He is not tolerating his formula feeds, has two episodes of bilious emesis, and has three episodes of bloody diarrhea. Physical exam reveals abdominal distention, visible loops of bowel, abdominal wall erythema, and absent bowel sounds. What is the most likely diagnosis?
(A) Hirschsprung's disease
(B) Duodenal atresia
(C) Esophageal atresia with tracheoesophageal fistula
(D) Necrotizing enterocolitis (NEC)
(E) Meconium ileus

cially in a full-term neonate who is otherwise healthy, is likely transient tachypnea of the newborn, which is benign and self-limited (C). Loops of small bowel in the left hemithorax suggest a congenital diaphragmatic hernia, as does a scaphoid abdomen (it indicates that bowel contents are elsewhere such as in the chest) (D–E).

13. Answer D

Given the history of polyhydramnios, bilious emesis, and Trisomy-21, the most likely diagnosis is duodenal atresia. Because of the duodenal obstruction, there would be no gas in the small bowel. Air–fluid levels on abdominal X-ray are characteristic of more distal intestinal obstruction (A). Inability to pass a nasogastric tube is suggestive of choanal atresia (B). Abdominal distention with erythema of the overlying skin is concerning for necrotizing enterocolitis (C). Narrowing of the distal rectum on GI contrast study is found in Hirschsprung's disease (E).

14. Answer D

In a premature neonate with rather sudden systemic illness, feeding intolerance, and bloody stools, necrotizing enterocolitis would be the most likely diagnosis. Visible loops of distended bowel and abdominal wall erythema are additional classic findings. Initial treatment is to place the infant nothing by mouth (NPO), stomach decompression, and administration of IV antibiotics. Surgical management is indicated for suspected perforation, as evidenced by free intraperitoneal air or progressive clinical deterioration (rising white blood cell [WBC] count, falling platelet count, worsening acidosis). Hirschsprung's disease would present with failure to pass stool at birth and not a sudden decompensation (A). Duodenal atresia presents with bilious vomiting, but due to the atresia, it presents at birth and with failure to pass meconium (B). Esophageal atresia with tracheoesophageal fistula would present with respiratory distress during feeding (D). Meconium ileus classically would present with failure to pass meconium at birth and raises concern for cystic fibrosis (E).

15. Answer C

Eviscerated bowel without a membrane covering it, with the abdominal wall defect to the right of the umbilicus, is termed gastroschisis. It is more common in young mothers and in those who smoke during pregnancy. Maternal serum AFP tends to be elevated in cases of abdominal wall defects, including both gastroschisis and omphalocele (evisceration though the umbilicus and with a membrane covering bowel). Typically, maternal serum AFP is greater in gastroschisis than in omphalocele. Maternal serum AFP is checked as part of the triple screen or quad screen that is performed. Elevated maternal serum AFP is seen in other conditions such as multiple gestation, neural tube defects, abruptio placentae, or endodermal sinus tumor, making this a nonspecific marker for abdominal wall defects. Gastroschisis is associated with intestinal atresia. Since the fetus may be unable to swallow amniotic fluid, it is associated with polyhydramnios.

16. Answer D

Gastroesophageal reflux is a common complaint in infants less than one year of age. In the first year of age, the pylorus is not fully developed and therefore not fully functional, leading to occasional episodes of reflux (also called spitting up). Gastroesophageal reflux *disease* (GERD) is not diagnosed until the infant is failing to gain weight. Treatment of GERD includes thickening the feeds, keeping the infant upright after feeds, and feeding smaller amounts at shorter intervals. Tracheoesophageal fistula typically presents at birth with inability to control secretions. A rare "H" type (fistula without esophageal atresia) often presents in a delayed fashion but would present with recurrent respiratory infections from aspiration and not vomiting (A). Duodenal atresia would present as bilious vomiting in the newborn period and the classic "double-bubble" sign on abdominal X-ray (B). Pyloric stenosis presents with non-bilious, projectile vomiting in the first few weeks of life and typically not at four months of age (C). In addition, it would progressively worsen with time. Malrotation would present with abdominal distension and bilious vomiting (E).

17. Answer C
Diffuse pulmonary interstitial and/or alveolar edema suggests transient tachypnea of the newborn, which is self-limited and resolves within one to two days. Loops of bowel in the left chest suggest a congenital diaphragmatic hernia (A). An orogastric tube that does not pass beyond the proximal esophagus suggests an esophageal atresia (B). Boot-shaped heart with upturned apex is found in infants with tetralogy of Fallot, a constellation of congenital cardiac anomalies, that specifically includes ventricular septal defect, pulmonary stenosis, large overriding aorta, and right ventricular hypertrophy (D). The double-bubble sign is found in duodenal atresia (E).

18. Answer D
This patient has gastroschisis. Since the intestines are outside of the abdominal cavity, insensible fluid losses will be much greater than in an infant without gastroschisis. Therefore, covering of the exposed intestine with moist gauze and IV fluid resuscitation are critical first steps in management. Hypothermia is also a common immediate risk due to exposed bowel and large surface area. While exposed intra-abdominal contents increase risk of infection and sepsis, this is not as immediate of a concern as is dehydration (A). After operative repair, patients may be paralyzed to allow the abdominal wall to relax and stretch to accommodate the intestines. If the abdominal cavity is not sufficiently large to accommodate the bowel, the bowel is covered with a silo temporarily. Attempting to forcefully reduce all the small bowels and close it under tension will result in abdominal compartment syndrome, bowel ischemia, and respiratory compromise (B). Cardiac anomalies are more of a concern in patients with omphalocele than gastroschisis, but regardless this is not an immediate concern (C). Urinary obstruction is not a typical feature of gastroschisis, though it could rarely occur if the bladder were also herniated through the abdominal wall (E).

Surgical Complications

Jeffry Nahmias

Contents

Postoperative Bleeding

Areg Grigorian, Christian de Virgilio, Dennis Y. Kim, and Jeffry Nahmias

Contents

C. de Virgilio, A. Grigorian (eds.), *Surgery*, https://doi.org/10.1007/978-3-032-09799-6_39

Case Study

A 50-year-old male is scheduled to undergo an elective inguinal hernia repair. He has noted pain in the hernia, which is reducible, for the past year. His past history is only significant for hypercholesterolemia and mild hypertension. He has had no prior surgery. He does not smoke and only drinks alcohol occasionally. Family history is positive for coronary artery disease. He takes aspirin and a statin. He takes no herbal remedies. On physical examination, he has no stigmata of portal hypertension or cirrhosis. Intraoperatively, the patient is noted to have diffuse oozing from all tissues in the operative field. Despite attempts at complete hemostasis, the patient develops a postoperative hematoma which requires evacuation on postoperative day 2. Laboratory values include a normal chemistry panel, normal hemoglobin and hematocrit, a platelet count of 250,000 cells/mL (normal 140,000–450,000 cells/ml), INR of 1.0, and a PTT of 42 seconds (normal 25-35 seconds). On further questioning, he reports a history of excessive bleeding when he had a wisdom tooth extracted 20 years ago.

Diagnosis

What Is the Differential Diagnosis of Bleeding in the Postoperative Setting? (◘ Table 39.1)

◘ **Table 39.1** Differential diagnosis of postoperative bleeding

Condition	Comments
Surgical bleeding	Bleeding from a major artery or vein that was missed during surgery (insufficient hemostasis) is the most common cause of postoperative bleeding in patients with no personal or family history of easy bleeding or bruising
Medications	Inquire about aspirin, clopidogrel, heparin, warfarin, or any other antiplatelet or direct oral anticoagulant (DOAC) medication and some herbal remedies
Inherited coagulation disorders	Patients with von Willebrand disease may have a history of excessive bleeding after minor procedures or very heavy menses; hemophilia A and B usually present in childhood with spontaneous hemorrhage into joints (hemarthrosis)
Liver disease	Reduced production of clotting factors
Renal failure	Uremia impairs platelet function
DIC	Seen with severe sepsis, malignancy, and childbirth complications; leads to bleeding and microthrombi; manifests with diffuse bleeding from wounds and surgical sites, hematemesis, digital cyanosis, renal insufficiency, and stroke
The bloody vicious cycle ("lethal diamond of death")	Refers to four factors (hypothermia, acidosis, coagulopathy, and hypocalcemia) that work in concert: More common after long operations, trauma, emergency general surgery, and in those who have had significant bleeding with massive transfusions

DIC disseminated intravascular coagulation

What Is the Most Likely Cause of the Bleeding in the Patient Described Above?

The bleeding is likely a medical bleed and not a surgical one. The finding of diffuse oozing at the time of operation together with a prolonged PTT would suggest an underlying bleeding disorder.

What Is the Differential Diagnosis for Prolonged PTT and the Common Features? (Table 39.2)

What Is the Most Likely Diagnosis?

The above patient has an isolated prolonged PTT. Antiphospholipid syndrome associated with SLE is paradoxically a *hypercoagulable* state as opposed to causing bleeding. An acquired antibody to factor VIII (acquired hemophilia) is rare and is most commonly associated with postpartum patients, rheumatic disease, and cancer. Hemophilia A and B are clinically indistinguishable. Hemoglobinopathies are diagnosed via hemoglobin electrophoresis. Those with severe factor deficiencies present early in childhood with spontaneous bleeding in the joints (hemarthrosis) or life-threatening hemorrhage following trauma. Von Willebrand disease (vWD) is not associated with a history of severe bleeding but rather with bleeding after minor surgical procedures or a history of excessive menses. Thus, the most likely diagnosis is vWD.

> **Watch Out**
> Sudden postoperative hypotension should be presumed to be caused by bleeding until proven otherwise. Other possibilities include under-resuscitation during surgery, medication side effects, postoperative myocardial infarction, and sepsis. Look for signs consistent with bleeding, including pallor, swelling, and ecchymosis at the surgical site.

Table 39.2 Differential diagnosis for prolonged PTT and common features

Condition	PT	PTT	BT	Acquired/congenital	Comments
Acquired factor VIII inhibitors	–	↑	–	Acquired	Occurs in postpartum patients, rheumatic disease, and malignancy; presents with purpura, hemarthroses, and soft tissue bleeding
Antiphospholipid syndrome (SLE)[a]	–	↑	–	Acquired	Young woman with malar rash, arthritis, photosensitivity, renal/cardiac symptoms, fevers, malaise, and recurrent first trimester pregnancy loss; associated with lupus; hypercoagulable despite prolonged PTT
Hemophilia A	–	↑	–	Congenital	X-linked recessive, factor VIII deficiency, males, present early in childhood with spontaneous bleeding in joints (hemarthroses) or life-threatening hemorrhage following minor trauma
Hemophilia B	–	↑	–	Congenital	Same as hemophilia A but factor IX deficiency
Heparin administration	–	↑	–	Acquired	Postoperative prophylaxis for DVT and PE, decreases post-MI thrombus risk
von Willebrand disease	–	–/↑	↑	Congenital, rarely acquired	Bleeding after minor surgical procedure or history of excessive menses

BT bleeding time, *DVT* deep vein thrombosis, *PE* pulmonary embolism, *MI* myocardial infarction, *PT* prothrombin time, *PTT* partial thromboplastin time, *SLE* systemic lupus erythematosus
[a]Antiphospholipid syndrome is a hypercoagulable state

39

History and Physical Examination

Why Is It Important to Ask About a History of Bleeding After Minor Trauma/Procedures?

A history of bleeding suggests a predisposition to a high bleeding risk. Important questions to ask include a family history of bleeding disorders, history of excessive bleeding in the mouth, epistaxis, bleeding into the muscle and joints (hemarthrosis), excessive menstrual bleeding, liver or kidney disease, and excessive bleeding after minor procedures (dental extraction, skin biopsy).

Why Is It Important to Ask About a Family History of Bleeding?

A family history of bleeding suggests there may be an inherited bleeding disorder.

What Medical Conditions Are Risk Factors for Bleeding?

Liver and renal diseases, as well as vitamin K deficiency, increase the risk of bleeding. Malabsorption syndromes, including short bowel syndrome and cystic fibrosis, lead to vitamin K deficiency. Cardiac disease, by virtue of the various antiplatelet and anticoagulation agents often prescribed (aspirin, clopidogrel, warfarin), increases the risk of bleeding.

Physiology/Pathophysiology

What Is the Difference Between Primary and Secondary Hemostasis Disorders?

Disorders of primary hemostasis are usually due to abnormalities in platelets, whereas disorders of secondary hemostasis are usually due to factor abnormalities. After primary hemostasis, the coagulation cascade (▪ Fig. 39.1) generates thrombin, which converts fibrinogen in the platelet plug to fibrin. The fibrin is then cross-linked by factor VIII to form a stable platelet-fibrin thrombus. Impairment in this cascade can lead to disorders of secondary hemostasis and is most often due to factor abnormalities.

What Is Coagulopathy?

This term is reserved for conditions that lead to an impairment of the body's ability to clot blood. Normal blood clotting involves as many as 20 different plasma proteins. When these proteins are missing or deficient,

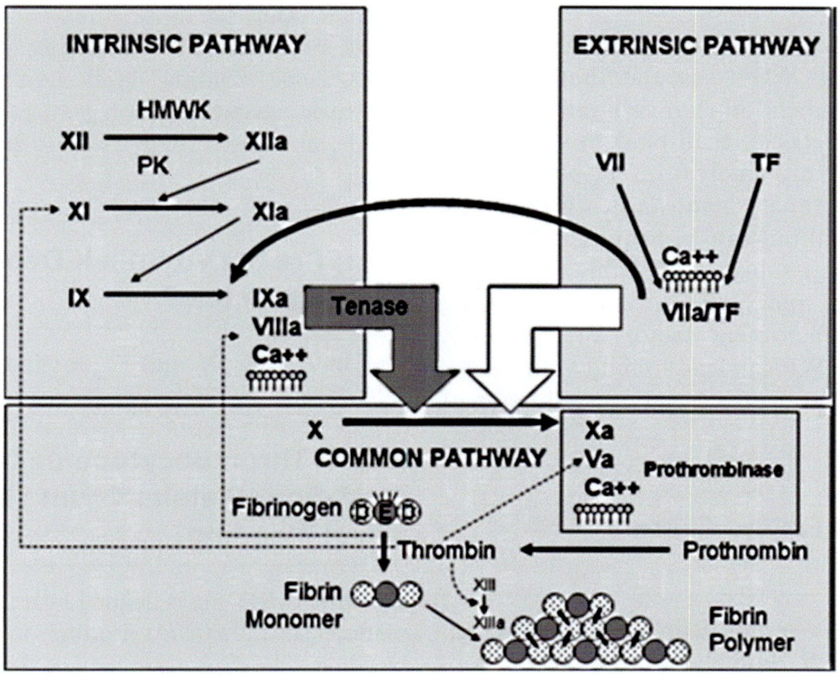

▪ **Fig. 39.1** Coagulation cascade. *HMWK* high molecular weight kininogen, *PK* prekallikrein, *TF* tissue factor. (From: Kottke-Marchant K. The role of coagulation in arterial and venous thrombosis. In: Contemporary Cardiology: Antithrombotic Drug Therapy in Cardiovascular Disease. Kottke-Marchant K, editor. © Humana Press, a part of Springer Science+Business Media, LLC 2010, reprinted with permission)

patients can present with bleeding symptoms that can range from mild to severe. This can occur spontaneously or following minor trauma. Metabolic acidosis and hypothermia exacerbate coagulopathy.

What Is Meant by a Medical Versus a Surgical Postoperative Bleed?

A surgical bleed refers to bleeding that should be corrected with surgery, for example, bleeding from a focal area (an artery or vein) that was inadequately ligated, cauterized, or sutured during the initial surgery. Insufficient hemostasis is the most likely cause of postoperative bleeding (or bleeding after biopsy) in patients with no family or personal history of easy bleeding or bruising. A medical bleed refers to diffuse bleeding caused by underlying coagulopathy. Since medical bleeding is diffuse and caused by a bleeding disorder, reoperation is not beneficial.

Watch Out
A postoperative neck hematoma should be promptly evacuated to avoid upper airway obstruction.

What Is the Pathophysiology of vWD? What Are the Subtypes?

von Willebrand factor (vWF) is a protein needed to form a platelet plug. When vascular tissue is damaged, the exposed subendothelial collagen is able to bind to vWF. Platelets can then bind to vWF using the GPIb receptor to ultimately form the platelet plug and thus complete primary hemostasis. vWD is most commonly congenital but can be acquired. The congenital form has three subtypes (◘ Table 39.3) causing both qualitative and quantitative defects. Since vWF is also a cofactor for factor VIII, severely decreased levels of vWF can lead to mildly prolonged PTT, depending on the degree of activity reduction of factor VIII.

39

◘ **Table 39.3** Subtypes of vWD

Type	Inheritance	Features
1	AD	The most common overall, often has mild symptoms; decreased amount of normally functioning vWF
2	AD	Often has moderate symptoms; normal to low-normal amount of vWF with decreased function
3	AR	Rare, causes the most severe symptoms; very low or absent vWF production

AD autosomal dominant, *AR* autosomal recessive

How Does Renal Failure Cause Coagulopathy?

End-stage renal disease results in uremic toxins circulating in the blood, which cause platelet dysfunction. This can initially be managed with the administration of desmopressin and/or hemodialysis.

How Does Liver Disease Cause Coagulopathy?

As liver disease worsens, so does the synthetic function of the liver, manifested by a prolonged PT and increased INR. The majority of patients have thrombocytopenia and decreased production of coagulation factors. The thrombocytopenia is caused by a combination of increased sequestration in the spleen, deficiency of thrombopoietin, and immune-mediated destruction of platelets.

Watch Out
Factor VIII is the only component of the clotting cascade not exclusively synthesized by the liver and remains at a normal (or higher) level during liver failure; all the other factor levels will decrease.

What Are the Vitamin K-Dependent Clotting Factors?

Factors II, VII, IX, and X, protein C, and protein S.

How Is Thrombocytopenia Defined? How Do Various Platelet Count Thresholds Affect Bleeding?

Thrombocytopenia is defined by a decreased number of platelets (<150,000/ul) leading to increased risk of bleeding. The clinical severity of thrombocytopenia has an inverse relationship with the platelet count (◘ Table 39.4).

■ **Table 39.4** Thrombocytopenia presentation based on platelet count

Laboratory finding	Clinical presentation
Platelets >100,000 cells/ml	Asymptomatic
Platelets 50,000 to 100,000 cells/ml	Occasional petechiae, 50,000 cells/ml is minimum to proceed with surgery
Platelets 10,000 to 50,000 cells/ml	Purpura after minor trauma
Platelets <10,000 cells/ml	Spontaneous intracerebral hemorrhage and bruising, bleeding gums

What Are the Causes of Thrombocytopenia? (■ Table 39.5)

■ **Table 39.5** Causes of thrombocytopenia

Etiology	Pathology	Labs	Management
Impaired production	Abnormal/reduced platelet precursor caused by drugs, infection, alcohol, mineral deficiency, malignancy	Bone marrow biopsy shows ↓ megakaryocytes	Stop offending agent, replace deficiencies, treat underlying disorder
Platelet pooling	Splenic platelet sequestration		If symptomatic, splenectomy may be required
HIT	Heparin forms complex with platelet factor 4 → produces IgG antibodies which destroy platelets; remnants activate remaining platelets → thrombus	Sudden decrease in platelet count >50%; typically, 5–10 days after administration of heparin	Stop heparin, switch to direct thrombin inhibitor such as dabigatran
ITP	Autoimmune production of IgG leading to platelet destruction	Platelets commonly <50,000	*Children*: Observe for spontaneous resolution, corticosteroids, and IVIG
			Adults: Corticosteroids, IVIG, and splenectomy
TTP	Platelets are consumed in the formation of microthrombi in small vessels, due to an enzyme deficiency (ADAMSTS13) that normally cleaves vWF multimers	↑ reticulocytes, blood smear shows evidence of hemolytic anemia (schistocytes)	Emergent plasmapheresis, corticosteroids, and splenectomy (severe cases)
DIC	Initial coagulopathy with widespread clot formation that quickly evolves to a state of pathologic consumption of platelets and coagulation factors	↑ INR, ↑ PTT, ↓ fibrinogen, ↑ fibrinogen split products, ↑ D-dimer, ↓ hemoglobin, ↓ hematocrit	Treat underlying disorder, platelets, FFP, and cryoprecipitate
HELLP syndrome	Pathogenesis unclear, sequela of eclampsia, and may be associated with aberrant placental development	↑ LFTs, ↓ hemoglobin, ↓ haptoglobin, schistocytes on blood smear	Methyldopa to reduce blood pressure, corticosteroids to speed lung maturity, induce labor if >34 weeks

DIC disseminated intravascular coagulation, *HIT* heparin-induced thrombocytopenia, *ITP* idiopathic thrombocytopenic purpura, *IVIG* intravenous immunoglobulin, *FFP* fresh frozen plasma, *TTP* thrombotic thrombocytopenic purpura, *HELLP* hemolysis, elevated liver (enzymes), low platelets

What Are the Two Types of HIT? What Is the Typical Timeline for HIT? (Table 39.6)

Watch Out

HIT should be suspected when the 4 T's are present: Thrombocytopenia, Timing within 5–10 days of heparin exposure, Thrombosis, and oTher causes of thrombocytopenia ruled out.

Watch Out

Although HIT leads to thrombocytopenia, it is considered a *hypercoagulable* state.

What Is the Mechanism of DIC?

DIC is caused by uncontrolled activation of the coagulation cascade, most commonly triggered by endothelial injury and the release of tissue factor. This leads to widespread intravascular fibrin deposition and the formation of microthrombi, which consume clotting factors, platelets, and fibrinogen—a process referred to as consumptive coagulopathy. Simultaneously, secondary activation of fibrinolysis occurs to break down these clots, which further depletes fibrinogen and other coagulation components and contributes to bleeding. Clinically, DIC is characterized by thrombosis and bleeding, which may manifest as organ dysfunction from ischemia, oozing at venipuncture sites, or mucosal hemorrhage. DIC can be differentiated from dilutional coagulopathy, which occurs following large-volume transfusion or resuscitation. In dilutional coagulopathy, fibrinogen and other clotting factors are diluted due to replacement of lost blood with fluids or packed red blood cells that lack coagulation components. Although fibrinogen can also be low in this setting, D-dimer levels are typically normal, and there is no evidence of systemic clot formation. In contrast, DIC is characterized by elevated D-dimer, prolonged PT and aPTT, thrombocytopenia, and low fibrinogen. The common causes of DIC can be remembered with the mnemonic DIC: delivery, infection, and cancer (Table 39.7). The primary treatment of DIC is to treat the underlying cause.

Watch Out

Continuous positive airway pressure (CPAP) can increase the risk of recurrent nosebleeds due to its drying effect on the nasal lining. Using humidification is a common and effective strategy to prevent CPAP-related epistaxis.

Table 39.7 Disseminated intravascular coagulation (DIC)

Etiology	Features
Delivery	Tissue thromboplastin in amniotic fluid activates the coagulation cascade
Infection	Sepsis can induce endothelial cells to make/release tissue factor; the most common mechanism involves TNF associated with gram-negative bacteria
Cancer	Auer rods in AML are potent activators of the coagulation cascade; mucin associated with adenocarcinoma can also activate the cascade

TNF tumor necrosis factor, *AML* acute myeloid leukemia

Table 39.6 Types of heparin-induced thrombocytopenia (HIT)

HIT	Timing	Presentation	Mechanism	Management
Type 1	1–4 days after heparin exposure	Mild, transient decrease in platelet count (~100 K/ μL) without clinical manifestations	Nonimmune-mediated platelet aggregation	Observation
Type 2	5–10 days after heparin exposure	Fall in platelet count >30–50%, thrombocytopenia (~20–60 K/ μL), arterial and venous thrombosis, necrosis at injection sites	Antibody mediated; heparin forms complex with platelet factor 4 → produces IgG antibodies which destroy platelets; remnants activate remaining platelets → thrombus	Stop heparin, start non-heparin anticoagulant (i.e., argatroban, bivalrudin, fondaparinux, apixaban)

39

What Is Hyperfibrinolysis? How Is It Classified?

Hyperfibrinolysis refers to excessive fibrin breakdown that leads to bleeding. It results from excess plasmin activity, which overwhelms antiplasmin mechanisms and consumes clotting factors. It is classified as primary or secondary. Primary hyperfibrinolysis is due to increased circulating tissue plasminogen activator and may occur in liver disease, severe trauma, or after cardiopulmonary bypass. Secondary hyperfibrinolysis occurs in response to widespread clot formation, as seen in DIC or sepsis, and also leads to excessive bleeding.

What Coagulation Factors Do INR and PTT Measure, and What Drug Therapies Can They Monitor? (Table 39.8)

Describe the Mechanism of the Commonly Used Antiplatelet and Anticoagulant Medications (Table 39.9)

Table 39.8 INR and PTT

	Measures	Coagulation factors	Monitors
INR	Extrinsic and common coagulation pathways	I (fibrinogen), II (prothrombin), V, VII, X	Warfarin
PTT	Intrinsic and common coagulation pathways	I, II, V, VIII, IX, X, XI, XII	Heparin

Table 39.9 Commonly used antiplatelet and anticoagulant medications

Medication	Mechanism of action	Reversible?
Aspirin	Irreversibly inhibits platelet cyclooxygenase enzymes, which results in decreased formation of PGE-2 and thromboxane-A2	No
Clopidogrel	Blocks ADP receptors to suppress fibrinogen binding to platelets and thus inhibits platelet aggregation	No
GP-IIb/GP-IIIa inhibitors (e.g., *abciximab*)	Inhibit platelet aggregation by binding to platelet GP-IIb/GP-IIIa receptors	No
Heparin	Activates antithrombin-III, activated antithrombin-III inactivates thrombin and factor Xa	Protamine sulfate
LMWH (e.g., *enoxaparin*)	Binds to factor Xa to prevent clot formation	Protamine sulfate
Direct thrombin inhibitor (e.g., *argatroban*)	Inhibits thrombin to suppress factor activity and decrease platelet aggregation	Idarucizumab; hemodialysis may help
Warfarin	Inhibits vitamin K epoxide reductase, an enzyme required for the production of factors II, VII, IX, and X	Prothrombin complex concentrate (rapid), fresh frozen plasma (slower), vitamin K (slowest)
Factor Xa inhibitors (e.g., *apixaban, rivaroxaban*)	Binds to factor Xa, preventing the activation of factor II (prothrombin) to factors IIa (thrombin)	Andexanet alfa

LMWH low molecular weight heparin

Workup

Prior to an Elective Operation, What Is the Best Method to Identify a Patient at Risk for Bleeding During Surgery? Is Routine Laboratory Screening for Bleeding Disorders Necessary?

Clinical history remains the gold standard for preoperative assessment of hemostasis. Specifically, a history of excessive bleeding after minor procedures is important. In addition, in most cases, INR, PTT, and platelet count are ordered preoperatively. No additional routine screening for bleeding disorders is necessary.

Management

What Is the First Step in the Management of a Patient with Suspected Postoperative Bleeding?

Always start with the A (airway), B (breathing), and C (circulation) of resuscitation. Make sure the patient has adequate IV access and that baseline labs have been sent, including a type and cross, complete blood count, INR, PTT, and lactate. Correct any observed coagulopathy.

At What Point Should Re-exploration Be Considered for a Patient Who Is Bleeding Postoperatively?

Postoperative bleeding, particularly after abdominal surgery, is sometimes difficult to recognize, as there are no visible signs on physical exam (such as an expanding hematoma), and the surgeon presumably closed the abdomen with good hemostasis. Bleeding should always be suspected in a patient who develops unexplained or sustained tachycardia and hypotension after surgery. However, if the bleeding is thought to be a medical bleed, the general recommendation is to correct the underlying coagulation problem first, as medical bleeds are unlikely to be corrected with surgery, and then re-explore if the bleeding continues.

How Is Bleeding Secondary to Uremia Corrected?

Although desmopressin can initially be used (increase vWF) for uremic bleeding, dialysis is considered the definitive management.

How Is Bleeding Secondary to Liver Disease Corrected?

Fresh frozen plasma, cryoprecipitate, coagulation factors, and platelet transfusion.

At What Threshold Should Platelets Be Administered?

The threshold for platelet transfusion remains controversial, but it is never recommended for platelet destructive processes (e.g., hemolytic uremic syndrome). For patients (bleeding or not) that will be undergoing an invasive procedure (e.g., surgery) and have platelet counts <50,000/ul, a prophylactic platelet transfusion is generally recommended. Prior to central line placement the recommended threshold is <20,000/ul. For all asymptomatic patients with platelet counts <10,000/ul, a platelet transfusion is also given to prevent *spontaneous intracranial bleeding*.

> **Watch Out**
> Patients undergoing surgery who are on anticoagulants should typically stop anticoagulation before surgery to prevent postoperative bleeding. For urgent or emergent surgery, PCC can be used in most cases to reverse coagulopathy. For warfarin, also administer IV vitamin K.

Complications

What Are the Different Types of Transfusion Reactions, Their Causes, and Management? (▫ Table 39.10)

> **Watch Out**
> An overlooked but common cause of fever in the first 6 h after surgery is a febrile nonhemolytic transfusion reaction if the patient received blood products during the case.

What Is the Leading Cause of Transfusion-Related Fatalities?

Transfusion-associated circulatory overload (TACO) is the leading cause of transfusion-related deaths. TACO occurs when rapid or excessive transfusion

Table 39.10 Types of transfusion reactions, causes, and management

Type	Timing	Pathology	Management
Anaphylactic	Rapid and sudden onset	Shock results from anti-IgA antibodies, occurs in patients with selective-IgA deficiency	Stop transfusion, epinephrine, intubation, fluid resuscitation
Febrile nonhemolytic	Minutes to hours after transfusion	The most common transfusion reaction; caused by cytokine accumulation in stored blood from donor leukocytes; presents with only fever and chills	Self-limited, acetaminophen can help
Allergic/urticarial	Minutes to hours after transfusion	Results from the plasma present in donor blood	Diphenhydramine
Transmitted bacterial infection	Within 30 min to hours	Most commonly from platelet transfusion as platelets are stored at room temperature to maintain function; presents with fever, tachycardia, hypotension, but no flank pain	Antibiotics
Acute hemolytic	Within 24 h of transfusion	ABO incompatibility leading to severe destruction of donor red blood cells by preformed host antibodies; presents with fever, flank pain, hemoglobinuria, DIC, and positive Coomb's test	Stop transfusion, IV fluids to induce diuresis
Delayed hemolytic	Days to weeks after transfusion	Rh antibodies leading to the destruction of donor red blood cells, requires sensitization (e.g., previous pregnancy); positive Coomb's test	Self-limited

leads to volume overload, increasing pulmonary hydrostatic pressure and causing pulmonary edema. It is most common in patients with underlying cardiac or kidney disease who receive a large volume of blood products over a short time. Clinical features include hypertension, elevated brain natriuretic peptide (BNP), jugular venous distension, and a net positive fluid balance. Treatment typically involves diuresis, which can effectively alleviate symptoms. In contrast, transfusion-related acute lung injury (TRALI) is the second leading cause of transfusion-related fatalities and is characterized by non-cardiogenic pulmonary edema. TRALI results from donor anti-leukocyte antibodies activating the recipient's neutrophils, leading to damage of the pulmonary microvasculature, diffuse endothelial dysfunction, and increased capillary permeability. Unlike TACO, TRALI presents with hypotension, diffuse pulmonary infiltrates (crackles on exam), and respiratory distress. Treatment is primarily respiratory supportive care.

What Are the Phases of Wound Healing?

Wounds proceed through four phases of healing: hemostasis, inflammation, proliferation, and maturation. Initial endothelial injury results in vasoconstriction, formation of a platelet plug (primary hemostasis), activation of the coagulation cascade, and eventual formation of a platelet-fibrin thrombus (secondary hemostasis). Next, the inflammatory phase is characterized by activation of the acute immune system, vasodilation, and increased vascular permeability. Chemotaxis and extravasation of neutrophils, monocytes, and macrophages allow for clearance of bacteria and foreign debris. Inflammatory cytokines and growth factors activate fibroblasts and epithelial cells for the proliferation phase. Epithelialization and collagen production begin during the proliferation phase. Type III collagen is synthesized first during the initial stages of wound healing. The maturation phase involves collagen remodeling and cross-linking, which are most responsible for the wound's final tensile strength. It typically takes at least 6 weeks for surgical wounds to regain most (~80%) of their original tensile strength; therefore, patients are often advised against strenuous activity during that period.

Areas You Can Get in Trouble

Failing to Stop Antiplatelets/Anticoagulants in a Timely Fashion Prior to Surgery

For most patients undergoing noncardiac surgery, aspirin should be stopped prior to surgery. Aspirin increases the risk of bleeding yet does not appear to lower the risk of perioperative myocardial infarction. Platelet aggregation is restored within 4 days of stopping aspirin, but clopidogrel must be stopped for 7 days to achieve normal platelet function. After stopping warfarin, the INR typically falls below 2.0 within 2–3 days and normalizes within 4–6 days. Once the INR is 1.5 or below, surgery can be performed with relative safety in most cases. Direct oral anticoagulants (i.e., apixaban, rivaroxaban, and dabigatran) may be stopped 24–48 h before surgery depending on the bleeding risk of surgery. Heparin is typically stopped 4–6 h prior to surgery.

Summary of Essentials

History and Physical Examination

39

- Surgical bleeds result from inadequate hemostasis and may require reoperation
- Risk factors for coagulopathy: copious IV fluids or transfusions, hypothermia, metabolic acidosis, liver or kidney disease, DIC, family history of bleeding, and anticoagulant/antiplatelet medications
- Beware of HIT in patients who have recently begun heparin therapy

Workup

- The most important diagnostic modality for coagulopathy is a clinical history
- Warfarin is monitored with INR; heparin is monitored with PTT
- Always check for signs of liver and kidney dysfunction

Management

- The treatments of uremic coagulopathy are desmopressin (acutely) and hemodialysis (more definitively)
- The treatment of hepatic coagulopathy is FFP
- Heparin can be reversed with protamine; warfarin can be reversed with PCC rapidly
- For most elective procedures, platelets >50,000/ul are sufficient
- Aspirin should be stopped before noncardiac surgery in most cases

Complications

- TACO is treated with diuresis and respiratory support
- TRALI is treated with IV fluids, vasopressors, and respiratory support

Acknowledgements The editors would like to acknowledge and thank the following authors for their contributions to the previous edition of the chapter: Paul N. Frank.

Suggested Reading

Cosmi B, Alatri A, Cattaneo M, et al. Assessment of the risk of bleeding in patients undergoing surgery or invasive procedures: guidelines of the Italian Society for Haemostasis and Thrombosis (SISET). Thromb Res. 2009;124:e6.

Douketis JD. Perioperative management of patients who are receiving warfarin therapy: an evidence-based and practical approach. Blood. 2011;117:5044.

Segal JB, Dzik WH, Transfusion Medicine/Hemostasis Clinical Trials Network. Paucity of studies to support that abnormal coagulation test results predict bleeding in the setting of invasive procedures: an evidence-based review. Transfusion. 2005;45:1413.

Postoperative Decreased Urine Output

Dennis Y. Kim, Christian de Virgilio, Areg Grigorian, and Jeffry Nahmias

Contents

C. de Virgilio, A. Grigorian (eds.), *Surgery*, https://doi.org/10.1007/978-3-032-09799-6_40

Case Study

A previously healthy 65-year-old female underwent an emergent sigmoid colectomy and proximal colostomy for perforated diverticulitis. Intraoperatively, the patient was found to have extensive fecal contamination of the peritoneal cavity with minimal blood loss. She received two liters of intravenous fluids during the operation. Twelve hours after surgery, the patient is found to have a blood pressure of 110/60 mmHg (supine), heart rate of 110/min, temperature of 37.8 °C, and respiratory rate of 14/min. Her mucous membranes appear dry, and skin turgor is decreased. She does not have jugular venous distention. Cardiac and respiratory exams are unremarkable. The patient is noted to have only produced 30 cc of dark yellow urine in the last 3 h. Postoperative laboratory values demonstrate a rising BUN of 34 mg/dl (normal 7–21 mg/dl) and a creatinine of 1.5 mg/dl (0.5–1.4 mg/dl) (preoperative creatinine 0.8 mg/dl). Hemoglobin and hematocrit are the same as preoperative at 11 g/dl (12–15.2 g/dl) and 33% (37–46%).

Diagnosis

What Is the Differential Diagnosis for a Rise in Creatinine in the Postoperative Setting? (Table 40.1)

What Is the Most Likely Cause for the Patient's Decreased Urine Output?

The most likely cause for the patient's decreased urine output is prerenal acute kidney injury (AKI) secondary to hypovolemia. Volume depletion and third-space losses are common following surgery, particularly in the setting of significant peritoneal inflammation. The patient is oliguric with tachycardia and physical exam findings consistent with volume depletion (dry mucous membranes and decreased skin turgor). There has also been an acute increase in her serum BUN and creatinine (>20:1), which is consistent with prerenal AKI.

History and Physical Exam

Why Is It Important to Review the Operative Record and the Anesthetic Record?

Checking the operative records can help identify the etiology of a decompensating patient. In patients who appear to be hypovolemic, checking the record for their estimated intraoperative blood loss, complications during the surgery that may increase suspicion for potential sites of postoperative bleeding, the administration of anticoagulants, the requirement of pressors or blood products, and the amount of fluids received is important in discovering the etiology.

Table 40.1 Differential diagnosis for a rise postoperative creatinine

Type	Causes	Pathophysiology
Prerenal	Hypovolemia (postsurgical bleeding, dehydration), decreased cardiac output (heart failure)	Inadequate perfusion for a normal functioning kidney
Intrinsic/ renal	Acute tubular necrosis (ATN) (e.g., renal artery occlusion; drugs: Radiocontrast agents, aminoglycosides; rhabdomyolysis); interstitial nephritis (penicillin, cephalosporins, sulfa drugs, NSAIDs)	Prolonged ischemia of the kidney or toxins leading to parenchymal injury
Postrenal	Obstruction of urine, benign prostate hypertrophy (BPH), prostate cancer, nephrolithiasis, bilateral ureteral ligation, urethral stricture	Increased nephron tubular pressure

What Is the Most Common Presentation of AKI?

The most common presentation of AKI is prerenal azotemia. Most patients are asymptomatic and present with only a rise in BUN and creatinine (azotemia) with a ratio >20:1. The earliest sign of AKI is oliguria (please see below).

What Is the Difference Between Oliguria and Anuria?

The normal urine output for an adult is 0.5–1.0 ml/kg/hour. For children, normal urine output is 1.0–2.0 ml/kg/hour. Oliguria describes decreased but not absent urine output and is defined as a urine output of less than 0.5 ml/kg/hour for two consecutive hours. When urine output becomes less than 50–100 ml over a 24-hour period, the patient is considered to be anuric. Producing absolutely no urine is unusual and may be a result of a technical error, especially in patients with a urinary catheter in place (clogged or kinked catheter).

What Are the Most Common Nephrotoxic Medications?

The most common nephrotoxic medications are intravenous contrast agents (contrast-induced nephropathy), aminoglycosides (e.g., gentamicin), ACE inhibitors, amphotericin, cisplatin, cyclosporine, and nonsteroidal anti-inflammatory drugs (NSAIDs).

Physiology/Pathophysiology

Which Patients Are at Greatest Risk for Intravenous Contrast-Induced AKI?

Patients with pre-existing renal damage (e.g., glomerulonephritis, diabetes) are at greatest risk. Contrast-induced nephropathy is widely defined as an absolute increase in serum creatinine of 0.5 mg/dl or a relative increase of 25% from the baseline value, assessed 48–72 h following intravascular administration of contrast media.

Watch Out

Pre- and post-hydration with normal saline has the most proven benefit in preventing contrast-induced nephrotoxicity in patients with pre-existing kidney disease.

What Is the Major Force Driving Filtration in the Kidney?

High hydrostatic pressure in the glomerular capillary is responsible for ensuring filtration in the nephron tubules. In situations where hydrostatic pressure in Bowman's space rises (postrenal AKI), filtering fluid becomes more difficult.

Watch Out

Increased BUN/creatinine ratio may be seen in conditions other than hypovolemia: upper gastrointestinal bleed (high protein absorption), increased urea production (steroid therapy), and/or low muscle mass (decreases serum creatinine creation).

Does Unilateral Ureteral Obstruction Lead to Renal Failure?

In most cases, this will not lead to renal failure unless the patient has a solitary kidney.

Is It Common to Have Oliguria Following Major Surgery? If So, Why?

Yes. This is a result of the response of the adrenal cortex and posterior pituitary to stress from surgery, leading to fluid loss and shifts. Aldosterone and antidiuretic hormone (ADH) released in the first 24 hours after surgery are primarily responsible for both salt and water retention (discussed in Sect. 40.5). Oliguria lasting longer than 24 h warrants investigation.

Watch Out

Postoperative bleeding can present as oliguria. Lab values such as hemoglobin and hematocrit may be misleading in detecting acute hemorrhage in the postoperative setting. It generally takes 8–12 h for interstitial fluid to redistribute into the vascular space, and blood concentration values will initially appear unchanged. In patients who receive fluid resuscitation, the hemoglobin will begin to drop over time as the fluid shifts into the plasma.

Can Prerenal AKI Lead to Intrarenal AKI and Eventually Renal Failure?

Yes. Prolonged periods of poor renal perfusion will directly damage the kidneys and lead to acute tubular necrosis (ATN), which will cause oliguria even after volume status and normal renal perfusion have been restored.

How Does General Anesthesia Affect Cardiac and Renal Function?

Most general anesthetics, commonly the inhaled volatile agents, result in myocardial depression and systemic vasodilation. This in turn can lead to a decrease in cardiac output and end-organ perfusion. In someone with no pre-existing medical conditions or comorbidities, patients usually tolerate temporary fluctuations in their blood pressure without considerable change to their renal and cardiovascular function. However, patients with renal disease at baseline are more susceptible to insults, which may result in worsening renal function.

Workup

What Is the Best Initial Test When Suspecting AKI?

The best initial tests are BUN and creatinine. A BUN/Cr ratio > 20:1 with a clear history of hypoperfusion or hypotension is consistent with prerenal AKI.

What Other Tests Can Help Distinguish Between the Three Major Categories of AKI?

Urine sodium, fractional excretion of sodium (FE_{Na}) (Table 40.2), and urine osmolality.

Table 40.2 FE_{Na}, U_{OSM}, U_{Cr}/P_{Cr}, and U_{Na}

	FE_{Na}	U_{OSM}	U_{Cr}/P_{Cr}	U_{Na}	BUN/Cr
Prerenal	<1%	>500	>40	<20	>20:1
Intrinsic renal	>1%	<350	<20	>40	<20:1
Postrenal	>4%	< 350	<20	>40	<20:1

UNa urine sodium, *UCr* urine creatinine, *PCr* plasma creatinine

FE_{Na} calculation

$$\text{FENa}\ (\%) = (\text{Urine Sodium} \times \text{Serum Creatinine}) / (\text{Serum Sodium} \times \text{Urine Creatinine}) \times 100$$

With prerenal AKI, decreased blood pressure and/or intravascular volume will increase aldosterone, which subsequently increases sodium reabsorption in the kidneys and results in a decreased FE_{Na}. Additionally, low intravascular volume results in an increase in ADH released from the posterior pituitary. This will lead to increased water reabsorption, increasing urine osmolality, and concentrating the urine to a dark yellow hue. The relevant laboratory values for AKI are presented in Table 40.2.

Watch Out

FE_{Na} is not reliable if the patient is receiving diuretics as they alter the renal excretion of sodium. In such a patient, the FE_{Urea} may be helpful.

What Are the Causes of Hyponatremia and how Does Urine/Serum Osmolality Help?

Hyponatremia can be classified based on serum osmolality. Hypotonic hyponatremia is the most common and can be further differentiated by urine osmolality and urine sodium. If urine osmolality is low (<100 mOsm/kg), it suggests excessive water intake (e.g., psychogenic polydipsia). If urine osmolality is high (>100 mOsm/kg), urine sodium helps differentiate hypovolemia (low urine sodium <20 mEq/L) from syndrome of inappropriate antidiuretic hormone secretion (SIADH) or renal failure (urine sodium >40 mEq/L). The administration of desmopressin, an analogue of ADH, can induce SIADH by impairing urinary water excretion and leading to hypotonic hyponatremia. SIADH can occur in response to stressors such as surgery, pain, neurologic injury, medications, or ectopic ADH production by neuroendocrine tumors, resulting in concentrated oliguria and hyponatremia.

Watch Out
Acute symptomatic hyponatremia (<48 h) should be treated with hypertonic saline to rapidly relieve symptoms, followed by gradual correction. Chronic hyponatremia requires slow correction to avoid central pontine myelinolysis.

How Do Specific Gravity and the Presence of Cells/Casts in a Urinalysis Help? (Table 40.3)

Watch Out
Urine dipstick is unable to differentiate between hemoglobin, myoglobin (rhabdomyolysis), and red blood cells.

What Are the RIFLE Criteria?

This allows clinicians to grade levels of kidney dysfunction based on serum creatinine, glomerular filtration rate (GFR), and urine output (Table 40.4).

What Imaging Is Useful in the Workup of Oliguria?

In cases of postoperative urinary retention, bladder ultrasound is the first step to assess for urinary retention. Ultrasonography of the bladder, ureters, and kidneys is useful to assess for obstructive pathology. Bilateral hydronephrosis with a BUN/Cr ratio less than 20:1 is highly suggestive of postrenal AKI. Doppler ultrasonography is a cost-effective means of evaluating renal perfusion.

Watch Out
In the postoperative setting, new-onset hydronephrosis with a clean urinalysis should raise suspicion for ureteral injury.

Table 40.3 Implications of urinalysis findings

Finding	Suggests
High specific gravity	Volume depletion
Red call casts	Glomerular disease
Hematuria	Renal emboli or stones
White blood cell casts	Infection or inflammation
Granular casts	Acute tubular necrosis

Table 40.4 RIFLE criteria

Grade	Serum creatinine	GFR	Urine output
Risk	1.5-fold increase	Decrease by 25%	<0.5 ml/kg per hour for 6 h
Injury	Twofold increase	Decrease by 50%	<0.5 ml/kg per hour for 12 h
Failure	Threefold increase	Decrease by 75%	<0.3 ml/kg per hour for 24 h or anuria for 12 h
Loss	Complete loss of kidney function for more than 4 weeks		
ESRD	Complete loss of kidney function for more than 3 months		

ESRD end-stage renal disease

Management

When Encountering Low Urine Output in a Patient with an Indwelling Foley Catheter, What Needs to Be Ruled Out First as an Easily Correctable Cause?

An obstructed urinary catheter needs to be ruled out first. One should first look for kinking in the tubing and flush the catheter to make sure it is not clogged.

What Should Be Done Next?

All medications should be reviewed, and all nephrotoxic drugs should be discontinued. In addition, all renally excreted drugs will need to be dose adjusted.

What Is a Fluid Challenge?

This involves giving an oliguric patient a bolus of isotonic crystalloid fluid such as normal saline (500–1000 ml) over a short amount of time (typically 30 min) in an effort to increase urine output. With a Foley catheter in place, urine output is recorded hourly. For patients with prerenal AKI due to hypovolemia with no other injuries to the kidney, urine output should increase. Raising the legs can simulate a fluid challenge (if the patient is hypotensive), but raising the legs is not therapeutic.

What if the Patient Does Not Respond to Repeat Fluid Challenges? How Do You Assess Fluid Responsiveness?

If repeated fluid challenges do not result in an improvement in urine output, the possibilities are either that the patient is still hypovolemic and needs additional fluid or the oliguria is not due to hypovolemia. The dilemma is whether to keep giving fluids and risk fluid overload. To help with this decision, a bedside ultrasound of the inferior vena cava (IVC) can be obtained to assess the diameter and collapsibility of the IVC with inspiration, as these findings correlate with volume status. Alternatively, a straight leg raise test can be performed, which transiently increases venous return; if this maneuver results in an increase in blood pressure or stroke volume, it suggests fluid responsiveness. Another option is the placement of a central venous catheter to measure the central venous pressure (CVP), with normal values ranging from 8 to 12 mmHg. Values below this range indicate persistently low intravascular volume and the need for additional fluid resuscitation. Once a normal CVP has been restored, if oliguria persists, postrenal and intrinsic renal causes must be considered.

What Should Be Done if the Patient Is Suspected of Having a Postrenal Obstruction?

Severe benign prostatic hypertrophy (BPH) can lead to postrenal obstruction. Insertion of a Foley catheter would be the first step in the management. If a Foley is already in place, replacing the catheter or irrigating it may be necessary. In elderly patients, urinary retention may be exacerbated by anticholinergic medications such as diphenhydramine, particularly in the setting of benign prostatic hyperplasia.

What Are the Indications for Urgent/Emergent Dialysis?

If the patient remains anuric and the renal failure persists, hemodialysis may be needed. Indications for emergent hemodialysis can be remembered with the AEIOU mnemonic: acidosis, electrolyte imbalance (hyperkalemia), intoxication (ethylene glycol), overload (fluid), and uremia (uremic encephalopathy, pericarditis, or platelet dysfunction).

What Is the Role of Diuretics in the Treatment of Oliguria?

Diuretics may be beneficial in the setting of cardiogenic oliguria (such as in association with decompensated congestive heart failure). Diuretics are otherwise not beneficial.

Area You Can Get in Trouble

MRI in Patient with Renal Failure

Patients with renal failure who undergo gadolinium-enhanced MRI are at risk for nephrogenic systemic fibrosis. Patients present with marked thickening and hardening of the skin in addition to fibrosis of internal structures, such as the muscle, fascia, lungs, and heart.

Areas of Controversy

Does Contrast-Induced Nephrotoxicity Actually Exist?

The concept of contrast-induced nephrotoxicity has traditionally been a major concern when considering intravenous contrast administration in patients with renal dysfunction. However, recent studies have questioned whether contrast exposure independently causes acute kidney injury. Newer evidence suggests that the risk of kidney injury is more strongly related to patient comorbidities such as baseline renal insufficiency and clinical conditions, such as hypotension and sepsis, rather than the contrast itself. As a result, in critically ill patients where imaging is needed to guide management, the benefit of contrast-enhanced studies often outweighs the theoretical risk of nephrotoxicity, provided that appropriate precautions, such as ensuring adequate hydration, are taken.

Summary of Essentials

History and Physical Exam

- AKI is often asymptomatic, with only decreased urine output as the presenting sign
- Physical exam findings such as dry mucous membranes, decreased skin turgor, and tachycardia suggest volume depletion
- Physical exam findings specific to AKI are rarely seen; the earliest sign is oliguria
- Oliguria: <0.5 ml/kg/h for two consecutive hours
- Anuria: <50 ml–100 ml/day

Physiology/Pathophysiology

- Three types of AKI:
- Prerenal: BUN/Cr ratio > 20:1, often with a history of hypotension/hypovolemia
- Intrinsic renal/intrarenal: sequelae of prerenal AKI, ATN, and interstitial nephritis
- Postrenal: obstruction secondary to BPH, obstructed urinary catheter, tumor, stone, or stricture
- The risk of contrast-induced nephropathy has traditionally been emphasized, but newer evidence suggests that hypotension, sepsis, and pre-existing renal insufficiency, rather than contrast exposure alone, are the primary contributors to AKI
- Aldosterone and ADH are primarily responsible for post-op oliguria

Workup

- The best initial tests are BUN and creatinine
- Urinalysis, urine sodium, fractional excretion of sodium (FE_{Na}), and urine osmolality
- FE_{Na} < 1% suggests prerenal AKI; values >1% suggest intrinsic renal injury, though FE_{Na} is unreliable in patients receiving diuretics; FE_{Urea} may be used instead
- RIFLE criteria to grade kidney dysfunction (serum creatinine, GFR, and urine output)
- Ultrasonography of the bladder, ureters, and kidneys is useful to assess for obstructive pathology

Management

- Flush Foley, discontinue nephrotoxic drugs, and perform a fluid challenge
- Use bedside ultrasound (IVC assessment) or straight leg raise testing to assess volume status if fluid responsiveness is uncertain
- Indications for urgent/emergent dialysis:
- AEIOU: acidosis, electrolyte imbalance (hyperkalemia), intoxication (ethylene glycol), overload, and uremia

Acknowledgement The editors would like to acknowledge and thank the following authors for their contributions to the previous edition of the chapter: Dean Spencer.

Suggested Reading

Galan A, Cowper SE, Bucala R. Nephrogenic systemic fibrosis (nephrogenic fibrosing dermopathy). Curr Opin Rheumatol. 2006;18:614.

Khwaja A. KDIGO clinical practice guideline for acute kidney injury. Kidney Int Suppl. 2012;2:8.

Nash K, Hafeez A, Hou S. Hospital-acquired renal insufficiency. Am J Kidney Dis. 2002;39:930.

Peerapornratana S, Manrique-Caballero CL, Gómez H, et al. Acute kidney injury from sepsis: current concepts, epidemiology, pathophysiology, prevention and treatment. Kidney Int. 2019;96(5):1083-1099. https://doi.org/10.1016/j.kint.2019.05.026. Epub 2019 Jun 7. PMID: 31443997; PMCID: PMC6920048.

Shortness of Breath 5 Days After Surgery

Christian de Virgilio, Areg Grigorian, and Jeffry Nahmias

Contents

C. de Virgilio, A. Grigorian (eds.), *Surgery*, https://doi.org/10.1007/978-3-032-09799-6_41

Case Study

Five days after a laparoscopic left colectomy for colon cancer, a 55-year-old female presents to the emergency department with shortness of breath for the past 6 h. She feels that she is breathing more rapidly and does not seem to be able to catch her breath. She denies any chest pain. Per report, the colon cancer was limited to the sigmoid colon, and the surgery was uneventful. She has no prior cardiac or pulmonary history. On physical exam, the patient has a temperature of 37.9 °C, respiratory rate of 26 cycles/min, heart rate of 110 beats/min, and blood pressure of 130/85 mmHg. Lungs are clear to auscultation without wheezing or rales. On cardiac exam, the patient has no murmurs or rubs. Her abdomen is soft and nontender. The wound appears to be clean without erythema or drainage. Her left leg appears to be swollen up to the knee with pitting edema. The left calf is not tender to palpation. The right leg is not swollen. Distal pulses are normal. O_2 saturation on room air is 92%. Arterial blood gas on room air reveals a pO_2 of 70 mmHg, a pCO_2 of 33 mmHg, a pH of 7.47, and an A-a gradient of 25. Laboratory studies reveal a leukocytosis of 10,600/mm^3, hemoglobin of 12 g/dL (12–15.2 g/dL), and hematocrit of 36% (37–46%). Chest X-ray (CXR) is normal. Electrocardiogram (ECG) demonstrates sinus tachycardia but is otherwise unremarkable.

Diagnosis

What Is the Differential Diagnosis for Postoperative Shortness of Breath? (Table 41.1)

Table 41.1 Differential diagnosis for postoperative shortness of breath

Diagnosis	History and physical	Comments
Pneumonia	Fever, dyspnea, dullness to percussion, productive cough, prolonged intubation, aspiration, PPI use	Most common cause of nosocomial mortality; can be caused by aspiration (right lower lobe if patient is upright, right upper lobe if patient is supine)
Pulmonary embolism	Recent travel (e.g., long airplane or car ride), immobilization, recent surgery, trauma or central line (within 3 months), cancer, history of DVT or PE, smoking, CVA, CHF, COPD	Usually from DVT in pelvic or leg veins, look for Virchow's triad (see below)
Myocardial infarction	History of MI, diabetes, CHF, CAD	Surgery creates proinflammatory state, leads to plaque rupture and thrombosis of coronary artery
Pneumothorax	Diminished/absent breath sounds, associated with central line placement	Air leak in pleura allows equalization of negative pleural pressure with ambient pressure
Cardiogenic pulmonary edema	Rales, JVD, S3 gallop, bilateral leg swelling, orthopnea	PCWP >18 mmHg
Noncardiogenic pulmonary edema	Sepsis, massive transfusion, trauma, pancreatitis; no rales, S3, or JVD	$PaO_2/FiO_2 < 200$, hypoxemia with respiratory alkalosis; bilateral infiltrates on CXR, includes ARDS
Pain/anxiety	Tachycardia, diaphoresis, shaking, shortness of breath, restless	Must rule out other causes first
Bleeding	Hypotension, tachycardia, decreased urine output	Most often in the first hours after surgery

ARDS acute respiratory distress syndrome, *CAD* coronary artery disease, *CHF* congestive heart failure, *COPD* chronic obstructive pulmonary disease, *CVA* cerebral vascular accident (i.e., stroke), *DVT* deep vein thrombosis, *JVD* jugular venous distention, *MI* myocardial infarction, *PCWP* pulmonary capillary wedge pressure, *PE* pulmonary embolism, *PPI* proton pump inhibitor

What Is the Most Likely Diagnosis?

The differential diagnosis for acute shortness of breath with hypoxia is extensive. The primary etiologies in the postoperative period are shown above. Pneumonia and cardiogenic pulmonary edema are high on the list; however, the absence of fluid overload (JVD, rales, or crackles) on exam points against cardiogenic pulmonary edema. Similarly, a normal lung exam and normal CXR make pneumonia, atelectasis, and noncardiogenic pulmonary edema very unlikely. The combination of hypoxia, hypocapnia, respiratory alkalosis, tachycardia, and a wide A-a gradient points to a pulmonary embolism (PE). This is further reinforced by a normal CXR and ECG demonstrating only sinus tachycardia. Finally, the unilateral leg swelling suggests that the source of the PE is a lower extremity deep vein thrombosis (DVT). DVT and PE both comprise venous thromboembolism (VTE) disease.

History and Physical Exam

What Is Virchow's Triad? Which Part of the Triad Can Be Invoked in the Patient?

At least one of Virchow's triad is generally present when a VTE event occurs. The triad includes *stasis*, *endothelial injury*, and a *hypercoagulable state* (◘ Table 41.2). The patient described above has two of the triad: cancer, which is a cause of hypercoagulability, and stasis from being immobile during and after the operation. Surgery, just like other types of trauma, also induces a hypercoagulable (prothrombotic) state. Stasis occurs during prolonged bed rest such as after an injury, a surgery, or a long plane flight or car ride. Walking permits the leg muscles to act as a pump to move blood back to the heart. In the immobile patient, venous blood will tend to collect in the legs, leading to stasis. Hypercoagulable states can be congenital or acquired. Venous endothelial injury can occur after a trauma (leg fracture) or an iatrogenic event (venous cannulation with a central line).

What Is the Wells Score for PE?

The Wells score is calculated by adding the points associated with clinical findings in ◘ Table 41.3. A score >4 points indicates a high likelihood of PE, whereas a score ≤4 points indicates a low likelihood of PE.

What Are the Main Clinical Findings Associated with a DVT?

The main clinical findings are leg swelling, calf pain, warmth of leg, mild redness of calf, and calf tenderness to palpation.

> **Watch Out**
> The left leg is 2× more commonly affected by DVT because the left iliac vein may be compressed by the right iliac artery crossing over it. This phenomenon is known as *May-Thurner syndrome*.

What Are the Five Classic Causes (Ws) of Postoperative Fever and When in the Postoperative Setting Would Each Be Expected to Occur? (◘ Table 41.4)

◘ **Table 41.2** Mechanisms of VTE and risk factors

Mechanism	Risk factors
Stasis	Immobilization, surgery
Endothelial injury	Trauma, central line within the last 3 months, history of DVT or PE
Hypercoagulability	Smoking, OCP use, history of DVT or PE, malignancy, inherited disorders (factor V Leiden, protein C deficiency)

DVT deep vein thrombosis, *PE* pulmonary embolism, *OCP* oral contraceptive

◘ **Table 41.3** Wells score

Finding	Points
Signs and symptoms of DVT	3
PE most likely diagnosis	3
HR >100	1.5
Prior DVT or PE	1.5
Immobilization within the last 4 weeks	1.5
Malignancy within the last 6 months	1
Hemoptysis	1

Table 41.4 Causes of postoperative fever

W	Etiology	Postoperative day
*W*ind	Atelectasis	1–2
*W*ater	Urinary tract infection	After 3
*W*ound	Wound infection	After 5
*W*alking	DVT/thrombophlebitis	7–10
*W*onder drugs	Drug fever (e.g., antibiotics)	Anytime

Watch Out

An often overlooked cause of fever in post-surgical patients is a febrile nonhemolytic blood transfusion reaction. This can occur within the first 6 h after transfusion. It is not uncommon to receive blood products during surgery (especially after trauma), and so a fever in the immediate postoperative setting can be related to this.

Pathophysiology

What Causes Atelectasis and How Does It Cause Alkalosis?

Atelectasis is the most common postoperative pulmonary complication and results from airway obstruction due to retained secretions, poor lung compliance, or inadequate deep breathing secondary to pain and/or sedation. Atelectasis leads to intrapulmonary shunting and ventilation-perfusion mismatch, which prompts an increase in respiratory rate and hyperventilation. This hyperventilation leads to the blowing off of CO_2, resulting in primary respiratory alkalosis. Prevention of atelectasis focuses on improving lung expansion and maintaining clear airways. Good postoperative pain control allows patients to take deep breaths more effectively. An incentive spirometer encourages deep breathing and lung recruitment, thereby reducing the risk of atelectasis.

41

Does Atelectasis Cause Postoperative Fever?

A common misconception is that atelectasis causes postoperative fever. Current evidence supports that most cases of early postoperative fever are actually the result of cytokine release as a response to tissue damage, not atelectasis. In support of this, patients undergoing minimally invasive surgery have lower risk of fever as compared to large open surgical procedures. Furthermore, in randomized studies, the use of an incentive spirometer has not been shown to reduce early postoperative fever.

What Are the Most Commonly Inherited Causes of Hypercoagulability (Thrombophilia)?

Factor V Leiden and prothrombin mutation are the first and second most common inherited thrombophilias. Less common inherited thrombophilias include protein C deficiency, protein S deficiency, antithrombin deficiency, and homocysteinemia.

Watch Out

Heparin-induced thrombocytopenia (HIT) may present as an acute (>50%) drop in platelet levels from baseline in a patient who initiated heparin or low molecular weight heparin (LMWH) therapy within the last 5–10 days. HIT is paradoxically a *hypercoagulable* state despite the thrombocytopenia.

What Are the Most Common Acquired Causes of Hypercoagulability?

Advanced age, pregnancy, malignancy, oral contraceptives, hormone replacement therapy, obesity, nephrotic syndrome, heparin-induced thrombocytopenia (HIT), and antiphospholipid antibody syndrome are common causes of acquired hypercoagulability. However, smoking is the most common acquired cause of hypercoagulability.

Watch Out

Factor V Leiden is the most common *inherited* cause of hypercoagulability and is associated with DVT. The most common *acquired* hypercoagulability is from smoking.

What if a Patient Has No Obvious Component of Virchow's Triad and Presents with VTE?

Always try to identify if the patient manifests any of the three parts of Virchow's triad. If there are no obvious risk factors (such as recent surgery, known malignancy, recent trauma, and plane flight), then a careful history and physical exam must be conducted to ascertain whether the patient has an undiagnosed malignancy or other hypercoagulable state.

What Is the Difference Between a Cardiac and Noncardiac Cause of Postoperative Pulmonary Edema?

Pulmonary edema is defined as excess fluid in the alveoli. There are both cardiac (i.e., cardiogenic) and noncardiac (i.e., noncardiogenic) etiologies. Noncardiogenic pulmonary edema is caused by inflammation that leads to an increased pulmonary capillary permeability secondary to cytokine signaling. Specific etiologies of noncardiogenic edema include pneumonia, acute respiratory distress syndrome (ARDS), pulmonary contusion, transfusion-related acute lung injury (TRALI), and fat embolism. Cardiogenic pulmonary edema arises from an increase in hydrostatic pressure within the capillaries of the lungs as a result of increased pulmonary venous pressure.

How Do You Distinguish Between Cardiogenic and Noncardiogenic Pulmonary Edema Based on History and Physical Exam?

Cardiogenic pulmonary edema typically occurs in the setting of an acute cardiac event, such as myocardial infarction (MI), left ventricular failure, dysrhythmias, or an acute exacerbation of chronic heart failure. History and physical examination often reveal findings indicative of acute heart failure and low cardiac output, including jugular venous distention, an S3 gallop, crackles on auscultation, and cool, pale extremities due to hypoperfusion. In contrast, noncardiogenic pulmonary edema is not related to heart failure and lacks these findings of a low-flow state. Instead, it is often associated with increased capillary permeability in conditions such as ARDS, sepsis, or inhalation injuries.

Why Is It Important to Distinguish Between Cardiogenic and Noncardiogenic Pulmonary Edema?

In cardiogenic pulmonary edema, the pulmonary capillary wedge pressure (PCWP) is elevated (>18 mmHg), reflecting increased left-sided heart pressures, whereas it is normal or low in noncardiogenic pulmonary edema. Distinguishing between these two diagnoses is important because the treatments differ significantly. Cardiogenic pulmonary edema is managed by reducing preload with diuretics, lowering afterload with vasodilators, and, in some cases, administering inotropes such as dobutamine to improve cardiac output. Noncardiogenic pulmonary edema is treated primarily with supportive care, including lung-protective ventilation. Accurate differentiation prevents inappropriate treatments that could worsen the patient's condition.

Watch Out

Cardiogenic pulmonary edema on postoperative day 3 can result from third-spacing fluid shifts. Large volumes of resuscitative intravenous (IV) fluids administered perioperatively equilibrate across body compartments but return to the vasculature around day 3. In elderly patients or those with poor cardiac function, the increased intravascular volume can overwhelm the heart, elevate ventricular filling pressures, and transmit to the pulmonary circulation, causing edema.

What Are the Three Routes by Which a Patient Develops Postoperative Pneumonia?

Postoperative pneumonia may be acquired via inhalation, aspiration, or hematogenous spread. After surgery, the cough reflex may be suppressed, and mucociliary transport may be inhibited by endotracheal intubation. Additionally, alveolar macrophage function may be inhibited by pulmonary edema. Accumulation of oral secretions in the airway is also a risk factor.

What Is an A-a Gradient? What Is the Differential of a Wide A-a Gradient?

A-a gradient refers to the difference in partial pressure of oxygen between the alveolar (P_{AO2}) and arterial blood (P_{aO2}). The A-a gradient can be calculated to help determine the cause of hypoxia. The differential diagnosis of a wide A-a gradient in the postoperative setting includes atelectasis, pneumonia, and pulmonary embolism. A normal A-a gradient is seen when there is no diffusion defect or ventilation-perfusion (V/Q) mismatch, such as in alveolar hypoventilation.

A simple normal value estimation can be calculated by

$$\text{normal A} - \text{a gradient} = \frac{\text{age in years}}{4} + 4$$

Workup

What Is the Full Diagnostic Algorithm for a Possible Pulmonary Embolism? (Fig. 41.1)

When There Is a High Suspicion of VTE, What Is the First Step in the Workup/Management?

If there are no major contraindications, start therapeutic anticoagulation right away *before* the diagnosis is even established. Following therapeutic anticoagulation, one should obtain a CT angiogram of the chest to evaluate the pulmonary arteries.

> **Watch Out**
> If a patient is found to have a PE, always rule out a lower extremity DVT by ordering a duplex ultrasound of the bilateral lower extremities.

When Suspicion of VTE Is Low, What Is the First Step in the Workup?

When suspicion of VTE is low (Wells score of 4 or less), the first step is to obtain a D-dimer assay. D-dimer is a product of the breakdown of fibrin by plasmin. There are many causes of elevated D-dimer levels, including VTE, recent surgery, malignancy, disseminated intravascular coagulation (DIC), infection, pregnancy, and renal and cardiovascular disease. Hence, D-dimer has very low specificity, particularly in the postoperative setting. That being said, D-dimer has a high negative predictive value. So, even though most postoperative patients will have an elevated D-dimer, a D-dimer level < 500 ng/mL effectively can rule out PE in low-risk patients. If D-dimer is elevated, the next step is to obtain a CT angiogram.

41

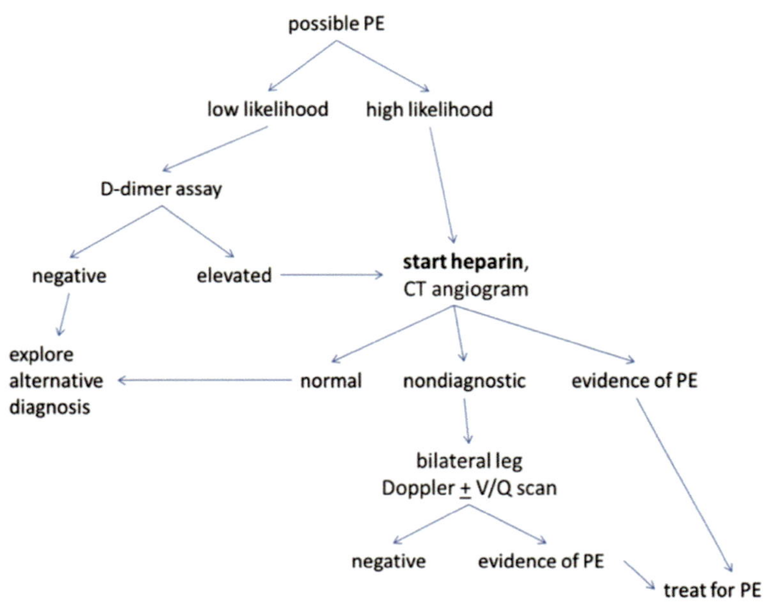

Fig. 41.1 Low likelihood is based on Wells score ≤4. D-dimer assay is considered normal if the D-dimer level is <500 ng/dL

In a Patient with PE, What Are the Most Common Findings on ABG, ECG, and CXR? (Table 41.5)

Table 41.5 Findings on ABG, ECG, and CXR in PE

Study	Most common finding
Arterial blood gas (*ABG*)	Acute respiratory alkalosis, hypoxemia, hypocapnia, increased A-a gradient
Electrocardiogram (*ECG*)	Sinus tachycardia
Chest X-ray (*CXR*)	Normal

What Are the Classic, Though Uncommon, Findings on CXR and ECG That Are Associated with PE?

Westermark's sign (focal/regional pulmonary oligemia distal to embolus) on CXR represents a region of decreased pulmonary blood flow secondary to PE. It is highly specific but has a very low sensitivity. Hampton's hump (wedge-shaped density at periphery of the lung) is another uncommon sign suggesting PE. The classic constellation of ECG findings is large S wave in lead I, large Q wave in lead III, and inverted T wave in lead III. This is seen in only 20% of patients and is a sign of right ventricular (RV) strain. The most common arrhythmia associated with PE is sinus tachycardia.

Since CXR and ECG Are Often Normal with a PE, How Do They Help?

CXR is quite useful in the diagnosis of PE, in that a normal CXR (no infiltrates, atelectasis, or fluid overload) in a hypoxic patient rules out other causes and strengthens the suspicion for PE. Likewise, a normal ECG (other than sinus tachycardia) helps to rule out cardiac causes (MI, arrhythmia) of shortness of breath.

What Are the Typical Findings on CT Angiography for PE? What Is the Sensitivity and Specificity?

CT angiography in PE (Fig. 41.2) will show a filling defect in the pulmonary arterial system. The sensitivity ranges from 91% to 100%, and the specificity ranges from 83% to 93%.

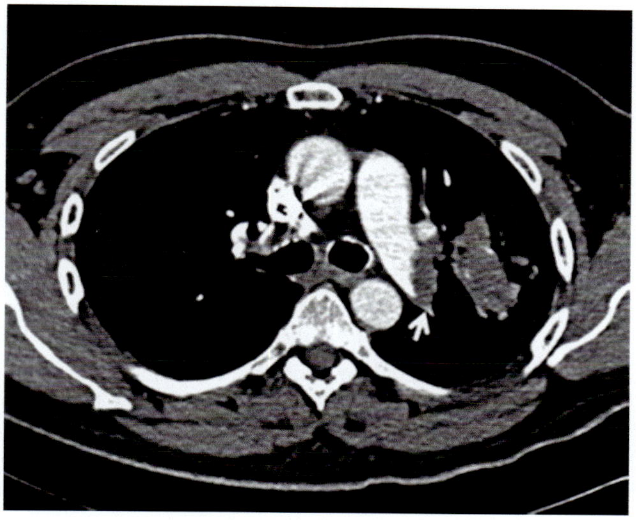

Fig. 41.2 Axial CT angiogram showing a filling defect in the left pulmonary artery consistent with pulmonary embolism

> **Watch Out**
> A large saddle embolus lodged in the common pulmonary artery can result in sudden death secondary to right heart failure.

How Does a V/Q (Ventilation/Perfusion) Scan Work? Why Has It Fallen Out of Favor for the Diagnosis of PE?

A V/Q scan uses inhaled and intravenous (IV) radionuclides to image lung ventilation and perfusion, identifying PE when perfusion deficits exist with normal ventilation. It has fallen out of favor due to its time demands, limited availability, and questionable predictive value.

If the Patient Is Critically Ill and Unable to Be Transported for CT Imaging, What Bedside Options Are There for the Indirect Diagnosis of PE?

Echocardiogram (ECHO) may show indirect evidence of PE, such as right heart strain (if the PE is large). Since most PE arise from DVT in the legs, a venous duplex (*Doppler ultrasound*) of the legs may demonstrate a venous thrombus. If a PE is suspected intraoperatively, a transesophageal ECHO can be performed.

How Is the Severity of PE Classified?

PE is classified into low-risk, submassive, and massive PE. The classification is important as it affects management and prognosis. A low-risk PE has no evidence of right ventricular (RV) dysfunction and no evidence of myocardial necrosis. A submassive PE has been defined as evidence of RV dysfunction on echocardiogram or myocardial necrosis, based on elevated troponin or brain natriuretic peptide (BNP) in the absence of systemic hypotension (systolic BP ≥90 mmHg). With a massive PE, there is the addition of sustained hypotension. The classification of PE to low-risk, submassive, and massive is not based on size, but rather determined by hemodynamic consequence.

Management

What Is the Initial Anticoagulant Management of PE?

The initial management of PE is therapeutic anticoagulation with subcutaneous low molecular weight heparin (LMWH) or intravenous unfractionated heparin. LMWH (e.g., enoxaparin) should be *avoided* in patients with renal dysfunction. In patients with a suspected high probability of PE, anticoagulation should be started immediately while the diagnostic workup is in progress, provided there are no contraindications to anticoagulation. Heparin is an anticoagulant—not a fibrinolytic. Hence, the purpose of heparin in VTE is not to dissolve the clot, but rather to prevent it from progressing/propagating. Unfractionated heparin is often favored initially due to its rapid onset and short half-life, allowing for quick discontinuation if an intervention or procedure is needed. Patients are typically transitioned to a direct oral anticoagulant (DOAC) before discharge for long-term management.

Watch Out
LMWH and unfractionated heparin are used for both therapeutic anticoagulation and VTE prophylaxis. The distinction lies in the doses, with higher doses used for treatment than for prophylaxis.

What If the Patient Has a History of or Suspected Heparin-Induced Thrombocytopenia (HIT)?

A non-heparin-based anticoagulant should be given such as argatroban or bivalirudin. These are direct thrombin inhibitors.

What Are the Four Options for the Subsequent Treatment of PE?

Once the diagnosis of PE is established, depending on the severity of the PE, patients may receive therapeutic anticoagulation alone, systemic tPA (tissue plasminogen activator; a thrombolytic agent), or endovascular (catheter directed tPA or suction thrombectomy) or open pulmonary embolectomy. In most patients (low-risk PE), therapeutic anticoagulation (i.e., heparin, LMWH, or DOAC) alone is sufficient.

When Should tPA Be Considered?

Intravenous tPA is indicated in patients with massive PE, should be considered in select patients with submassive PE, and is not indicated in low-risk PE. Contraindications to tPA include surgery within the last 2 weeks (such as in the patient described above), intracranial hemorrhage or malignancy, ischemic stroke within the last 3 months, suspected aortic dissection, active bleeding (other than menses), significant closed head trauma within 3 months, and severe hypertension (>185/110 mmHg). The greatest risk of tPA is fatal hemorrhage, including intracranial hemorrhage.

When Should Pulmonary Embolectomy Be Considered?

Pulmonary embolectomy, either by endovascular suction thrombectomy or open surgical approach, should be considered in patients with massive pulmonary embolism who have contraindications to thrombolytic therapy or who fail to respond to it.

What If the Patient Has a Contraindication to Anticoagulation?

If the patient has a contraindication to anticoagulation, such as ongoing bleeding or recent intracranial hemorrhage, placement of an inferior vena cava (IVC) filter is indicated to lower the risk of additional PEs. Patients with an IVC filter have a higher risk of developing a lower extremity DVT but lower risk of developing a PE.

What Is the Recommendation for Long-Term Anticoagulation After First-Time VTE?

For initial management of VTE, heparin or LMWH should be used until any planned interventions are completed and the patient is stable for discharge. At that point, patients are transitioned to a DOAC, such as apixaban, rivaroxaban, or dabigatran, which do not require frequent blood monitoring. Warfarin is now rarely used except in select cases, such as patients with mechanical heart valves or severe renal dysfunction, due to its need for regular blood draws and careful monitoring to maintain an INR (international normalized ratio) of 2–3. Anticoagulation therapy should continue for at least 3 months after a provoked VTE and may be extended indefinitely in patients with recurrent or unprovoked VTE or persistent risk factors such as cancer.

Watch Out
Rivaroxaban is renally cleared so should be avoided in patients with renal dysfunction.

Areas Where You Can Get in Trouble

Anticoagulation During Pregnancy

PE is a significant cause of maternal death in the United States, so aggressive therapy is warranted. Anticoagulation with LMWH or unfractionated heparin should be used to treat VTE in pregnancy, and continued for 6 weeks post-partum. Warfarin is a teratogen and should not be given during pregnancy.

Summary of Essentials

History and Physical Exam

- Look for Virchow's triad (stasis, hypercoagulability, and endothelial injury)
- Check for sudden onset of dyspnea, pleuritic chest pain, and/or tachycardia
- Calculate Wells score
- Look for evidence of DVT: leg swelling, calf pain, warmth of leg, mild redness of calf, and calf tenderness to palpation

Pathophysiology

- DVT is most likely to form in the leg or pelvic veins, also at the site of intravenous catheter insertion, and less commonly in the arms

Differential Diagnosis

- Patients with shortness of breath and pleuritic chest pain should also be evaluated for pulmonary edema (cardiogenic and noncardiogenic), myocardial infarction, and pneumonia

Diagnosis

- If there is high suspicion of PE, start anticoagulation immediately, even before the workup is completed
- Patients with high suspicion of PE should undergo CT angiography
- D-dimer, BNP, and troponin labs should be sent
- Echocardiogram may be used to assess for evidence of right heart strain (particularly if hypotensive or troponin elevated)
- ECG will most commonly show sinus tachycardia in patients with PE
- Order a duplex ultrasound of the bilateral lower extremities to evaluate for lower extremity DVT

Management

- IV heparin or subcutaneous LMWH
- Submassive PE-IV heparin or subcutaneous LMWH + consider tPA
- Massive PE—tPA vs. pulmonary embolectomy
- IVC filter—only if contraindication to anticoagulation
- Recent surgery contraindication for tPA

Special Conditions

- VTE in pregnancy—avoid warfarin
- VTE with HIT—direct thrombin inhibitors (e.g., argatroban)

Acknowledgement The editors would like to and thank the following authors for their contributions to the previous edition of the chapter: Jacquelyn L. Phillips, Paul N. Frank.

Suggested Reading

Anand SS, Wells PS, Hunt D, et al. Does this patient have deep venous thrombosis? JAMA. 1998;279(14):1094–9.

Jaff M, McMurtry M, Archer S, et al. Management of massive and submassive pulmonary embolism, iliofemoral deep vein thrombosis, and chronic thromboembolic pulmonary hypertension a scientific statement from the American Heart Association. Circulation. 2011;123:1788–830.

Johnson CM, Mureebe L, Silver D. Hypercoagulable states: a review. Vasc Endovasc Surg. 2005;39:123–33.

Nieuwdorp M, Stroes ES, Meijers JC, Buller H. Hypercoagulability in the metabolic syndrome. Curr Opin Pharmacol. 2005;5(2):155–9.
Niimi R, Hasegawa M, Sudo A, et al. Evaluation of soluble fibrin and D-dimer in the diagnosis of postoperative deep vein thrombosis. Biomarkers. 2010;15(2):149–57.
Ortel TL, Neumann I, Ageno W, et al. American Society of Hematology 2020 guidelines for management of venous thromboembolism: treatment of deep vein thrombosis and pulmonary embolism. Blood Adv. 2020;4(19):4693–4738. https://doi.org/10.1182/bloodadvances.2020001830

Surgical Complications

Question Set: Surgical Complications

Questions

1. A 38-year-old male undergoes an elective laparoscopic cholecystectomy under general anesthesia. The operation is uneventful. However, 30 minutes after arriving in the post-anesthesia care unit, the patient develops a temperature of 39.7 °C, a heart rate of 128/min, and respiratory rate of 30/min. He is noted to have generalized muscle rigidity, including tightness of the jaw, and dark-colored urine is observed in his Foley bag. Oxygen saturation is 95% on room air. Arterial blood gas shows pH 7.26, partial pressure of carbon dioxide ($PaCO_2$) 55 mmHg, and partial pressure of oxygen (PaO_2) 98 mmHg. Which of the following is the most likely diagnosis?
   (A) Neuroleptic malignant syndrome
   (B) Alcohol withdrawal
   (C) Malignant hyperthermia
   (D) Serotonin syndrome
   (E) Sepsis

2. What is the most common initial acid/base abnormality seen in patient with a pulmonary embolus (PE)?
   (A) Respiratory alkalosis
   (B) Respiratory acidosis
   (C) Metabolic alkalosis
   (D) Metabolic acidosis
   (E) Combined respiratory alkalosis and metabolic acidosis

3. A 60-year-old female returns to the emergency department for right leg swelling one week after undergoing a right colectomy for cecal adenocarcinoma. Duplex scan confirms a deep vein thrombosis (DVT) and the patient is started on intravenous (IV) heparin. The patient's hospital course is further complicated by a urinary tract infection and pneumonia. On hospital day 7, the morning laboratory study shows a platelet count of 55,000 cells/mL, down from a baseline of 140,000 cells/mL. What is the next immediate step?
   (A) Stop heparin
   (B) Stop heparin and start a direct thrombin inhibitor
   (C) Stop heparin and switch to low molecular weight heparin (LMWH)
   (D) Transfuse two units of platelets
   (E) Start corticosteroids

4. A 68-year-old female presents to the emergency department three days after total hip replacement. She became suddenly short of breath two hours ago. Her vitals include a blood pressure of 100/60 mmHg, heart rate of 120 beats/min, and respiratory rate of 30 cycles/min. On physical examination, lung sounds are clear. Chest X-ray is normal. Arterial blood gas shows a pH of 7.53, $PaCO_2$ 28, PaO_2 70, and HCO_3 25. Oxygen is given by nasal cannula. Which of the following is the next best step in the management?
   (A) Spiral CT angiogram of the chest
   (B) Intravenous heparin
   (C) Intravenous thrombolytic infusion
   (D) Venous duplex scan of both legs
   (E) Echocardiogram

addition, the smaller volume of PCC required to reverse INR will help avoid fluid overload in this patient with end-stage renal disease. Fresh frozen plasma can also help reverse INR but will work slower than PCC (B). Holding warfarin is not acceptable as it would take three to four days for reversal (A). Oral vitamin K takes about 24 hours, whereas IV vitamin K takes about 8–12 hours (D). Such strategies would be acceptable if surgery was not urgent. Cryoprecipitate has high levels of fibrinogen and von Willebrand factor but is not effective for warfarin reversal (E).

13. Answer C

Virchow's triad (hypercoagulability, immobility, endothelial injury) is a common risk factor for PE. Patients can present with dyspnea, pleuritic chest pain, cough, tachycardia, and/or hemodynamic instability. Most patients with PE have a normal chest X-ray. If present, the most common abnormality is a peripheral wedge-shaped opacity (Hampton's hump) or pleural effusion, but these are seen in a minority of cases (D). Westermark's sign (focal/regional pulmonary oligemia distal to embolus) is even more rare and only seen in cases of saddle embolus (E). Consolidation of an entire lobe is more consistent with lobar pneumonia (A). Fluffy bilateral infiltrates seen on plain films are suggestive of pulmonary edema (B).

14. Answer D

The most common ECG finding in patients with PE is sinus tachycardia. S1Q3T3 (C) refers to a deep S wave in lead I, Q wave in III, and inverted T wave in III, and although it is considered a "classic" finding for PE, it is neither sensitive nor specific and found in only 20% of patients. When pulmonary arterial pressures get high, ECG findings may demonstrate right ventricular strain (A). The remaining answer choices can all occur in patients with PE but appear infrequently (B–C, E).

15. Answer A

There are four types of operative wounds. These are used to predict the likelihood of a postoperative wound infection and to guide the use of preoperative antibiotics. Clean wounds (class-I) are those that do not involve entering an organ or cavity that is known to harbor bacteria (such as the alimentary, genitourinary, or reproductive tracts). Examples would be skin, eye, brain, and elective orthopedic surgery or hernia repair. Clean-contaminated (class-II) wounds are those in which an aseptically made wound enters the alimentary, respiratory, or genitourinary tracts (e.g., elective bowel resection, caesarean section) (B). Contaminated (class-III) wounds occur secondary to trauma, breaks in sterile technique, or gross spillage from the gastrointestinal tract (e.g., penetrating wound to the bowel) (C). Dirty-infected (class-IV) wounds are those involving a preoperative infection (drainage of an abscess) or perforated viscera (e.g., abscess) (D). Elective wound is not a recognized type of wound (E). Patients that have optimized oxygen delivery to tissue are most likely to have normal wound healing. Factors known to increase the risk of wound infections include wound ischemia, diabetes, low albumin, steroids, poor arterial flow (e.g., peripheral arterial disease), smoking, and hypothermia.

16. Answer B

Deep vein thrombosis (DVT) occurs more commonly in the left leg than the right due to the fact that the right common iliac artery often compresses the left common iliac vein (this condition is termed May-Thurner syndrome). The risk of DVT is further increased in pregnancy due to the gravid uterus causing further compression. The other sites listed are less common locations of DVT (A, C–E). Note that pregnant women cannot be treated with warfarin due to its teratogenicity.

17. Answer E

The patient is in shock. The most likely etiology of the shock in this setting is hypovolemic shock, most likely from bleeding (in this case most likely the ligation of the splenic artery has come off). Massive postoperative bleeding after surgery is rare and can be difficult to recognize. It can present as oliguria and differentiating bleeding from other causes of hypotension and oliguria can be difficult. Lab values such as hemoglobin and hematocrit are not useful in detecting acute hemorrhage in the postoperative setting. It generally takes 8–12 hours for interstitial fluid to redistribute into the vascular space, and blood concentration will initially appear unchanged. This patient's hemoglobin/hematocrit has shown a significant drop, and in combination with his thirst, pale skin, mechanism of injury, and hemodynamic instability, he is most likely suffering from internal bleeding and will need to return to the operating room. CT scan would be inappropriate for a patient with hemodynamic instability (A). An ECG, DPL, or a chest X-ray (the breath sounds are clear) is unlikely to be of value (B–D). Failure to recognize bleeding has fatal consequences. An adjunct while preparing for immediate return to the operating room would be to perform a bedside ultrasound (to look for fluid), if available.

18. Answer D

The patient is in shock. Given the high cardiac output, and low systemic vascular resistance, septic and anaphylactic shock are the most likely. However, since the patient has not had any medications or unusual exposures and is breathing normally, it is most likely septic shock. Patients with difficult urinary catheterizations may have subsequent bacteremia which can result in septic shock. After identifying septic shock based on the hemodynamic profile, the most immediate treatment is aggressive IV fluid resuscitation. This is best accomplished with crystalloids such as lactated Ringer's or normal saline. Early fluid administration helps increase preload and improve organ perfusion. Vasopressors like norepinephrine are initiated only if hypotension persists after adequate volume resuscitation. Norepinephrine (E) is considered as the first-line vasopressor for septic shock (E). Additionally, vasopressin can be used in combination with norepinephrine. Epinephrine is also used for septic shock, but after the above two. Dopamine was initially believed to increase renal perfusion in patients with shock, but studies have failed to consistently demonstrate this (B). It is not typically recommended for patients with septic shock (except for the rare patient with associated bradycardia). Phenylephrine is not recommended for septic shock except in highly selected patients (A). All patients with septic shock should also receive blood cultures, ideally before starting broad-spectrum antibiotics (but this should not delay initiation of antibiotics) (C).

Trauma

Jeffry Nahmias

Contents

Abdominal Pain Following Motor Vehicle Collision

McKensie Hammons, Areg Grigorian, Christian de Virgilio, and Dennis Y. Kim

Contents

C. de Virgilio, A. Grigorian (eds.), *Surgery*, https://doi.org/10.1007/978-3-032-09799-6_42

Case Study

A 35-year-old unrestrained male driver is brought in by paramedics following a motor vehicle collision (MVC). There was extensive passenger space intrusion and significant steering wheel deformity. On arrival to the emergency department, the patient is conscious and responsive. His blood pressure is 80/40 mmHg and heart rate is 110/min. His pupils are equal, round, and reactive to light. His breathing is shallow but he is able to protect his airway. Breath sounds are clear bilaterally. His abdomen is distended and mildly tender to palpation, without rebound or guarding. He has blood at the urethral meatus. There are no obvious deformities in his extremities.

Diagnosis

Is This Patient in Shock? What Are the Different Types of Shock?

Yes. Shock is a state in which there is inadequate utilization of oxygen needed for aerobic metabolism, leading to hemodynamic instability and end-organ dysfunction. Although there is no precise blood pressure cutoff that defines shock, hypotension (a blood pressure below 90 mmHg) in a trauma patient is due to hypovolemic/hemorrhagic shock until proven otherwise. Other less common causes of shock (Table 42.1) in the trauma patient are obstructive shock and neurogenic shock.

Table 42.1 Types of shock in the *trauma* setting

Type of shock	Clinical scenario	Mechanism	CVP	SVR	CO	PCWP
Hypovolemic	Any blunt or penetrating trauma with hemorrhage; burns	Decreased blood and plasma volume	Low	High	Low	Low
Obstructive	Blunt cardiac injury, cardiac tamponade, tension pneumothorax, pulmonary embolus	Failure of myocardial pump (blunt cardiac injury), decreased preload (cardiac tamponade, tension pneumothorax)	High	High	Low	High
Neurogenic	High cervical spinal cord injury, warm well-perfused extremities, normo–/bradycardic (different from other types of shock), priapism	Autonomic dysfunction (loss of sympathetic tone) with peripheral vasodilation	Low	Low	Low	Low

CVP central venous pressure, *SVR* systemic vascular resistance, *CO* cardiac output, *PCWP* pulmonary capillary wedge pressure

History and Physical Exam

What Are the Clinical Manifestations of Hypovolemic Shock?

Clinical manifestations of shock include tachycardia (*initial sign*), hypotension, pale and cool extremities, weak peripheral pulses, prolonged capillary refill (>2 seconds), low urine output, and altered mental status.

Watch Out

Pediatric patients can have significant hypovolemia from hemorrhage but still maintain normal blood pressure, owing to a strong vascular tone; tachycardia may be only clue. Older patients can be in hypovolemic shock but still maintain a seemingly normal blood pressure (as they may be hypertensive at baseline) and heart rate (as they may be receiving beta blockers).

Watch Out

A pregnant trauma patient who presents with hypotension should be placed in left lateral decubitus position to alleviate compression of the inferior vena cava (IVC) from the gravid uterus and improve venous return.

What Is the Significance of Blood at the Urethral Meatus?

Blood at the urethral meatus in men, in the setting of blunt trauma, is highly suggestive for a urethral injury as a result of a pelvic fracture. Other signs of urethral injury include perineal ecchymosis, scrotal hematoma, and a high-riding (non-palpable) prostate on digital rectal examination. Placing a urinary catheter (Foley) is contraindicated due to the risk of worsening a partial or complete urethral injury. Radiographic imaging (via a retrograde urethrogram [RUG]) should be performed to confirm that the urethra is intact. However, if pelvic vascular injury is suspected, CT angiogram (CTA) of the pelvis should be performed first as contrast used during RUG can confound CTA interpretation.

Watch Out

In women with a pelvic fracture, the fracture can lacerate the vagina, creating an open fracture. Do not assume vaginal blood is due to menses. Such an injury can easily be overlooked without a pelvic exam.

What Is the Significance of Gross Hematuria?

Gross hematuria following blunt trauma strongly suggests an injury to the kidney or bladder. Intraperitoneal rupture of the dome of the bladder can occur in the absence of a pelvic fracture. Such patients typically are involved in a high-speed MVC and have a full bladder (e.g., drinking at the bar). An injury to the bladder is best determined by a CT cystogram. Intraperitoneal bladder injuries are generally managed with open repair (as they are usually large blow out injuries and urine leaks into the peritoneum), whereas extraperitoneal injuries are mostly smaller (associated with pelvic fractures) often managed nonoperatively with bladder catheter (Foley) drainage alone, typically for 2 weeks. Renal injury can be ruled out by obtaining a CT of the abdomen/pelvis with IV contrast.

Pathophysiology

How Much Blood Loss Is Necessary to Cause Hypotension (As in the Patient Above) in the Supine Position?

Hypotension in the supine position implies the patient has lost at least 30–40% of his blood volume (Class III shock; see ◘ Table 42.2), which represents 1500–2000 mL of blood.

What Are the Five Main Sources of Major Blood Loss in Blunt Trauma?

The main sources are chest, abdomen, pelvis/retroperitoneum, long bones, and "street" or external.

What Are the Most Likely Injuries in Each of These Locations That Would Lead to Major Blood Loss?

Hypotension in the supine position typically indicates a blood loss of 1500–2000 mL. In the chest, this is most often due to a massive hemothorax caused by lung laceration or intercostal artery injury, commonly from rib fractures. In the abdomen, the liver is the most frequently injured organ in blunt trauma, but the spleen is the most common source of life-threatening hemorrhage. Retroperitoneal bleeding is often due to pelvic fractures, which can tear branches of the internal iliac artery or pelvic veins. Renal trauma may also cause sig-

Table 42.2 Shock classes I–IV

	Class I	Class II	Class III	Class IV
Blood loss (% blood volume)	Up to 750 mL (<15%)	750–1500 mL (15–30%)	1500–2000 mL (30–40%)	>2000 mL (>40%)
Heart rate	Normal	Tachycardia (100–120/min)	Tachycardia (>120/min)	Tachycardia (>120/min)
Blood pressure	Normal	Normal to minimal change	Significantly decreased (SBP < 90 mmHg)	Significantly decreased (SBP < 90 mmHg)
Pulse pressure	Normal or increased	Decreased	Decreased	Decreased (<25 mmHg)
Respiratory rate	Normal	Tachypnea	Tachypnea	Tachypnea

SBP systolic blood pressure

nificant bleeding. Blunt abdominal vascular injuries to the abdominal aorta or inferior vena cava are very rare. In the extremities, each femur fracture can result in the loss of approximately 500–1000 mL of blood, so bilateral femur fractures may lead to shock. Additionally, scalp lacerations, despite being external, can cause substantial blood loss due to the scalp's rich vascular supply and should not be overlooked.

Watch Out

Although blunt injuries to the abdominal aorta are rare, the descending thoracic aorta is prone to transection with rapid deceleration injuries. The tear typically occurs just distal to the ligamentum arteriosum (as the aorta is tethered there). This injury is often fatal. It should be suspected if the mediastinum is wide on chest X-ray. The next step would be a CTA of the chest.

What Cavity Should Not Be Considered to Be the Source of Hemorrhagic Shock and Why?

A closed-head injury should not be considered the source of hypovolemic shock as one cannot lose that much blood into the cranium. In fact, a severe closed head may induce the *Cushing reflex* (hypertension, bradycardia, irregular respirations) via a sympathetic response causing peripheral vasoconstriction in order to maintain adequate blood pressure and regulate perfusion to the brain. As a result of the vasoconstriction, the baroreceptors respond with increased parasympathetic stimulation of the heart, causing bradycardia. This reflex is seen in patients with increased intracranial pressure (ICP) and often heralds brain herniation.

Initial Management

What Are the ABCDE of Trauma Patient Management?

The ABCDEs form the primary survey in trauma and prioritize life-threatening conditions. Although presented sequentially, many steps occur simultaneously. **A**irway with cervical spine protection is first, as airway obstruction can rapidly lead to hypoxia. Any patient with a Glasgow Coma Scale (GCS) ≤8 requires intubation ("8 or less, intubate"). **B**reathing assessment follows, focusing on chest movement, breath sounds, and signs of trauma such as crepitus or deformity. **C**irculation is next, beginning with pulse assessment. A palpable radial pulse suggests a systolic pressure ≥80 mmHg; carotid or femoral pulses indicate ≥60 mmHg. Establish two large-bore intravenous (IVs) and begin fluid resuscitation if needed. **D**isability refers to a quick neurologic exam using the GCS, which assesses eye, verbal, and motor responses. **E**xposure and environmental control involves fully exposing the patient to assess for hidden injuries while using warming measures to prevent hypothermia.

What Type of Airway Is Recommended in the Trauma Setting?

Orotracheal intubation is the most common method of securing an airway. In the trauma setting, this is performed using rapid sequence intubation (RSI) with C-spine protection. RSI is designed to prevent aspiration in patients who have not been fasting. Rather than slowly titrating drugs to effect while utilizing bag-valve-mask ventilation ("bagging"), RSI involves administering immediate weight-based doses of sedatives (etomidate) and neuromuscular blocking agents in quick succession without "bagging." Since the trauma patient should be presumed to have a C-spine injury until proven otherwise, intubation must be performed with strict in-line cervical immobilization. This is a two-person technique.

What Are the Two Types of Surgical Airways? Which One Is More Appropriate in the Emergent Trauma Setting?

The two surgical airways are cricothyrotomy (also called cricothyroidotomy) and tracheostomy. Cricothyrotomy is the surgical airway of choice in the emergency setting because it is easier and faster to perform. Indications include severe facial trauma, angioedema, failed orotracheal intubation, and upper airway obstruction. An incision is made through the cricothyroid membrane, which is located between the thyroid (superior) and cricoid (inferior) cartilages. Cricothyrotomy is not generally a good long-term airway, as there is a tendency to develop subglottic stenosis. Tracheostomy (through the tracheal rings) is more time-consuming to perform, requires significant expertise, and is therefore performed in a more elective setting. It is the surgical airway of choice for long-term management. Indications include malignancies causing upper airway obstruction and long-term need for mechanical ventilation (due to inability to wean).

Why Is Nasotracheal Intubation Not Recommended in the Trauma Setting?

Trauma patients may have facial and basilar skull fractures. Attempts at nasotracheal intubation may lead to inadvertent intracranial passage of the nasotracheal tube.

How Does One Confirm Proper Intubation?

Clinical indicators (e.g., condensation of tube with ventilation, adequate breath sounds on auscultation) alone cannot be relied upon to confirm proper endotracheal placement. Confirmation of proper endotracheal tube placement is done by end-tidal CO_2 determination (capnography) and considered the gold standard. A chest X-ray is subsequently performed to confirm that the endotracheal tube is not advanced too far in the tracheobronchial tree (i.e., past the carina).

Watch Out

End-tidal CO_2 determination is not accurate for ensuring proper endotracheal tube placement if a patient is in cardiac arrest. In such cases, the only practical option is to confirm placement by auscultating breath sounds.

What Is the First Step in the Management of the Patient Presented?

This patient is hypotensive following blunt trauma with a secure airway, raising concern for hemorrhagic shock. Initial management includes establishing two large-bore IVs and initiating balanced blood product resuscitation rather than large volumes of crystalloid. A FAST (focused assessment with sonography for trauma) exam should be performed to rapidly assess for intra-abdominal bleeding or cardiac tamponade without delaying definitive management. The operating room (OR) should be notified early, as this patient will likely require emergent exploratory laparotomy. Endotracheal intubation should be avoided unless absolutely necessary, as induction agents can blunt sympathetic tone and precipitate cardiovascular collapse in hypotensive patients.

Where Should the Peripheral IV Lines Be Placed?

Preferably large-bore (14–16 gauge) IVs should be placed in each antecubital fossa. However, the placement should take into consideration potential sources of active hemorrhage. For example, if a patient has significant arm trauma, the IVs should be placed in a non-injured upper and/or lower extremity.

Is a Central Line Preferred over a Peripheral IV for Trauma Patients?

Peripheral IVs are preferred over central lines in the setting of trauma. Central lines (subclavian, internal jugular) require more time to place and are associated with more risks (iatrogenic pneumothorax), especially in the hypovolemic patient (central veins are collapsed). Peripheral IVs provide less resistance to flow, given the shorter length of the catheter. A large bore and shorter central line (called a sheath introducer or cordis) is indicated if peripheral access is problematic and in the hemodynamically unstable patient. It is generally placed in the femoral vein.

> **Watch Out**
> If peripheral access is unobtainable, a line can be placed in an intraosseous location (preferably tibial).

What Is the Ideal Fluid Resuscitation in Trauma?

In hemorrhagic trauma patients, the preferred resuscitation strategy is early administration of balanced blood products rather than large volumes of crystalloid. Balanced transfusion typically refers to a 1:1:1 ratio of packed red blood cells, fresh frozen plasma, and platelets. In patients with controlled bleeding or those awaiting definitive hemostasis, permissive hypotension may be appropriate to reduce ongoing blood loss. Rather than targeting a specific blood pressure, the goal is to maintain sufficient perfusion, typically assessed by preserved mental status or the presence of a palpable radial pulse.

Why Are Excessive Crystalloid Infusions Avoided in Trauma Patients?

Excessive crystalloid use can dilute clotting factors, worsen coagulopathy, and increase the risk of complications such as abdominal compartment syndrome.

What Is Colloid? What Is the Theoretical Benefit? Is There Any Actual Benefit in Trauma Resuscitation?

Colloids contain larger molecules that are insoluble, such as albumin, in addition to water and electrolytes. The theoretical benefit is that such large molecules do not freely diffuse across a semipermeable membrane, thus preserving intravascular osmotic pressure. In actuality, however, colloids have not been shown to be of benefit, are more expensive, and, in patients with traumatic brain injury, have been shown to be harmful.

Why Are Large Doses of K^+ Not Given in the Initial Resuscitation?

Due to severe hemorrhage, trauma patients may be in shock, which leads to a decreased renal perfusion, a decreased glomerular filtration, and, therefore, a decreased ability to excrete excess potassium. Trauma patients are at risk of developing hyperkalemia due to crush injuries. Since potassium is the main intracellular ion, such injuries may result in muscle cells releasing potassium. Of note, the amount of K^+ in lactated ringers is considered physiologic and is therefore considered acceptable.

What Is the Role of Tranexamic Acid (TXA)?

TXA competitively and irreversibly binds to lysine residues on plasminogen, preventing the formation of plasmin. This prevents the degradation of fibrin by plasmin, stabilizing the fibrin clot and preventing further hemorrhage. The administration of TXA reduces mortality in adult trauma patients with significant bleeding without increasing the risk of thromboembolic events. However, the benefit is only seen in patients administered TXA within 3 hours of injury.

> **Watch Out**
> A hemodynamically unstable trauma patient should be presumed to be bleeding until proven otherwise. The immediate focus should be on resuscitation (with blood) and quickly determining the bleeding source.

After Appropriate Fluid Resuscitation Is Started, What Must Be Done Next?

Once resuscitation has begun, the source of bleeding must be rapidly identified and controlled. If a trauma patient remains hypotensive despite blood product resuscitation, they should be taken to the operating room for hemorrhage control. In most cases, the source is intra-abdominal, warranting an exploratory laparotomy. Additionally, signs of peritonitis following trauma indicate a likely bowel injury and are also an indication for immediate laparotomy without further diagnostic workup.

What Is Included in the Secondary Survey of Trauma Patients?

The primary survey should be done completely and quickly before moving on to diagnostic adjuncts and the secondary survey (history and detailed physical examination). If the patient is conscious and able to speak, a quick AMPLE history should be obtained (*A*llergies, *M*edications, *P*ast medical history, *L*ast meal, *E*vents preceding the trauma). A careful and systematic head-to-toe physical exam should be done to ensure that nothing has been overlooked and to identify all major injuries.

What Imaging Adjuncts Are Used as Part of the Secondary Survey in Blunt Trauma?

A focused assessment with sonography for trauma (FAST scan) is primarily used in the setting of blunt trauma to rapidly identify free fluid in the peritoneal, pericardial, or pleural spaces. It is most useful when evaluating hypotensive patients after blunt injury, where likelihood of intra-abdominal bleeding is high. In addition, an X-ray of the chest is obtained to look for a massive hemothorax. In such a case, a tube thoracostomy (chest tube) is inserted. A pelvic radiograph is obtained to determine if there is a pelvic fracture as it may indicate pelvic bleeding.

Is FAST Scan Useful in Hemodynamically Stable Blunt Trauma Patients, and in Penetrating Trauma?

The FAST scan is routinely used as part of the secondary survey in most blunt trauma patients whether they are stable or not, as it has become essentially an extension of the physical exam. However, in hemodynamically stable blunt trauma patients, the sensitivity of FAST scan is low. As such, additional imaging is typically warranted as there is a significant false-negative rate. In penetrating trauma, FAST is useful to detect pericardial effusion. However, it is not useful to rule out significant abdominal injury as there is greater risk of bowel injury, and FAST may not detect these injuries.

Watch Out

FAST scan sensitivity in identifying intraperitoneal hemorrhage can vary significantly by multiple factors such as equipment type, operator expertise and patient body habitus, and the hemodynamic stability of the patient. Its sensitivity for intraperitoneal bleeding is high in hypotensive blunt trauma patients but is low in normotensive ones. Injuries to retroperitoneal structures are not commonly visualized on FAST exam.

What Are the Next Steps After a FAST, and What Injuries Can Be Missed?

If the FAST scan is positive and the patient is hemodynamically stable, the next step is a CT scan to further characterize intra-abdominal injuries and guide management. If the FAST scan is negative in a hemodynamically stable patient, a CT scan is still typically obtained to rule out a false-negative FAST. Despite its utility, FAST has limitations and may miss injuries that do not produce large fluid collections. Examples include duodenal hematoma, which involves an intramural bleed without free fluid; pancreatic transection, which may only cause a small retroperitoneal fluid collection; and traumatic diaphragmatic hernia, which may be overlooked unless abdominal contents are clearly visualized in the chest. FAST is also poor at visualizing retroperitoneal injuries and bleeding. In unstable patients, a positive FAST typically warrants immediate operative intervention.

Subsequent Management

What Is the Management of Intra-Abdominal Bleeding Due to Splenic Injury?

The most common cause of intra-abdominal bleeding following blunt trauma is splenic injury (◘ Fig. 42.1) (the most commonly injured organ is the liver). For hemodynamically stable patients with evidence of a splenic injury (based on CT scan) and no other indication for exploratory laparotomy, the management depends on the severity of the splenic injury. Low-grade injuries can be managed with observation. Higher-grade injuries (active extravasation) are best managed with splenic embolization, if the appro-

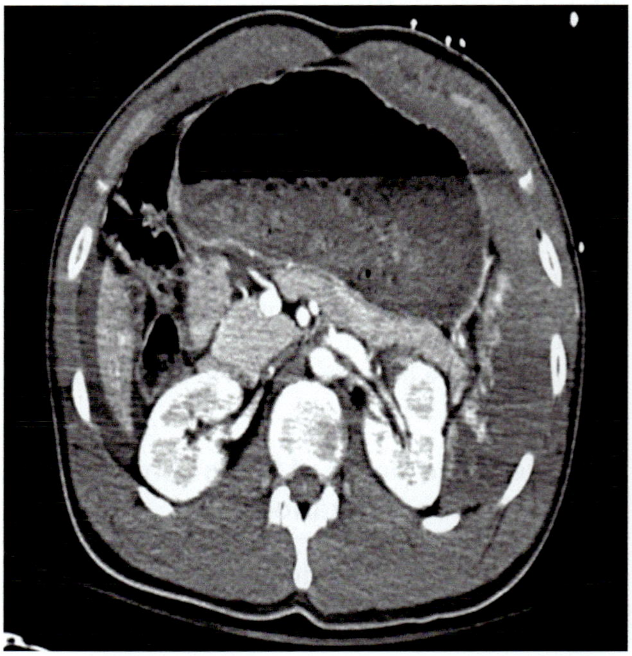

◘ **Fig. 42.1** Axial CT showing a ruptured spleen with free fluid around the liver from blunt abdominal trauma

priate interventional radiology personnel and resources are available. For hemodynamically unstable patients, the recommended management is surgical exploration with splenectomy or splenorrhaphy (repair of the spleen).

Watch Out

Kehr's sign is an acute referred pain in the left shoulder due to splenic injury.

What Is the Management of Intra-Abdominal Bleeding Due to Liver Injury?

The most commonly injured organ after blunt trauma is the liver (▪ Fig. 42.2). Most patients with liver injury can be managed nonoperatively. If the patient is stable but demonstrates ongoing bleeding, embolization via interventional radiology is an accepted therapeutic adjunct. If the patient is unstable, surgical exploration is necessary. Bleeding from most liver injuries can be stopped intraoperatively using a combination of perihepatic packing (with laparotomy pads), cauterization, and/or suturing. This may stabilize the patient sufficiently to then perform embolization. If bleeding cannot be stopped, the laparotomy packs are sometimes left in situ for 24–48 hours.

Watch Out

During surgery for liver injury, the Pringle maneuver (clamping the portal triad) is utilized to temporarily control bleeding from hepatic artery or portal venous sources. Failure of the Pringle maneuver to stop bleeding implies that the bleeding is coming from the hepatic veins.

What Are the First Steps in the Management of Patients with a Pelvic Fracture? What Is the Subsequent Management?

Initial management includes blood product resuscitation if there are signs of hemorrhagic shock. In cases of an open book pelvic fracture, a pelvic binder or sheet should be applied around the greater trochanters to reduce pelvic volume and tamponade bleeding. This intervention is only appropriate for open book fractures, as binders can worsen bleeding in other fracture patterns. If no other sources of bleeding are identified (negative FAST and chest X-ray), the patient should undergo angiography with possible embolization for further control of pelvic hemorrhage.

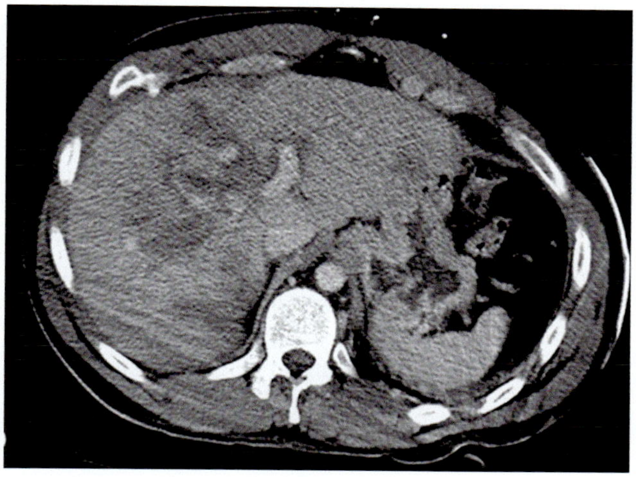

▪ **Fig. 42.2** Axial CT showing severe blunt liver trauma as evidenced by regions of hypoenhancement suggesting laceration and/or vascular compromise

Areas You Can Get in Trouble

Failing to Recognize the Significance of Free Fluid in the Peritoneal Cavity When There Is No Solid Organ Injury

After blunt trauma, the presence of free fluid in the abdomen is most commonly due to splenic or liver injury. In the absence of solid organ injury, free fluid should raise concern for an occult hollow viscous (bowel) injury.

Treating Hypovolemic Shock Initially with Vasopressors

The early use of vasopressors in the management of hemorrhagic shock is not recommended and may even be harmful in patients that have not been adequately resuscitated. Hypotension in the setting of trauma is usually due to hemorrhagic shock. Treatment is to give volume and identify and stop the source of hemorrhage. Patients with hypovolemic shock have a very high systemic vascular resistance due to vasoconstriction, which decreases perfusion to vital organs. Adding a vasopressor early on will only serve to aggravate the situation.

Infection After Splenectomy

Elevated white blood cell and platelet counts are an expected physiologic response post-splenectomy. However, it is essential to distinguish this from early infection, as asplenic patients are at high risk for fulminant sepsis due to encapsulated organisms. Overwhelming post-splenectomy infection (OPSI) is a life-threatening condition that requires prompt recognition and treatment. On or after postoperative day 5, a white blood cell count greater than 15,000 and a platelet-to-WBC ratio less than 20 may indicate infection rather than a reactive process. To prevent OPSI, patients should be vaccinated against *Streptococcus pneumoniae*, *Haemophilus influenzae* type-b, and *Neisseria meningitidis*, ideally 2 weeks after surgery. However, in trauma patients with unreliable follow-up, vaccination prior to discharge is acceptable and often preferred. Daily antibiotic prophylaxis may also be considered in high-risk groups, such as children under 5 years of age and immunocompromised individuals.

Jaundice and Hematemesis After Liver Injury

In the setting of abdominal (hepatic) trauma, jaundice and hematemesis in the postoperative period should raise concern for hemobilia (bleeding into or from the hepatobiliary tract). This is due to a traumatic fistula between a hepatic artery and a bile duct. Liver enzymes may demonstrate a post-hepatic (cholestatic) pattern (due to blood clots in the bile ducts impairing bile flow). The "classic triad" of hemobilia, right upper quadrant pain, jaundice, and gastrointestinal (GI) bleeding, is seen in a minority of patients. Diagnosis can be made by upper endoscopy that demonstrates blood emanating from the ampulla of Vater and/or CT scan demonstrating a pseudoaneurysm within the liver. Treatment often consists of embolization of a hepatic artery branch by interventional radiology.

Management of a Pelvic Fracture in a Hemodynamically Unstable Patient

Most surgeons recommend angiographic embolization for ongoing bleeding from a pelvic fracture. However, if the patient is truly in severe shock, they may not be able to wait until an interventional radiologist is called in to perform such a procedure. As such, some trauma surgeons recommend taking the patient to the operating room for preperitoneal packing (to temporarily tamponade bleeding) followed by angiographic embolization or alternatively, ligation of bilateral internal iliac arteries is another option in lieu of angiographic embolization.

Blood Loss in Trauma (▫ Fig. 42.3)

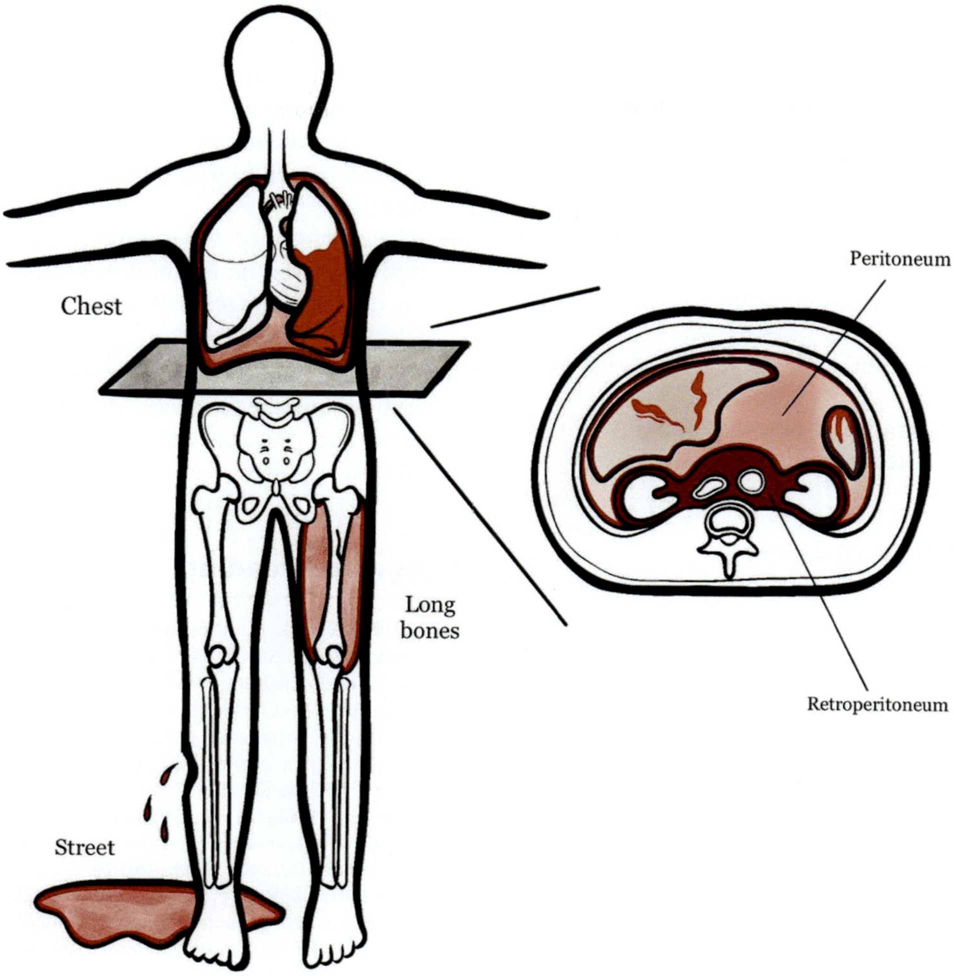

Fig. 42.3 Sources of bleeding in trauma: Potential sources of major blood loss after blunt trauma include the chest, abdomen, retroperitoneum, long bones, and external wounds ("the street")

Summary of Essentials

Diagnosis

- Types of shock in the trauma setting:
  - Hypovolemic: blunt/penetrating trauma with hemorrhage, burns
  - Cardiogenic: blunt cardiac injury, arrhythmias, cardiac tamponade
  - Neurogenic: high cervical spinal cord injury, warm well-perfused extremities

History and Physical Exam

- Clinical manifestations of shock: tachycardia, hypotension, pale and cool extremities, weak peripheral pulses, prolonged capillary refill, low urine output, altered mental status.
- Blood at urethral meatus may indicate urethral injury; Foley catheter contraindicated.

Pathophysiology

- Hypotension in supine position indicates 30–40% loss of blood volume (Class III).
- Five main sources of blood loss: chest, abdomen, pelvis/retroperitoneum, long bones, and "street" or external.
- Closed-head injury should not be considered a source of hypovolemic shock.

Initial Management

- Start with ABCs
- Orotracheal intubation using RSI and C-spine protection is the preferred method of securing an airway

- Nasotracheal intubation is not recommended
- Cricothyrotomy is the emergent surgical airway of choice
- Peripheral IVs are preferred over central lines in setting of trauma
- Ideal fluid resuscitation is a 1:1:1 ratio of packed RBCs, fresh frozen plasma, and platelets
  - Large-volume crystalloids increase risk of coagulopathy and hypothermia
- TXA in patients with significant bleeding if within 3 hours of injury
- FAST scan to evaluate unstable patient, CT scan in stable patients
  - If hemodynamically unstable and FAST (+) go directly to OR for exploratory laparotomy

Subsequent Management

- Splenic injury:
  - Observation if stable and not bleeding
  - Splenic embolization for hemodynamically *stable* patients with blush on CT
  - Surgical exploration and splenectomy or splenorrhaphy for hemodynamically *unstable* patients with splenic injury (vaccinate for encapsulated bacteria two weeks postoperatively)
- Liver injury:
  - Most are managed nonoperatively
  - Hemodynamically stable with ongoing bleeding require embolization
  - Hemodynamically unstable with ongoing bleeding require surgical exploration
- Pelvic fracture:
  - Pelvic angiography and embolization if ongoing bleeding

Watch Out

- Free fluid in abdomen without solid organ injury may represent bleeding from a more occult source (such as a mesenteric artery), enteric contents (from a small bowel injury), or urine (from a bladder rupture).
- The early use of vasopressors is not recommended and may even be harmful in patients who have not been adequately resuscitated.

Acknowledgement The editors would like to acknowledge and thank the following authors for their contributions to the previous edition of the chapter: Alexis L. Woods.

Suggested Reading

Ahmed N, Vernick JJ. Management of liver trauma in adults. *J Emerg Trauma Shock*. 2011;4(1):114–119.

CRASH-2 trial collaborators, Shakur H, Roberts I, et al. Effects of tranexamic acid on death, vascular occlusive events, and blood transfusion in trauma patients with significant haemorrhage (CRASH-2): a randomised, placebo-controlled trial. *Lancet*. 2010;376(9734):23–32.

Okabayashi T, Hanazaki K. Overwhelming postsplenectomy infection syndrome in adults - a clinically preventable disease. *World J Gastroenterol*. 2008;14(2):176–179.

Weng J, Brown CV, Rhee P, et al. White blood cell and platelet counts can be used to differentiate between infection and the normal response after splenectomy for trauma: prospective validation. *J Trauma*. 2005;59(5):1076–1080.

Penetrating Abdominal Trauma

James McDermott, Jeffry Nahmias, Areg Grigorian, and Dennis Y. Kim

Contents

C. de Virgilio, A. Grigorian (eds.), *Surgery*, https://doi.org/10.1007/978-3-032-09799-6_43

Case Study

A 24-year-old male is brought to the emergency room following a gunshot wound (GSW) to the left lower abdomen. On initial examination his blood pressure is 80/65 mmHg, heart rate is 140/min, and respiratory rate is 26/min. He is pale, diaphoretic, and writhing in pain. The patient's airway is patent, and breath sounds are equal bilaterally. He has a rigid abdomen with diffuse tenderness, guarding, and rebound. There is a single GSW to the left lower quadrant. Palpation of the patient's groin reveals pulses are bilaterally weak but symmetrical. Despite starting blood product transfusion, he continues to remain hypotensive.

Diagnosis

What Is the Most Likely Diagnosis?

Given that this patient presents with penetrating abdominal trauma, he is most likely in hemorrhagic shock secondary to bleeding in the peritoneal cavity. This is supported by his hemodynamic instability (decreased systolic blood pressure, narrowed pulse pressure [defined as $\leq$30 mmHg], and tachycardia). Peritonitis on physical exam (e.g., rigid abdomen, diffuse tenderness, rebound) supports the presence of a hollow viscus or bowel injury.

History and Physical

What Three Physical Exam Findings Independently Mandate Immediate Operative Intervention in Patients with Penetrating Abdominal Trauma?

The three physical exam findings are shock, peritonitis, and evisceration. Prior to surgery, chest and abdominal X-rays can be performed to learn more about the trajectory or path of bullets and potential injuries. However, this should only occur in a hemodynamically stable patient. This patient has two indications for emergent exploratory laparotomy: shock and peritonitis.

Watch Out

Careful exposure and examination of the entire patient is critical to avoid missing penetrating injuries, including rolling the patient to look at their back (while maintaining C-spine precautions). The perineum and axilla should always be examined for evidence of occult injury.

What Is a Tangential GSW?

A tangential GSW is an injury in which a bullet grazes the surface of the body, resulting in superficial entry and exit wounds without evidence of penetration into deeper structures. These injuries occur when a bullet grazes the body rather than traversing or embedding into it. However, tangential GSWs should not be dismissed as benign. They can be associated with significant blast effects or fragmentation, which may cause delayed injuries to underlying tissues, vessels (e.g., pseudoaneurysm), and organs.

Do Patients with Findings of a Tangential GSW Require Any Further Workup?

Yes, patients with tangential GSWs should undergo additional evaluation. This typically includes a contrast-enhanced CT scan to assess for occult injuries along with serial physical examinations. This approach ensures that any potential injury is promptly identified and managed.

Anatomy

What Are the Borders of the Anterior Abdomen, Flank, Back, and Thoracoabdomen? (▫ Table 43.1)

What Is the Significance of Injuries to the Thoracoabdominal Region?

Thoracoabdominal injuries can affect thoracic structures, abdominal organs, and the diaphragm. On the left side, CT imaging is often insufficient to detect diaphragm injuries. Therefore, delayed diagnostic laparoscopy (>8

Table 43.1 Borders of the anterior abdomen, flank, back, and thoracoabdomen

Location	Borders
Anterior abdomen	Xiphoid and costal margins superiorly, the anterior axillary lines laterally, and the inguinal ligaments and pubic symphysis inferiorly
Flank	Between anterior and posterior axillary lines from the level of the sixth intercostal space to the iliac crest
Back	Tips of the scapular superiorly, posterior axillary lines laterally, and the iliac crests inferiorly
Thoracoabdomen	Nipple (fourth intercostal space) to costal margin, anterior to posterior axillary lines

hours) is indicated for left thoracoabdominal injuries, assuming no immediate indications for surgery. The delay allows time to identify bowel injuries (based on laboratory trends, vitals, and exam), which may not be apparent initially but can influence the operative approach.

What Three Distinct Regions Comprise the Internal Abdomen?

The three distinct regions of the internal abdomen are the peritoneal cavity, the pelvis, and the retroperitoneum.

Watch Out

A penetrating wound below the fourth intercostal space (nipple line) may traverse the diaphragm and the peritoneal cavity, as such laparoscopy and/or laparotomy are generally indicated.

Why Is It Difficult to Diagnose Injuries to Retroperitoneal Organs in Trauma Patients?

43

Injuries to retroperitoneal organs may not manifest with signs of peritonitis due to their protected location. In addition, the focused assessment with sonography for trauma (FAST) exam is not able to identify retroperitoneal bleeding.

Retroperitoneal Organs/Structures

- Duodenum (second to fourth parts)
- Pancreas
- Kidneys
- Ureters
- Ascending colon (posterior wall)
- Descending colon (posterior wall)
- Rectum (distal)
- Aorta, inferior vena cava, iliac veins

What Is the Zone Classification for Retroperitoneal Hematomas and How Does the Location Affect Management?

Retroperitoneal hematomas are classified into three zones to serve as a reminder as to what vascular structures may be injured and helps guide intraoperative management. The ultimate decision as to whether to explore a retroperitoneal hematoma is based upon the hemodynamic status of the patient, the mechanism of injury, the zone location, and in some instances whether it is expanding or pulsatile (Table 43.2).

What Are the Two Most Common Organs Injured Following a Penetrating Abdominal Injury?

The two most common organs injured are the small bowel and the liver.

What Injuries Must Be Ruled Out with GSWs That Travel Across the Pelvis?

Transpelvic GSWs are associated with vascular (iliac vessels), genitourinary (bladder, ureters, uterus, vagina), and gastrointestinal (small bowel, colon, rectum) injuries. In stable patients with a transpelvic GSW, a contrast-enhanced CT scan of the abdomen and pelvis should be performed. Consideration should be given to

Table 43.2 Retroperitoneal zones

	Zone 1	Zone 2	Zone 3
Location	Upper midline/central	Upper lateral	Lower midline/pelvic
Vascular structures	Aorta and its branches (celiac, SMA, proximal renal artery), IVC, SMV	Renal artery and vein	Common/internal/external iliac arteries and veins
Mechanism			
Blunt	Always explore	Selective	Do not explore[a]
Penetrating	Always explore	Explore[b]	Explore

SMA superior mesenteric artery, *IVC* inferior vena cava, *SMV* superior mesenteric vein
[a]In patients with shock or hemodynamic instability and evidence of an expanding or pulsatile Zone 3 hematoma following blunt trauma, consideration may be given to exploring the hematoma (with or without bilateral internal iliac artery ligation)
[b]If non-expanding, and directly over kidney, these can sometimes be observed, as exploration and opening Gerota's fascia may lead to more bleeding

performing a proctoscopy to rule out injury to the rectum, particularly if there is blood in the rectal vault on digital rectal exam. Females should undergo a vaginal examination.

Workup

What Initial Workup Is Recommended for the Above Patient?

No workup is needed in this patient as he has clear indications for surgical intervention (both peritonitis and hemodynamic instability/shock following penetrating trauma). He should be taken directly to the operating room (OR) for a laparotomy.

In the Absence of Shock, Peritonitis, or Evisceration, What Imaging Is Recommended for a Patient with Penetrating Abdominal Trauma?

CT of the abdomen and pelvis with intravenous contrast. If concern exists for multi-cavitary torso trauma, a CT chest should also be obtained.

Is a FAST Exam Helpful for Patients with Penetrating Abdominal Trauma?

The FAST exam is primarily used for patients following blunt trauma. Its primary utility in penetrating abdominal trauma is to rule out cardiac tamponade in thoracoabdominal injuries. It has poor utility in predicting the need for a laparotomy because there is a high likelihood of bowel injury. FAST has a low sensitivity for detecting these injuries as one needs at least 250–500 cc of free fluid for a FAST to be positive, which is unlikely to occur after a bowel injury.

Watch Out
The FAST exam is not helpful in identifying injury to retroperitoneal structures.

Is There a Role for Local Wound Exploration for Penetrating Abdominal Injury?

Local wound exploration may be undertaken in patients with anterior stab wounds (not flank) by an experienced surgeon, but only if the patient does not have an indication for immediate surgery. The goal of local wound exploration is to determine if the injury has penetrated the anterior fascia. If it has not, surgery can be avoided. Violation of the anterior fascia is an indication for either an exploratory laparotomy or diagnostic laparoscopy to assess for peritoneal violation and rule out injury to the abdominal viscera.

Initial Management

What Are the First Steps in the Management of This Patient?

Initial management of the trauma patient always begins with the primary survey to identify and treat immediately life-threatening conditions. The primary survey involves assessing the ABCDEs (*a*irway with cervical spine precautions, *b*reathing, *c*irculation [with hemorrhage control], *d*isability, and *e*xposure/environment). With penetrating injuries, attention should be directed to identifying the presence and location of all wounds. If the patient is stable, it may be helpful to place radiopaque markers over these sites prior to radiologic imaging to help reconstruct the path or trajectory of bullets.

What Is a Massive Transfusion Protocol (MTP)?

MTP is an institutional protocol activated for patients with life-threatening hemorrhage. Its purpose is to rapidly deliver blood products, typically in a 1:1:1 or 1:1:2 ratio of plasma, platelets, and red blood cells, to prevent dilutional coagulopathy and hypovolemia. Whole blood is now preferentially used when available. MTP replaces traditional resuscitation methods that relied heavily on crystalloids followed by red blood cells.

When Should MTP Be Initiated?

MTP initiation is based on clinical judgment. The ABC score aids this decision, recommending activation if a patient has any two of the following: penetrating mechanism, systolic blood pressure $\leq$ 90 mmHg, heart rate $\geq$ 120/min, or a positive FAST.

43

What Is Permissive Hypotension?

In a hemorrhaging patient, the goal of fluid resuscitation is to achieve permissive hypotension rather than aggressive normalization of blood pressure. The primary objective is to maintain sufficient perfusion to ensure normal mentation, without aiming to restore a normal systolic blood pressure. This strategy minimizes the risk of exacerbating hemorrhage, as the bleeding is often temporarily contained by vasoconstriction and clot formation. Excessive fluid resuscitation before surgical control of the bleeding can disrupt these clots, raise systolic blood pressure, and dilute coagulation factors, all of which can worsen bleeding and reduce the chances of survival.

Watch Out

Permissive hypotension is only applicable to patients with penetrating torso trauma (as well as ruptured abdominal aortic aneurysm (AAA)). This strategy should not be employed in patients with blunt trauma, especially in the presence of a head injury.

Should Empiric Antibiotics Be Routinely Administered to All Patients with Penetrating Trauma?

No. There is no indication to administer empiric antibiotics to patients with penetrating trauma not requiring operative intervention. Patients going to the operating room after penetrating trauma, however, should receive preoperative antibiotics to cover skin and bowel flora.

Should Tetanus Vaccines or Tetanus Immunoglobulin Be Routinely Administered to Patients with Penetrating Trauma?

No. Only patients with <3 doses of tetanus toxoid vaccine or if immunization status is unknown along with a tetanus-prone wound (e.g., obvious soil contamination, >6 hours old) should receive tetanus

Table 43.3 Tetanus prophylaxis recommendations

Immunization status	Clean wound	Contaminated wound
Immunized (3 or more lifetime doses)	Tetanus toxoid vaccine only if last dose was more than 10 years ago	Tetanus toxoid vaccine only if last dose was more than 5 years ago
Not immunized (less than 3 lifetime doses) or unknown	Tetanus toxoid vaccine only	Tetanus toxoid vaccine and tetanus immunoglobulin

immunoglobulin. Patients who have not been fully immunized, or have not had a recent tetanus toxoid vaccine, should receive a tetanus toxoid vaccine (◘ Table 43.3).

How Do You Manage a Patient Who Presents with Impalement?

Patients who present with an impaled object (e.g., knife, arrow, and rebar) should be assessed in the same manner as other patients with penetrating trauma. No attempt should be made to remove the impaling object until the anatomy of the injury has been identified on imaging studies. These objects are best removed in the operating room under controlled conditions.

Subsequent Management

What Are the Management Options in Patients with Penetrating Abdominal Trauma?

Depending on the patient's hemodynamic stability (hypotensive vs. stable), mechanism of injury (GSW vs. stab), and physical exam (peritonitis vs. benign abdomen), the options vary. For patients with peritonitis, hemodynamic instability, or evisceration, one should directly proceed to exploratory laparotomy. For stable patients without peritonitis or evisceration, there are several options. One is to perform a diagnostic laparoscopy. Another is to perform local wound exploration (particularly for anterior stab wounds). Finally, another option is nonoperative management via admission for close observation and serial abdominal examinations.

When Is It Appropriate to Consider Nonoperative Management of Patients with Penetrating Abdominal Trauma?

Nonoperative management of penetrating abdominal wounds may be appropriate in a certain subset of patients. In order to be considered for nonoperative management, five essential criteria must be met (◘ Table 43.4). Selective nonoperative management is employed to reduce the incidence of nontherapeutic laparotomies and the complications associated with these operations. In general, most patients with penetrating abdominal trauma are managed with an exploratory laparotomy.

◘ **Table 43.4** Criteria for nonoperative management of penetrating abdominal trauma

Criteria for nonoperative management
Hemodynamically stable patient
No peritonitis
Reliable clinical exam (normal mental status)
CT scan demonstrating no intra-abdominal injury
Absence of bowel evisceration

Why Are Trauma Patients Prepped and Draped from Chin to Knees in the Operating Room?

Trauma patients taken to the OR should be prepped widely to allow for access to all critical areas of the body. Immediate access to the left chest is crucial should a trauma patient lose vital signs and require a resuscitative left anterolateral thoracotomy to maintain cardiocerebral perfusion. Access to the thighs allows for the harvesting of saphenous vein should a vascular conduit be required at the time of initial operation.

What Is the Traditional Mainstay of Surgical Management for Patients with Penetrating Abdominal Trauma?

A full midline exploratory laparotomy is the traditional mainstay of surgical management for patients with penetrating abdominal trauma.

What Is the "Lethal Triad of Death" in Trauma? What Is the Lethal Diamond?

The lethal triad of death (◘ Fig. 43.1) refers to the three key interrelated factors, which if left uncorrected could lead to death in the trauma patient. More recently, the terms "acute traumatic coagulopathy" or "coagulopathy of trauma" have been employed to describe the multitude of factors resulting in widespread and uncontrollable hemorrhage in severely injured patients. Some trauma surgeons have added hypocalcemia (lethal diamond) to the triad, recognizing that hypocalcemia is frequent in trauma patients due to the combination of massive blood loss and transfusions (citrate in blood products binds to calcium). Hypercalcemia can worsen coagulopathy and cardiac function.

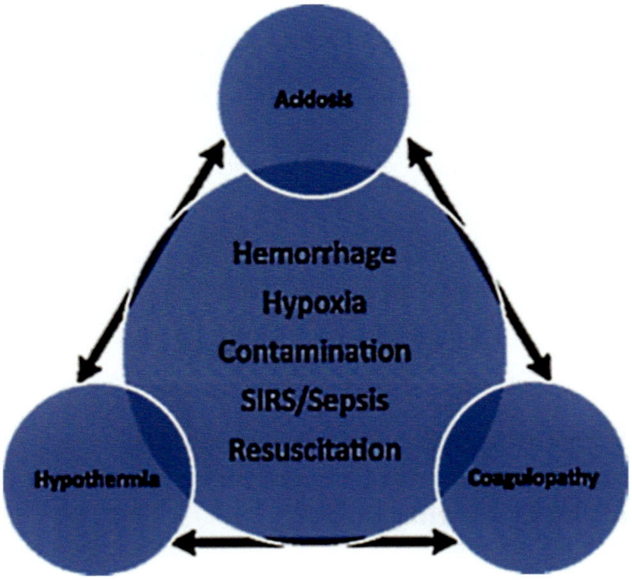

Fig. 43.1 Lethal triad of death in the trauma patient. (Source: From Grabo and Beekley (2017). © Springer Nature 2017, Reprinted with permission)

What Is Damage Control Surgery?

Patients with massive hemorrhage and multiple injuries are at high risk of death once hypothermia, coagulopathy, and acidosis develop intraoperatively. At that point, the surgeon must make the decision to stop surgery (even if every injury is not repaired) and transport the patient to the intensive care unit (ICU), with a plan to re-explore the patient after correction of these physiologic derangements. This approach is called *damage control surgery*. It involves limiting surgery to addressing life-threatening hemorrhage, and temporarily controlling gastrointestinal contamination (such as by stapling off bowel without establishing continuity), and transferring to the ICU for ongoing resuscitation. Typically, in this instance the abdomen is left open and covered with a negative pressure wound vacuum. Once patients are adequately resuscitated in the ICU, they are brought back to the operating room to undergo definitive repair of the injuries (typically within 12–24 hours).

How Long Should Antibiotics Be Continued for Following a Trauma Laparotomy?

A single dose of antibiotics administered preoperatively is usually adequate, although some physicians may elect to continue antibiotics for up to 24 hours postoperatively. Even in the presence of a colon injury, a longer duration of antibiotics is not associated with a decreased incidence of infections and may predispose to the development of resistant organisms.

Do Patients with Small Bowel or Colon Injuries Require a Stoma?

Almost all small bowel injuries can either be repaired primarily or a resection performed with primary anastomosis. With colonic injuries, there is more concern about leakage following repair. Nevertheless, today it is rare that a colon injury require a stoma. The majority of both small and large bowel injuries can be repaired primarily or undergo a resection with primary anastomosis.

Complications

What Is Abdominal Compartment Syndrome? Who Is at Risk?

Patients with multiple traumatic injuries, particularly intra-abdominal or retroperitoneal, who have received large volume of fluids and blood products are at risk of developing intra-abdominal hypertension (IAH) that can progress to abdominal compartment syndrome (ACS). Bladder pressures should be measured as a surrogate of intra-abdominal pressure. IAH is defined as sustained intra-abdominal pressures ≥12 mmHg, whereas ACS is intra-abdominal pressures ≥20 mmHg with associated organ dysfunction. Elevated intra-abdominal pressure compresses the inferior vena cava, thereby reducing preload and overall cardiac output. The subsequent malperfusion results in end organ damage. ACS should be suspected in any severely injured patient who demonstrates decreased urine output, increased peak airway pressures on the ventilator, and increased vasopressor support, in the absence of another identifiable cause. The treatment is to take the patient to the operating room and perform a decompressive laparotomy by reopening the abdominal fascia and leaving the wound open.

Watch Out

In the case of ACS secondary to ascites, a therapeutic paracentesis can be performed first to decrease IAH. If this does not resolve ACS, decompressive laparotomy needs to be performed.

Special Situations/Circumstances

Thoracoabdominal Penetrating Wounds

Penetrating injuries to this area can present a challenge as there may be concomitant injuries to the thoracic cavity, mediastinum, heart, diaphragm, retroperitoneum, and abdominal cavities. Determining which cavity to address first—chest or abdomen—depends on clinical findings. In most cases, the abdomen is the source of hemorrhage, especially if a chest X-ray does not reveal a large hemothorax. Even if a nonoperative approach is planned, penetrating wounds to the left thoracoabdominal area still require a delayed diagnostic laparoscopy to rule out an occult left-sided diaphragm injury. If such an injury is missed, the patient may later develop a diaphragmatic hernia (the liver protects the right side from bowel contents entering a hernia defect).

Summary of Essentials

History and Physical Exam

- GSWs and stab wounds are the most common mechanisms of penetrating injury.
- Every effort should be made to identify all wounds (look in axilla and perineum).
- Assess for hypotension, peritonitis, or evisceration.

Anatomy

- The peritoneal cavity, pelvis, and retroperitoneum comprise the internal abdomen.
- Injuries to retroperitoneal structures are difficult to diagnose.
- Liver and small bowel are the most commonly injured organs following penetrating abdominal trauma.

Initial Management

- Start with ABCs.
- Initiate massive transfusion protocol in all unstable patients with suspected major blood loss.
- Consider permissive hypotension in patients with penetrating torso trauma.
- FAST useful to rule out cardiac tamponade; it is not useful in penetrating trauma to determine if laparotomy is needed.

Subsequent Management

- Immediate operative exploration if either: hypotensive, peritonitis, or evisceration
- If hemodynamically stable with no peritonitis or evisceration:
  - Local wound exploration (if anterior abdominal stab wound)
  - CT (chest, abdomen, pelvis) and if negative, serial abdominal exams
    - Nonoperative management of penetrating abdominal trauma is the exception rather than the rule
- Diagnostic laparoscopy (particularly for left lower thoracic or upper abdomen wounds)

Subsequent Management

- Damage control surgery
- Minimize operating time
  - Control hemorrhage
  - Temporary control of gastrointestinal injuries

Complications

- ACS is diagnosed by an elevated bladder pressure in conjunction with low urine output and elevated airway pressures.

Suggested Reading

Como JJ, Bokhari F, Chiu WC, et al. Practice management guidelines for selective nonoperative management of penetrating abdominal trauma. *J Trauma*. 2010;68(3):721–733. https://doi.org/10.1097/TA.0b013e3181cf7d07.

Grabo D, Beekley AC. Initial management priorities: beyond ABCDE. In: Martin MJ, Beekley AC, eds. *Front line surgery*. Springer, New York, 2017

Nicholas JM, Rix EP, Easley KA, et al. Changing patterns in the management of penetrating abdominal trauma: the more things change, the more they stay the same. J Trauma. 2003;55:1095.

Velmahos GC, Demetriades D, Toutouzas KG, et al. Selective nonoperative management in 1856 patients with abdominal gunshot wounds: should routine laparotomy still be the standard of care? Ann Surg. 2001;234:395.

Wray JP, Bridwell RE, Schauer SG, et al. The diamond of death: Hypocalcemia in trauma and resuscitation. Am J Emerg Med. 2021 Mar;41:104–109. https://doi.org/10.1016/j.ajem.2020.12.065. Epub 2020 Dec 28. PMID: 33421674.

Zafar SN, Rushing A, Haut ER, et al. Outcome of selective nonoperative management of penetrating abdominal injuries from the North American National Trauma Database. Br J Surg. 2012;99(Suppl 1):155.

Pedestrian Struck by Motor Vehicle

McKensie Hammons, Areg Grigorian, Christian de Virgilio, and Dennis Y. Kim

Contents

C. de Virgilio, A. Grigorian (eds.), *Surgery*, https://doi.org/10.1007/978-3-032-09799-6_44

Case Study

A 30-year-old male is struck by a car while crossing the street. He is brought in by paramedics with a blood pressure (BP) of 130/70 mmHg, heart rate of 80/min, and a right knee deformity. He is awake and alert and complaining of severe right knee pain. His airway is intact and breath sounds are equal bilaterally. Abdominal and pelvic exams are unremarkable. There is swelling and an obvious deformity of his right knee. His right foot is pale and cool, with a 6 s capillary refill, whereas the left foot is pink and warm with <2 s capillary refill. Pulse examination reveals normal 2+ pulses in his left femoral, popliteal, dorsalis pedis (DP), and posterior tibial (PT) arteries. On the right, there is a 2+ femoral pulse. Doppler signals on the left foot are triphasic, whereas on the right they are monophasic. Due to severe knee pain, neither the right knee nor the popliteal pulse can be examined. The right dorsalis pedis and posterior tibial artery pulses are non-palpable. Sensory and motor function is intact bilaterally. There is no tenderness or deformity in the right thigh or in the tibia or ankle. The right lower extremity ankle–brachial index (ABI) is 0.20, whereas the left is 1.0.

Diagnosis

What Is the Most Likely Diagnosis?

Given the mechanism of injury, deformity of the right knee, pale and cool right foot, and absence of distal pulses, this patient most likely has a right popliteal artery injury secondary to a posterior knee dislocation.

History and Physical Exam

What Are "Hard" and "Soft" Signs of Vascular Injury?

Hard signs are specific, overt physical exam findings that, if present, confirm the suspected injury or disease. In general, if a hard sign of vascular injury is present, the thought is that further imaging is unnecessary and would delay definitive treatment. As such, *immediate* operative intervention is recommended when hard signs are present. Soft signs increase the index of suspicion for a vascular injury but are not sufficient for immediate surgery, and thus their presence on exam should prompt further investigation (◘ Table 44.1).

Do All Patients with Hard Signs Need to Go Emergently to the OR?

The hard signs of vascular injury were created at a time when formal transfemoral arteriography was needed to diagnose arterial injuries, and this would delay definitive management by several hours, potentially leading to irreversible ischemia. Today CT angiogram (CTA) can be obtained within minutes at a trauma center. As such, patients with a palpable thrill or bruit may have time to undergo imaging to better delineate the injury. Similarly, those with an absent pulse often undergo CTA as well provided there is no evidence of acute limb ischemia. Those with arterial bleeding, shock, expanding hematoma should still go directly to the operating room (OR) without imaging.

What Are the Ps of Acute Limb Ischemia?

Pain, pallor, paresthesia, paralysis, pulselessness, and poikilothermia.

◘ **Table 44.1** Signs of vascular injury

Hard signs	Soft signs
Arterial/pulsatile bleeding	History of hemorrhage in the field
Persistent hemorrhage with shock	Small, stable, non-pulsatile hematoma
Expanding or pulsatile hematoma	Unexplained hypotension
Palpable thrill	Penetrating wounds in proximity to major vessels
Audible bruit	Associated nerve deficit
Absent pulse	Diminished or unequal pulses

What Is the Implication of an Audible Bruit/ Palpable Thrill Near an Artery in Association with Trauma?

These are highly suggestive of a traumatic arteriovenous fistula. This needs to be worked up with CTA.

What Are the Principles of the Physical Examination of an Injured Extremity?

The physical exam should include an assessment of vascular, neurologic, musculoskeletal, and soft tissue integrity of the entire limb, including the joints above and below the site of injury. Comparison of potentially abnormal findings to the contralateral extremity should be done.

Pathophysiology

What Is the Mechanism of Popliteal Artery Injury?

The popliteal artery is susceptible to traction and transection injuries due to its fixed course across the knee joint. The artery is tethered at both its superior border, as the superficial femoral artery exits the adductor hiatus, and its inferior border at the tendinous arch of the soleus. Along its course, the popliteal artery forms a weak anastomotic network around the knee by giving off paired geniculate branches. Posterior dislocation of the knee stretches the relatively fixed popliteal artery, leading to intimal disruption. The most common presentation of popliteal artery injury is thrombosis with acute distal limb ischemia.

What Are the Classic Orthopedic Fractures/ Dislocations That Are Associated with Arterial Injury? (▣ Table 44.2)

Why Is It Important to Promptly Reduce a Dislocation?

Dislocations that are left unreduced for a prolonged period are associated with poorer long-term outcomes, including limited functional recovery. In the short term, these injuries are associated with significant pain and discomfort, which are improved with reduction. Prompt reduction allows for near-normal range of motion and use. Furthermore, unreduced dislocations can compress blood flow to the joint, increasing the risk of osteonecrosis of the involved bone. Occasionally, the dislocation can lead to stretching or kinking of the artery, and reduction can improve or restore blood flow.

▣ Table 44.2 Classic orthopedic fractures/ dislocations associated with arterial injury

Injury	Artery involved	Features
Shoulder girdle dislocation	Axillary artery	*Anterior* dislocations are more common and present with axillary nerve *or* artery injuries; *posterior* dislocations result from seizures and have an increased risk of axillary nerve injury
Clavicle fracture	Subclavian artery	Patients may have associated pneumothorax and/or hemothorax
Supracondylar humerus fracture	Brachial artery	Occurs more commonly in children; may result in Volkmann's contracture if left untreated
Pelvic fracture	Branches of internal iliac artery (superior gluteal and internal pudendal)	Arterial bleeding in the presence of severe *posterior* fractures is more likely to be due to an injury to the superior gluteal artery; severe *anterior* fractures may result in injury to the internal pudendal artery; both can result in hemorrhagic shock (major source of blood loss)
Hip dislocation	Femoral artery	*Posterior* dislocations present with an internally rotated and adducted leg with an increased risk of sciatic nerve injury; *anterior* dislocations present with externally rotated and abducted legs with an increased risk of femoral artery injury; risk of avascular necrosis if combined with femoral head fracture
Knee dislocation	Popliteal artery	Arterial injuries occur more frequently in patients with *posterior* dislocation than with anterior
Tibial plateau fracture	Popliteal artery	Arterial injuries occur more frequently in patients with *medial* injuries and less with lateral

> **Watch Out**
> Always examine a patient's vascular and neurological status both *before* and *after* performing reduction as it can change post reduction.

What Is a Minimal Vascular Injury?

Minimal vascular or arterial injuries refer to clinically silent injuries that are discovered on radiographic studies such as angiography or ultrasonography. These injuries usually have a benign or self-limited course. They involve small intimal flaps or irregularities.

What Is Suggested by Numbness of the Skin Overlying the Lateral Shoulder After Shoulder Dislocation?

Numbness to the skin overlying the lateral shoulder suggests injury to the axillary nerve. This occurs most commonly with anterior shoulder dislocation but can also occur with posterior shoulder dislocation (excessive abduction and external rotation of the glenohumeral joint). Patients may also have poor function of the deltoid muscle with weakened shoulder abduction. While anterior shoulder dislocations can also present with axillary artery injury, this is uncommon in posterior dislocations.

Workup

Should the Knee Be Tested for Ligamentous Injury?

No. In the acute setting of a severe knee injury, testing for ligamentous injury should not be done as the patient will be in severe pain, imaging has not yet been obtained to rule out fractures, and manipulating the knee may worsen the arterial injury.

What Noninvasive Bedside Test Provides Objective Evidence of a Vascular Injury? How Is It Performed?

The ankle–brachial index (ABI) is a noninvasive bedside test that provides objective evidence of a vascular injury. It is measured with the patient in a supine position. A handheld Doppler and a blood pressure (BP) cuff are needed to measure ABI. The BP cuff is inflated at the ankle, while the Doppler is held on the dorsalis pedis (DP) artery. The cuff is inflated until the Doppler signal disappears. The cuff is slowly deflated until the signal returns. The systolic pressure at which the signal returns is recorded. The process is repeated with the posterior tibial (PT) and bilateral brachial arteries. The ABI is the ratio of the highest systolic pressure measured at the foot (of the side in question) over the highest brachial systolic pressure (of right *or* left side). A normal ABI is between 1.0 and 1.2. An ABI of <0.90 is highly sensitive and specific for arterial injury following both blunt and penetrating injuries.

> **Watch Out**
> In trauma, the arterial-pressure index (API) is often used instead of ABI. API compares the blood pressure in the injured extremity to the contralateral non-injured extremity, whereas the ABI compares the ankle pressure to the arm (brachial) pressure.

If the ABI Is Abnormal, What Additional Vascular Imaging Study Is Recommended?

If the ABI or API is <0.9, additional vascular imaging is recommended. If the patient is hypothermic or hypotensive when the initial ABI is taken, it should be repeated 10–15 minutes after resuscitation and warming. CTA is currently the test of choice due to its availability, rapidity, and noninvasive nature.

What Additional Radiologic Imaging Study Is Recommended for a Posterior Knee Dislocation?

Postreduction films should be obtained to assess for the adequacy of reduction and to rule out a periarticular fracture.

In Penetrating Trauma, Should an Angiogram Be Performed If the Bullet/Stab Wound Is Close to an Artery, Even If There Are No Signs of Injury and the ABI is Normal?

No. So-called proximity injuries should raise the level of suspicion for vascular injury, but no further workup is warranted in the patient with a normal ABI.

What Is the Mangled Extremity Severity Score and How Is It Used?

In certain situations, particularly those involving extensive soft tissue or musculoskeletal injury of an extremity, with or without associated neurovascular trauma, the limb is so severely injured that the likelihood of salvaging the limb may be in doubt. The Mangled Extremity Severity Score (MESS) is one of the most commonly used scoring systems to quantify injury severity in patients with severe trauma of the extremities (see below). It is designed to help surgeons decide whether to attempt limb salvage or proceed directly to amputation. A limb may be considered "mangled" if at least three out of four components (bone, soft tissue, blood vessels, and nerves) are damaged. However, efforts to validate this scoring system prospectively have demonstrated poor predictive value for amputation. As such the decision to proceed directly to amputation should optimally be done via multidisciplinary consultation between trauma, vascular, orthopedic, and plastic surgeons.

Mangled Extremity Severity Score Components
- Patient age
- Mechanism/energy of injury
- Presence of hypotension or shock
- Severity of ischemia
- Ischemia duration (>6 hours)

Management

What Are the First Steps in the Management of This Patient?

Initial management (Fig. 44.1) of the trauma patient begins with the primary survey to identify and treat immediately life-threatening conditions. The primary survey involves assessing the *ABCDE*s (airway with C-spine precautions, breathing, circulation with hemorrhage control, disability, and exposure/environmental control). Among patients with extremity vascular

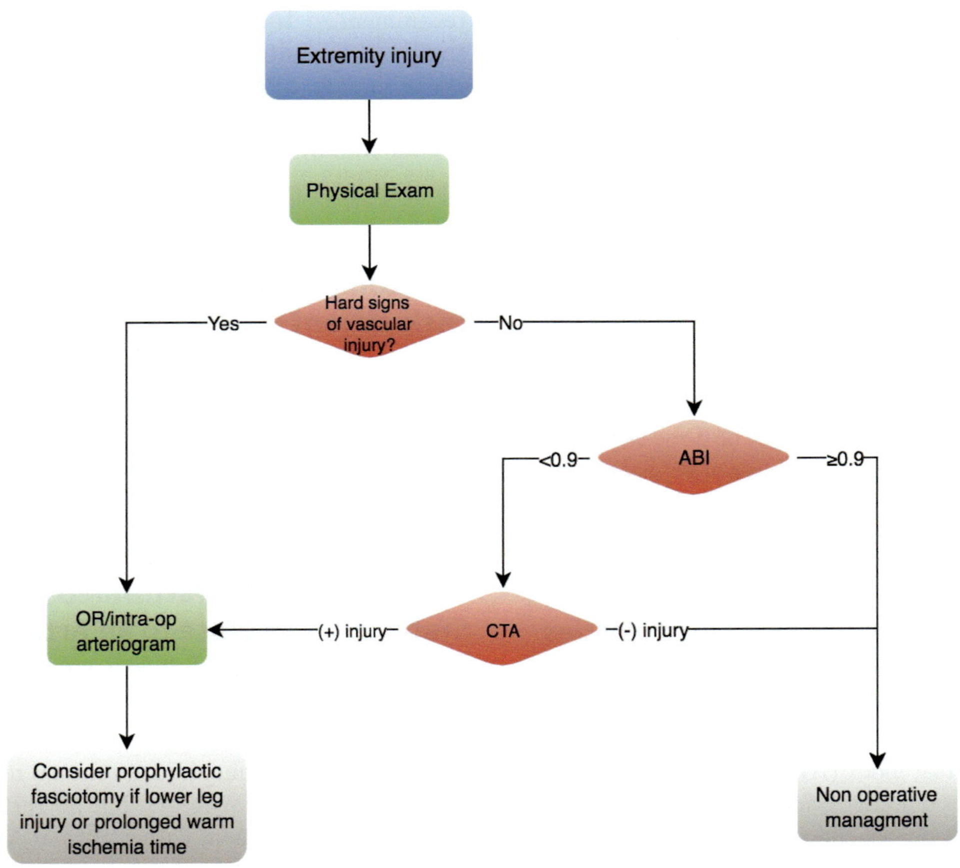

Fig. 44.1 Algorithm for extremity injury management

trauma, aggressive efforts should be directed toward identifying and controlling bleeding. The secondary survey is performed only after completing the primary survey and consists of a detailed head-to-toe examination to identify all wounds and injuries not detected during the primary survey.

Is There a Role for Tourniquets in Patients with Life-Threatening Hemorrhage of an Extremity?

Recent literature and guidelines support the use of tourniquets for exsanguinating extremity trauma when application of direct pressure is not successful or feasible. These may be placed in the prehospital/field setting and emergency or operating rooms. Improper placement of tourniquets may result in paradoxical bleeding if the pressure applied to the affected limb does not arrest arterial inflow while occluding venous outflow. The solution to paradoxical bleeding is to increase the tourniquet pressure to obtain arterial occlusion.

What Is the Next Step in the Management of a Knee Dislocation?

Immediate reduction of the right knee dislocation is indicated in an ischemic limb. Early orthopedic consultation should be obtained.

What Is the Next Step Following Reduction?

Recheck the neurovascular status. If there is still no pulse, emergency surgery will be needed. However, most trauma surgeons would get a CTA first to localize the injury. If pulse returns, check the ABI. If ABI is <0.9, obtain a CTA. If the CTA confirms arterial injury, take the patient to the operating room.

What Are the Principles of Operative Management of a Popliteal Artery Injury in This Setting?

The focus of operative management is restoration of circulation. Definitive management within 6 hours of injury offers the best chance of limb salvage with minimal neurologic deficits in the ischemic limb. However, recent studies indicate that the risk of limb loss increases for every hour delay.

If a Conduit Is Needed to Replace the Injured Artery, Where Is It Taken From?

Autogenous vein grafts offer better long-term patency compared to prosthetic grafts and lower risk of infectious complications following repair in contaminated wounds. The proximal greater saphenous vein is harvested from the contralateral, uninjured leg (and must be reversed due to valves). This approach is preferred to preserve collateral venous circulation of the injured leg in the context of a possible popliteal venous injury.

Watch Out

In general, a conduit is chosen from the *contralateral* extremity in trauma patients, whereas the conduit in a patient with peripheral arterial disease undergoing bypass is chosen from the *ipsilateral* extremity.

What If the Popliteal Vein Is Also Injured?

The vein should be repaired if it can be done easily and if the patient is stable. If repair is not practical, ligation is acceptable. Combined arterial and venous injuries significantly increase the risk of compartment syndrome. In such cases, prophylactic four-compartment fasciotomy is often recommended, although recent evidence supports close monitoring as an alternative in select patients.

What If There Is a Combined Orthopedic and Vascular Injury? Which Is Repaired First?

This depends on the severity of ischemia to the limb. The issue is as follows: if the bone is fixed first, and the patient has severe arterial ischemia, a prolonged orthopedic procedure may lead to irreversible muscle and nerve ischemia. Alternatively, if the artery is repaired first, and then the orthopedic injury is repaired after, the required manipulation of the bone may disrupt the arterial repair. Thus, if the limb is markedly ischemic, it is recommended to insert a shunt proximal and distal to the injured artery so as to restore flow. This permits a less rushed orthopedic surgery. The artery can then be fixed afterward. If the arterial injury has not caused limb ischemia, the orthopedic injury is fixed first, followed by the arterial repair.

Does Heparin Administration Help?

The benefit of heparin for penetrating arterial trauma is somewhat controversial. However, in the setting of blunt popliteal injury (and in particular with an ischemic limb), systemic heparin administration is recommended. It is thought to reduce rates of amputation by preventing microvascular thrombosis in the setting of low-flow arterial circulation. Contraindications to heparinization include active hemorrhage, intracranial injury, and coagulopathy.

What Is the Risk of Limb Loss with a Posterior Knee Dislocation and Popliteal Injury?

This injury has a high risk of limb loss, ranging from 30% to 50%. This is largely due to the poor collateral blood supply around the knee, associated extensive arterial thrombosis, associated venous injury, and risk of postoperative compartment syndrome. Early recognition of compartment syndrome from reperfusion injury is essential.

Area Where You Can Get in Trouble

Assuming There Is No Arterial Injury Because You Think You Feel Palpable Pulses

The pulse exam is very unreliable in adequately assessing vascular injury. It is not uncommon for the examiner to feel their own pulse. Thus, always measure the ABI in conjunction with the pulse exam to confirm normal blood flow.

Area of Controversy

The Role of Endovascular Repair

The use of endovascular techniques to repair extremity vascular trauma has increased over the last decade. Good candidates for endovascular repair are those who are hemodynamically stable with a wound location that is difficult to access surgically (proximal limb injuries with extension into the chest or abdomen, so-called junctional injuries). Patients at risk for compartment syndrome or those requiring embolectomy are not good candidates for endovascular repair.

Summary of Essentials

History and Physical Exam

- Always start with the ABCs
- Suspect popliteal artery injury with posterior knee dislocation
- Look for hard signs of vascular injury
- Assess the neurologic and vascular function with any extremity injury

Diagnosis

- No testing is needed if hard signs are present; expedited operative repair is required.
- ABI testing is sensitive and specific for significant extremity vascular injury.
- CTA if soft signs of injury or abnormal ABI.
- Vascular imaging is not needed with a normal pulse and normal ABI ($\geq$0.9).

Management

- Immediately reduce the dislocated joint
- Reassess neurovascular function after reduction
- Hard signs of vascular injury are indications for surgery
- Start heparin in the pulseless extremity with no contraindications to anticoagulation
- Repair the injured artery with reverse saphenous vein from contralateral leg

Prognosis

- Mangled Extremity Severity Score
- Risk of limb loss depends on duration of limb ischemia, patient age, hemodynamic status, severity of neurovascular injury, and severity of soft tissue injury

Acknowledgement The editors would like to acknowledge and thank the following authors for their contributions to the previous edition of the chapter: Zane W. Ashman.

Suggested Reading

Johnson CA. Endovascular management of peripheral vascular trauma. Semin Intervent Radiol. 2010;27(1):38–43.

Rowe VL, Pourrabbani S, Weaver FA. Blunt popliteal artery injuries. In: Stanley JC, Veith FJ, Wakefield TW, editors. Current therapy in vascular and endovascular surgery. 5th ed. Philadelphia: Elsevier; 2014. https://www.clinicalkey.com/dura/browse/bookChapter/3-s2.0-C20110000303.

Vogel TR, O'Donnell PL, Trauma JGJ, injuries t. Injuries to the peripheral blood vessels. In: Ashley SW, editor. ACS surgery [online]. Philadelphia: Decker Intellectual Properties; 2012.

Gunshot Wound to the Left Neck

Sebastian D. Schubl, Christian de Virgilio, and Dennis Y. Kim

Contents

C. de Virgilio, A. Grigorian (eds.), *Surgery*, https://doi.org/10.1007/978-3-032-09799-6_45

Case Study

A 30-year-old male presents to the emergency department with a single gunshot wound (GSW) to the left neck. The patient is hemodynamically stable, with a blood pressure of 120/70 mmHg, heart rate of 100/min, respiratory rate of 16/min, and a Glasgow Coma Scale (GCS) score of 15. He is able to speak and states that his voice sounds normal to him. There is no stridor or odynophagia. He denies any weakness or numbness in his arms or legs. On physical examination, he is awake and alert. There is a single wound in the left mid-neck between the cricoid cartilage and the angle of the mandible with no bleeding. There is a small but nonexpanding hematoma overlying the injury with no other wounds seen. There is no palpable crepitus or audible bruit. Neurological examination is normal.

History and Physical Examination

What Are the Most Important Parts of the History and Physical Examination for a Patient with a Neck Injury?

Mechanism of injury (e.g., penetrating vs blunt), location of injury, and clinical exam findings.

What Are Hard Signs of Vascular Injury?

"Hard signs" are physical exam findings that indicate the presence of a significant vascular injury. They include active arterial bleeding, pulsatile or expanding hematoma, the presence of shock, a palpable thrill, audible bruit, and neurological deficits that indicate a possible stroke. The presence of one of these findings (particularly the first three) is an indication for *immediate* surgical exploration.

What Are Other Nonvascular Hard Signs That May Warrant a Surgical Exploration?

In addition to the vasculature, there are "hard signs" for the aerodigestive system that also prompt most trauma surgeons to consider *immediate* operative exploration. These include massive hemoptysis or hematemesis, bubbling or food particles in the wound, and respiratory distress.

What Is the Significance of the Following Signs/Symptoms? (Table 45.1)

What Is the Diagnosis in This Patient?

The patient has a penetrating neck injury without hard signs of injury. Despite the lack of hard signs, injury to critical structures needs to be ruled out. Although

Table 45.1 Significance of various signs/symptoms following penetrating neck trauma

Sign/symptom	Significance
Stridor	A sign of upper airway obstruction caused by compression of the trachea from a large hematoma, soft tissue swelling, direct laryngeal injury, or bilateral recurrent laryngeal nerve injury; it warrants immediate attention to the airway, usually in the form of endotracheal intubation
Odynophagia	Pain with swallowing is suggestive of an injury to the oropharynx or esophagus
Horner's syndrome	Ptosis, miosis, and anhidrosis; due to injury to sympathetic fibers that innervate the pupil, eyelid, and skin surrounding the eye that travel along the course of the common carotid and internal carotid arteries; may indicate carotid injury
Thrill/Bruit	Indicates an arteriovenous fistula, most likely between carotid/jugular and subclavian artery/vein; the fistula leads to turbulent blood flow causing vein to vibrate, leading to palpable rumble or a whooshing sound on auscultation
Crepitus	A sign of subcutaneous emphysema (air trapped under the skin) secondary to injury of the aerodigestive tract (trachea, bronchus, or esophagus) or lungs
Hoarse voice	Dysfunction of the vocal cord either because of direct trauma or damage to the vagus or recurrent laryngeal nerve causing ipsilateral vocal cord paralysis

- If primary anastomosis is not possible, place interposition graft.
- Ideal conduit is autogenous graft (greater saphenous vein from the thigh).

Acknowledgment The editors would like to acknowledge and thank the following authors for their contributions to the previous edition of the chapter: Alexis L. Woods.

Suggested Reading

Bell RB, Osborn T, Dierks EJ, et al. Management of penetrating neck injuries: a new paradigm for civilian trauma. J Oral Maxillofac Surg. 2007;65:691.

Brywczynski JJ, Barrett TW, Lyon JA, Cotton BA. Management of penetrating neck injury in the emergency department: a structured literature review. Emerg Med J. 2008;25:711.

Van Waes OJ, Cheriex KC, Navsaria PH, et al. Management of penetrating neck injuries. Br J Surg. 2012;99(Suppl 1):149.

Stab Wound to the Chest

Patrick T. Delaplain, Christian de Virgilio, Areg Grigorian, and Dennis Y. Kim

Contents

C. de Virgilio, A. Grigorian (eds.), *Surgery*, https://doi.org/10.1007/978-3-032-09799-6_46

Case Study

A 20-year-old male is brought in by paramedics after suffering two stab wounds to his chest. In the emergency department, the patient is awake but combative. He responds to questions by stating his name but is flailing his arms and shouting to leave him alone. His breath smells of alcohol. On physical examination, his blood pressure is 88/70 mmHg, heart rate is 110/min, and respiratory rate is 20/min. His airway is patent. Breath sounds are absent on the left and clear on the right. He has two stab wounds to the left chest, one just above and one just below the nipple. There is no bubbling of air from the wounds. There is palpable crepitus over the left chest. His neck veins appear to be distended. His trachea is midline. The heart sounds are difficult to hear, but the rate is regular but fast, without murmurs. The abdomen is soft and non-tender. The patient is log-rolled and no other injuries are identified.

Diagnosis

What Are Considered the "Lethal Six" Injuries of Thoracic Trauma? (◘ Table 46.1)

Watch Out
The most common cause of airway obstruction occurs in patients with diminished airway reflexes in which a relaxed tongue falls back against the rear of the pharynx.

What Are Considered the "Hidden Six" Injuries of Thoracic Trauma? (◘ Table 46.2)

Watch Out
The "lethal six" and "hidden six" make up the "deadly dozen" of thoracic trauma.

Watch Out
Do not assume that a combative trauma patient's behavior is due to intoxication; it may represent an underlying physiologic derangement such as hypoxia or hemodynamic collapse.

How Is the Diagnosis of Tension Pneumothorax Established?

This is a clinical diagnosis without a need for X-ray confirmation, which will delay treatment. Suspect tension pneumothorax in patients with hypotension, dyspnea, tachypnea, jugular venous distention, unilaterally absent breath sounds, and tracheal deviation away from the injury.

How Is the Diagnosis of Cardiac Tamponade Established?

This is also considered a clinical diagnosis and requires prompt intervention. Patients who present with Beck's triad (hypotension, distended neck veins, and muffled heart sounds) should be suspected of having tamponade. The diagnosis is supported by an immediate bedside FAST—Focused Assessment with Sonography for Trauma—(ultrasound) scan demonstrating fluid in the

◘ **Table 46.1** The lethal six injuries of thoracic trauma

Lethal six	Characteristics
Airway obstruction	Laryngeal trauma, foreign body aspiration, stridor, expanding neck hematoma, and gurgling
Tension pneumothorax	Hemodynamic instability, tracheal shift away from injury, and one-way valve in injured lung
Open pneumothorax	Associated with open chest wall injury; air enters pleural cavity through the skin
Massive hemothorax	Lung parenchymal or intercostal artery injury; total whiteout of lung field
Flail chest	Two or more contiguous ribs fractured in two sites leading to paradoxical motion of chest wall; often have underlying lung contusion
Cardiac tamponade	Beck's triad (hypotension, distended neck veins, and muffled heart sounds)

Table 46.2 The "Hidden six" injuries of thoracic trauma

Hidden six	Characteristics
Blunt aortic injury	High-energy rapid deceleration injury (e.g., fall from greater than 10 feet, high-speed motor vehicle accident, aviation accident); widened mediastinum; left-sided hemothorax; deviation of the trachea to the right on chest X-ray
Esophageal injury	Penetrating trauma; subcutaneous air
Tracheobronchial injury	Massive subcutaneous emphysema
Diaphragmatic rupture	Due to sudden rise in intra-abdominal pressure, the stomach and colon are the most frequently herniated structures; penetrating thoracoabdominal injuries; delayed diagnosis (may be asymptomatic)
Blunt cardiac injury	Ranging from arrhythmias (tachycardia or bundle branch block) to cardiac rupture; associated with sternal fracture and hemopneumothorax
Pulmonary contusion	Develops within first 24 hour; often not seen on initial chest X-ray

pericardial sac. Patients may also exhibit pulsus paradoxus (decrease in systolic blood pressure [SBP] $\geq$10 mmHg with inspiration).

Watch Out

In cases of exam findings suggestive of acute cardiac tamponade (hypotension, distended neck veins, and muffled heart sounds), the chest X-ray will typically be *normal.* A normal cardiac silhouette will often be seen with no other obvious cause for the hypotension (e.g., tension pneumothorax).

What Is the Most Likely Diagnosis in This Patient?

Given that the patient has sustained a penetrating chest injury to the cardiac box in association with Beck's triad, there is a high suspicion for cardiac tamponade. The cardiac box is defined as the area of the anterior chest wall bounded by the sternal notch and clavicles superiorly, the nipples laterally, and the subcostal margin inferiorly. Up to a third of patients with a penetrating wound in this area may have an associated cardiac injury. He also has absent breath sounds on the left. Given this and his hypotension, a tension pneumothorax is also possible.

History and Physical

What Is the Differential Diagnosis for a Combative Trauma Patient?

While alcohol or drug intoxication is a common cause of combativeness in trauma patients, it is a diagnosis of exclusion. Hypoxia, shock, and hypoglycemia must be ruled out immediately, as they can all present with altered mental status. In cases of blunt trauma, traumatic brain injury should also be considered. Other possibilities include postictal states and pain-related agitation.

What Is the Differential Diagnosis of the Absent Breath Sounds on the Left?

Pneumothorax or massive hemothorax.

What Is the Implication of a Penetrating Injury to the Chest That Is Above Versus Below the Nipple?

The diaphragm is a dome-shaped muscle that peaks at an imaginary line between the nipples. A penetrating injury above the nipple line likely only involves injury to the thoracic structures. Penetrating injuries below the nipple line (typically at the level of the fourth intercostal space) are considered thoracoabdominal because they may traverse the diaphragm and involve both thoracic and abdominal cavities. The thoracoabdominal region extends from the nipple line (anteriorly) or inferior scapular tip (posteriorly) down to the costal margin. Injuries in this zone can affect thoracic structures, abdominal organs, or the diaphragm itself, and therefore require evaluation of all three compartments.

Why Is It Important to Know the Type of Weapon Used in a Penetrating Injury?

While the path of stab wounds can normally be traced, ballistic injuries can be unpredictable in their path. This makes it essential to determine the trajectory of a bullet so an injury is not missed. All wounds should be identified. If there is an odd number of wounds, the bullet must be located radiographically. On rare occasions, bullets may enter an artery and embolize.

What Is the Concern Given That the Systolic and Diastolic Pressures in the Patient Presented Are So Close to Each Other?

A pulse pressure (systolic minus diastolic blood pressure) less than 30 mmHg is considered narrow and is indicative of reduced left ventricle stroke volume. In the trauma setting, the differential diagnosis for a narrow pulse pressure is typically reduced preload (e.g., hemorrhagic/hypovolemic shock) or obstructive shock (e.g., pericardial tamponade, tension pneumothorax). A narrow pulse pressure often precedes hypotension and is an early indicator of cardiovascular collapse without prompt resuscitation.

Why Is It Important to Roll the Patient Over?

In all patients with penetrating trauma, it is important to check for wounds to the back that may otherwise be missed. The axilla and perineum are two other areas that should be examined in patients with penetrating mechanisms of injury. In general, cervical spine immobilization in patients with penetrating injuries is not required given the extremely low incidence of unstable cervical spine fractures.

What Is the Significance of Air Bubbling from a Penetrating Chest Wound?

This is also referred to as a sucking chest wound, a type of open pneumothorax (Table 46.3). An open pneumothorax indicates there is an injury to the lung or bronchial tree that connects directly to the atmosphere. With a sucking chest wound, the chest wall defect is so large (at least 2/3rd the diameter of the trachea) that inspired air takes the path of least resistance and enters the chest cavity through the wound instead of through the trachea.

Watch Out

Always order a chest X-ray after inserting a central line to make sure you did not cause an iatrogenic pneumothorax. Hypotension or shortness of breath after central line placement should be presumed to be a pneumothorax until proven otherwise.

What Is Subcutaneous Emphysema?

The word emphysema is derived from Greek and means trapped air, which in this case is within the subcutaneous tissues. Crepitus refers to the crunchy sen-

Table 46.3 Types of pneumothorax

Type	Population	Etiology
Primary spontaneous pneumothorax	Young, tall, thin, male, smokers	Spontaneous rupture of apical alveolar blebs
Open	All trauma patients	Free communication between the atmosphere and pleural space through a large chest wound communicating with the pleural space
Simple	All trauma patients	Jagged rib fracture punctures lung; stab or gunshot wound
Tension	All trauma patients	Lung injury or chest wall injury creates one-way valve
Iatrogenic	Patients with central line or thoracentesis	Direct needle injury to the lung

sation on palpation of the skin in the presence of subcutaneous air. In the trauma setting, subcutaneous emphysema is caused by a pneumothorax until proven otherwise.

Pathophysiology

Why Is a Tension Pneumothorax Dangerous?

Tension pneumothorax is considered the most dangerous type of pneumothorax because the injury creates a one-way valve effect. With each inspiration, air leaks out of the lung and into the pleural cavity or is sucked in from the environment. However, the air is unable to leave the pleural space because of the one-way valve effect. This leads to compression of the vena cava resulting in decreased preload, severe reduction in cardiac output, and eventual hemodynamic collapse.

What Is the Implication of Distended Jugular Veins?

Distended jugular veins are suggestive of elevated jugular venous pressure, an indirect measure of central venous pressure. In the trauma patient, it should raise the suspicion of either cardiac tamponade or tension pneumothorax.

Watch Out

Consider a large hemothorax in a patient with hemorrhagic shock, contralateral tracheal deviation, decreased breath sounds, and dullness to percussion.

What Causes Hypotension in Cardiac Tamponade?

Cardiac tamponade occurs when pericardial fluid accumulates under pressure, compressing the heart. Because the pericardium is noncompliant, even a small increase in volume can significantly raise intrapericardial pressure. As this pressure approaches and eventually exceeds the intracardiac filling pressures, diastolic filling becomes impaired. This reduces stroke volume and cardiac output, resulting in hypotension.

What Are the Hemodynamic Findings in Cardiac Tamponade?

Cardiac catheterization typically reveals elevated and *equalized* diastolic pressures across all chambers, including the right atrium, right ventricle, and pulmonary capillary wedge pressure (PCWP). Echocardiography is the diagnostic modality of choice and should be performed urgently if tamponade is suspected. In contrast, pulmonary embolism usually presents with elevated right-sided pressures but normal or low PCWP due to reduced left atrial filling.

What Is the Most Important Factor in the Development of Cardiac Tamponade?

The rate of accumulation of fluid is the most important factor. If fluid accumulates slowly (such as with uremia), the pericardial sac is better able to accommodate by stretching, and volumes of up to 1 liter can potentially be asymptomatic. However, volumes as small as 150 mL in *acute* cardiac tamponade (such as in penetrating trauma) can reduce cardiac output.

Does a Normal Abdominal Examination Rule Out an Intra-Abdominal Injury? Why or Why Not?

No. A penetrating injury to the colon or small bowel may not immediately create peritonitis (it may take several hours to manifest). A reliable physical examination also requires a cooperative and reliable patient. Intoxication, a depressed mental status, and associated "distracting" injuries may all interfere with the accuracy of the abdominal examination. Since the patient described has an injury below the nipple, intra-abdominal injuries need to be ruled out.

Why Are Penetrating Chest Trauma Patients at Increased Risk of Air Embolism? How Would It Present?

Air embolism can occur in both the venous and arterial systems and are potentially life-threatening. If air were to enter the coronary arteries, blood flow to the heart could be interrupted resulting in myocardial infarction. Concomitant injury to a bronchus and pulmonary vein may result in an air embolism. Stab wounds or gunshot wounds near the hilum are the most common mechanism of such injuries as this is where these two structures lie in close proximity. Symptoms of air embolism can manifest in the cardiovascular (chest pain, arrhythmia, right-sided heart failure), respiratory (dyspnea, hypoxia, hypercarbia), and central nervous (confusion, altered mentation, stroke) systems.

Why Would a Trauma Patient Lose Pulses (Cardiac Arrest) After Induction or Intubation During General Anesthesia?

Trauma patients with significant, life-threatening injuries may be relying on the sympathetic surge occurring after trauma to keep vital organs perfused. Induction agents used in general anesthesia notoriously disrupt this sympathetic surge, and, if coupled with decreased preload (e.g., hypovolemia, obstructive shock), this can result in circulatory collapse. In addition to the induction agents used in general anesthesia, after endotracheal intubation the patient is subjected to *positive end-expiratory pressure (PEEP)*, which increases intrathoracic pressure. Similarly, in the setting of decreased preload, the initiation of mechanical ventilation with PEEP can also result in a loss of cardiac output and subsequent cardiac arrest.

Watch Out

A tension pneumothorax is rapidly exacerbated by positive-pressure ventilation. Thus, a tension pneumothorax should be decompressed immediately with a needle decompression/aspiration followed by a chest tube as soon as it is suspected.

Initial Management

What Is the First Step in Management?

The management of any trauma patient always starts with the primary survey (ABCDE: airway, breathing, circulation, disability, exposure). The first question one should always ask is whether the patient needs to be intubated. This decision is usually not based on a specific criterion but rather based on the clinician's best judgment. The above patient is able to talk and his airway is not obstructed; he does not need to be intubated.

Watch Out

Do not intubate and institute positive-pressure ventilation in a patient with suspected cardiac tamponade unless ready to treat the tamponade (prepped and draped in the operating room). Positive-pressure ventilation results in reduced cardiac filling, which can exacerbate the already compromised cardiac output seen in cardiac tamponade.

What Is the Next Step?

The patient has absent breath sounds on the left and is hemodynamically unstable. In the setting of trauma, this raises concern for a tension pneumothorax. Imaging should not delay treatment. According to advanced trauma life support (ATLS) protocol, the next step is immediate needle decompression, followed by tube thoracostomy. Although in-hospital practice often favors immediate tube or finger thoracostomy, needle decompression remains the correct answer on the shelf exam.

What Is a Needle Thoracostomy? What Is the Indication for Placement? Where Is It Placed? Why Is That Location Chosen? What Needs to Follow After It Is Placed?

Needle thoracostomy is a temporizing measure used to relieve tension pneumothorax in unstable patients. It is performed by inserting a large-bore needle into the fifth intercostal space at the anterior axillary line, just above the rib to avoid the neurovascular bundle. This location is preferred due to a thinner chest wall and more consistent decompression success. A rush of air confirms entry into the pleural space. Because this is only a temporary intervention, it must be followed by definitive tube thoracostomy.

What Is a Tube Thoracostomy? What Is the Indication for Placement? Where Is It Placed?

Tube thoracostomy, or chest tube insertion, involves placing a hollow plastic tube between the fourth or fifth intercostal space at the midaxillary line into the chest to decompress a hemothorax and/or pneumothorax.

When Does a Hemothorax Mandate Going to Surgery (Thoracotomy)?

Most patients with a traumatic hemothorax do not need surgery, as the bleeding stops. Classic indications for immediately transporting the patient to the operating room (OR) for a thoracotomy include initial chest tube output ≥1.5 liters or continued bleeding ≥150–200 mL/h for 3 or more hours. However, the most important indication is persistent hemodynamic instability despite blood product resuscitation, which should prompt immediate exploratory thoracotomy regardless of output volume.

> **Watch Out**
> Tube thoracostomy is used to drain blood (hemothorax) or air (pneumothorax) from the pleural space, while a resuscitative thoracotomy is a surgical procedure in which the chest is opened in an arrested patient to perform lifesaving and invasive resuscitation maneuvers including release of tamponade, cross-clamping of the descending thoracic aorta, internal cardiac massage, and hemorrhage control.

Should Prophylactic Antibiotics Be Given for Chest Tube Placement?

In trauma patients, a single pre-procedural dose of prophylactic antibiotics is recommended at the time of chest tube placement to reduce the risk of empyema. Routine extended antibiotic courses are not indicated. In non-trauma cases, such as spontaneous pneumothorax, prophylactic antibiotics are generally not used.

Does a Larger Chest Tube Allow for Better Evacuation of Air or Blood?

Not necessarily. For pneumothorax, small-bore chest tubes (typically 14–20 Fr) or even pigtail catheters are usually sufficient and are better tolerated by patients. For hemothorax, large-bore tubes (28–36 Fr) have traditionally been used, but recent data suggest that moderate-sized tubes (24–28 Fr) are often equally effective. Tube size should be selected based on the clinical scenario, but larger tubes do not always result in better drainage and may increase patient discomfort.

What Are the Goals and Guidelines for Resuscitative or Emergency Department Thoracotomy (EDT)?

EDT is performed to resuscitate trauma patients who present with a recent or witnessed traumatic full arrest. It is typically performed through a left anterolateral thoracotomy at the fifth intercostal space. The primary goals of resuscitative thoracotomy include decompression of cardiac tamponade, facilitation of cardiac massage, cross-clamping of the descending thoracic aorta to restore perfusion to the brain, and temporary control of cardiac or thoracic bleeding. If ROSC (return of spontaneous circulation) is achieved, the patient is then transported to the OR for definitive management of injuries. Outcomes are best in patients who have suffered penetrating thoracic injuries. ◘ Table 46.4 discusses the indications and contraindications for EDT.

What Is the Next Step?

Circulation is next. Palpate the central and peripheral pulses. If radial or femoral pulse is verified and is normal and no external bleeding is noticed, circulation can be considered stable temporarily. Two large-bore (14 or 16 gauge) intravenous (IV) catheters, one in each arm, are placed, and blood is drawn. If there is any sign of external bleeding, manual pressure should be applied. If there are no central pulses, an immediate decision needs to be made as to whether to perform an EDT. In the case

◘ **Table 46.4** Indications and contraindications for EDT

Indications	Contraindications
Penetrating trauma with <15 min of prehospital CPR	Penetrating trauma with CPR >15 min and no signs of life (e.g., respiratory effort, pupillary response, motor activity)
Blunt trauma with <5 min of prehospital CPR	Blunt trauma with CPR >5 min and no signs of life or asystole
Persistent severe postinjury hypotension (SBP ≤ 60 mmHg) or patient in extremis	

CPR cardiopulmonary resuscitation, *SBP* systolic blood pressure

of severe or ongoing blood loss, the patient should be transfused with type O or uncrossed blood.

Watch Out
IV catheters should be placed in an extremity above and opposite the site of truncal injury. The most important laboratory study to send in a trauma patient presenting in extremis is a type and cross.

Following the Primary Survey, What Is the Next Step in the Management?

In this hemodynamically unstable patient, the source of instability needs to be quickly ascertained. A FAST scan should be performed to look for fluid around the pericardium. Fluid around the pericardium, coupled with the patient's hemodynamic instability, is highly suggestive of cardiac tamponade.

Once Cardiac Tamponade Is Highly Suspected, What Is the Next Step?

Increasing a patient's preload via intravenous fluids or blood can temporarily overcome tamponade. However, definitive management requires opening the pericardium (to relieve the pressure) and repairing the underlying cardiac injury. Ideally this is performed via a median sternotomy, but an EDT would be indicated in patients with a non-palpable pulse or loss of vital signs. Pericardiocentesis is *not recommended* in trauma patients because it is unreliable, does not allow for evacuation of clotted blood, and delays definitive surgical management. The patient presented is hemodynamically unstable, and there is strong evidence of cardiac tamponade. Thus, the patient should be taken directly to the operating room for a median sternotomy.

What Is the Role of a Subxiphoid Window?

Subxiphoid window is an open surgical diagnostic procedure that is performed in a stable patient in whom cardiac tamponade is suspected but not certain (e.g., ultrasound is unavailable or equivocal). The premise behind the technique is that if no blood is found upon opening the pericardium, a full median sternotomy can be avoided. Whereas if blood is found, a full median sternotomy is performed to adequately drain the pericardium and repair any associated cardiac injury. In the unstable patient, a subxiphoid window is contraindicated, as it will delay adequately decompressing and repairing the source of the tamponade.

Are Vasopressors Recommended in the Management of Traumatic Cardiac Tamponade?

No. Most pressors will increase systemic vascular resistance (afterload), which will exacerbate myocardial dysfunction in the setting of traumatic pericardial tamponade.

Subsequent Management

What Should Be Immediately Ordered in All Patients That Present with Combative Behavior?

A rapid serum glucose measurement (e.g., finger-stick glucose), pulse oximetry, and a complete set of vital signs should be obtained in all such patients. Be careful not to quickly attribute combative behavior to alcohol or drug intoxication.

How Much Pleural Fluid Can the Diaphragm "Hide" in an Upright Chest Radiograph?

Up to 500 mL of pleural fluid can be hidden by overshadow of the diaphragm.

What Is the Classic Description for Cardiac Tamponade on Chest Radiograph?

The "water bottle sign" is classically described for diagnosing cardiac tamponade on chest radiography, where the heart has an enlarged and elongated silhouette. However, chest X-ray in acute tamponade is *typically normal*.

How Does a Chest Tube Drainage System Work, and How Do You Look for a Leak?

Chest tube drainage devices are composed of three chambers (◘ Table 46.5). One can look for leaks by checking the water seal chamber. Large leaks will be obvious and are evidenced by bubbles passing through the water seal fluid. If one suspects a small leak but no air bubbles are present, remove the suction, ask the patient to cough, and look for the air bubbles.

Table 46.5 Chambers of chest tube drainage system

Chamber	Purpose	Connects
Collection	Collects fluid, blood, and pus and measures the volume	Water seal chamber to chest tube
Water seal	One-way valve allows air to be removed from the pleural space but does not allow air to enter the pleural cavity	Suction control chamber to the collection chamber
Suction control	Controls the amount of suction	Wall suction and the water seal chamber

Does Inspiring 100% O_2 Help to Resolve a Pneumothorax?

It is debatable. Breathing 100% oxygen reduces the alveolar partial pressure of nitrogen, creating a diffusion gradient that favors reabsorption of intrapleural air into the pulmonary circulation. This can modestly accelerate the resolution of a pneumothorax. However, while physiologically sound, this method alone is insufficient for managing large or symptomatic pneumothoraces (they require drainage), and the clinical effect is limited. Breathing 100% oxygen for prolonged periods may cause oxygen toxicity. Conversely, in selected, stable patients with small, uncomplicated pneumothoraces, chest tube drainage may not be needed. In these small pneumothoraces, oxygen may not be needed.

How Is a Sucking Chest Wound Managed?

Prehospital treatment of a sucking chest wound involves covering the chest wall defect with an occlusive dressing that is taped on three sides. This prevents air from entering the pleural space on inspiration while allowing air to escape during expiration, thereby resulting in re-expansion of the lung while minimizing the risk of developing a tension pneumothorax. In the emergency department, an occlusive dressing followed by tube thoracostomy is recommended.

How Is Flail Chest Managed?

Flail chest results from fractures of three or more contiguous ribs in at least two locations, creating a free-floating segment that moves paradoxically with respiration. This impairs the generation of negative intrathoracic pressure, leading to ineffective ventilation, hypoxia, pulmonary contusion, and atelectasis. Management begins with adequate analgesia to prevent splinting and improve respiratory mechanics. Options include systemic opioids, thoracic epidural, paravertebral, or intercostal nerve blocks. If oxygenation or ventilation is compromised, endotracheal intubation and mechanical ventilation may be necessary.

What Is the Most Important Management in Patients with Rib Fractures?

Pain control with a multimodal pain regimen is the most important management in these patients as it helps prevent poor inspiratory effort, hypoventilation, atelectasis, and pneumonia. While thoracic epidurals were historically favored, especially in elderly patients with multiple rib fractures, they are now less commonly used due to logistical challenges, contraindications (e.g., anticoagulation), and availability of effective alternatives.

When Should Patients Undergo Rib Fixation?

Rib fixation is indicated in patients with flail chest who require mechanical ventilation or have persistent respiratory compromise despite optimal pain control. It is also considered in patients with three or more severely displaced rib fractures, especially if they have difficulty with ventilation, refractory pain, or inability to wean from the ventilator. Fixation can reduce ventilator days, ICU (intensive care unit) length of stay, and pulmonary complications. Routine use in nondisplaced or minimally symptomatic fractures is not recommended.

How Would You Manage a Traumatic Air Embolus?

Echocardiogram can be diagnostic for air embolus. However, treatment should not be delayed in patients suspected of having an air embolism. When recognized, patients should be placed in Trendelenburg position with the left side down (Durant's maneuver) and air aspirated from a central venous catheter. This positioning allows the air embolus to move into the apex of the right ventricle.

What Can Increase the Risk of Developing an Air Embolism in a Patient Arriving with Penetrating Chest Trauma?

Patients that are intubated with high positive-pressure ventilation can develop air emboli if a concurrent bronchial and pulmonary vein injury is present. The high pressures favor movement of air from the bronchus into the pulmonary vein and eventually into the left atrium and the systemic arterial circulation.

What Are the Classic Mechanisms and Imaging Findings for Aortic Injury?

Patients with complete aortic transection die in the field. Those with a partial transection or contained rupture may make it to the hospital alive. The classic mechanisms involve an acceleration–deceleration injury, most commonly a fall greater than ten feet or a high-speed motor vehicle accident. The classic chest X-ray findings are a wide mediastinum with or without a left-sided hemothorax. The most common location for blunt aortic injury is just distal to the origin of the left subclavian artery as the aorta is tethered here by the ligamentum arteriosum. Treatment depends on the injury grade, and involves endovascular placement of a stent graft.

Complications

What Is the Most Dangerous Complication Following Pericardiocentesis?

Laceration of a coronary vessel is the most dangerous complication of pericardiocentesis and can lead to worsening of cardiac tamponade.

What Nerve Is at Risk When Opening the Pericardium During EDT?

Left phrenic nerve innervating the diaphragm. It passes longitudinally over the posterior aspect of the pericardium of the left ventricle. To avoid injury, the pericardium should be opened anterior and parallel to the phrenic nerve.

How Is a Recurrent or Persistent Hemothorax Managed if Chest Tube Drainage Fails?

In stable patients with a retained hemothorax not adequately drained by chest tube, early video-assisted thoracoscopic surgery (VATS) within 48–72 hours is recommended. Leaving a hemothorax undrained is not recommended, as the lung will not completely re-expand (trapped lung or fibrothorax) and creates a risk of empyema (infected hemothorax), and VATS has been shown to be superior to attempting a second chest tube.

What Should You Consider in Patients with a Pneumothorax That Continue to Have a Large Air Leak Following Chest Tube Placement?

Most traumatic pneumothoraces are due to a superficial lung injury. The lung typically seals itself and air stops leaking. If an air leak persists, make sure the chest tube is in the proper location and that there are no mechanical obstructions (e.g., kinking, clot in tube) or leaks in the system. If the chest tube is properly inserted and functioning, the most likely etiology of a persistent air leak is a major airway injury such as disruption of the tracheobronchial tree. Patients with such injuries typically also have massive subcutaneous emphysema on exam and pneumomediastinum on imaging. Unstable patients require immediate intubation. Diagnosis is confirmed with bronchoscopy and repair entails a thoracotomy.

Areas Where You Can Get in Trouble

Long-Term Consequence of Missing a Diaphragm Injury

A missed diaphragmatic injury after penetrating trauma to the left thoracoabdominal region can result in herniation of abdominal contents into the thoracic cavity. This is due to positive intra-abdominal pressure and the absence of a protective organ like the liver on the left side. In contrast, right-sided injuries rarely lead to herniation because the liver acts as a physical barrier and tamponade, often masking or preventing clinical consequences. Diaphragmatic injuries are often occult and may not be detected on imaging. CT scan lacks sensitivity for identifying small diaphragm defects. In stable patients with left-sided thoracoabdominal stab wounds, diagnostic laparoscopy is recommended, but typically delayed for at least 8 hours. This observation period allows time for serial abdominal exams and laboratory monitoring to identify signs of hollow viscus injury, which would require exploratory laparotomy instead of laparoscopy. If a diaphragmatic injury is missed, the defect can enlarge and present months or years later with chest pain, respiratory symptoms, or bowel obstruction due to herniated abdominal contents. Surgical repair is required and can be performed via an abdominal or thoracic approach.

> **Watch Out**
> A classic chest X-ray finding in a patient with diaphragm rupture is curling of the nasogastric tube in the thoracic cavity.

Do All Patients with Pneumothorax Require a Chest Tube?

No. In cases where patients have a small pneumothorax (e.g., small apical pneumothorax on chest X-ray) or an occult pneumothorax (one that is only seen on CT scan and not on chest X-ray), it can be treated with observation, supplemental oxygen, and repeat chest X-ray. If the patient becomes hemodynamically unstable or develops respiratory distress, needle decompression followed by a chest tube is indicated.

Missed Esophageal Injury

Esophageal perforation is a rare but life-threatening complication of penetrating trauma to the chest or neck. A classic clue is the presence of green, food-like, or foul-smelling material in the chest tube output, suggesting communication with the gastrointestinal tract. This finding should raise immediate suspicion for esophageal injury. Failure to recognize this can lead to mediastinitis, sepsis, and rapid clinical deterioration. When suspected, the diagnostic test of choice is a CT esophagogram using water-soluble contrast, which is more sensitive than plain esophagography and allows evaluation of the surrounding mediastinum. Traditional contrast esophagography may still be used, but CT is preferred in most trauma centers due to its broader diagnostic utility. Emergent surgical consultation is mandatory, as early recognition and operative management are critical to patient survival.

Areas of Controversy

How Accurate Is Focused Assessment with Sonography for Trauma (FAST) in the Setting of Penetrating Trauma?

Most of the trauma literature has focused on the role of FAST in blunt trauma. The utility of FAST in penetrating trauma is limited except for diagnosing cardiac tamponade and pneumothorax. Its greatest value is evidenced by the fact that it helps the clinician concentrate their efforts on cardiac, thoracic, or intraperitoneal injuries within minutes of the patient's presentation.

Special Situations/Circumstances

Following Chest Tube Placement for a Traumatic Pneumothorax/Hemothorax, When Is It Appropriate to Remove It? What Is the Main Risk During Removal?

To minimize the risk of infection, chest tubes should be removed as soon as it is safe to do so. Removing the chest tube is appropriate when there are no air leaks present and the lung is fully expanded, as evidenced on a chest radiograph. The main risk during the chest tube removal is air being inadvertently reintroduced into the pleural cavity, resulting in recurrent pneumothorax. Therefore, it is recommended to remove the chest tube either at the end of expiration or at peak inspiration and to immediately cover the wound with an occlusive dressing.

Initially Stable Patient with Multiple Rib Fractures Has Increasing Oxygen Requirements and Respiratory Distress

Patients with multiple rib fractures can have a flail chest and/or underlying pulmonary contusion, which is not always apparent on the initial chest X-ray and can "blossom" over the first few days. Pulmonary contusions can present with hypoxia, tachycardia, and shortness of breath. A chest X-ray will oftentimes demonstrate opacity over the lung parenchyma (alveolar infiltrate) under the rib fracture. An arterial blood gas should be obtained, and, if indicated, early intubation should be considered.

Lethal Six Injuries of Thoracic Trauma (Fig. 46.1)

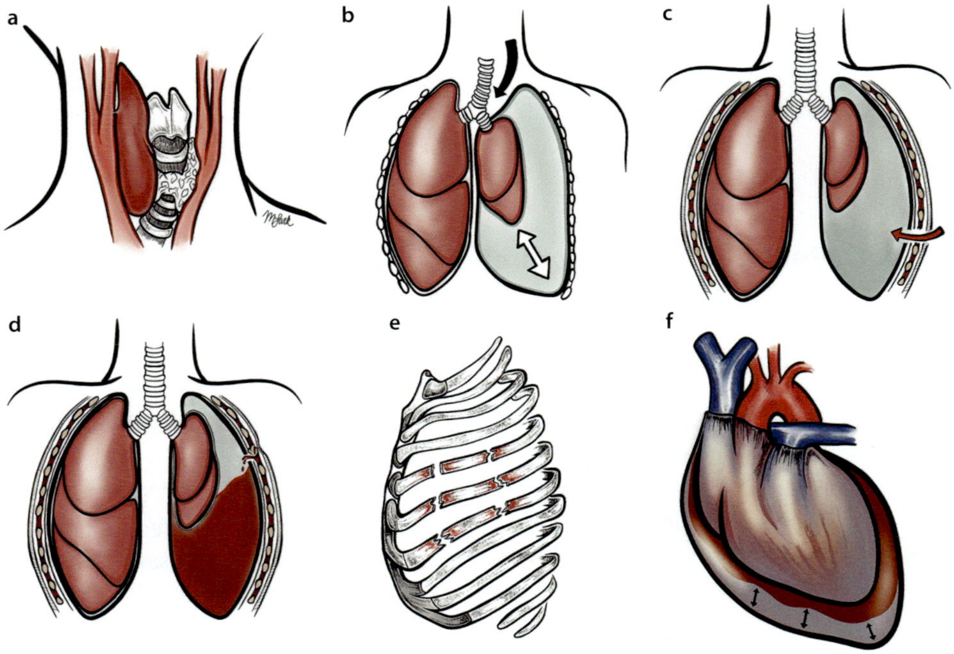

Fig. 46.1 These illustrations demonstrate the lethal six injuries of thoracic trauma. 1. Airway obstruction **a**—more likely to be due to blood in context of trauma 2. Tension pneumothorax **b**—increased pressure from pneumothorax leads to mediastinal shift and results in decreased preload in the heart and cardiovascular collapse 3. Open pneumothorax **c**—air is drawn into the pleural space during inhalation, leading to respiratory collapse 4. Massive hemothorax **d**—resulting from a bleeding vessel from thoracic trauma (ex rib fracture) 5. Flail chest **e**—multiple adjacent rib fractures resulting in a free segment of chest wall that moves paradoxically and impairs adequate ventilation 6. Cardiac tamponade **f**—blood accumulation in the pericardial sac, which in turn impairs the heart's ability to fill and pump, resulting in hypotension and shock

Summary of Essentials

History and Physical

- Tension pneumothorax is a clinical diagnosis that should not be delayed for imaging.
- Suspect cardiac tamponade based on location of injury and presence of hypotension (Beck's triad often not all present).
- Penetrating injury above nipple line likely only involves thoracic structures while below the nipple line can involve thoracic structures, abdominal structures, or the diaphragm.
- A narrow pulse pressure (<30 mmHg) suggests reduced stroke volume and may precede overt hypotension.

Differential Diagnosis

- The "deadly dozen" thoracic injuries include the *lethal six* and *hidden six*:
  - Lethal six: airway obstruction, tension pneumothorax, open pneumothorax, massive hemothorax, flail chest, and cardiac tamponade.
  - Hidden six: blunt aortic injury, esophageal injury, tracheobronchial injury, diaphragmatic rupture, blunt cardiac injury, and pulmonary contusion.

Pathology/Pathophysiology

- Tension pneumothorax can compress superior vena cava/inferior vena cava (SVC/IVC) and result in decreased CO.
- Pericardial pressure exceeds ventricular filling pressure in cardiac tamponade resulting in hypotension.
- The most important factor in cardiac tamponade is the rapid accumulation of fluid.
- The underlying mechanism in air embolism is the traumatic creation of a fistula between an injured bronchus and pulmonary vein.

Management

- Always start with primary survey: airway, breathing, circulation, disability, and exposure.
  - Follow with FAST to look for fluid around the pericardium in patient suspected of having cardiac tamponade.
- All combative patients in emergency room should get rapid serum glucose, pulse oximetry, and set of vitals.
- Suspected tension pneumothorax requires immediate needle thoracostomy, placed at the fifth intercos-

tal space in the anterior axillary line, followed by tube thoracostomy.

- EDT indications include:
  - Penetrating trauma with <15 min of prehospital cardiopulmonary resuscitation (CPR).
  - Blunt trauma with <5 min of prehospital CPR.
  - Persistent severe postinjury hypotension (SBP ≤60 mmHg) due to cardiac tamponade, air embolism, or hemorrhage (intrathoracic, intra-abdominal, extremity, or cervical).
- Traumatic cardiac tamponade is treated with median sternotomy.
  - Subxiphoid window can be considered when the diagnosis is uncertain.
- Sucking chest wound is treated with occlusive dressing and chest tube.
- Rib fixation is indicated in patients with flail chest requiring mechanical ventilation or in those with three or more severely displaced rib fractures with persistent respiratory compromise.

Suggested Reading

ACS-COT Subcommittee on Outcomes Practice management guidelines for emergency department thoracotomy. JACS. 2001;193:303.

ATLS Subcommittee; American College of Surgeons' Committee on Trauma; International ATLS working group. Advanced trauma life support (ATLS®): the ninth edition. J Trauma Acute Care Surg. 2013;74(5):1363–6.

Freeman JJ, Asfaw SH, et al. Antibiotic prophylaxis for tube thoracostomy placement in trauma: a practice management guideline from the Eastern Association for the Surgery of Trauma. Trauma Surg Acute Care Open. 2022 Oct 25;7(1):e000886. https://doi.org/10.1136/tsaco-2022-000886. PMID: 36312819; PMCID: PMC9608538.

Mowery NT, Gunter OL, Collier BR, Diaz JJ Jr., et al. Practice management guidelines for management of hemothorax and occult pneumothorax. J Trauma Acute Care Surg. 2011;70(2):510–8.

Schoen FJ. The heart. In: Kumar V, Abbas AK, Fausto N, editors. Robbins and Cotran pathologic basis of disease. 7th ed. Philadelphia: Elsevier Saunders; 1999. p. 555–618.

Burns to the Face, Trunk, and Extremities

Areg Grigorian, Christian de Virgilio, and Dennis Y. Kim

Contents

C. de Virgilio, A. Grigorian (eds.), *Surgery*, https://doi.org/10.1007/978-3-032-09799-6_47

Case Study

A 25-year-old woman arrives to the emergency department an hour after sustaining burn injuries in a house fire. She weighs 70 kilograms. She is awake but appears confused and disoriented. She complains of a severe headache and sounds stridorous. At initial exam, her temperature is 38.3 °C, blood pressure is 90/74 mmHg, heart rate is 120/min, respiratory rate is 26/min, and oxygen saturation is 89%. She has blistering, painful burns to the entire face with singed nasal hairs and carbonaceous sputum. She has burns on her entire chest, abdomen, and back, which are painless, circumferential, white, dry, and leathery. The bilateral upper extremities are also burned with painful, swollen, mottled areas with blisters that appear to have open weeping surfaces. The remainder of her skin that is not burned has a cherry-red appearance. She also has sunken eyes, a dry tongue, and slow capillary refill.

Diagnosis

What Is the Diagnosis and What Are the Associated Complications in This Patient?

She has sustained major burn injuries (i.e., >20% total body surface area [TBSA]) involving the face, trunk, and extremities. She has second-degree burns to the face and bilateral upper extremities and third-degree burns to the chest, abdomen, and back. Singed nasal hairs and exposure to fire in an enclosed space are risk factors for smoke inhalation injury. The presence of carbonaceous sputum coupled with her low oxygen saturation is a hard sign of inhalation injury and should be addressed immediately by securing the airway via intubation and administration of 100% O_2. The cherry-red appearance of her skin along with her confusion and disorientation is concerning for carbon monoxide (CO) poisoning. Additionally, she is in hypovolemic shock secondary to endothelial damage and increased capillary permeability.

History and Physical

What Are the Risk Factors for Burn Injuries?

Extremes of age (very young or old), alcohol or substance use, smoking, violence, and low socioeconomic status.

How Does One Determine the Severity of a Burn Injury?

Calculating the total body surface area (TBSA) affected by second- or third-degree burns will allow one to determine the severity of a patient's burn injuries (Table 47.1). This can be approximated using the rule of nines (Fig. 47.1). The body is divided into regions whose surface areas are multiples of nine: head, 9%; each arm, 9%; anterior torso, 18%; posterior torso, 18%; each leg, 18%. In areas of patchy involvement, the clinician can use the size of the palmar surface of the *patient* (including fingers) to estimate the surface area of the burn. The adult palmar surface area represents ~1% body surface area.

Table 47.1 Severity of burn injuries

Degree	Involves	Presentation
First (superficial)	Epidermis only	Similar to sunburn; localized, painful, dry, blanching redness with no blisters
Second (superficial partial thickness)	Epidermis and part of the dermis (papillary)	Very painful, swollen, warm, pink, moist, blanching *with blisters*
Second (deep partial thickness)	Epidermis and part of the dermis (papillary and reticular)	Painful, paler with little to no blanching; may have mottled areas that appear to have open weeping surfaces (hemorrhagic)
Third (full thickness)	All of the skin (epidermis and dermis)	Painless and insensate, white/brown/black, dry, leathery, and do not blanch with pressure
Fourth	All of the skin and underlying bone, tendon, adipose, or muscle	Similar to third degree as deep injury may not be obvious on the surface; however, some may be extensive and disfiguring

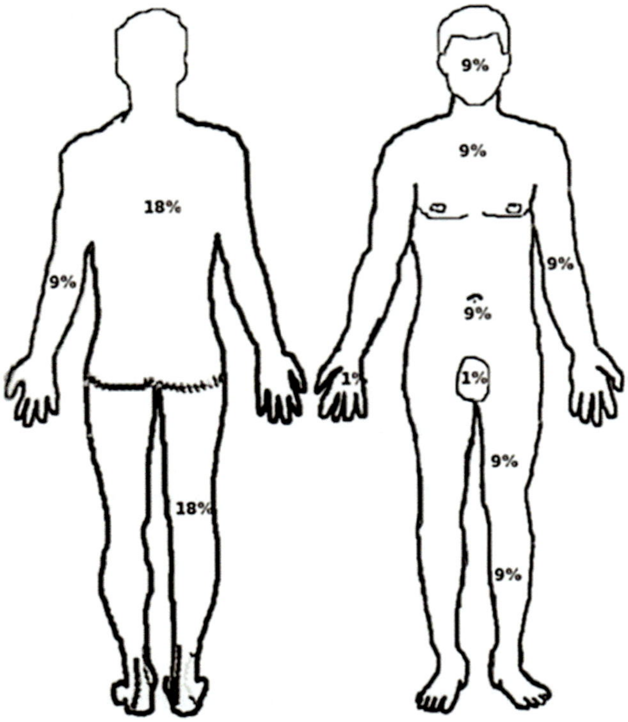

■ **Fig. 47.1** Rule of 9s in adults

> **Watch Out**
> The presence of pain is an easy way to differentiate superficial partial-thickness burns (presents with pain) from full-thickness burns (decreased sensation) due to destruction of nerve endings.

What Is the Significance of Carbonaceous Sputum?

Carbonaceous sputum indicates possible inhalational injury. There should be a high index of suspicion for inhalation injury in patients who present after burn injuries within enclosed areas and with singed nasal hairs or significant facial burns. Changes in voice quality, stridor, and carbonaceous sputum are hard signs of inhalational injury. There are three components of inhalational injury: supraglottic (upper airway inflammation/edema), infraglottic (e.g., acute respiratory failure secondary to a chemical pneumonitis from the products of combustion), and carbon monoxide poisoning (i.e., systemic toxicity for gases). If significant supraglottic edema develops, the patient may lose their airway.

What Is the Significance of Cherry-Red Skin in a Patient Rescued from a House Fire?

This is a classic sign for carbon monoxide poisoning and typically occurs in patients with prolonged exposure to smoke (e.g., house fires or the exhaust from a running car or gas heater). The cherry-red skin discoloration occurs because carbon monoxide binds tightly to hemoglobin to form carboxyhemoglobin, which gives the blood a bright red color and causes the skin to appear unusually flushed. Patients initially present with headaches and other nonspecific constitutional symptoms such as nausea (carboxyhemoglobin level 10–20%) and dizziness (>20%). If severe or left untreated, carbon monoxide poisoning may progress to seizures, coma, multiorgan failure, and death.

What Is the Significance of a Circumferential Burn in the Extremity? How About If on the Chest?

Circumferential full-thickness burns in the extremity *significantly* increase the risk of developing compartment syndrome. Patients with circumferential extremity full-thickness burns and evidence of compromised distal perfusion should undergo escharotomy. Circumferential burns of the chest can compromise a patient's respiratory efforts due to the inflexible eschar and underlying tissue edema, which can prevent chest wall motion and, thus, limit ventilation. These patients should also be considered for chest escharotomy.

Pathophysiology

What Are the Different Mechanisms of Burn Injury? (■ Table 47.2)

> **Watch Out**
> Direct current (DC) electrocution (e.g., lightning) puts patients at risk for asystole, while alternating current (AC) electrocution (e.g., wall socket) puts patients at risk for ventricular fibrillation.

Table 47.2 Mechanisms of burn injury

Cause	Comments
Thermal	May be from flame, contact with a hot surface, or hot liquid; the most common cause of burn injuries is fire/flame. In children, the most common cause is scalding, typically from hot water.
Chemical	Alkali burns are more damaging than acidic burns owing to their ability to penetrate tissues more deeply. Acid burns cause *coagulation necrosis*, whereas alkali burns cause *liquefactive necrosis*.
Electrical	Immediate life-threatening complication is cardiac arrhythmia. Injuries are often out of proportion to the size of the external burn wound. Patients may also sustain other systemic injuries to organs, such as muscle necrosis, posterior shoulder dislocations, long bone fractures, and acute kidney injury (myoglobinuria due to rhabdomyolysis).

What Are the Physiologic Manifestations of a Burn?

In the first 24 hours, cardiac output is decreased to 40–60% of normal as a result of decreased plasma volume, increased systemic vascular resistance, and direct reduction in myocardial contractility. Cardiac output then returns to normal over the ensuing 24 hours. The decrease in plasma volume, which occurs primarily from endothelial damage resulting in capillary leakage, subsequently leads to hypovolemia and a decrease in central venous pressure. The capillary leak also results in sequestration of proteins in the interstitial space. Together, this leads to edema in both burned *and* non-burned tissue. Severe burn injury results in a profound hypermetabolic response manifested by a marked rise in plasma catecholamines, cortisol, and inflammatory cells. Due to the release of catecholamines, the circulating glucose concentration is increased during the first 24 hours following thermal burn injury (stress hyperglycemia). However, the hypermetabolic state can last up to 2 years.

Why Are Burn Patients at Increased Risk for Severe Volume Depletion?

The skin acts as a protective barrier and plays an essential role in fluid and temperature regulation of the body. When the integrity of this protective layer is compromised, the skin becomes unable to regulate body temperature or prevent fluid from seeping out of the body. This can lead to hypovolemic shock if enough intravascular volume is lost.

Why Are Burn Patients at Higher Risk for Gastrointestinal Ulcers?

Diminished intravascular volume leads to decreased perfusion of the gastrointestinal tract and subsequent mucosal ischemia. In the stomach, this leads to mucosal atrophy and loss of protective barrier function, increasing the risk for gastric and duodenal ulcer formation. This is known as a Curling's ulcer.

What Organisms Are Classically Involved in Burn Wound Infections?

The most common organisms in burn wound infections are *Staphylococcus* and *Pseudomonas*. In the first several days after the initial burn, the most likely organism in a burn wound infection is a Gram-positive organism. Burn wound infections occurring five or more days from the initial injury are more likely to be infected with Gram-negative organisms and fungi. Infections in burn patients can be problematic for multiple reasons. They may delay wound healing and encourage scarring, lead to burn wound conversion, and can result in burn wound sepsis with resultant bacteremia.

Workup

What Is the First Step in the Evaluation of This Patient?

As with any trauma patient, one should begin with the airway, breathing, circulation (ABCs). It is important to maintain cervical spine precautions and evaluate for concomitant traumatic injuries if the mechanism of injury warrants it. In this patient with hard signs of inhalational injury (stridor, carbonaceous sputum, and hypoxia), securing the airway via endotracheal intubation is essential. Intravenous lines for fluid resuscitation may be placed through burned skin initially if needed.

How Is Inhalational Injury Definitively Diagnosed?

In the absence of stridor and hypoxia, bronchoscopy remains a standard component of the assessment for inhalation injury. Inhalational injury is suspected in the setting of facial burns, singed nasal hairs, and history of injury in an enclosed space. Other diagnostic features include carboxyhemoglobin >10% and oxygen saturation <90%. Chest X-rays are usually negative initially and have little value in diagnosing inhalational injury.

What Is the Best Way to Evaluate for Carbon Monoxide Poisoning? How Does CO Lead to Death?

Checking for an elevated carboxyhemoglobin level is the best way to evaluate for CO poisoning. However, this is not always available. Standard pulse oximetry is more readily available but is not always reliable since standard devices *are unable to differentiate* between oxygen and carbon monoxide bound to hemoglobin. Arterial blood gases will demonstrate a normal PaO_2 and decreased SaO_2, and CO–Hb levels may be directly obtained from both arterial and venous blood sampling. Carbon monoxide has nearly 200× more affinity for hemoglobin than oxygen. Thus, the hemoglobin–oxygen dissociation curve shifts to the left as more carbon monoxide binds to hemoglobin. This interferes with oxygen delivery in two ways. First, displacement of oxygen by hemoglobin leads to decreased bound oxygen in circulation. Second, the leftward shift results in increased affinity of oxygen to hemoglobin, decreasing the ability to release bound oxygen to the tissues.

> **Watch Out**
> Standard pulse oximetry (SpO_2) cannot distinguish between oxygen and carbon monoxide and therefore is not useful in diagnosing carbon monoxide poisoning.

How Do You Diagnose a Burn Wound Infection?

Burn wound infections comprise a spectrum of states from wound colonization to actual invasive infection with cellulitis and even necrotizing skin and soft tissue infection. Diagnosis of burn wound infections by clinical signs and symptoms alone is difficult and variable but include factors such as burn wound conversion, surrounding erythema, suppuration, and systemic manifestations (e.g., fevers and tachycardia). Patients with large burns (>20% TBSA) have higher risk for burn wound infection. Quantitative culture of a punch biopsy demonstrating $>10^5$ bacteria/g of tissue is considered to be the "gold standard" to diagnose a burn wound infection.

Management

When Should You Consider Immediately Intubating a Burn Patient?

Early intubation should be performed in patients with suspected inhalational injury. The inhalation of hot gases can create thermal injury, leading to upper airway edema that can cause a sudden loss of the airway. Indications for intubation include extensive full thickness facial burns, stridor, respiratory distress, altered mentation, hypoxia/hypercarbia, hemodynamic instability, and singed facial hair. If a patient is intubated for suspected inhalational injury, a bronchoscopy should be performed to suction out any debris and to characterize the degree and severity of airway trauma.

What Type of Fluid Should Be Used Acutely in a Burn Patient?

Lactated Ringer's is the fluid of choice. Some clinicians choose to use colloids (albumin and fresh frozen plasma) for patients not responding to crystalloid alone in an effort to restore intravascular volume and reduce the risks associated with excessive fluid volumes. However, more research is needed to delineate the role and timing of colloids.

How Do You Calculate the Appropriate Volume of Fluid Resuscitation for a Burn Victim in the First 24 Hours?

While several burn resuscitation formulas and adjuncts exist, the Parkland formula is commonly used to calculate the amount of volume resuscitation necessary for a patient with second- or third-degree burns involving more than 20% TBSA. One-half of the total fluid volume should be administered in the first 8 hours *from the time of injury* and the second half in the subsequent 16 hours. However, the more important principle is to titrate fluids based on end markers of resuscitation such as urine output.

- **Parkland Formula**

$$\text{Total fluid volume} = 4\text{cc}/\text{kg} \times \text{weight}(\text{kg}) \times \text{TBSA}(\%)$$

Watch Out

Urine output is a well-established parameter for guiding fluid management. The rate of fluid administration is titrated to a urine output of 0.5–1 mL/kg/h in adults and 1–1.5 mL/kg/h in children. Hourly monitoring and appropriate titration of fluid is important for successful burn resuscitation.

What Is the Management for CO Poisoning?

They should all be started on 100% oxygen via non-rebreather face mask.

Watch Out

Normal saline is not recommended for burn resuscitation. With 154 mEq/L of Na^+ and Cl^-, the high volumes needed will lead to hyperchloremia and metabolic acidosis (as $HCO3^-$ will be excreted to balance the excess Cl^-).

What Electrolyte Abnormality Must Be Closely Monitored in Burn Patients?

Burn patients should be monitored for hyponatremia and hyperkalemia. Although hyponatremia can be related to the burn itself, it is often iatrogenic. While the Parkland formula can help calculate the fluid needs in burn patients, it cannot account for the subsequent compartmental fluid shifts that disrupt normal electrolyte levels. Hyponatremia can increase the risk of developing seizures in burn patients. Hyperkalemia can develop from the destruction of cells and tissues and can lead to cardiac conduction abnormalities.

Watch Out

Succinylcholine should not be used for rapid sequence intubation in patients with significant burn or crush injuries. These injuries cause an upregulation of acetylcholine receptors in skeletal muscle, leading to an exaggerated efflux of potassium when succinylcholine binds and depolarizes the muscle membrane. The resulting hyperkalemia can be life-threatening. In such patients, nondepolarizing neuromuscular blocking agents such as rocuronium or vecuronium should be used instead.

What Should Be Considered as a Potential Cause of Deteriorating Respiratory Status in a Patient with a Circumferential Third-Degree Chest Burn? How Do You Treat It?

Third-degree burns cause the skin to lose its elasticity. If the patient has a circumferential chest burn, they may lose the ability to expand their chest cavity, leading to respiratory compromise. Treatment is an immediate chest escharotomy (cutting through the burned skin). This is performed by incising the constricting eschar, thereby improving chest wall compliance and respiration. Unlike a fasciotomy (which incises through skin, fat, and fascia), escharotomy only involves incisions through the burned skin, into the superficial fat, and not the deeper underlying structures. This procedure is relatively painless as the nerve endings in the dermis are already damaged by the burn injury. In emergent circumstances, it can be done at the bedside.

Can Circumferential Extremity Burns Cause Compartment Syndrome?

Yes. Extremity escharotomies should also be considered in patients with full-thickness circumferential burns with evidence of compartment syndrome and neurovascular compromise of the extremity (e.g., tense extremity, decreased capillary refill, sensory and/or motor deficits).

What Things Can Be Done to Reduce the Hypermetabolic Response Seen in Severe Burn Injuries?

Several things can be done including early excision of the eschars caused by third-degree burns and skin grafting, early initiation of enteral nutrition, and administration of various pharmaceutical agents including beta blockers.

How Do You Manage Burn Wounds?

Following the institution of resuscitative measures, local treatment of burn wounds involves cleansing, non-excisional debridement, and application of antimicrobial agents and dressings. Tangential excision of full thickness burns is indicated and is typically performed within 24–72 hours after the injury. Skin grafting (autografting) is performed for wounds too large to heal by contraction or primary closure after the wound bed is deemed clean and viable. Skin grafts may be partial-thickness or full-thickness (depending on several cosmetic and functional factors). Skin grafts are contraindicated if there is evidence of infection.

Should Burn Patients Be Started on Prophylactic IV Antibiotics?

No. Studies have failed to demonstrate efficacy of prophylactic intravenous (IV) antibiotics in reducing burn wound infections. Instead, they are thought to select for resistant organisms.

What Topical Burn Agents Are Commonly Utilized in Burn Patients? (Table 47.3)

What Medication Should All Burn Patients Be Started on to Prevent Curling's Ulcers?

Proton pump inhibitors or H_2 blockers.

Can Patients with Severe Burn Injuries Be Fed Orally? Why or Why Not?

In general, the enteral route is the *preferred* method of delivery of nutrition. Early initiation of enteral nutritional support (within 12 hours after injury) is recommended if the patient is hemodynamically stable. There is evidence of improved tolerance to feeding and amelioration of the hypermetabolic response with early initiation. Intragastric feeding is acceptable though enteral feeding into the small intestine is preferred, especially for patients with very large burn injuries (causes gastric stasis). In patients in whom enteral tube feedings are not tolerated, parenteral nutrition should be considered.

Table 47.3 Topical burn agents

Agent	Comments
Silver sulfadiazine (Silvadene)	Commonly used topical burn agent; may result in granulocyte reduction (neutropenia and thrombocytopenia); poor deep tissue penetration and *ineffective* against *Pseudomonas*
Sulfamylon or mafenide acetate	Dispensed in a cream and a solution; it functions as a carbonic anhydrase inhibitor and may result in *metabolic acidosis*; deep tissue penetration and *effective* against *Pseudomonas*; may be painful in application
Silver nitrate	Poor deep tissue penetration and *ineffective* against *Pseudomonas*; brown staining of skin is common; electrolyte abnormalities (hyponatremia, hypokalemia) and methemoglobinemia may occur

What Are the Principles of Management for Chemical Burns?

Protection of others from exposure and removal of patients from area of exposure. Following removal of all clothing, dry chemicals should be brushed off the patient. With few exceptions, copious irrigation with water is the most important principle in the management of chemical burns. The longer the acid/alkali material stays in contact with the patient's body, the worse the prognosis is.

What Is the Key Management Principle for Patients with Electrical Burns?

Cardiac monitoring for 12–24 hours to look for arrhythmias, particularly when a high-voltage injury (>1000 V) is suspected. In general, patients with a normal electrocardiogram after *low*-voltage exposure do not require 24 hours of cardiac monitoring.

Areas You Can Get in Trouble

Cyanide Poisoning

Cyanide toxicity is a rare and lethal condition associated with inhalation injury. Domestic fires are the most common cause, as cyanide is released from the combustion of common household nitrogen-containing products, such as plastics, synthetic rubber, vinyl, wool, and silk. Cyanide toxicity leads to an increase in lactate and profound anion gap metabolic acidosis. Patients may report detecting an almond odor or metallic taste. They may present with tachycardia, flushing, headache, nausea, anxiety, confusion, seizures, abdominal pain, and vomiting. Diagnosis relies on a high level of clinical suspicion, as blood cyanide levels are often not immediately available. First-line treatment is with hydroxocobalamin, a form of vitamin B12 that will bind cyanide and facilitate its excretion in the urine.

Child Abuse

Burn injuries account for a minority of child abuse cases but should be considered for all children presenting with burn marks characterized by sharply demarcated margins (e.g., submersion in hot water) or deep localized contact injury (e.g., cigarette burn). The majority of children with non-accidental burns are less than 2 years of age. Toilet training is a particularly vulnerable time. Caregivers in this setting may provide inconsistent histories or conflicting accounts of how their child received the burn injury.

Chronic Non-Healing Wound

Patients with chronic non-healing wounds are at increased risk for the development of squamous cell carcinoma of the skin (Marjolin's ulcer). All chronically non-healing wounds should be evaluated with a skin biopsy.

Frostbite

Frostbite is caused by tissue injury due to cold-induced cell death and subsequent reperfusion injury after exposure to subfreezing temperatures. Initial management includes removing cold or wet clothing, and rapid rewarming by immersing the affected area in warm (not hot) water. This process is often painful and requires opioid analgesics. After rewarming, the extent of injury is assessed by the degree of cyanosis, depth of tissue involvement, and presence of blisters. Severity may be difficult to determine early, and additional tissue damage may become evident over time. In severe cases, early thrombolysis using tissue-type plasminogen activator (tPA) with adjunct intravenous heparin can improve perfusion and reduce the risk of amputation.

Summary of Essentials

History and Physical

- First degree (superficial), second degree (superficial and deep partial thickness), third degree (full thickness), and fourth degree
- Second degree (painful) and third degree (little or no pain)
- Severity of burns determined by TBSA approximated by rule of 9s:
  - Head, 9%; each arm, 9%; anterior torso, 18%; posterior torso, 18%; each leg, 18%
  - Only count second- or third-degree burns (not first)
- Carbonaceous sputum, burns to the face, and singed nasal hairs indicate possible inhalational injury

Pathophysiology

- Thermal, chemical, and electrical
- Initially results in decreased plasma volume from capillary leak, increased systemic vascular resistance, and decreased myocardial contractility
- Loss of skin barrier increases risk of fluid and temperature disregulation:
  - Hypovolemic shock
  - Infection
- Hypermetabolic response

Workup

- Inhalational injury:
  - Clinical suspicion by presence of facial burns, singed nasal hairs, and history of injury in an enclosed space
  - Fiberoptic bronchoscopy for definitive diagnosis

Management

- Parkland formula:
  - Total fluid volume = 4 mL/kg × weight (kg) × TBSA (%); administer 1/2 total in first 8 hours; use lactated Ringer's.
  - Titrate urine output to 0.5–1 mL/kg/h in adults and 1–1.5 mL/kg/h in kids.
- Non-excisional debridement and topical antibacterial agents for initial wound care.
- Reducing hypermetabolic response
  - Early serial tangential excision and grafting for full-thickness burns
  - Early enteric feeding
  - Propranolol

Acknowledgement The editors would like to acknowledge and thank the following authors for their contributions to the previous edition of the chapter: Victor C. Joe.

Suggested Reading

Alvarado R, Chung KK, Cancio LC, Wolf SE. Burn resuscitation. Burns. 2009;35:4–14

Cartotto R, Johnson LS, Savetamal A, et al. American Burn Association Clinical Practice Guidelines on Burn Shock Resuscitation. *J Burn Care Res*. 2024;45(3):565–589. https://doi.org/10.1093/jbcr/irad125

Foncerrada G, Culnan DM, Capek KD, et al. Inhalation injury in the burned patient. Ann Plast Surg. 2018;80:S98–S105

Rowan MP, Cancio LC, Elster EA, et al. Burn wound healing and treatment: review and advancements. Crit Care. 2015;19:243–55.

Vercruysse GA, Alam HB, Martin MJ, et al. Western Trauma Association critical decisions in trauma: Preferred triage and initial management of the burned patient. J Trauma Acute Care Surg. 2019;87(5):1239–1243. https://doi.org/10.1097/TA.0000000000002348

Wibbenmeyer L, Lacey AM, Endorf FW, et al. American Burn Association Clinical Practice Guidelines on the Treatment of Severe Frostbite. J Burn Care Res. 2024;45(3):541–556. https://doi.org/10.1093/jbcr/irad022

Severe Right Leg Pain After Tibia Fracture

Chantal Creighton, Areg Grigorian, Christian de Virgilio, and Dennis Y. Kim

Contents

C. de Virgilio, A. Grigorian (eds.), *Surgery*, https://doi.org/10.1007/978-3-032-09799-6_48

Case Study

A 30-year-old male is brought to the emergency department by paramedics after a motorcycle accident. He has an obvious deformity of the right lower extremity below the knee. Imaging reveals a fracture of the tibia and fibula. He is taken to the operating room for an open reduction and internal fixation (ORIF). Approximately eight hours after surgery, the patient complains of severe pain in his right leg. On physical examination, the right leg is tensely swollen. He endorses severe tenderness on palpation, especially lateral to the tibia. When his ankle is passively dorsiflexed, he grimaces in pain. His foot appears pink and well perfused. Pulses in the dorsalis pedis and posterior tibial are 2+, and Doppler interrogation demonstrates biphasic signals in both arteries. Sensory exam of the right foot is intact except for numbness in the first web space.

Diagnosis

What Is the Differential Diagnosis? (◘ Table 48.1)

What Is the Most Likely Diagnosis?

In a patient presenting with a tense leg following ORIF, with pain on passive dorsiflexion and tenderness upon palpation of the compartments, the most likely diagnosis is a lower extremity compartment syndrome.

◘ **Table 48.1** Differential diagnosis for clinical presentation

Diagnosis	Comments
Compartment syndrome	Pain out of proportion to exam, particularly with passive motion of the ankle; tense leg edema, recent trauma, pulse usually present
Necrotizing soft tissue infection (NSTI)	Acute infection of the skin, fascia, or muscle, often with exam findings of crepitus, bullae, and necrosis of subcutaneous tissue; often mixed bacterial flora
Cellulitis	Superficial infection of the skin presenting with redness and erythema
Deep vein thrombosis	Calf pain, leg edema; risk factors include prolonged stasis, hypercoagulable state, and endothelial injury *(Virchow's triad)*
Acute limb ischemia	Pain, pallor, pulselessness (pulse always absent), paresthesias, paralysis, and poikilothermia; history of claudication, arterial insufficiency or atrial fibrillation, trauma (posterior knee dislocation, tibial fracture)

History and Physical

What Are the Ps of Compartment Syndrome?

Compartment syndrome occurs when elevated pressure within a closed tissue compartment compromises blood flow and tissue perfusion, leading to ischemia of muscles and nerves. Various references use either 5 or 6 Ps, and differ slightly. The Ps of compartment syndrome are **p**ain (often described as out of proportion to the injury and pain on passive motion), **p**aresthesia (tingling or numbness), **p**allor (paleness of the skin), **p**aralysis (weakness or inability to move the affected limb), **p**ulselessness (absent pulses, a late finding), and **p**ressure (a swollen or tense extremity or compartment). Others add another P, poikilothermia, defined as a change in temperature or coolness. These signs and symptoms arise due to increased intracompartmental pressure impairing capillary perfusion.

What Is the Implication of Pulselessness in the Setting of Compartment Syndrome?

The increase in compartmental pressure required to develop compartment syndrome is not generally sufficient to occlude arterial flow. Thus, pulselessness is not a common feature of compartment syndrome. An absent pulse in the setting of compartment syndrome would imply extremely high compartment pressures and likely very advanced, irreversible tissue ischemia.

What Are Considered Early Symptoms/Signs of Compartment Syndrome?

As compartment pressures increase, the first symptom that manifests is pain, especially with passive range of motion. Continually elevated compartment pressures will result in tense swelling (pressure) and nerve ischemia, producing a sensory deficit (paresthesia) that usually precedes motor deficits. As capillary refill continues to diminish, pallor and paralysis may occur.

What Is Meant by Pain Out of Proportion to the Physical Exam Findings?

The tense swelling of muscles in a compartment may eventually lead to ischemic necrosis, which manifests as marked pain in the affected extremity. However, the physical exam and clinical scenario may be deceptively benign. The foot itself often appears pink and well perfused. Pulses are almost always present (as in the present case). Thus, an unsuspecting clinician may be falsely reassured that the pain is simply from the injury (bone fracture). Compartment syndrome remains a clinical diagnosis, and severe extremity pain after injury mandates careful evaluation.

How Do the Ps Differ from Acute Limb Ischemia?

Pain is a prominent feature of both acute limb ischemia and compartment syndrome. However, acute limb ischemia differs in its progression and underlying cause. Acute limb ischemia typically results from sudden arterial occlusion, leading to rapid loss of perfusion. Thus, in acute limb ischemia, pulselessness is an early finding. In contrast, pressure from a tensely swollen limb is characteristic of compartment syndrome, whereas in acute limb ischemia, the affected limb is usually soft

Can Patients with Acute Limb Ischemia Also Develop Compartment Syndrome?

Yes. Following acute limb ischemia, compartment syndrome can occur when blood flow is restored to previously ischemic or hypoxic muscle. Reperfusion can result in an influx of inflammatory markers and cytokines, which increase capillary permeability. As a result, there is an increase in the fluid in the interstitial space, which may cause increased compartment pressures and result in compartment syndrome. Release of reactive oxygen species from ischemic areas may cause further tissue damage.

> **Watch Out**
> Pain out of proportion to the exam is also a feature of acute mesenteric ischemia, classically due to an embolus to the superior mesenteric artery in the setting of atrial fibrillation. Early in bowel ischemia, the patient complains of severe abdominal pain, but the exam may be relatively benign.

Anatomy

How Many Compartments Are There in the Upper Leg (Thigh)? Lower Leg? Upper Arm? Forearm? (Table 48.2)

Table 48.2 Compartments of the leg and arm

Extremity	Number	Names
Upper leg (thigh)	3	Anterior, medial, posterior
Lower leg	4	Anterior, lateral, superficial posterior, deep posterior
Upper arm	2	Anterior, posterior
Forearm	3	Dorsal, volar, mobile wad

Pathophysiology

How Are the Etiologies of Compartment Syndrome Classified?

They are broadly categorized into those that reduce compartment size and those that increase intra-compartmental volume within the confines of a noncompliant fascial compartment. Causes that reduce compartment size include external compression from tight dressings, splints, casts, or circumferential third-degree burns, all of which physically constrain the compartment. In contrast, causes that increase compartment volume involve accumulation of fluid or swelling within the compartment, such as bleeding from vascular injury, bone fractures, crush injuries, blast injuries, electrical burns, or reperfusion injury following prolonged ischemia. Regardless of the mechanism, the final common pathway is elevated compartment pressure that compromises capillary perfusion, leading to tissue ischemia.

What Is the Pathophysiology of Compartment Syndrome?

Compartment syndrome typically occurs after an extremity injury, such as a crush, burn, fracture, or reperfusion event. These injuries trigger inflammation, increasing capillary permeability and causing fluid accumulation, or they may lead to bleeding into the compartment. Both processes elevate compartment pressure above the normal range of 5–10 mmHg. As pressure rises, venules collapse, causing venous hypertension and a reduction in the arterial-venous pressure gradient. This compromise in capillary perfusion leads to tissue ischemia. Without timely intervention, tissue necrosis can occur, resulting in permanent neurological damage or systemic complications.

> **Watch Out**
> Compartment syndrome can cause muscle cell injury and death, leading to massive release of potassium (arrhythmias), acid (metabolic acidosis), and myoglobin (rhabdomyolysis, acute kidney failure).

What Is the Significance of First Web Space Numbness?

Numbness in the first web space (between the first and second toes) is a significant clinical finding because it indicates potential ischemia of the deep peroneal nerve, which runs within the anterior compartment of the lower leg. This compartment is the most commonly affected in compartment syndrome. The deep peroneal nerve provides motor function to the extensor muscles of the foot and cutaneous sensation to the first web space. Early recognition of this sensory deficit is important, as it may be one of the first signs of compartment syndrome.

What Is Volkmann's Ischemic Contracture?

Volkmann's ischemic contracture is a sequela of untreated compartment syndrome. It is classically seen in children following a supracondylar fracture that leads to marked swelling of the forearm muscles. An associated brachial artery injury from the fracture may lead to ischemia and subsequently, compartment syndrome. Untreated, compartment syndrome leads to ischemic muscle that becomes fibrosed and contracted. The eventual result is a clawlike hand with flexion of the hand at the wrist as well as damaged and insensate nerves.

> **Watch Out**
> After surgical intervention for acute limb ischemia, reperfusion injury may occur. Inflammatory response results in increased vascular permeability, compartment edema, and may cause compartment syndrome.

What Is Abdominal Compartment Syndrome? What Are the Risk Factors?

The abdominal cavity, like the extremities, is contained in a fascial envelope and is therefore susceptible to elevated pressures. Patients with multiple traumatic injuries, particularly intra-abdominal or retroperitoneal, who have received a large volume of fluids and blood products, are at risk of developing intra-abdominal hypertension (IAH), which can progress to abdominal compartment syndrome (ACS). ACS should be suspected in any severely injured patient who demonstrates decreased urine output, increasing peak airway pressures on the ventilator, and increasing vasopressor requirements, in the absence of another identifiable cause. Untreated it can lead to multiorgan failure and death.

Workup

How Is the Diagnosis of Extremity Compartment Syndrome Established?

The diagnosis of extremity compartment syndrome is chiefly clinical and is based on the aforementioned findings of tense, tender, and swollen compartments with pain on passive motion. With the classic history and physical examination, no further workup is necessary.

What Is the Role of Measuring Compartment Pressures with Suspected Extremity Compartment Syndrome?

Compartment pressures should be measured in situations where either the clinical exam is not definitive or in patients who are unable to provide a reliable exam (e.g., obtunded or intoxicated). Both absolute compartment pressures and the delta pressure (the difference between diastolic blood pressure and the compartment pressure) are used in decision-making. A normal compartment pressure is 5–10 mmHg. Absolute thresholds of >25–30 mmHg are often cited as indications for decompression. However, many clinicians prefer using the delta pressure. A delta pressure $\leq$30 mmHg suggests compromised perfusion and is a more sensitive indicator for intervention.

How Is Abdominal Compartment Syndrome Diagnosed?

Abdominal compartment syndrome is not reliably defined on physical exam, as patients with this condition are often intubated. Indirect measurement of abdominal pressures may be performed by transducing a bladder pressure. Intra-abdominal hypertension (a precursor to compartment syndrome) is defined by pressure $\geq$ 12 mmHg, while abdominal compartment syndrome is defined by pressure $\geq$ 20 mmHg associated with new organ dysfunction, such as oliguria.

Management

What Is the Treatment of Extremity Compartment Syndrome?

Treatment is immediate decompressive fasciotomy of all the compartments of the affected limb.

If Compartment Syndrome Is Suspected in Only One Compartment of the Lower Leg, Why Is Fasciotomy Performed for All Four Compartments?

It is difficult to reliably rule out the absence of compartment syndrome in one compartment if another is affected. Furthermore, compartment syndrome may not be fully manifested in other compartments at the time of surgery but may develop later. Therefore, fasciotomy of *all compartments* of the affected limb should be performed.

What Compartment in the Lower Leg Is Most Often Missed During Fasciotomy?

The deep posterior compartment is the most difficult to release and is most often missed. Decompression of this compartment is vital for long-term foot function, as it contains both the posterior tibial and peroneal arteries and the tibial nerve.

Watch Out
The superficial peroneal nerve is the most common nerve injured during lower extremity fasciotomy, resulting in the inability to evert the foot. This can be avoided by ending the lateral fasciotomy about 5 cm below the fibular head.

What Is the Treatment of Abdominal Compartment Syndrome?

Treatment is urgent decompressive laparotomy, with maintenance of an open abdomen and temporary coverage with a vacuum-assisted closure device. Delayed closure of the abdomen is accomplished when acute edema improves, and fascial closure can be accomplished without reproducing intra-abdominal hypertension. In cases of ascites leading to compartment syndrome, it is reasonable to attempt paracentesis first.

Complications

What Are the Consequences of Delayed Recognition of Compartment Syndrome?

Delays in diagnosis lead to a dramatic increase in the risk of permanent motor/sensory deficits, limb loss, and even death.

What Complications Can Occur from Lower Leg Fasciotomy? (Table 48.3)

Areas of Controversy

Should Patients at High Risk for Getting Compartment Syndrome Undergo Prophylactic Fasciotomies?

Given the devastating consequences of the delay in recognition of compartment syndrome, some surgeons advocate for performing prophylactic fasciotomies in patients deemed at high risk. However, the procedure itself can result in significant morbidity as outlined above, and most patients deemed high risk may not have ever developed compartment syndrome. Thus, more surgeons are leaning away from prophylactic fasciotomy in favor of close postoperative surveillance.

Compartments of the Lower Leg (Fig. 48.1)

Table 48.3 Complications of lower leg fasciotomy

Complication	Comments
Wound infection	This is the most common complication and can occur in as many as 40% of cases, likely multifactorial due to tissue necrosis and open wound
Superficial peroneal nerve injury	Passes superficially in the lateral compartment and is easily injured during the procedure, resulting in the inability to evert the foot
Incomplete fasciotomy	Inadequate fascial incisions causing incomplete decompression of the compartment; generous skin and fascial openings are needed to fully decompress the leg
Chronic swelling	Can contribute to diminished limb function

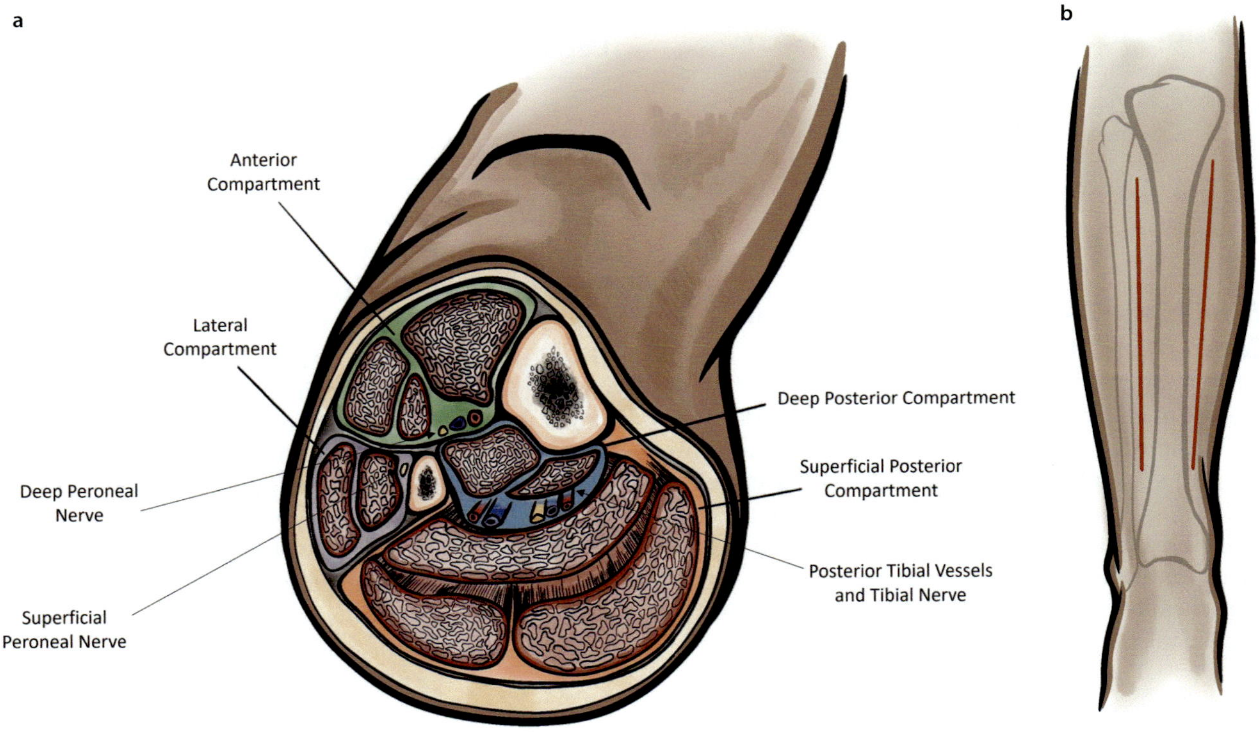

Fig. 48.1 Four compartments of the lower leg include **a** (1) Anterior compartment—contains the deep peroneal nerve. (2) Lateral compartment—contains the superficial peroneal nerve. (3) Superficial posterior compartment. (4) Deep posterior compartment—contains the tibial nerve and posterior tibial artery. To perform a four-compartment fasciotomy, two incisions are made on the lower leg—one 2 cm medial to the tibia, and one 1 cm medial to the fibula **b**.

Summary of Essentials

History and Physical

- Severe pain, tense, swollen compartments.
- Pain worsens with passive motion.
- Pain out of proportion to clinical exam.
- The six Ps: pain, paresthesia, pressure, pallor, paralysis, and pulselessness.
  - Pulselessness is a very late sign in compartment syndrome.
  - The six Ps are not consistently present.

Pathophysiology

- Decreased compartment size
  - Casts, circumferential burn, compression dressing, anti-shock garments, and splints
- Increased compartment volume
  - Trauma (bleeding, muscle swelling)
  - Ischemia/reperfusion

Workup

- In the presence of a classic history and physical examination, no further workup is needed.
- Measure compartment pressures only if the diagnosis is in doubt.
  - Normal pressure is 5–10 mmHg.
  - Intervention if >25–30 mmHg.

Management

- Immediate decompressive fasciotomy of all the compartments of the affected area of the limb

Prognosis

- Delayed recognition/treatment may lead to limb loss, hyperkalemia, acidosis, and renal failure.

Acknowledgement The editors would like to acknowledge and thank the following authors for their contributions to the previous edition of the chapter: Austin R. Dosch.

Suggested Reading

Amendala A, Rorabeck CH. In: Welsh RP, Shepard RJ, editors. Current therapy in sports medicine Chronic exertional compartment syndrome. Toronto: BC Decker; 1985. p. 250–2.

Grigorian, Areg, Nii-Kabu Kabutey, Christian de Virgilio, Michael Lekawa, Sebastian Schubl, Matthew Martin, Jeffry Nahmias. "Combined arterial and venous lower extremity injury." JAMA surgery 158, no. 12 (2023): 1346–1347.

Matsen FA 3rd. Compartmental syndrome. An unified concept. Clin Orthop Relat Res. 1975;113:8–14.

Trauma

Question Set: Trauma

Questions

1. A 49-year-old man is brought to the emergency department after crashing his bicyscle into a parked car. He was not wearing a helmet and struck the handlebars with his chest. On arrival, his vital signs are: temperature 36.9 °C, heart rate 110/min, blood pressure 102/68 mmHg, and respiratory rate 18/min. He is alert and oriented. Physical examination reveals mild anterior chest wall tenderness but is otherwise unremarkable. Chest CT shows no great vessel injury or intrathoracic bleeding. While under observation, cardiac monitoring shows frequent premature ventricular contractions. What is the most appropriate next step in management?
   (A) Discharge home with follow-up
   (B) Stress test
   (C) Echocardiography
   (D) Intravenous (IV) beta-blocker therapy
   (E) Coronary angiography
2. A 32-year-old female is stabbed in the right lateral neck 1 cm above the clavicle. There is an expanding hematoma in her neck, and she is having great difficulty speaking. Breath sounds are absent on the right. Subcutaneous air is noted in her neck. What is the next step in management?
   (A) Intubation
   (B) Chest tube placement
   (C) Duplex ultrasound of the carotid
   (D) Operative repair
   (E) Esophagoscopy
3. A 58-year-old intoxicated man presents to the emergency department after getting struck by a vehicle. His blood pressure on arrival was 98/55 mmHg with a pulse of 120/min. Following fluid resuscitation, his blood pressure increases to 120/70 mmHg, and pulse decreases to 80/min. His abdomen is distended and mildly tender, and he has no obvious source of blood loss. A CT scan of the abdomen and pelvis shows no intraperitoneal fluid but demonstrates bilateral pelvic fractures and a large pelvic fluid collection adjacent to the fracture with a contrast blush within it. What is the best next step in management?
   (A) Military anti-shock trousers (MAST)
   (B) External pelvic fixation
   (C) Open reduction and internal fixation of pelvic fracture
   (D) Exploratory laparotomy
   (E) Emergency angiography with embolization
4. A 30-year-old male presents to the emergency department with a gunshot wound to the right chest, just above his right nipple. He complains of shortness of breath and severe right chest pain. His blood pressure is 110/70 mmHg, heart rate is 100/min, and respiratory rate is 20/min. His breath sounds are slightly diminished on the right. The trachea is midline. Neck veins are flat. The abdomen is non-tender. Upper extremity pulses are equal. A chest X-ray demonstrates a moderate right hemo- and pneumothorax. The bullet is seen in the upper chest. A chest tube is inserted into the right chest with an immediate output of 500 cc of dark blood, with no significant ongoing bleeding. What is the next step in the management?
   (A) Exploratory right thoracotomy
   (B) Video-assisted thoracoscopic surgery (VATS)
   (C) Admit to ICU for observation

(D) Repeat chest X-ray
(E) CT of the chest and abdomen

5. A 28-year-old man arrives to the emergency department following a high-speed motor vehicle collision. He is in severe pain and breathing rapid shallow breaths. His blood pressure is 80/60 mmHg, heart rate is 120/min, and respiratory rate is 30/min. A segment of his right anterolateral chest wall exhibits paradoxical inward motion on inspiration. Despite supplemental oxygen, the respiratory rate remains the same. Breath sounds are equal bilaterally. The trachea is midline. What is the next best step in management?
(A) 2 L bolus of normal saline
(B) Insert a right needle thoracostomy
(C) Endotracheal intubation
(D) Transfuse two units of O-negative blood
(E) Place tube thoracostomy (chest tube) on the right

6. Which of the following parameters would be most consistent with acute carbon monoxide poisoning?
(A) Hemoglobin decreases
(B) Partial pressure of oxygen (PaO_2) decreases
(C) Oxygen content of blood decreases
(D) Oxidized hemoglobin increases
(E) Increased alveolar ventilation

7. Which of the following clinical scenarios is the best indication for four-compartment lower extremity fasciotomies?
(A) After a crush injury with an open tibia and fibula fracture
(B) After successful revascularization of a leg that was ischemic for six hours
(C) After repair of a femoral artery injury due to a gunshot wound to the leg
(D) After repair of a combined popliteal artery and vein injury due to a gunshot injury
(E) After an electrical burn, with a tensely swollen and tender leg and numbness in the first web space

8. A 30-year-old male arrived via paramedics after getting struck in the abdomen by a golf cart while vacationing with his family. He had no head trauma and only complained of mild abdominal pain. His vitals were normal and stable. A CT scan revealed no abnormal findings, and he was discharged on the same day. Three days later, he comes back to the emergency department complaining of fevers, nausea, poor appetite, and abdominal pain. A repeat CT scan shows a laceration at the neck of the pancreas with disruption of the pancreatic duct. What is the best next step in management?
(A) Order serum amylase
(B) Endoscopic retrograde cholangiography (ERCP)
(C) CT-guided drainage
(D) Magnetic resonance cholangiopancreatography (MRCP)
(E) Exploratory laparotomy

9. A 40-year-old man involved in a motor vehicle collision with a drunk driver on the freeway is brought to the emergency department. He has a dark bruise from his seat belt across the left side of his neck. On physical examination, he is neurologically intact. However, his left eyelid is drooping, and his left pupil is constricted as compared to his right. CT scan with contrast demonstrates dissection of the left internal carotid that extends into the base of the skull. CT of the head and abdomen is negative. Which of the following would be the most appropriate management?
(A) Left neck exploration
(B) Low molecular weight heparin administration
(C) Carotid stenting
(D) Thrombolytic therapy
(E) Observation

10. A 22-year-old male arrives to the emergency department by paramedics with a gunshot wound in the right upper quadrant of his abdomen. He is anxious and complains of pain near his wound. His temperature is 37.8 °C, blood pressure is 114/78 mmHg, and pulse is 90/min. His abdomen is soft, and he has no rebound or guarding. A portable chest X-ray

is normal, and nasogastric tube (NG) tube demonstrates clear fluid with no blood. His rectal examination shows no blood. What is the most appropriate next step in management?

(A) Serial physical examination
(B) Exploratory laparotomy
(C) CT scan of the abdomen
(D) Diagnostic peritoneal lavage (DPL)
(E) Focused assessment with sonography for trauma (FAST)

11. A 62-year-old man with atrial fibrillation presents to the emergency department with a painful right lower leg. He has refused warfarin in the past. His physical exam is significant for an irregularly irregular heart rate and a painful right leg that is cool to touch with absent distal pulses. Pulses in the left foot are normal. He has significant motor weakness and sensory deficit in the right foot. Duplex scan reveals an occlusion of the right popliteal artery. He receives heparin and undergoes open surgical embolectomy. Following the procedure, his motor and sensory deficit dramatically improves. The next day, he experiences intense pain in the right calf. His right calf is swollen and tense, and the pain is worsened with passive dorsi- and plantar flexion of his right foot. He has palpable distal pulses. What is the most likely underlying etiology for his acute condition?

(A) Compartment syndrome
(B) Recurrent embolization
(C) Deep vein thrombosis (DVT)
(D) Atherosclerotic plaque
(E) Lymphedema

12. Burn patients are at risk for multiple infections. What is the most common organism to cause infection in burn patients?

(A) Klebsiella
(B) Streptococcus pyogenes
(C) Streptococcus agalactiae
(D) Pseudomonas aeruginosa
(E) Candida albicans

13. A 10-year-old boy presents to the emergency department with severe abdominal pain after falling over his bicycle handles while attempting a trick. A CT scan shows oral contrast extravasation into the retroperitoneum that is coming from the posterior aspect of the duodenum. Which of the following is the best management recommendation?

(A) Laparoscopy
(B) Exploratory laparotomy
(C) Observation
(D) Upper endoscopy to confirm injury
(E) CT-guided drainage

14. A 40-year-old with alcohol use disorder presents to the emergency department with a markedly swollen right forearm that is diffusely tender. He states that following an alcohol and heroin binge, he fell asleep on his arm for 12 hours. He woke up to find his hand completely numb and unable to move it. On physical exam, he has normal brachial and radial pulses. His heart has a regular rate and rhythm. He is unable to extend his wrist when the hand is palm down. Electrocardiogram reveals peaked T-waves, and creatine kinase level is 20,000 IU/L (normal, 60–400 IU/L). What is the next step in management?

(A) Propranolol
(B) Insulin + dextrose
(C) Calcium gluconate
(D) Kayexalate (sodium polystyrene)
(E) Furosemide

15. An 18-year-old man presents to the emergency department after a stab wound to the chest. He is combative and with severe shortness of breath. His blood pressure is 94/76 mmHg with a pulse of 120/min and respiratory rate of 28/min. Physical exam reveals a 2 cm stab wound on the left chest. Lung fields on the left have decreased breath sounds and are hyperresonant to percussion. His neck veins are distended. A needle

is placed in the left second intercostal midclavicular line and aspirated until a gush of air is heard escaping the chest wall. A liter of normal saline is given, and blood pressure improves to 120/70 mmHg, and pulse decreases to 100/min. What is the best next step in management?

(A) Transfuse O-negative blood
(B) Tube thoracostomy
(C) Chest X-ray
(D) CT scan of the chest
(E) Transport to the operating room for exploratory thoracotomy

16. A 25-year-old male suffers a gunshot wound to his right mid-thigh. On physical examination, there is no hematoma, no palpable thrill, and no bleeding from the wound. He has diminished but present pedal pulses on the right and normal pulses on the left. Neurological exam is normal. Ankle–brachial index (ABI) on the right is 0.8 and 1.0 on the left. What is the next step in the management?

(A) Surgical exploration of the leg
(B) CT angiography
(C) Formal angiography
(D) Observation
(E) Systemic heparinization

17. A 25-year-old male arrives to the emergency department with a stab wound lateral to his umbilicus after being involved in a drunken fight at a local bar. You can smell alcohol on his breath, and he is uncooperative during the exam. His temperature is 37.8 °F, blood pressure is 90/60 mmHg, and pulse is 120/min. His abdomen is soft, non-tender with no rebound or guarding. What is the most appropriate next step in management?

(A) Exploratory laparotomy
(B) Local wound exploration
(C) CT scan of the abdomen
(D) Serial physical examination
(E) Focused assessment with sonography for trauma (FAST)

18. In a patient presenting with acute limb ischemia in the right leg, what is the first structure to develop ischemic changes?

(A) Fat
(B) Sensory nerve
(C) Muscle
(D) Skin
(E) Motor nerve

19. A 25-year-old football player presents to the emergency department after sustaining a devastating tackle and hyperextension of his right knee. The knee appears to be posteriorly dislocated and the leg is swollen. Pedal pulses on the right appear to be diminished but present, whereas they are normal on the left. The remainder of his exam does not reveal any obvious signs of bleeding. What is the appropriate next step in management?

(A) Fasciotomy of all four compartments of the lower leg
(B) CT angiography
(C) Immediate heparinization
(D) Plain film of the knee, followed by reduction in the dislocation
(E) MRI of the knee

20. A 30-year-old unrestrained driver is brought in by paramedics after a high-speed motor vehicle collision. In the emergency department, his heart rate is 110/min and blood pressure is 104/75 mmHg and decreases to 92/68 mmHg during inspiration. His tachycardia and hypotension persist despite aggressive fluid resuscitation. He appears pale, and his neck veins are distended. He has multiple bruises on his chest and abdomen. His chest X-ray is unremarkable. What is the most likely diagnosis?

(A) Aortic transection
(B) Cardiac tamponade
(C) Severe lung contusion

(D) Tension pneumothorax
(E) Diaphragm injury

21. A 38-year-old obese construction worker arrives to the trauma bay after accidentally getting struck by a bulldozer at his job site. In the emergency department, his mental status is altered, with a Glasgow Coma Scale (GCS) score of 10. His blood pressure is 80/66 mmHg with a pulse of 112/min. He is given 2 L of intravenous fluids, but his blood pressure and pulse remain the same. A focused assessment with sonography for trauma (FAST) is inconclusive. A portable chest X-ray is negative, and a pelvic X-ray demonstrates bilateral pubic rami fractures. What is the best next step in management?
(A) Diagnostic peritoneal aspiration (DPA)
(B) Pelvic angiography with possible embolization
(C) Exploratory laparotomy
(D) Head CT scan
(E) Abdominal CT scan

22. A 25-year-old male is at a pool party and is heavily intoxicated. He dives into the shallow end of the pool and is subsequently found to be floating face down in the pool. He is rushed to the emergency department by paramedics in a cervical collar. He opens his eyes, nods his head appropriately to questions, and his pupils are equally round and reactive to light. However, he is not moving his arms or legs. There is no evidence of external bleeding. His blood pressure is 85/45 mmHg, and his heart rate is 70/min. Which of the following would most likely be seen in association with the injury described?
(A) Low cardiac output
(B) Elevated systemic vascular resistance (SVR)
(C) Priapism
(D) Parasympathetic blockade
(E) Lumbar spine injury

23. A 45-year-old male construction worker is digging a trench when he cuts his arm on a rusty nail in the soil. He has not been to the doctor since he was a teenager, but he is confident he received all of his vaccinations up to the age of 18 years. What is the next step in treatment?
(A) Tetanus immunoglobulin only
(B) Tetanus vaccination only
(C) Tetanus immunoglobulin and vaccination
(D) Primary wound closure
(E) Clindamycin for three weeks

24. A seven-year-old boy presents to his pediatrician with a tense, painful, weak, and shortened forearm with a claw-like deformity of the hand. The mother states that one year earlier, the child fell backward on his outstretched hand and suffered a supracondylar fracture that was treated with closed reduction and casting. The most likely explanation for the current physical exam findings is:
(A) Nerve entrapment
(B) Suppurative tenosynovitis
(C) Ischemia/necrosis of forearm muscles
(D) Complex regional pain syndrome
(E) Improperly reduced fracture

25. A 65-year-old former firefighter arrives for follow-up for chronic wound in his right leg from a burn he suffered 25 years earlier. The wound has failed to heal despite repeat skin grafting. Recently, the wound has become more painful and larger, measuring 2 × 2 cm, and continuously drains. Multiple biopsies of the wound are taken. Which of the following is the most important contributing factor to this patient's presenting condition?
(A) Radiation exposure
(B) Excess ultraviolet (UV) light exposure
(C) Work-related exposure to heavy metals
(D) Genetic predisposition
(E) Chronic inflammation

26. A 25-year-old man arrives to the emergency department following a motor vehicle collision with multiple abrasions on his abdomen. His blood pressure is 90/60 mmHg, and his pulse is 120/min. After a primary survey, a focused assessment with sonography for exam is performed. Which of the following is a focused assessment with sonography for trauma (FAST) poor at detecting?
(A) Pericardial effusion
(B) Single pneumothorax
(C) Free peritoneal fluid in the hepatorenal space (Morrison's pouch)
(D) Laceration of the kidney with perinephric fluid
(E) Free peritoneal fluid in the perisplenic space

27. A 23-year-old male is rushed to the emergency department by paramedics after sustaining a gunshot wound to the lateral neck at the level of the thyroid cartilage. The patient is hemodynamically stable and is able to speak. Physical exam shows no signs of hematoma, pulsatile bleeding, thrill, or bruit. Which of the following is the next step in management?
(A) Surgical exploration
(B) Wound closure
(C) CT angiography
(D) Intubation
(E) Formal angiography

28. A 41-year-old patient presents to the emergency department following a stab wound to the chest, just above the left nipple line. On initial exam, his blood pressure is 94/70 mmHg, and respiratory rate is 16/min. He has distended neck veins, and his heart sounds are muffled. A focused assessment with sonography for trauma (FAST) demonstrates fluid in the pericardial sac. Which of the following is considered the earliest finding associated with this condition?
(A) Electrical alternans
(B) Impaired diastolic filling
(C) "Water-bottle" shape on chest radiograph
(D) Left ventricle cavity becomes smaller
(E) Distended neck veins

29. A pregnant woman in her second trimester arrives to the emergency department after a minor motor vehicle collision. She has no injuries or complaints but is worried that her pregnancy is in danger. She has a nonstress test that shows two accelerations of fetal heart rate, each at least 15 beats per minute above baseline and lasting at least 15 s. She has no contractions, vaginal bleeding, or abdominal pain. A focused assessment with sonography for trauma (FAST) is negative. What is the next best step in management?
(A) Monitor the patient overnight
(B) Biophysical profile
(C) Discharge and follow-up in two weeks
(D) CT of the abdomen
(E) MRI of the abdomen

30. A 40-year-old policeman is brought to the emergency department having suffered burns after helping to rescue a woman from a burning warehouse. His temperature is 37.9 °C, blood pressure is 100/70 mmHg, pulse is 95/min, and respiratory rate is 24/min. On physical examination, he has 40% total body surface area deep partial and full-thickness burns to his face, arms, and back as well as a circumferential burn of his neck. He has singed nasal hairs, and there is carbonaceous sputum coming out of his mouth. His lungs are clear to auscultation bilaterally. Electrocardiogram demonstrates premature ventricular contractions. What is the most appropriate next step in management?
(A) Broad-spectrum antibiotics
(B) Endotracheal intubation
(C) IV fluid resuscitation
(D) Cardiac enzymes and serial electrocardiogram
(E) Bronchoscopy

31. A 40-year-old depressed and schizophrenic man jumps off a three-story window onto the street. Paramedics arrive on scene within five minutes, and he is rushed to the emergency department but loses vitals in the field and is dead on arrival (DOA). What is the most likely cause of death?
    - (A) Thoracic aortic transection
    - (B) Tension pneumothorax
    - (C) Abdominal aortic transection
    - (D) Ruptured spleen
    - (E) Pulmonary artery transection secondary to a jagged rib edge

Answers

1. Answer C
   Blunt cardiac injury (BCI) should be suspected in patients with blunt chest trauma and new electrocardiographic changes, arrhythmias, or unexplained tachycardia. This patient has frequent premature ventricular contractions after a high-impact chest injury, which raises concern for myocardial contusion. In a hemodynamically stable patient with no signs of major vascular injury on chest CT, the next step in management is admission for cardiac monitoring and transthoracic echocardiography to evaluate for wall motion abnormalities or pericardial effusion. Continuous telemetry is important, as BCI can progress to more serious arrhythmias or heart failure. Discharge is inappropriate due to the risk of decompensation (A). Stress testing is contraindicated in the setting of possible cardiac trauma (B). Beta-blockers are not used empirically for trauma-related arrhythmias before cardiac function has been evaluated (D). Coronary angiography is not indicated unless there is evidence of ischemia or suspected coronary dissection (E).

2. Answer A
   This patient has likely sustained damage to several structures of zone-1 of the neck. The first steps in management are always ABC. Given that there is an expanding hematoma and she is having difficulty speaking, there is concern that her airway is compromised, so she should be intubated. Since the apices of the lungs are contained within zone 1 of the neck, and she has absent breath sounds, she likely has a pneumothorax and will also need a chest tube (B). Duplex ultrasound of the carotid is not necessary since there is a hard sign of vascular injury (C). The patient requires operative repair, but the airway should be protected first (D). This patient may have sustained esophageal injury that will require repair as well, but esophagoscopy should not be performed since she has a hard sign of vascular injury (E).

3. Answer E
   This patient's mechanism of injury and blood pressure drop are highly suggestive of hemorrhagic shock. Given that the patient responded well to IV fluids, it is appropriate to obtain CT imaging to look for the source of bleeding. If the source was intra-abdominal bleeding, the next step would be exploratory laparotomy (D). However, the CT indicates that the source is pelvic bleeding, likely from the pelvic fracture. Such bleeding is best managed via emergent pelvic angiography, which could be diagnostic and therapeutic (with embolization). MAST suits were at one time popular as the compression was thought to tamponade bleeding (A). However, they have not been shown to be effective. External pelvic fixation can reduce and stabilize fractures and thus lead to a slowing of bleeding but is not considered as effective as angiographic embolization (B). Open reduction and internal fixation are the definitive treatment for a pelvic fracture (C). But given the technical difficulty and long length of such an operation, it is not recommended acutely and especially not in someone who is actively bleeding. Pelvic packing is emerging as an alternative to angiography for pelvic bleeding.

4. Answer D

This patient presents with a right hemo- and pneumothorax, and tube thoracostomy was able to evacuate 500 cc of dark blood. The most appropriate next step in management is to perform a repeat chest X-ray to ensure that the tube thoracostomy is in the right position and that the hemo- and pneumothorax have resolved. Patients with penetrating chest trauma who are hemodynamically stable and have a self-limited hemothorax should be closely monitored in the ICU (C). Exploratory right thoracotomy would be indicated only if the initial output after chest tube placement was >1500 cc or if the patient continued to bleed briskly (>200 cc/hour for 3 hours) (A). VATS is indicated if the chest tube has inadequately drained the hemothorax and should be done early (within 2 days) to prevent an empyema (B). CT of the chest is generally not needed if the chest X-ray shows that the hemothorax is resolved, and CT of the abdomen is unnecessary at this time as the bullet entered just above the nipple (and thus above the diaphragm) and is visualized in the chest, thus sparing the abdominal cavity (E).

5. Answer C

This is concerning for a flail chest, most commonly caused by blunt trauma. Although the diagnosis is made clinically with a paradoxical inward motion of the chest wall during inspiration, it is supported by imaging studies demonstrating two or more consecutive ribs broken at two or more sites. The primary morbidity related to flail chest is the frequent underlying *pulmonary contusion* that accompanies it and compromises adequate respiration. Oftentimes, this does not manifest until 12–24 hours when the pulmonary contusion "blossoms." Furthermore, severe pain may also affect respiration. Pain control is a crucial component of the management of patients with rib fractures. However, always start with the ABCs of trauma. The best course of management for the above patient (given the marked tachypnea and flail chest) is to first ensure an airway with endotracheal intubation. This can be followed by two large bore IVs and fluids (A). Blood products may be needed if he does not respond to fluids and continues to remain hemodynamically unstable (D). There is no indication for a needle thoracostomy or chest tube given that the breath sounds are equal (B). Chest tube may be indicated if the patient had a concurrent pneumothorax on subsequent chest X-ray (E).

6. Answer C

Acute carbon monoxide (CO) poisoning affects the organs with the highest oxygen demand first. Patients will present in the early stages with neurologic complaints (e.g., headaches, dizziness, confusion) and cardiac symptoms (e.g., chest pain, arrhythmias). All these patients should be started on 100% oxygen via nonrebreather facemask. CO has nearly 250× more affinity for hemoglobin than oxygen. Thus, the hemoglobin–oxygen dissociation curve shifts to the left and more hemoglobin is bound by CO than it is by oxygen. This decreases both the hemoglobin saturation (of oxygen) and the oxygen content in the blood despite normal PaO_2, which is measured as dissolved oxygen and not affected by CO. The arterial partial pressure of oxygen is not affected in CO poisoning, and so a compensatory increased alveolar ventilation would not be expected (B, E). CO poisoning is not a consumptive or destructive process, and so hemoglobin would not be expected to change (A). Oxidized hemoglobin, also known as *methemoglobin*, has a higher affinity for cyanide, and so patients with cyanide poisoning are oftentimes given nitrates to induce the oxidization of hemoglobin to help bind the cyanide for renal clearance.

7. Answer E

Electrical burns are deceptive as, at the skin level, there may be a relatively minor burn wound. Yet, the electrical current can penetrate deep into the soft tissues, leading to extensive injury to the soft tissues and muscle. Thus, electrical burns are associated with the development of compartment syndrome. The best indication for fasciotomy is in the presence of compartment syndrome. Choice E is the only choice in which there is an *absolute indication* for fasciotomy as the patient has clear evidence of compartment syndrome. Numbness of the first web space is the classic finding of anterior compartment syndrome, as the deep peroneal nerve travels within it, and it supplies sensation to the first web space. Options B, C, and D are relative indications for prophylactic fasciotomy, as they place the patient at increased risk of subsequently developing compartment syndrome. A crush injury by itself is not considered an indication for prophylactic fasciotomy (A). Fasciotomy is most beneficial when performed early, before irreversible muscle and nerve damage occurs.

8. Answer E

The diagnosis of isolated pancreatic injury is often delayed as it is notoriously known to be missed initially on CT. If there is no associated splenic injury to cause bleeding or bowel injury to cause peritonitis, initial physical examination findings may be unremarkable. In addition, a serum amylase level is neither specific nor sensitive for pancreatic injury (A). However, if there is pancreatic duct disruption, the release of enzymes will eventually lead to symptoms as in the patient presented above. Surgery is recommended for such major injuries and may require a distal pancreatectomy. Minor pancreatic injuries without pancreatic duct disruption can be managed nonoperatively. In such cases, ERCP is more sensitive and specific than MRCP for ductal injury (B, D). CT-guided drainage (C) will not address the underlying pancreatic injury and would not be appropriate for this patient.

9. Answer B

The patient has sustained a blunt injury to the carotid artery as evidenced by a dissection in the left internal carotid artery. Such an injury should be suspected whenever there is high-energy force to the head and/or neck. He is exhibiting evidence of Horner's syndrome (ptosis, meiosis, anhidrosis), as sympathetic nerve fibers can be interrupted with carotid injury. A dissection is a partial-thickness tear in an artery that begins in the intima and extends into the media. It can narrow or occlude the lumen. Most blunt carotid injuries are managed nonoperatively with antiplatelets or low molecular weight heparin (provided there is no contraindication). Thus, observation alone would be inappropriate for such a patient (E). Since the dissection extends to the base of the skull, it would be impossible to access and repair through a standard neck incision (A). Although some dissections may heal spontaneously, early anticoagulation has been shown to reduce stroke risk, and is indicated even in asymptomatic patients if there are radiographic findings of dissection. Carotid stenting has a risk of causing a stroke and would not be appropriate for a dissection that extends to the base of the skull (C). Thrombolysis is contraindicated in a patient with a carotid dissection and in patients with trauma causing acute vascular injury (D).

10. Answer C

Immediate exploratory laparotomy is recommended in the majority of patients with a gunshot wound to the abdomen, particularly if the patient is hemodynamically unstable, has evidence of peritonitis, or has bowel evisceration. However, cooperative patients with gunshot wounds to the abdomen that are hemodynamically stable, with no evidence of peritonitis, are candidates for nonoperative management. They should be evaluated further for injuries requiring surgical repair with an abdominal CT scan. This approach may avoid an unnecessary exploratory laparotomy that carries significant morbidity (B). CT scan should be done even for patients with wounds that appear to only be superficial. If the CT scan is normal, the patient can be managed with serial physical exams and serial laboratory exams (e.g., white blood count) (A). NG tube can help identify gastric injuries, while rectal examination can help identify rectal or colon penetration by the bullet. Though occasionally utilized for penetrating trauma, DPL and FAST are more appropriate for blunt trauma (D–E).

11. Answer A

It is important to note that acute limb ischemia (in this instance due to embolization of atrial thrombus secondary to atrial fibrillation), followed by reperfusion, is a well-recognized risk for the subsequent development of compartment syndrome. Ischemia/reperfusion results in an increase in vascular permeability to plasma proteins and progressive interstitial edema. This leads to an increase in interstitial pressure. When interstitial pressure exceeds capillary perfusion pressure, muscle ischemia and necrosis ensue. It is important to note that palpable pulses do not rule out compartment syndrome. Pain with passive stretch, as seen here, is often the earliest and most specific clinical finding of compartment syndrome and should prompt immediate fasciotomy. The lymph system is not involved in the development of acute compartment syndrome (E). A recurrent embolus would not be expected to present with a swollen leg and palpable distal pulses (B). DVT can present with calf tenderness that is worsened with passive extension (Homan sign) (C). However, the temporal relation to his presenting problem and the physical exam findings are more supportive for compartment syndrome. Atherosclerotic plaque would be expected in a patient presenting with claudication secondary to peripheral arterial disease (D).

12. Answer D

Infections in burn patients can be problematic for multiple reasons. They may delay wound healing and encourage scarring, lead to burn wound conversion, and can result in burn wound sepsis with resultant bacteremia. *Pseudomonas aeruginosa* is a gram-negative bacillus and is considered to be the most common cause of infections in burn patients. Methicillin-resistant *Staphylococcus aureus* is also commonly seen in burn patients and difficult to treat due to a large number of virulence factors. *Klebsiella* is also commonly seen in burn wounds. *Streptococcus pyogenes* is more of a concern in pediatric burn patients because they may have colonization of *Streptococcus pyogenes* in their oropharynx (B). *Streptococcus agalactiae* is not an organism thought to infect burn patients (C). This organism can colonize the genitourinary tract and be transmitted to the neonate during birth which may result in bacteremia, pneumonia, or meningitis. Fungal infections tend to occur in burn patients during the later stages of recovery because by this time the majority of bacteria have been eliminated by the use of antibiotics. The most common cause of fungal infection in burn patients is by *Candida albicans* (E).

13. Answer B

Duodenal injury following blunt abdominal trauma is rare. When it does occur, it is usually accompanied by other abdominal injuries. Isolated duodenal injuries are even more uncommon. In children, they have classically been reported following a direct blow to the epigastrium such as a bicycle handlebar injury. The retroperitoneal location of some portions of the duodenum may lead to a delay in diagnosis, as enteric contents spilling from the injury may not cause peritonitis. Contrast-enhanced CT scan of the abdomen can help confirm the diagnosis by detecting extravasation of oral contrast, the presence of retroperitoneal air, or a paraduodenal hematoma. Some duodenal injuries can be managed nonoperatively. Specifically, a duodenal wall hematoma, without contrast extravasation, does not require surgery. On the other hand, the presence of contrast extravasation confirms a full-thickness injury that mandates exploratory laparotomy. Depending on the extent of injury, primary repair can be performed. Because of the close relationship of the duodenum to the pancreas and the bile duct, resection of the duodenum is often not possible. Upper endoscopy would be contraindicated in the presence of bowel perforation (D). CT-guided drainage will not address the underlying duodenal injury and would not be appropriate for this patient (E). Laparoscopy would not likely be able to adequately assess and repair the duodenal injury (A).

14. Answer C
This patient has evidence of compartment syndrome that has led to muscle necrosis as evidenced by high creatine kinase and hyperkalemia (peaked T-waves). Though compartment syndrome is mostly thought of as caused by severe bleeding after trauma, there are many other causes. In this case, it occurred secondary to prolonged compression of the forearm muscles due to his alcohol and drug binge. This resulted in ischemia, followed by reperfusion, and then swelling and death of the muscles. An alcohol binge can also lead to *Saturday night palsy*, a colloquial term referring to radial neuropathy from falling asleep with one's arm hanging over a park bench (compressing the spiral groove which houses part of the radial nerve). Hyperkalemia is a known complication of muscle necrosis from compartment syndrome and, if left untreated, can result in fatal arrhythmias. Although all the options listed (A–B, D–E) are appropriate management options for hyperkalemia, calcium gluconate should be administered *first* to stabilize cardiac myocytes and prevent further damage, particularly because the electrolyte imbalance has already begun to affect the heart (e.g., peaked T-waves).

15. Answer B
This patient has a left-sided tension pneumothorax as confirmed by hypotension, distended neck veins, decreased breath sounds, and hyperresonant left chest. Immediate treatment is with needle thoracostomy, allowing for immediate thoracic decompression. This is preferred in the setting of a tension pneumothorax as it is faster than a chest tube but provides only *temporary* relief. All these patients require a tube thoracostomy (chest tube) immediately following needle thoracostomy. Operative management is not routinely indicated for patients with tension pneumothorax as needle decompression and subsequent tube thoracostomy are able to resolve most cases (E). If he had a significant hemothorax that continued to hemorrhage despite tube thoracostomy, surgical management could be considered as well as blood products (A). Tension pneumothorax is considered a clinical diagnosis, and confirmation with imaging is not recommended as it delays definitive care in the unstable patient (C–D).

16. Answer B
Penetrating trauma to the extremities should be assessed for neurovascular injuries. Prompt surgical exploration would be indicated if the patient had *hard signs* of vascular injury (e.g., pulsatile bleeding, expanding hematoma) (A). It is important to note that a diminished pulse is considered a soft sign while an absent pulse is considered a hard sign. In the absence of hard signs, an ABI should be checked. If the ABI is <0.9, suspicion for an arterial injury is high, and as such, imaging with CT angiography is the most appropriate management option. Formal angiography can be considered if CT results are equivocal (C). Observation would be appropriate if he had a normal ABI (D). Systemic heparinization is sometimes used during the course of arterial repair if the injury led to thrombosis and an interposition vein graft is used (E).

17. Answer A
This patient has a penetrating abdominal wound which is concerning for an intraperitoneal injury. Immediate exploratory laparotomy is recommended in patients with a penetrating injury to the abdomen if the patient is hemodynamically unstable, has evidence of peritonitis, has bowel evisceration, or is uncooperative (e.g., intoxicated). Further workup can be considered for patients that are hemodynamically stable, with no evidence of peritonitis (B–E).

18. Answer C
The muscle is the *first structure* to be affected by ischemic changes in acute limb ischemia, and since it is the primary mass of the tissue in the extremity, the extent and duration of muscle damage are the most critical aspects of limb reperfusion syndrome and subsequent compartment syndrome. The muscle can be tolerant of isch-

emia for up to four hours. Irreversible nerve damage occurs after eight hours of ischemia (B). Sensory nerves are more vulnerable to ischemia than motor nerves. Fat changes remain reversible for up to 13 hours and the skin up to 24 hours, while the bone damage does not typically occur until after four days of ischemia (A, D–E).

19. Answer D
A dislocated limb has the potential of compromising arterial blood flow. As such prompt reduction is essential. However, prior to reduction, the first step is to obtain a plain film of the limb to confirm the dislocation and to rule out associated fractures. Following reduction, a postreduction film is needed to confirm proper alignment. Fasciotomy would be indicated if there is concern for compartment syndrome (pain in calf muscles on passive motion, tense swelling, paresthesias); however, reduction in a dislocated knee would still take priority (A). CT angiography would be performed after reduction if there is concern for arterial injury (ankle–brachial index <0.9) (B). Heparinization would be initiated after limb ischemia is diagnosed (e.g., cold, pulseless limb) (C). MRI of the knee is seldom indicated in the acute setting for knee injuries (E).

20. Answer B
Patients with blunt chest trauma that present with persistent hypotension, tachycardia, and elevated jugular venous pressure (e.g., distended neck veins) should be suspected of having an injury to the heart. Furthermore, this patient had a drop ≥10 mmHg in systolic blood pressure during inspiration (*pulsus paradoxus*) which supports a diagnosis of cardiac tamponade. Although cardiac tamponade classically causes a globular appearance of the heart on chest X-ray, the cardiac silhouette is *frequently normal*. A lung contusion would cause respiratory distress but not features of tamponade (C). An aortic transection presents with a wide mediastinum and would not cause neck vein distention (A). Tension pneumothorax may have distended neck veins, but the collapsed lung would be apparent on chest X-ray combined with tracheal deviation (D). Diaphragmatic injury can occur following blunt abdominal trauma and often present with gastrointestinal (GI) and respiratory complaints though they may initially be asymptomatic (E).

21. Answer A
Hypotension after blunt trauma should be considered due to hemorrhage until proven otherwise. Head injury should not be considered the source of hypotension. The most likely sources of bleeding are the abdomen, pelvis, and chest. However, major chest bleeding has been ruled out by the negative chest X-ray. In the stable patient, an abdominal CT is the best test to rule out bleeding (E). However, the patient's hemodynamic instability precludes such a study. FAST scan is the test of choice in the unstable patient, but its utility is often limited in obese patients because of poor image quality. In equivocal cases, the next best choice is to perform a diagnostic peritoneal aspiration (DPA) to detect blood in the peritoneum, which would be an indication for exploratory laparotomy. This is likely the only clinical indication in the modern era where DPA would be appropriate as it allows for a determination of the source of bleeding. Proceeding directly to exploratory laparotomy would be appropriate if the patient manifested peritoneal signs (C). However, if the source of his bleeding was from the pelvis, an exploratory laparotomy may decompress this and result in free hemorrhage from the pelvis into the peritoneum. The appropriate management for an unstable patient with bleeding in the pelvis is to perform pelvic packing. Additionally, his altered mental status precludes a proper physical examination. If the DPA was negative, one would then pursue pelvic angiography to definitively rule out pelvic bleeding (B). Given the GCS of 10, a head CT is indicated, but this would not take precedence over identifying the source of hemorrhagic shock first (D).

22. Answer C

The patient is displaying evidence of neurogenic shock with hypotension and an *inappropriately* normal heart rate. Neurogenic shock may also present with bradycardia and is associated with a high cervical spinal cord injury (not lumbar spine injury {E}). Priapism (a sustained erection due to unopposed parasympathetic tone) is often a presenting sign of acute spinal cord injury. Neurogenic shock would be expected to present with a normal/high cardiac output, decreased SVR, and sympathetic blockade (A–B, D). Treatment is with intravenous fluids first and, if needed, pressor support (typically norepinephrine).

23. Answer B

This patient has a dirty wound but has likely had all three tetanus vaccinations. Since he received his complete primary vaccination series as a child, he only requires a tetanus toxoid booster if it has been more than five years since his last dose. The correct treatment is tetanus vaccination only. Tetanus immunoglobulin is indicated only for patients who have never been vaccinated or whose vaccination history is unknown (A, C). Antibiotics are not indicated since the patient is not infected (E). Primary closure of a contaminated wound is generally avoided; instead, the wound should be irrigated, debrided, and left open to heal by secondary intention or delayed primary closure (D).

24. Answer C

Children with supracondylar fractures are at risk for acute compartment syndrome. There are three mechanisms as to why this occurs: (1) the fracture is often associated with an unrecognized brachial artery injury that leads to ischemia in the compartments of the arm; (2) if the subsequent cast is placed too tightly, this may contribute to compartment syndrome; and (3) initial bleeding and muscle damage/edema cause high pressures in the compartments of the arm leading to compartment syndrome. Compartment syndrome presents with the "six Ps": pain, pallor, paresthesias, paralysis, poikilothermia, and pulselessness (late sign). *Volkmann's contracture* is the manifestation of unrecognized and untreated compartment syndrome. This occurs because prolonged ischemia can lead to muscle death and subsequent fibrotic changes within the tissue. Volkmann's contracture presents with a tense, painful, weak, and shortened forearm with a claw-like deformity of the hand. Nerve entrapment is more likely to present acutely after the injury and will have deficits consistent with the distribution of a particular nerve (A). Suppurative tenosynovitis is characterized by the four cardinal signs (Kanavel signs): flexor tendon sheath tenderness, fusiform swelling (sausage-shaped digits), pain with passive extension, and a semi-flexed posture of the involved digit (B). Complex regional pain syndrome is a poorly understood phenomenon that occurs in patients that have had a crushing or soft tissue injury, typically to the distal extremities (D). They can present within days or months with intermittent pain, difficulty using the extremity, neglect-like symptoms, and rapid fatigability. An improperly reduced fracture would have been recognized earlier and corrected and would be unlikely to result in the deficits seen in this patient.

25. Answer E

Cutaneous squamous cell carcinoma arising from a chronic non-healing wound (such as a burn) is known as *Marjolin's ulcer*. Although all the answer choices are considered independent risk factors for skin cancer, chronic inflammation is the most important contributing factor in Marjolin's ulcer and can be seen in burn wounds, scars, chronic ulcers, or sinus tracts (A–D). Carcinoma develops on average 20–30 years after the original burn. Persistent non-healing wounds, especially those with new-onset drainage, ulceration, or pain, should raise concern for malignant transformation. All chronic wounds that fail to heal after a long period should undergo a skin biopsy to rule out malignancy.

26. Answer D

The FAST scan is a bedside ultrasound that is used to detect free fluid in the peritoneal cavity, around the pericardium, and in the thorax. The four areas of focus in a FAST exam are the hepatorenal space, perisplenic space, pouch of Douglas/rectovesical pouch, and pericardial space (C, E). FAST exam cannot distinguish blood from ascites and/or enteric content, is unable to detect retroperitoneal bleeds (from, for instance, a renal laceration with perinephric fluid), and is oftentimes limited by obesity. FAST exam will be able to detect bowel perforation if there is free fluid and only if the bowel is within the peritoneum (so would miss injuries to parts of the duodenum, posterior walls of cecum, sigmoid). For detecting pericardial effusion, the sensitivity approaches nearly 100% (A). Although bilateral pneumothoraces may limit comparison of sides, a single pneumothorax has a sensitivity of 95% and specificity approaching 100% (B). In contrast, retroperitoneal injuries such as renal lacerations or bleeding into the perinephric space are typically not visible on FAST, making CT the imaging modality of choice if suspected.

27. Answer C

Penetrating neck trauma may result in injury to major blood vessels, the pharynx, esophagus, trachea, and/or cervical spine. Immediate surgical exploration would be indicated if there were hard signs of vascular injury such as a pulsatile bleeding from the wound or rapidly expanding hematoma (the latter only after intubation first to prevent airway compression) (A, D). In the absence of hard signs of vascular injury, immediate surgical exploration is not necessary. Since physical examination is unreliable in terms of ruling out major injury, further imaging with CT angiogram should be obtained. CT angiogram has largely replaced formal angiography which was once considered the gold standard (E). Formal angiogram is invasive (requires a femoral artery catheterization), time-consuming, and costly and is only useful to rule out arterial injuries. Wound closure would only be appropriate for injuries that *do not penetrate* the platysma (B).

28. Answer B

In a patient presenting with hypotension, distended neck veins, and muffled heart sounds (Beck's triad) following a stab wound to the chest, the most likely diagnosis is cardiac tamponade. The earliest physiological abnormality is impaired diastolic filling, which leads to reduced preload and decreased cardiac output. Distended neck veins, although part of Beck's triad, are not the earliest sign (E). Electrical alternans is characterized by varying alterations in the amplitude of the QRS complex between beats (A). It can occur in various other conditions and is not always present in patients with cardiac tamponade. Radiographic images are often negative initially, but some may develop the characteristic "water-bottle" shape later in the course of the disease (C). In patients that have hemorrhage after trauma (hemorrhagic shock), the left ventricular cavity becomes smaller as the ejection fraction increases above 75% (D).

29. Answer C

Many worried pregnant patients arrive to the emergency department following minor trauma. Most patients do not have any significant clinical findings. Her nonstress test showed a normal strip. The criteria to discharge pregnant patients following minor trauma include contractions no more than every 10 minutes, no vaginal bleeding, no abdominal pain, and a normal fetal heart tracing. This patient meets the discharge criteria and does not need to be monitored overnight (A). Biophysical profile is indicated in patients with an abnormal nonstress test (B). CT of the abdomen should not routinely be done in a pregnant patient because of the high radiation risk to the fetus (D). Although there have been no ill effects reported from MRI use during pregnancy, there are no indications to warrant MRI use in this patient (E).

30. Answer B

Do not forget the ABCs of trauma. The airway should always be addressed first in the primary survey. Burn victims are at high risk of respiratory compromise since the supraglottic airway is susceptible to direct thermal injury and does not have the protection afforded to the infraglottic airway via the reflexive closure of vocal cords to intense heat. Circumferential burns of the neck further increase the risk of respiratory compromise by way of inelastic, circumferential eschars that may constrict the airway. Endotracheal intubation should be performed for all burn patients with acute respiratory distress, circumferential neck burns, full-thickness burns of the face or oropharynx, supraglottic edema, and progressive hoarseness, stridor, or wheezing. Broad-spectrum antibiotics are not routinely recommended for the management of burn victims (A). Burn patients are also at risk of severe intravascular collapse and require significant volume replacement with IV fluid resuscitation (C). However, this should be addressed *after* securing the airway. Premature ventricular contractions are usually benign (D). If the patient did not have indications for immediate intubation (circumferential neck burn), bronchoscopy would be indicated in the presence of singed nasal hairs and carbonaceous sputum to determine the presence of thermal damage to the airway (E).

31. Answer A

High-energy rapid deceleration chest trauma is most commonly caused by a fall from greater than two stories or from a motor vehicle accident (e.g., steering wheel striking the chest). This mechanism of injury is known to cause aortic injuries which may lead to aortic transection and ultimately death. The most common cause of immediate death from high-speed blunt trauma is thoracic aortic transection. Overall, immediate mortality is greater than 70%. The majority of patients die instantly of exsanguination. Of those who survive, 50% will die within 24 hours. Patients will present with a widened mediastinum, deviation of the trachea to the right, and left-sided hemothorax on chest radiographs. They may also have fractures of bones (e.g., first rib, sternum, scapula) that are uncommonly broken as high energy is required to break them. The aortic tear is usually at the ligamentum arteriosum, located just distal to the left subclavian take off, as the aortic arch is relatively fixed to that point. CT angiogram can confirm the diagnosis, and definitive management includes operative repair. Although a ruptured spleen can lead to significant blood loss, instant death is highly unlikely (D). The remaining choices can all cause instant death, but they occur in less frequency than thoracic aortic transection with this mechanism of injury (B, E). Abdominal aortic transection is extremely rare following blunt trauma as it is more mobile than the thoracic aorta (C).

Upper Gastrointestinal Bleeding

Brian R. Smith

Contents

Bloody Emesis

Areg Grigorian, Christian de Virgilio, and Brian R. Smith

Contents

C. de Virgilio, A. Grigorian (eds.), *Surgery*, https://doi.org/10.1007/978-3-032-09799-6_49

Case Study

A 50-year-old male presents to the emergency department with a three-hour history of bloody emesis. He has no such prior history. The vomiting was not preceded by retching. He states that the blood was bright red. He currently feels slightly dizzy. He has no history of alcohol use. He has noted intermittent epigastric pain for the past 2 weeks that is relieved by taking oral antacid pills. On review of systems, the patient notes that he injured his knee a month ago and has been taking ibuprofen daily for pain relief. Physical exam reveals a blood pressure of 100/60 mmHg and a heart rate of 110/minute. There are no signs of jaundice, and the abdomen is flat. No hepatosplenomegaly, caput medusa, or spider veins are appreciated. Laboratory values reveal a hematocrit of 40%. Liver function tests are normal, as are international normalized ratio (INR) and partial thromboplastin time (PTT). Blood urea nitrogen (BUN) is 36 mg/dL, and creatinine is 1.0 mg/dL.

Diagnosis

What Is the Differential Diagnosis for an Upper GI Bleed (UGIB)? (Table 49.1)

Table 49.1 Differential diagnosis for case presentation

Diagnosis	Comments
Gastritis	Nausea, bloating, dyspepsia, NSAID use, *Helicobacter pylori*, alcohol use
Gastric ulcer	Epigastric pain with eating, *Helicobacter pylori*, hematemesis is more common than melena
Duodenal ulcer	Epigastric pain with an empty stomach is relieved two hours after eating, possible weight gain, *Helicobacter pylori*; melena is more common than hematemesis
Erosive esophagitis	Associated with infections (herpes simplex virus, cytomegalovirus, *Candida*), GERD, and drug ingestion (potassium chloride, NSAID, tetracycline)
Mallory-Weiss tear	History of forceful emesis and/or retching (after alcohol binge); partial tear into mucosa/submucosa, self-limited
Esophageal varices	History of alcohol use disorder; stigmata of liver disease, including jaundice, spider angiomas, gynecomastia, ascites, caput medusa, palmar erythema, asterixis, encephalopathy
Gastric cancer	Involuntary weight loss, dysphagia, bloating, early satiety, cachexia
Stress-related mucosal damage (ulcers and gastritis)	Critically ill patients, severe trauma, severe burns (Curling ulcer), increased intracranial pressure (Cushing ulcer), shock; likely due to an inability to maintain the integrity of the gastric mucosal barrier
Angiodysplasia	Degeneration of previously healthy small vessels, associated with chronic renal failure, valvular heart disease, and CHF
Sinistral/left-sided hypertension	Splenic vein thrombosis after acute pancreatitis leading to large isolated gastric varices at risk for rupture and bleeding
Aortoenteric fistula	Prior aortic surgery with graft eroding into the distal duodenum; massive hemorrhage, often with a "herald" bleed
Osler-Weber-Rendu disease	Epistaxis, red nodules, and starry telangiectasias on the lips, nodular angiomas/telangiectasias in the small bowel, migraines

NSAID nonsteroidal anti-inflammatory drug, *GERD* gastroesophageal reflux disease, *CHF* congestive heart failure

What Are the Most Likely Diagnoses in This Patient?

With an upper gastrointestinal (GI) bleed, assumptions about the source of bleeding should not be made without performing an endoscopy. That being said, given the absence of stigmata of cirrhosis/portal hypertension, the absence of alcohol use, no history of retching, and a history of recent NSAID use, the most likely diagnoses are either acute gastritis or peptic ulcer disease. The question stem does not give any antecedent dyspepsia or prior symptoms to suggest a history of gastritis. NSAID use may mask the symptoms of dyspepsia.

History and Physical

What Information Can the Color and Texture of Stool or Emesis Provide?

The color and texture of stool or emesis (◘ Table 49.2) can provide clues to the location of the GI bleed, and may influence the workup and management. Iron in the red blood cells, when exposed to gastric acid, becomes oxidized, resulting in a coffee-ground appearance. This oxidized iron can also be excreted in the stool, producing a tarry, blackened stool known as *melena*. Ninety percent of melena comes from an upper GI source. Coffee-ground emesis and melena are both classic signs of chronic UGIB, whereas emesis of bright red blood or clots suggests rapid bleeding. Bright red or maroon-colored stools, also known as *hematochezia*, are more suggestive of bleeding in the lower GI tract (colon).

If a Patient Presents with Bright Red Blood per Rectum, Is It Always a Lower GI Bleed?

No. Massive UGI bleeding may cause such a rapid transit of the blood through the GI tract that it does not have time to be subjected to digestive enzymes, resulting in bright red blood per rectum. These patients typically have a significant amount of blood loss, enough to cause hypotension.

Pathophysiology

What Are Esophageal Varices?

Esophageal varices are dilated, tortuous veins located in the submucosa of the distal third of the esophagus that form as a result of portal hypertension, causing back pressure in vessels that have a systemic connection. Given their size, high pressure, and superficial location, they are highly prone to erode and cause life-threatening bleeding into the lumen of the esophagus. The primary venous drainage of the esophagus is via the esophageal veins that empty into the superior vena cava. However, distal veins within the submucosa empty into the left gastric vein (also known as the coronary vein), which normally drains into the portal

◘ **Table 49.2** Color and texture of stool and emesis

Emesis or stool	Likely location of the lesion
Bright red bloody emesis	UGI (moderate to severe, acute)
Coffee-ground emesis	UGI (more limited, chronic)
Black, tarry, foul-smelling stool (*melena*)	UGI (probable), LGI (possible)
Bright red bloody stool (*hematochezia*)	UGI (possible), LGI (probable)
Maroon-colored stool	UGI (possible), LGI (probable)

UGI upper gastrointestinal, *LGI* lower gastrointestinal

vein. In the presence of cirrhosis and impeded portal flow through the liver, the portal vein has much more difficulty draining its blood into the scarred liver. Blood is forced to flow in a retrograde direction, under high pressure, toward the tributaries of the portal vein, leading to varices.

What Is Acute Gastritis?

Acute gastritis is an *erosive*, superficial inflammation in the lining of the stomach secondary to the dysfunction of mucosal defenses. These defense mechanisms include the production of prostaglandins, bicarbonate, and somatostatin. All three reduce the inflammatory effects that gastric acid can have on the gastric mucosa. NSAIDs, which are COX-1 and COX-2 inhibitors, reduce the production of prostaglandins, thereby limiting their protective mechanisms on the stomach lining. Consumption of corrosive materials (e.g., household cleaners, pesticides, gasoline, cosmetics) can also lead to acute gastritis.

What Is Chronic Gastritis?

Chronic (atrophic) gastritis is a *nonerosive* inflammation of the gastric mucosa (◘ Table 49.3). Type A or fundus-dominant chronic gastritis is associated with pernicious anemia, in which the body produces autoantibodies to parietal cells, leading to megaloblastic anemia and vitamin B12 deficiency. Type B or antral-dominant chronic gastritis is the most common form and is frequently caused by a *Helicobacter pylori* infection leading to peptic ulcer disease and an increased risk of gastric cancer and mucosa-associated lymphoid tissue (MALT) lymphoma.

What Is Dieulafoy's Lesion?

Dieulafoy's lesion is a rare cause of acute UGIB. This is a congenital dilated submucosal tortuous artery, often located on the lesser curvature of the stomach, that erodes the gastric epithelium in the absence of a primary ulcer and is thus exposed to gastric secretions that may lead to massive upper GI hemorrhage. The classic finding on endoscopy is a small, pinpoint defect in the normal-appearing surrounding gastric mucosa with a visible, raised, large vessel that erodes through the mucosa. These lesions are identified endoscopically (if bleeding) and described as a visible vessel without an underlying ulcer present. If not actively bleeding, they may be easily missed.

◘ **Table 49.3** Acute versus chronic gastritis

	Acute gastritis	Chronic gastritis
Erosive	Yes	No
Etiology	NSAID abuse, alcohol, steroids, and uremia	Pernicious anemia, *H. pylori* infection
Pathogenesis	Decreased integrity of the mucosal barrier	Inflammation related to autoantibodies or *H. pylori* infection

◘ **Table 49.4** Bleeding vessels in peptic ulcer disease

Branch of the celiac	Type of ulcer	Location
Splenic artery	Gastric	Posterior wall of the stomach
Left gastric artery	Gastric	Lesser curvature of the stomach/gastric cardia
Gastroduodenal artery (comes off common hepatic artery)	Duodenal	Posterior wall of the first portion of the duodenum (D1)

What Are the Important Anatomic Correlations for Peptic Ulcer Disease?

The branches of the celiac trunk (◘ Table 49.4) may be subject to erosion, leading to severe hemorrhage if an ulcer penetrates through the gastrointestinal mucosa and into the vessel.

Workup

Why Might the Hemoglobin/Hematocrit Be Normal in Spite of a Major GI Bleed?

Hemoglobin and hematocrit may initially remain normal in acute GI bleeding because both plasma and red cell volume are lost proportionally. Since these are concentration measures, the hematocrit does not decrease immediately, potentially misleading the clinician. A drop in hematocrit typically becomes evident 12–24 hours later as the kidneys retain sodium and water. Further dilution occurs with IV fluid resuscitation, leading to a progressive decrease in hemoglobin. However, significant blood loss is usually indicated earlier by signs of hypovolemic shock, including tachycardia, low urine output, hypotension, and a narrowed pulse pressure.

Watch Out

A patients blood pressure may not drop until 30–40% of their blood volume is lost, by which point they are already in significant shock and at risk for end-organ damage secondary to hypoperfusion.

What Happens to the BUN/Creatinine Ratio During an UGIB?

The BUN/creatinine ratio *increases*. In the absence of renal insufficiency, a decreased hemoglobin/hematocrit combined with a BUN/creatinine ratio greater than 36 (normal <20) suggests an UGIB. This increase is a result of absorption of degraded blood products during intestinal transit and prerenal azotemia secondary to hypovolemia. BUN/creatinine ratio correlates positively with the likelihood of an UGIB, and isolated increases in BUN can be a subtle indicator of an UGIB.

What Part of the GI Tract Is Considered an UGIB?

From the oropharynx to the distal duodenum (where it crosses the ligament of Treitz), which marks the transition from the retroperitoneal duodenum to the intraperitoneal jejunum. Bleeding distal to the ligament of Treitz is considered a lower GI bleed.

What Is the Difference Between Occult and Obscure GI Bleeding?

An occult GI bleed is one that is not visible to the patient. It is discovered by either fecal occult blood testing or by noting a microcytic iron deficiency anemia on blood testing. The majority of causes of both upper and lower GI bleeding present as occult bleeding. Obscure bleeding refers to bleeding for which the source is not able to be identified after initial endoscopy.

What Is a Common Cause of GI Bleeding and/or Anemia Unique to Patients with a Hiatal Hernia?

A Cameron's ulcer. This is a gastric mucosal ulceration in which the herniated stomach slides up and down across the diaphragm. The presence of anemia and a Cameron's ulcer is an indication for repair of the hiatal hernia (once all other sources of GI bleed have been ruled out). The ulcer heals quickly after hernia repair and is rarely seen preoperatively on endoscopy.

Management

What Are the First Steps in the Management of This Patient?

The first step involves addressing the ABCs. Vital signs should be checked for evidence of major blood loss (hypotension, tachycardia) (▪ Fig. 49.1). All patients with hemodynamic instability or active bleeding should receive two large-bore IV lines and be typed and crossed for blood. Adequate resuscitation and stabilization are essential prior to upper endoscopy, which will determine the source of bleeding.

Watch Out

If a patient has massive ongoing UGIB, the first step is to secure the airway to prevent aspiration, followed by fluid resuscitation.

What Is the Role of Placing an NG Tube?

In the past, a nasogastric (NG) tube was sometimes used to lavage the stomach, or in the setting of melena, to help determine if the bleeding was an UGIB or LGIB. However, NG tubes have not been shown to be effective as either a diagnostic or therapeutic tool and have largely been replaced by early upper endoscopy.

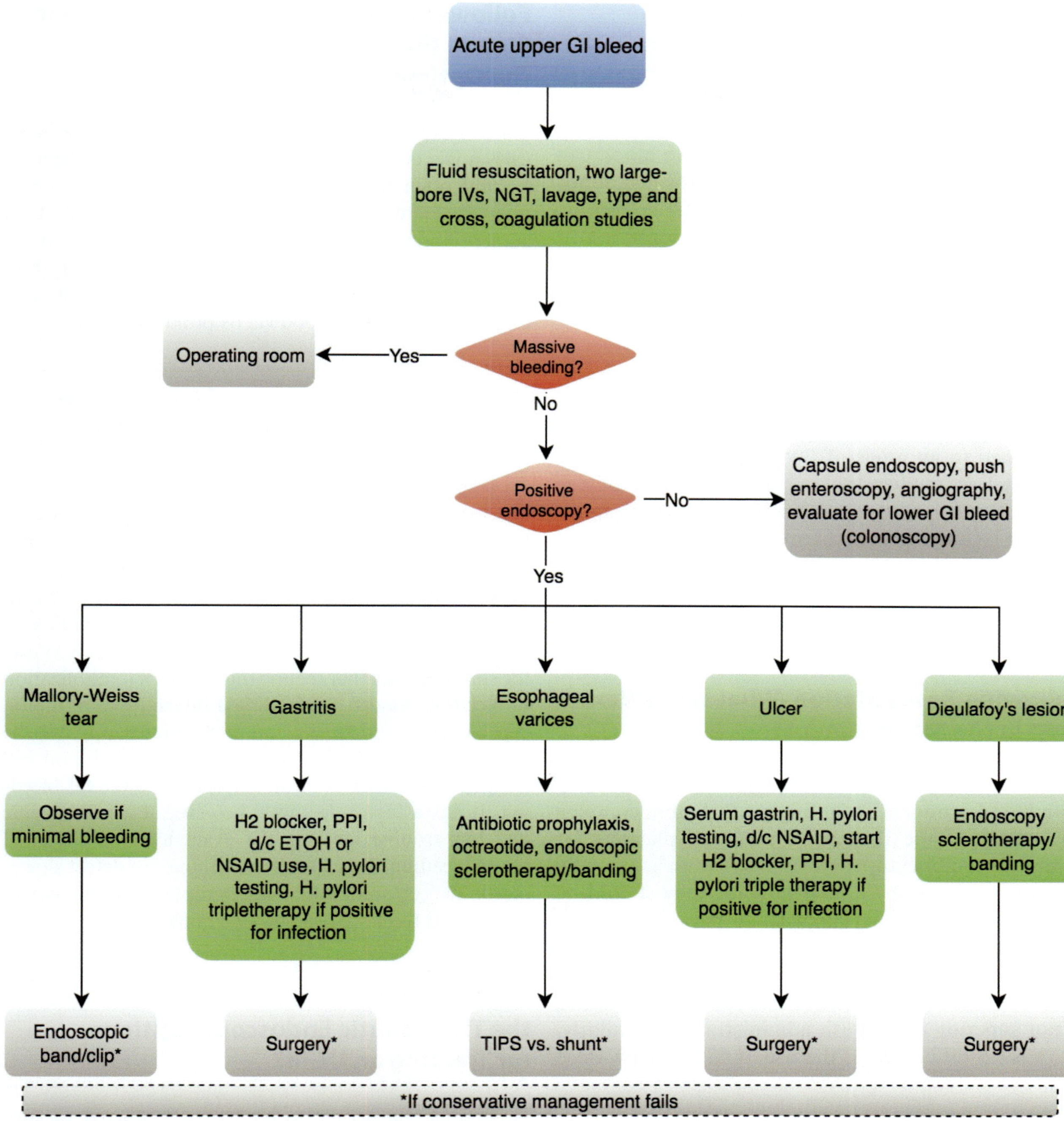

Fig. 49.1 Management algorithm of UGIB

What Is the Difference Between a "Type and Screen" and a "Type and Cross"? Which One Is More Appropriate in This Setting?

A type and screen is done when a transfusion is possible but unlikely, such as in elective surgery. It determines ABO and Rh status and screens for alloantibodies that could react with donor blood. If the screen is positive, further testing is needed to identify clinically significant antibodies. A type and cross is ordered when a transfusion is likely, as in this case. It includes a crossmatch, where the recipient's blood is tested against donor red cells to check for reactions. This ensures compatible blood is available if needed.

What If the Patient Needs Blood Immediately?

In emergent cases, if the patient is exsanguinating and time constraints preclude a type and cross (typically a 30–45 minute process), O-negative blood can be administered. Type O blood is the universal donor because it does not contain A or B antigens, so the recipient will not mount an immune response to it.

How Should the Bed Be Positioned in a Patient Who Is Vomiting Blood?

Provided that there are no contraindications (ongoing hypotension), it is recommended to elevate the head of the bed to an angle of 30° to prevent aspiration. Nevertheless, studies looking at the efficacy of the reverse Trendelenburg position in minimizing aspiration are lacking. If the patient is at high risk of aspiration or if the patient's mental status is altered, intubating the patient is far more important to protect the airway.

Following Resuscitation, What Is the Next Step in the Management?

Any coagulopathy should be aggressively corrected with blood products, including prothrombin complex concentrate if the INR is elevated and platelets for severe thrombocytopenia (<50,000/mm^3). If the patient is taking any anticoagulants, they should be actively reversed. The majority of patients with an UGIB are typically started on an intravenous proton pump inhibitor (PPI) such as pantoprazole, lansoprazole, and esomeprazole. A continuous infusion of PPI is not superior to IV push administration. Similarly, there is no difference in the use of high or low-dose PPI.

In What Setting Should the Patient with an UGIB Be Managed?

Unstable patients with an UGIB have a high mortality and should be managed in the ICU. Blood volume should be maintained using blood products and intravenous fluids. The patient will need continuous monitoring, which may include a central venous line for central venous pressure monitoring, an arterial line to continuously monitor blood pressure, and an indwelling Foley catheter to monitor urine output.

Following Stabilization, What Is the Next Step in the Management? What Is the Optimal Timing?

Gastroenterology should be consulted to perform an early upper endoscopy as the next step. It is both diagnostic and often therapeutic. Endoscopy within 24 hours improves outcomes by reducing hospital stay, need for surgery, and mortality, making it the most useful tool for both diagnosis and treatment of an UGIB. Oral erythromycin can be administered prior to endoscopy as it helps clear the stomach of blood via its prokinetic effects.

What if Upper Endoscopy Fails to Show the Source of a GI Bleed? What Other Imaging Might Be Useful?

Colonoscopy should be performed for patients with hematochezia after a negative upper endoscopy. The next step depends on the severity of the bleeding. CT angiography may help in identifying the source of bleeding. Formal angiography with interventional radiology is recommended if the bleeding is ongoing, as it allows for simultaneous therapeutic intervention (embolization of bleeding vessels). If bleeding is intermittent or minor, capsule video endoscopy and push enteroscopy may be considered. A technetium-99 m-labeled red blood cell (tagged RBC) scan is more helpful for lower GI bleeding. It has a high sensitivity; however, it is not specific and has trouble locating the exact location of small bowel bleeding. Tagged RBC scanning can detect slower bleeds (0.5 cc/min), while angiography will only detect more rapid bleeding (rate of 1 cc/min).

In the Absence of Varices, What Are the Therapeutic Endoscopic Options for Treating an UGIB?

Numerous endoscopic techniques are utilized to stop bleeding in the stomach and duodenum, including injection of epinephrine, bipolar electrocautery, heater probe coagulation, argon plasma coagulator, laser photocoagulation, application of hemostatic materials, and use of endoscopic clips.

What Are the Indications for Surgery in a Patient with an UGIB?

- Failure of endoscopic therapy (usually after two attempts)

- Persistent hemodynamic instability despite aggressive resuscitations
- Cardiovascular disease with a predictive poor response to hypotension
- Hemorrhagic shock

What Are the Surgical Options for a Bleeding Ulcer that Fails Medical Management?

For bleeding duodenal ulcers, the most common source is the gastroduodenal artery eroding through the posterior duodenal wall. If medical management fails (which is rare today), surgical intervention involves a longitudinal duodenotomy with oversewing of the ulcer in three quadrants to ensure proper ligation of the artery. All patients should be treated for *H. pylori* postoperatively if they test positive (approximately 90%). Historically, acid-reducing surgeries such as truncal vagotomy with pyloroplasty or highly selective vagotomy (HSV) were performed to prevent recurrence. However, with the advent of PPIs, these procedures are rarely needed today. Vagotomy reduces acid secretion by decreasing vagal stimulation of parietal cells. For bleeding gastric ulcers, partial gastrectomy with ulcer excision may be necessary due to the higher risk of malignancy. Approximately 80% of gastric ulcers will test positive for *H. pylori* and should be treated accordingly.

Special Management Circumstances

If an Ulcer or Gastritis Is Found on Endoscopy, What Additional Studies/Therapies Are Recommended?

H. pylori infection is present in the majority of uncomplicated gastric or duodenal ulcers. Leaving this untreated can result in recurrent ulcers, which may lead to perforation. In addition, there is an increased risk for the development of lymphoma in the stomach (MALToma, mucosa-associated lymphoid tissue lymphoma) as well as gastric adenocarcinoma as a consequence of long-standing infection. After confirmation of infection with *H. pylori* (see section below), the standard first-line therapy consists of "triple therapy" with a proton pump inhibitor such as omeprazole, along with clarithromycin and amoxicillin. Most patients are treated with triple therapy for 2 weeks. If a gastric ulcer is found, a biopsy should be taken, as it may represent a malignancy.

How Do You Test for *H. pylori* Eradication?

Because of the increasing presence of antibiotic-resistant *H. pylori*, it is recommended to confirm eradication of infection in all patients 4–6 weeks following treatment. The best test is the urea breath test. The urease produced by *H. pylori* can hydrolyze urea to produce CO2 and ammonia, which can be traced using a radiolabeled carbon isotope given by mouth to the patient. The patient should be off proton pump inhibitors for 2 weeks prior to the test because it can result in a false negative. Other options to confirm eradication include stool antigen testing or endoscopy with biopsy (the most invasive option). Serologic testing demonstrates prior exposure to *H. pylori* by detecting IgG antibodies, but it is a poor choice to test for eradication.

How Does the Management of UGIB Differ for Esophageal Varices?

Variceal bleeding requires additional interventions beyond standard UGIB management. Short-term antibiotic prophylaxis is given to reduce infection risk and improve survival. Somatostatin analogs (e.g., octreotide) reduce portal blood flow and are preferred over vasopressin, which causes systemic vasoconstriction and is contraindicated in coronary artery disease. Endoscopic band ligation is the best approach to stop the bleeding varices, with repeat endoscopy in 48 hours to address remaining varices. If combination therapy and repeat endoscopic therapy fail to control bleeding, transjugular intrahepatic portosystemic shunting (TIPS) may be considered to lower portal pressure. In unstable patients, balloon tamponade (e.g., Sengstaken-Blakemore tube) can provide temporary control.

What Is the Best Way to Prevent Recurrent UGI Bleed from Esophageal Varices?

For esophageal varices, long-term nonselective ß-blocker (nadolol or propranolol) use has been shown to decrease the likelihood of rebleeding. ß-Blockers are not helpful in the acute setting as they do not stop bleeding.

How Does the Management of UGI Bleeding Differ for a Mallory-Weiss Tear?

Mallory-Weiss tears are linear erosions in the gastroesophageal mucosa and submucosa that result from a sudden increase in intra-abdominal pressure. Precipitating factors include vomiting, retching, straining during defecation, heavy lifting, or violent coughing. The typical patient is middle-aged with a history of binge drinking and retching without blood, prior to the onset of bloody emesis. The bleeding is almost always self-limited, and the erosions heal rapidly.

Following Gastrectomy, Why Would Patients Develop Nausea, Dizziness, and Flushing?

Patients with bleeding gastric ulcers may require a partial gastrectomy. The most common complication from this surgery is dumping syndrome, which occurs in early and late forms. Early dumping (30 minutes after eating) presents with GI symptoms including nausea, emesis, bloating, and explosive diarrhea, as well as cardiovascular symptoms including diaphoresis, dizziness, and flushing. The etiology for this is related to the release of serotonin, bradykinins, and enteroglucagon. Late dumping occurs three hours after eating and presents with symptoms consistent with hypoglycemia (diaphoresis, confusion, and tachycardia). This is related to a large amount of carbohydrates suddenly entering the duodenum, leading to a surge in insulin secretion.

Areas Where You Can Get in Trouble

Assuming That UGIB in a Patient with Alcohol Use Disorder Is Due to Esophageal Varices

Although alcohol use disorder is associated with cirrhosis and portal hypertension, it is crucial to rule out other etiologies by performing an endoscopy. A Mallory-Weiss tear should be considered if the patient presents with a history of retching prior to bleeding. A careful history should be taken to determine if NSAIDs may have played a role or if the patient has a known history of ulcers.

Sequelae of Ingesting Harmful Liquids

Patients with suicidal ideations or young children can mistakenly ingest harmful household substances. Acidic liquids (e.g., hydrochloric acid) can cause a chemical burn to the esophagus and gastric mucosa and increase the risk of ulceration and perforation. Alkaline substances (e.g., liquid detergents, cleaning liquids) are more commonly ingested and produce more widespread and severe injuries (acidic liquids burn the mouth and therefore limit the volume of ingestion). In the acute setting, EGD is used to visualize the extent of esophageal and gastric injury, but the endoscope should not traverse the affected area as this increases the risk of perforation. Weeks to months after acidic/alkaline ingestion, patients may develop strictures either in the esophagus or near the pylorus. Esophageal strictures will present with dysphagia, while pyloric strictures will present with symptoms suggestive of gastric outlet obstruction (nausea, emesis, early satiety, bloating, and weight loss).

Summary of Essentials

History and Physical Exam

- Do not forget to ask about alcohol and NSAID use
- Always inquire about any known *H. pylori* status
- Look for stigmata of cirrhosis

Pathology/Pathophysiology

- UGIB is proximal to the ligament of Treitz.
- About 75% of GI bleeding is from the upper GI tract.
- Most common cause of melena (LGIB) is UGIB.
- An occult bleed is defined by fecal occult blood positivity and/or iron deficiency anemia.

Differential Diagnosis

- Consider stress ulceration in a critically ill ICU patient
- Consider an aortoenteric fistula if the patient has a history of aortic surgery; work up with endoscopy and CT (gas/stranding around graft)
- Consider Mallory-Weiss tear if bleeding follows forceful vomiting

Diagnosis

- When it is unclear whether the bleed is upper or lower GI, start with upper endoscopy.
- UGI bleeding can increase the BUN/creatinine ratio.

Management

- Start with ABCs (airway, breathing, circulation), two large-bore IVs, and type and cross

- With a massive bleed, consider intubation to protect the airway
- Liberal blood transfusion policy not helpful; restrict blood unless the hemoglobin drops below 7 g/dL
- Start PPI early
- Triple therapy for *H. pylori* eradication
- Admit to a monitored setting
- Perform upper endoscopy within 24 hours
- Most bleeding is successfully treated with endoscopic techniques
- Surgery only if endoscopy fails: duodenal ulcer (open duodenum, three-point ligation of ulcer) and gastric ulcer (excise and close for acute vs distal gastrectomy for chronic history of ulcer disease)
- For variceal patients with cirrhosis, calculate the Model for end-stage liver disease (MELD) score

Special Management Situations

- Esophageal varices—start antibiotics and octreotide, band varices, TIPS
- With isolated gastric varices along the greater curve, consider splenic vein thrombosis from prior pancreatitis; splenectomy is curative
- Gastric varices are more difficult to treat than esophageal varices and do not respond well to banding or sclerotherapy
- Mallory-Weiss tear: bleeding usually stops spontaneously

Prevention

- Use proton pump inhibitors in patients on long-term NSAID therapy (e.g., rheumatoid arthritis) to prevent ulcers.
- Propranolol helps prevent recurrent bleeding from esophageal varices; it is not helpful in an acute bleeding episode.

Acknowledgements The editors would like to acknowledge and thank the following authors for their contributions to the previous edition of the chapter: Viktor Gabriel.

Suggested Reading

Laine L, Barkun AN, Saltzman JR, Martel M, Leontiadis GI. ACG Clinical Guideline: Upper Gastrointestinal and Ulcer Bleeding [published correction appears in Am J Gastroenterol. 2021 Nov 1;116(11):2309.https://doi.org/10.14309/ajg.0000000000001506.]. Am J Gastroenterol. 2021;116(5):899–917. https://doi.org/10.14309/ajg.0000000000001245

Meltzer AC, Klein JC. Upper gastrointestinal bleeding: patient presentation, risk stratification, and early management. Gastroenterol Clin North Am. 2014;43(4):665–75.

Rockey, Don C., Chul Ahn, et al. Randomized pragmatic trial of nasogastric tube placement in patients with upper gastrointestinal tract bleeding. J Invest Med. 65, no. 4 (2017): 759-764.

Saltzman JR, Tabak YP, Hyett BH, Sun X, Travis AC, Johannes RS. A simple risk score accurately predicts in-hospital mortality, length of stay, and cost in acute upper GI bleeding. Gastrointest Endosc. 2011;74(6):1215–24.

Simon TG, Travis AC, Saltzman JR. Initial assessment and resuscitation in nonvariceal upper gastrointestinal bleeding. Gastrointest Endosc Clin N Am. 2015;25(3):429–42.

Severe Epigastric Abdominal Pain

Flora Park and Brian R. Smith

Contents

C. de Virgilio, A. Grigorian (eds.), *Surgery*, https://doi.org/10.1007/978-3-032-09799-6_50

Case Study

A 61-year-old male with a history of gastroesophageal reflux disease (GERD), hypertension, and diabetes presents to the emergency room complaining of severe abdominal pain. The patient reports epigastric pain on and off for months, but with a sudden and severe worsening over the last 8 h. He states that the chronic pain has been a "gnawing" pain that is relieved by eating. He typically takes antacids for relief. He denies smoking, alcohol, or nonsteroidal anti-inflammatory drug (NSAID) use. Late last night, the pain suddenly became excruciating, and he is now having trouble moving. On physical exam, blood pressure is 130/70 mmHg, heart rate is 120/min, and temperature is 39.1 °C. He appears to be in severe distress secondary to pain. His mouth appears dry. Bowel sounds are absent. He has diffuse tenderness to palpation, with guarding and rebound tenderness. Laboratory values reveal a white blood cell count of 18,000/μL (normal 4.1–10.9 × 10^3/μL), blood urea nitrogen (BUN) of 40 mg/dL (7–20 mg/dL), creatinine of 1.8 mg/dL (0.5–1.4 mg/dL), serum amylase of 130 μ/L (30–110 μ/L), and lipase of 60 μ/L (7–60 μ/L). An upright chest x-ray demonstrates free air under the right diaphragm.

Diagnosis

What Is the Differential Diagnosis? (Table 50.1)

What Is the Most Likely Diagnosis?

The free air under the diaphragm indicates that the patient has a perforated viscus. This is supported by evidence of diffuse peritonitis on physical exam (exquisite tenderness to palpation, abdominal guarding, and rigidity). The most common causes of free air under the diaphragm are perforated ulcers and perforated diverticulitis. Given the patient's long-standing history of epigastric pain relieved by antacids, the most likely diagnosis is a perforated peptic ulcer.

History and Physical

What Are the Most Common Symptoms in a Patient with Peptic Ulcer Disease (PUD)? How Might One Distinguish Gastric from Duodenal Ulcers?

The most common presenting symptoms and signs are well-localized, non-radiating mid-epigastric abdominal pain and tenderness, respectively. However, the description and location of the pain can vary and be vague. A comparison of duodenal and gastric ulcers can be seen in Table 50.2. Patients with gastric ulcers often have pain that begins 30 min after eating (food releases stomach acid). As such, they may avoid eating and lose weight. Patients with duodenal ulcers report relief of pain with eating (food releases bicarbonate in the duodenum), so

Table 50.1 Differential diagnosis of case presentation

Diagnosis	History and physical
Acute cholecystitis	Persistent postprandial right upper quadrant (RUQ) pain, radiating to the scapula, positive Murphy's sign; fever
Acute pancreatitis	Severe epigastric pain radiating straight through to the back in a patient with a history of cholelithiasis or alcohol abuse
Acute cholangitis	Persistent RUQ pain, fever, jaundice (*Charcot's triad*)
Perforated gastric or duodenal ulcer	History of peptic ulcer disease (PUD), *Helicobacter pylori* or chronic NSAID use; tachycardia, epigastric abdominal pain radiating to the shoulder; guarding, rigidity, and rebound tenderness suggestive of peritonitis
Diverticulitis	Can present with signs of peritonitis; pain is usually located in the left lower quadrant (LLQ)
Small bowel obstruction	Severe abdominal pain and marked abdominal distention; extensive nausea/vomiting and failure to pass flatus

NSAID nonsteroidal anti-inflammatory drug

Table 50.2 Comparison of duodenal and gastric ulcers

Duodenal ulcer	Gastric ulcer
Increased acid	Normal or low acid
Pain may be relieved by food, but may return 3 h later	Pain exacerbated by food
Wake up at night with pain	No pain at night
May gain weight	May lose weight
Malignancy very rare	Malignancy occasionally seen
If it bleeds, it usually presents as melena	If it bleeds, it usually presents as hematemesis

they may gain weight or develop pain 2–3 h postprandially (so they may wake up at night with pain). Other signs and symptoms include nausea, vomiting, hematemesis (more common with gastric ulcers), and melena.

What Is the Typical Presentation for a Perforated Peptic Ulcer?

Patients will classically present with a triad of acute onset abdominal pain, tachycardia, and abdominal rigidity. They may occasionally complain of shoulder pain secondary to diaphragm irritation (referred pain from the phrenic nerve), right lower quadrant pain secondary to fluid tracking along the right paracolic gutter, and abdominal distension and vomiting. Approximately a third of patients will have a known history of PUD, and 5–10% will present with septic shock. Depending on the duration of symptoms, the patient may have evidence of marked hypovolemia secondary to a combination of peritonitis, poor oral intake, and/or vomiting. Laboratory findings may be benign, other than leukocytosis with left shift and elevated BUN/creatinine ratio secondary to hypovolemia. Due to the location of the pain, pancreatitis should be in the differential diagnosis. Amylase and lipase should be ordered and will likely be within normal limits. However, a posterior ulcer can cause elevation of serum amylase secondary to peripancreatic inflammation or spillage of amylase-rich luminal fluid. Late-presenting perforated ulcers (>12 h) may present in septic shock, which may be accompanied by a metabolic lactic acidosis. However, the acidosis can be masked by respiratory compensation or by the loss of acid via extensive vomiting.

Pathophysiology

How Common Are Peptic Ulcer Perforations and How Often Do They Result in Death?

PUD is one of the most common gastrointestinal disorders worldwide, but the rate of peptic ulcer perforation has dramatically decreased since the introduction of medical therapy for *H. pylori* (antibiotics and proton pump inhibitors). However, ulcers continue to be a common cause of perforated viscus resulting from the ongoing use of aspirin and NSAIDs. Gastroduodenal perforations occur in up to 10% of patients with PUD and account for more than 70% of deaths associated with PUD. Duodenal ulcers are more likely to perforate than gastric ulcers.

What Is the Most Common Cause of Peptic Ulcers?

Peptic ulcers are a result of an increase in destructive factors (hypersecretion of hydrochloric acid), a decrease in protective factors (hyposecretion of mucus and bicarbonate), or a combination of the two. *H. pylori* accounts for more than 90% of duodenal ulcers and up to 80% of gastric ulcers. In addition to producing toxic mediators that degrade mucus, *H. pylori* induces a local inflammatory reaction. The inflammatory reaction induces a hypersecretion of gastrin, which leads to increased acid secretion. This leads to the development of antral gastritis. The production of prostaglandins, bicarbonate, and somatostatin has been recognized to decrease in patients with *H. pylori* but normalizes once the bacteria are eradicated.

How Do NSAIDs Lead to Peptic Ulcers?

By inhibiting both COX-1 and COX-2 production, NSAIDs inhibit prostaglandin synthesis, which negatively impacts mucosal defenses. Prostaglandins stimulate mucin and bicarbonate production by gastric epithelium, reduce acid production by the parietal cells of the stomach, and enhance mucosal blood flow by inducing local vasodilation. Chronic NSAID use results in the unopposed secretion of acid and a reduction in mucosal defense and blood flow.

What Are Some Other Factors That May Lead to the Presence of Peptic Ulcers?

Other factors include smoking, alcohol, steroids, and stress. Cigarette smoking has been found to double the risk of developing PUD compared to nonsmokers. Smoking results in an imbalance between mucosal apoptosis and proliferation. Additionally, cigarette smoke inhibits prostaglandin and mucus production, resulting in a decrease in defense mechanisms. Alcohol damages the gastric mucosa and stimulates gastrin secretion. Cushing and Curling stress ulcers occur in head trauma and burn patients, respectively. Gastrin-secreting tumors of the pancreas may also lead to recurrent ulceration as part of Zollinger-Ellison syndrome.

What Are the Five Types of Gastric Ulcers and How Are They Categorized? (▫ Table 50.3)

▫ **Table 50.3** Types of gastric ulcer

Type	Location	Acid hypersecretion?
I	Lesser curvature (most common)	No
II	Pyloric channel (often in combination with a duodenal ulcer)	Yes
III	Prepyloric	Yes
IV	Gastric cardia	No
V	Any location in the stomach (NSAID use)	No

Watch Out

Only Type II and III gastric ulcers would benefit from an acid-reduction surgery, if one is indicated, as these are the only ones resulting from acid hypersecretion.

How Does Vomiting Change a Patient's Acid/Base Balance?

Vomiting results in the loss of fluid rich in potassium and hydrochloric acid. The loss of acidic fluid relative to bicarbonate leads to a metabolic alkalosis. If the vomiting continues, the patient will also start losing sodium, and renal perfusion will decrease. The macula densa cells of the kidneys will sense this decrease in sodium, activating the renin-angiotensin-aldosterone system. This results in reabsorption of sodium and water within the renal tubules at the expense of potassium cations. To avoid severe hypokalemia, which can lead to fatal arrhythmia, the kidneys begin to secrete hydrogen ions instead of potassium, resulting in *paradoxical aciduria* in the context of *contraction alkalosis*.

Workup

How Is the Diagnosis of Perforated PUD Established?

The diagnosis is usually made with clinical examination (peritonitis) and confirmed by radiologic findings (free air under the diaphragm). These findings can be masked in patients with extensive subcutaneous fat. The majority of patients will exhibit guarding with palpation and significant muscle rigidity, as well as evidence of a systemic inflammatory response (leukocytosis, tachypnea, fever, tachycardia).

What Laboratory Studies Should Be Sent?

Initial labs should include a complete blood count, basic chemistries, liver function tests, amylase, and lipase. Common abnormalities include leukocytosis with left shift, elevated C-reactive protein (CRP), low albumin (a poor prognostic indicator), and an elevated BUN/creatinine ratio suggestive of hypovolemia. Liver enzymes help rule out biliary causes of epigastric pain. Amylase and lipase are obtained to exclude pancreatitis. A serum gastrin level is warranted in cases of recurrent or refractory ulcers to evaluate for Zollinger-Ellison syndrome. All patients should be tested for *H. pylori*, and those previously treated should undergo confirmation of eradication using a urea breath test, fecal antigen test, or endoscopic biopsy at least 4 weeks after completing therapy.

What Additional Diagnostic Studies Are Recommended for a Patient with a Suspected Perforated PUD?

The classic finding on an acute abdominal series or upright chest x-ray is pneumoperitoneum (free air)—a hyperlucent area under one or both hemidiaphragms (although free air under the left diaphragm alone can be difficult to distinguish from the gastric air bubble). However, the absence of pneumoperitoneum does not exclude the diagnosis of perforation. For posterior gastric ulcers, care must also be taken to evaluate for retroperitoneal air. In this subset of patients, their abdominal exam may not be impressive due to little or no peritoneal soilage despite a significant and potentially life-threatening perforation.

What Is the Role of a CT Scan?

A CT scan of the chest and upper abdomen with oral contrast is useful in the diagnosis of a perforated ulcer. It offers excellent sensitivity and can identify extraluminal air, fluid collections, and contrast extravasation. In some cases, the perforation may have sealed, and free air without contrast leak may be the only finding. CT also assists in excluding alternative diagnoses such as pancreatitis, aortic dissection, or other causes perforated viscus (such as diverticulitis).

What Is the Role of an Upper GI Study (UGIS)?

While historically considered the gold standard, UGIS with water-soluble contrast is now used less frequently due to the widespread availability and superior anatomic detail provided by CT. UGIS may still be helpful in cases where CT findings are equivocal or in follow-up to assess for persistent leakage after nonoperative management.

Watch Out

It is important to note that if a perforated peptic ulcer is suspected, using barium in an upper GI study is contraindicated, as this can cause barium peritonitis. Additionally, an upper endoscopy is a relative contraindication as insufflation of air may exacerbate a perforation.

Management

What Is the Basic Principle of Surgical Treatment for Perforated Peptic Ulcer?

Sepsis has been found to occur in up to 20% of patients with a peptic ulcer perforation; therefore, adequate volume resuscitation to provide organ perfusion and careful ICU monitoring are necessary. A nasogastric tube should also be placed to decompress the stomach and attempt to decrease the amount of spillage into the abdominal cavity. Additionally, the patient should be given IV broad-spectrum antibiotics and antifungals. Antibiotics should cover gram-negatives, anaerobes, mouth flora, and fungi. If the patient is not already on an intravenous PPI, this should also be started, as well as triple therapy if *H. pylori* positive (clarithromycin, amoxicillin, or metronidazole and a PPI for 2 weeks).

How Should a Perforated Peptic Ulcer Be Repaired?

For a perforated duodenal ulcer, the hole is repaired with through-and-through sutures at the site of the perforation, which are then tied over a pedicled piece of omentum (known as an omental/Graham patch). The omentum produces high levels of tissue factor, leading to fibrin formation to seal GI tract perforations and stop bleeding, and acts as a nidus for an inflammatory reaction. If proper *H. pylori* treatment and antisecretory therapy are given postoperatively to patients with a perforation, primary closure with omental patch is all that is necessary in the vast majority of cases. For perforated gastric ulcers, there is greater concern for malignancy, so ulcer closure alone is not sufficient. As such, a biopsy or a full-thickness primary ulcer excision is needed, as this approach assures a tissue biopsy to rule out malignancy.

Is Conservative (Nonoperative) Management in Perforated PUD Ever Appropriate?

Yes. One may consider a nonoperative management if all of the following conditions are met: (a) the patient is hemodynamically stable, (b) the abdominal exam is benign without peritonitis, and (c) there is radiologic confirmation that the perforation has sealed. In addition, some surgeons will only consider nonoperative management if the patient is <70 years old or has associated comorbidities that make the surgery too high-risk.

What Are the Principles of Nonoperative Management?

Nasogastric decompression, antibiotics, initiation of a PPI, and close observation have been reported in the literature as a successful alternative to surgery in a specialized group of patients with a perforated ulcer that has already spontaneously sealed (occurs in 40–80% of cases). Conservative therapy is successful in about 70% of patients with a sealed perforation. It affords comparable morbidity and mortality while avoiding an operation and its associated complications. If the patient deteriorates or fails to improve within the first 12 h of conservative management, then surgery is indicated.

Can Perforated Peptic Ulcers Be Treated Laparoscopically?

Laparoscopic repair is a reasonable initial approach in hemodynamically stable patients with early presentation, minimal contamination, and anterior perforations, particularly duodenal ulcers. Benefits include less postoperative pain, shorter hospital stay, fewer pulmonary complications, and lower wound infection rates. However, open repair may be preferred in cases of hemodynamic instability, posterior ulcers, or diffuse peritonitis. Laparoscopic repair should be performed by an experienced surgeon and is not recommended in patients with prior extensive abdominal surgery.

Summary of Essentials

History and Physical

- Sudden onset of severe epigastric pain that becomes diffuse, suggestive of a perforated viscus
- History of PUD, *H. pylori*, smoking, alcoholism, and chronic steroid or NSAID use
- Abdominal guarding, rigidity, and rebound tenderness

Pathophysiology

- Acid hypersecretion or mucosal defense hyposecretion
- Five types of gastric ulcers
  - Type I ulcers are on the lesser curve of the stomach.
  - Type II ulcers are in the stomach and duodenum.
  - Type III ulcers are prepyloric.
  - Type IV ulcers are located proximal by the cardia.
  - Type V ulcers are anywhere secondary to NSAID use.

Workup

- Acute abdomen with diffuse peritonitis
- Leukocytosis with left shift
- Upright CXR: free air under diaphragm
- CT with oral Gastrografin if plain films are nondiagnostic

Management

- Duodenal perforation
  - Primary closure with an omental patch
- Gastric perforation
  - Primary closure, biopsy, and omental patch vs. wedge resection and closure
  - Must rule out malignancy
- Triple therapy: clarithromycin, amoxicillin, or metronidazole and a PPI for 2 weeks to eradicate *H. pylori*
- Additional acid-reduction surgery is rarely needed.

Acknowledgements The editors would like to acknowledge and thank the following authors for their contributions to the previous edition of the chapter: Viktor Gabriel, Sahil Aggarwal.

Suggested Reading

Bertleff MJ, Lange JF. Perforated peptic ulcer disease: a review of history and treatment. Dig Surg 2010;27(3):161–9.

Chey WD, Leontiadis GI, Howden CW, Moss SF. ACG clinical guideline: treatment of helicobacter pylori infection. Am J Gastroenterol 2017;112:212–38.

Chung KT, Shelat VG. Perforated peptic ulcer—an update. World J Gastrointestinal Surg 2017;9(1):1–12.

Dellinger RP, Levy MM, Rhodes A, Annane D, et al. Surviving sepsis campaign guidelines committee including the Pediatric Subgroup. Surviving sepsis campaign: international guidelines for management of severe sepsis and septic shock, 2012. Intensive Care Med 2013;39(2):165–228.

Tan S, Wu G, Zhuang Q, Xi Q, Meng Q, Jiang Y, et al. Laparoscopic versus open repair for perforated peptic ulcer: a meta analysis of randomized controlled trials. Int J Surg (London, England). 2016;33 Pt A:124–32.

Weight Loss and Early Satiety

James McDermott and Brian R. Smith

Contents

C. de Virgilio, A. Grigorian (eds.), *Surgery*, https://doi.org/10.1007/978-3-032-09799-6_51

Case Study

A 73-year-old female presents with complaints of abdominal pain, weight loss, and early satiety. She states that she has been experiencing a "gnawing" pain in the mid-epigastrium. The pain started 8 months ago. She attributed it to "indigestion." She took an over-the-counter proton pump inhibitor (PPI) and calcium carbonate, which initially improved the pain. The pain has progressively worsened, and now she is experiencing early satiety. Over the past 4 months, she has lost 25 lbs., is easily fatigued, and unable to perform daily tasks around the house. The patient has a 50 pack-year history of smoking. She denies more than the occasional alcoholic beverage. She moved to the United States 10 years ago from Japan. Family history includes her father passing away of "some type of cancer" and "ulcers" among two of her siblings. Physical exam reveals a cachectic female with tenderness to deep palpation in the mid-epigastrium, with no rebound or guarding. Laboratory findings include a hemoglobin of 8.5 g/dL (normal 12–15 g/dL) and hematocrit of 27% (36–47%) and mean corpuscular volume (MCV) of 65 μm^3 (80–94 μm^3). All other routine lab findings were within normal limits. A fecal occult blood test is positive.

Diagnosis

What Is the Differential Diagnosis for a Patient with Vague Abdominal Pain? (Table 51.1)

What Is the Most Likely Diagnosis?

In an elderly patient with abdominal pain, significant weight loss, a low MCV (iron deficiency) anemia, and a positive fecal occult blood test, the diagnosis is cancer until proven otherwise. Gastric cancer is uncommon in the United States but is one of the most common can-

Table 51.1 Differential diagnosis for a patient with vague abdominal pain

Diagnosis	Pertinent positives and negatives
Peptic ulcer disease (PUD)	Burning abdominal pain, nausea, vomiting, bloating; history of PPI or H_2-blocker use; pain presents postprandially (gastric) or improved with eating (duodenal) and usually self-limited; not likely to have significant weight loss; history of *H. pylori* and/or chronic NSAID use
Gastroesophageal reflux disease (GERD)	Postprandial abdominal and chest pain (heartburn); bitter taste in the mouth, regurgitation, bloating
Pancreatitis	Midepigastric pain; significant tenderness to palpation; elevated pancreatic enzymes; history of alcohol use disorder or cholelithiasis
Cholelithiasis	Right upper quadrant or midepigastric pain, often postprandial and intermittent (colicky); associated with fatty foods; may have elevated LFTs; ultrasound positive for stones
Hiatal hernia	Sliding and paraesophageal hernias may cause upper abdominal pain, anemia, and chest pain with or without GERD symptoms; may need immediate surgical intervention if signs of incarceration or strangulation (pain with nausea/vomiting) are present
Gastric outlet obstruction	Persistent nausea/vomiting and abdominal discomfort and bloating, early satiety
Small bowel obstruction	Nausea/vomiting with vague abdominal pain and distention; absent flatus and stool; history of abdominal surgery; most common cause in US is adhesions from prior surgery
Gastric cancer	Vague abdominal pain or discomfort, involuntary weight loss, early satiety, dysphagia, iron deficiency anemia, cachexia
Colon cancer	Iron deficiency anemia (right colon), change in stool caliber, bright red blood per rectum (left colon)
Pancreatic cancer	Painless jaundice, weight loss, acholic stools, new-onset diabetes

PPI proton pump inhibitor, *NSAID* nonsteroidal anti-inflammatory drug, *LFT* liver function test, *GERD* gastroesophageal reflux disease

cers worldwide, particularly in Asia and Latin America. In the United States, colon cancer is much more prevalent. However, due to the location of the pain (epigastric), the weight loss, and the patient's Japanese origin, gastric cancer is most likely.

Watch Out

It is important to consider gastric cancer as part of the differential in any patient that presents with upper abdominal pain and weight loss. In the United States, approximately 50% of gastric cancers have already spread past the confines of surgical resectability at the time of diagnosis, resulting in a high mortality rate.

History and Physical

What Is the Prevalence of Gastric Cancer and What Causes It?

Gastric cancer is common in Asia, particularly Japan, Korea, and China where it is one of the leading causes of cancer-related death. Gastric adenocarcinoma accounts for approximately 90% of all gastric cancers and is uncommon in the United States. This is predominately due to the identification and eradication of endemic *Helicobacter pylori*, with triple therapy (amoxicillin, clarithromycin, and omeprazole) as well as dietary habits, as in some Asian countries there is a higher rate of smoked, salted, and pickled foods that are associated with gastric cancer.

What Are the Risk Factors for the Development of Gastric Cancer?

Positive family history, familial polyposis, smoked meats, pickled foods, high nitrates/salts, gastric adenomas, *Helicobacter pylori* infection (atrophic gastritis, intestinal metaplasia, and dysplasia), tobacco use, Ménétrier's disease, Type A blood, BRCA-1 and BRCA-2, HER2 gene overexpression, Peutz-Jeghers syndrome

Watch Out

Peutz-Jeghers syndrome is characterized by hamartomatous (benign) polyps throughout the GI tract and risk of multiple cancers. Children develop small dark-colored spots on the lips and mouth and small bowel obstruction from polyp intussusception.

Watch Out

Risk factors for the development of gastric cancer are multifactorial. There is a synergism between *H. pylori* infections and other risk factors leading to a higher rate of gastric dysplasia and metaplasia.

Why Is the Mortality Rate So High for Gastric Cancer?

Patients present in a delayed fashion due to a combination of vague and nonspecific symptoms. The large size of the stomach lumen permits tumors to grow for a long period of time before causing symptoms. Typically, patients are diagnosed at a late stage when the tumor extends beyond locoregional confines. These findings exemplify the importance of diagnostic esophagogastroduodenoscopy (EGD) in patients that are high risk.

What Are the Most Common Symptoms/Signs for a Patient with Gastric Cancer? What Are "ALARM" Symptoms/Signs?

The challenge of diagnosing gastric cancer is that the early symptoms are the same as those seen in common benign diseases such as gastritis, peptic ulcer disease, or simply indigestion. These symptoms, termed dyspepsia (indigestion), include upper abdominal fullness, heartburn, nausea, belching, or upper abdominal pain. A key to the diagnosis of cancer is that these "benign" symptoms fail to resolve after 6 weeks of antacid therapy or the presence of dyspepsia *in combination* with so-called "ALARM" symptoms/signs:

ALARM Symptoms

- Anemia (iron deficiency) due to slow intermittent bleeding of the tumor
- Loss of weight
- Anorexia
- Recent onset of progressive symptoms
- Melena/hematemesis
- Dysphagia
- Dyspepsia and age >55 years

Watch Out

Patients with "ALARM" symptoms are more likely to have gastric cancer, more likely to have advanced cancer at diagnosis, and more likely to have shorter survival. The presence of "ALARM" symptoms mandates upper endoscopy.

Are There Specific Findings on Physical Exam for Gastric Cancer?

Physical exam findings are usually nonspecific and often absent. If the patient does have physical findings, it is likely they also have advanced, incurable disease. These include a palpable epigastric mass, palpable left (not right) supraclavicular adenopathy (Virchow's node), periumbilical lymphadenopathy (Sister Mary Joseph node), and left axillary adenopathy (Irish's node).

Pathophysiology

What Is the Vascular Supply to the Stomach?

There are four major arteries: the left and right gastric arteries on the lesser curve and the left and right gastroepiploic arteries along the greater curve, all of which are derived from the celiac artery. The left gastric is a direct vessel off the celiac artery. The right gastric most commonly is a branch of the common hepatic artery. The left and right gastric arteries communicate on the lesser curvature of the stomach. The right gastroepiploic artery is a branch from the gastroduodenal artery which originates from the common hepatic artery, and the left gastroepiploic artery is a branch of the splenic artery. These two communicate and supply blood to the greater curvature of the stomach. Additionally, the short gastric arteries come off the splenic artery and supply the greater curvature.

What Is an Intestinal-Type Gastric Adenocarcinoma?

This well-differentiated cell type arises from the gastric mucosa and is usually located in the distal stomach. It is more commonly seen in the patient that has exposure to environmental factors such as poor diet, smoking, and alcohol. This type has decreased with the eradication of *H. pylori* and other detrimental risk factors. Intestinal type accounts for 50% of all gastric adenocarcinomas and has a stepwise histologic pattern of progression starting from an *H. pylori*-induced inflammatory reaction (acute gastritis) and ultimately leading to gastric carcinoma in 10–20 years.

What Is a Diffuse-Type Gastric Adenocarcinoma?

This is a poorly differentiated tumor, believed to originate from the lamina propria of the stomach and grows in an infiltrative, submucosal pattern. Contrary to the intestinal type, the unorganized growth pattern does not lead to a discrete mass but rather to gastric thickening. Diffuse-type gastric adenocarcinomas are most often found in the proximal stomach near the cardia. These patients do not follow the typical histologic progression of atypia, instead jumping directly from chronic atrophic gastritis to adenocarcinoma and can do so relatively rapidly as compared to the intestinal type. As such, it is seen in younger patients as compared to the intestinal type.

What Is Linitis Plastica?

Diffuse-type gastric cancer (◘ Table 51.2) is highly metastatic and aggressive, leading to its rapid progression. It can filtrate the entire gastric wall, known as "linitis plastica" (plastic lining) named after the stiff, non-distensible gastric wall that develops after it is infiltrated with tumor. This pattern of diffuse submucosal spread lowers the accuracy of endoscopy biopsies and thus presents a diagnostic challenge.

What Is a Gastrointestinal Stromal Tumor (GIST)?

GISTs are mesenchymal tumors of variable malignant potential that originate from the interstitial cells of Cajal (gastrointestinal pacemaker cells) within the GI tract. They are smooth submucosal masses with regular borders. There is near-universal expression of c-KIT and CD-117 by GISTs. Biopsy is not necessary or recommended if there is a high endoscopic or radiographic suspicion for this tumor. Unlike adenocarcinomas, GISTs rarely spread through lymphatics, making a

◘ **Table 51.2** Types of gastric adenocarcinoma

Intestinal	Diffuse
Well differentiated	Poorly or undifferentiated
Distal stomach	Anywhere, but most often proximal stomach
Secondary to environmental factors	Secondary to congenital disorders such as hereditary diffuse gastric cancer (HDGC)
Decreasing in incidence	No change in incidence
Discrete mass	Generalized gastric hypertrophy
Progressive evolution to cancer over years	Aggressive and rapid progression

lymph node dissection or major gastrectomy frequently unnecessary.

Does Lymphoma Occur in the Stomach?

The stomach is the *most common site* for a gastrointestinal lymphoma. The two most common types are lymphoma of the mucosa-associated lymphoid tissue (MALT) and diffuse large B-cell lymphoma. They account for nearly 90% of all gastric lymphomas. MALT is most commonly associated with an *H. pylori* infection and can be completely treated with triple therapy against *H. pylori*. CHOP chemotherapy (cyclophosphamide, doxorubicin, vincristine, and prednisone) followed by radiation is the therapy of choice for high-grade lymphoma or that which does not respond to *H. pylori* therapy alone.

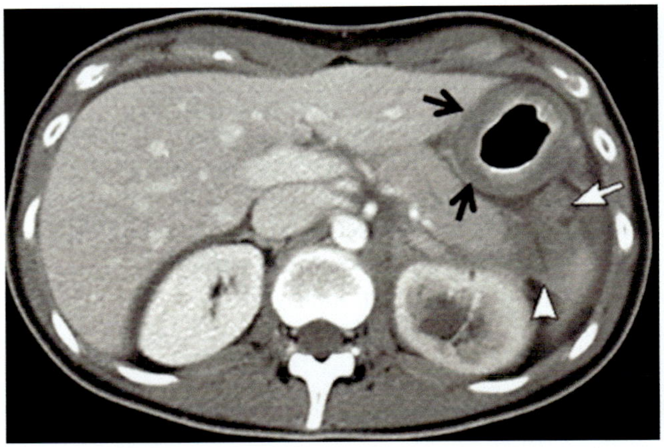

Fig. 51.1 Axial CT of gastric adenocarcinoma showing a thickened stomach wall and a metastatic gastrosplenic mass. *Black arrows: thickened stomach. White arrows: gastrosplenic mass*

Workup

What Is the Best Way to Work Up a Patient with Suspected Gastric Cancer?

Upper endoscopy is the diagnostic procedure of choice. It allows for direct visualization of the gastric mucosa, localization of the tumor for operative planning, and the ability to biopsy suspicious lesions.

Is Screening for Gastric Cancer Recommended in Asymptomatic Patients?

In high prevalence countries such as Japan and South Korea, screening for gastric cancer via endoscopy is recommended and performed. However, in the United States due to the low prevalence, the data do not support screening as it is not cost-effective.

Once the Diagnosis of Gastric Cancer Is Established, What Further Staging Is Recommended?

Endoscopic ultrasound (EUS) is performed to determine if the tumor is locally invasive. EUS provides a more accurate assessment of tumor size, depth, and locoregional lymph node involvement as compared to radiographic imaging. CT scan of the chest/abdomen/pelvis is performed to rule out metastasis (liver, distant suspicious lymph nodes) which may have been missed on EUS and would preclude a curative resection (Fig. 51.1). Positron emission tomography scan (PET scan) has been proven to be highly accurate in detecting small metastases and lymph node involvement and is often utilized to further evaluate for metastatic disease. Finally, diagnostic laparoscopy is helpful in staging, as it can directly evaluate the surface of the liver and peritoneum for disease that may have been missed on imaging. Peritoneal washings and cytology may be performed to evaluate for occult disease when no obvious disease is seen.

> **Watch Out**
> In patients with locally advanced gastric cancer, chemotherapy is effective when used prior to surgery. However, surgery is still considered first-line therapy when curative resection can be achieved and not otherwise precluded.

Management

How Is Gastric Cancer Treated?

The management of gastric adenocarcinoma is dependent on how advanced the tumor is. Surgical resection (gastrectomy) is the only curative therapy. However, a multi-therapeutic approach is becoming increasingly recommended for locally advanced tumors. This includes neoadjuvant (preoperative) chemotherapy, then surgical resection, followed by adjuvant (postoperative) chemotherapy, or chemoradiation. Chemotherapy has been proven to be effective both the pre- and postoperatively. The MAGIC trial was the first study to show the effectiveness of perioperative chemotherapy prior to surgical resection, with improved outcomes and survival (Fig. 51.2).

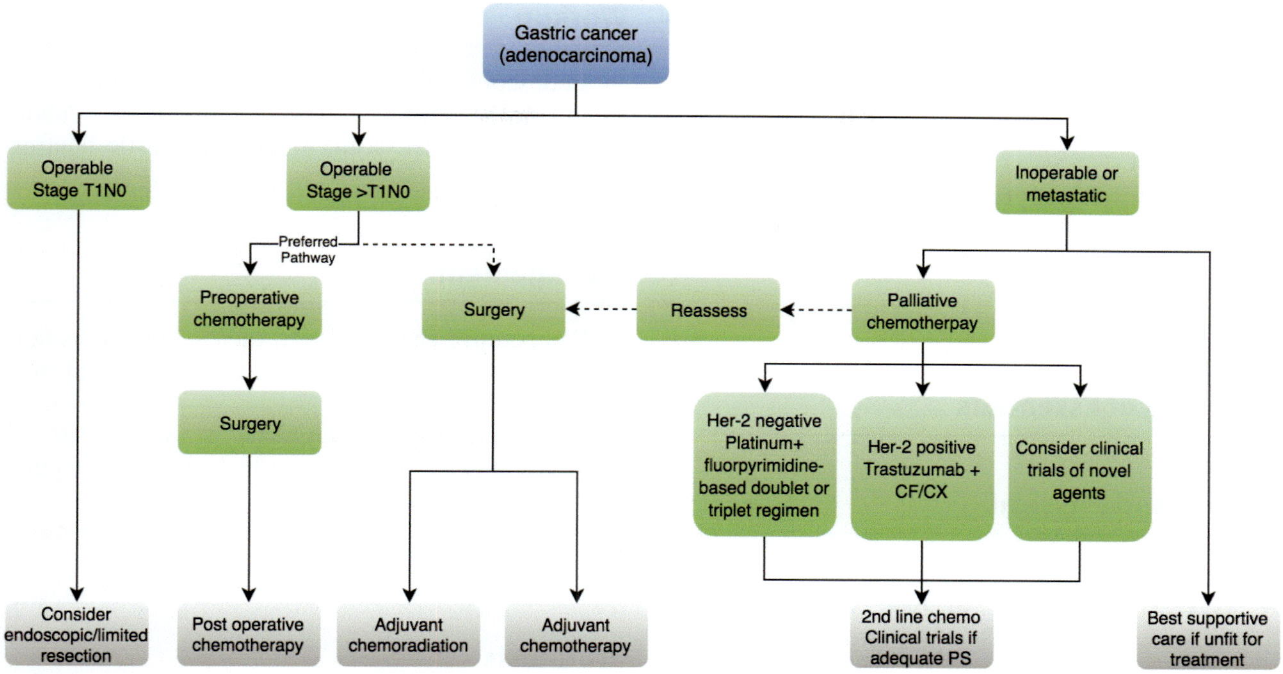

Fig. 51.2 Algorithm for gastric cancer

> **Watch Out**
> At least 16 lymph nodes are necessary for adequate staging of gastric adenocarcinoma.

What Is the Role of HER2 Gene Amplification and Chemotherapy?

HER2 overexpression has been recognized as a molecular abnormality that increases the aggressive nature of breast cancer. More recently, evidence reveals the role of HER2 overexpression in gastric cancer patients leading to poorer outcomes and more aggressive disease. Similar to breast cancer, the HER2 gene has been recognized to respond to certain chemotherapy agents, such as trastuzumab, and therefore, patients with gastric cancer should have genetic testing for the HER2 gene prior to the induction chemotherapy.

How Is GIST Treated?

The standard treatment of GIST is surgical resection. For patients with tumors that are large, not amenable to resection, or have a high risk of recurrence, a tyrosine kinase inhibitor (e.g., imatinib) may be prescribed in the neoadjuvant or adjuvant setting.

Complications

What Are the Common Complications That Can Occur After a Gastric Resection?

Diarrhea, early satiety, dumping syndrome, anastomotic leak, afferent limb syndrome, internal hernia, small bowel obstruction and marginal ulceration.

How Are Anastomotic Leaks Identified and Treated?

Patients with anastomotic leaks in the gastrointestinal tract will present with abdominal pain and varying degrees of peritonitis, fever, tachycardia, leukocytosis, and sepsis if not treated rapidly. If the patient is stable with no signs of peritonitis and there is concern for a gastric leak, an upper GI study with gastrografin can confirm the diagnosis. The primary treatment in any patient that has an anastomotic leak is source control. This typically involves percutaneous drainage and supportive care (bowel rest, antibiotics), though surgical washout and drainage may be required.

> **Watch Out**
> The initial management of a gastrointestinal anastomotic leak is source control with CT-guided drainage and NPO (nothing by mouth; not resection and/or diversion).

51

Summary of Essentials

History and Physical

- Gastric cancer is more common in men than women
- ALARM symptoms: anemia, loss of weight, anorexia, recent onset of progressive symptoms, melena/hematemesis or mass, swallowing difficulty, dyspepsia with age >55 years
- Often diagnosed late
- Once symptoms are present, cancer is already advanced

Pathophysiology

- The most common type: adenocarcinoma
- Two types of gastric adenocarcinoma: intestinal and diffuse
- More common in Asian countries
- The most common cause: *H. pylori* infection
- Intestinal-type gastric cancer occurs in the distal stomach and is usually associated with environmental factors
- Diffuse type is poorly differentiated, occurs most often in the proximal stomach, and is often related to congenital disorders
- Linitis plastica is the infiltration of the entire gastric wall with cancer in the submucosal plane (high mortality rate)
- GIST tumors are smooth, submucosal tumors that express c-KIT and CD-117

Workup

- Endoscopy is the study of choice for diagnosis
- Further staging with EUS, CT of the chest/abdomen/pelvis, PET scan, and/or diagnostic laparoscopy

Management

- Preoperative chemotherapy, then surgical resection, followed by postoperative chemotherapy, or chemoradiation
- Low-grade MALT lymphoma is treated with *H. pylori* eradication; high-grade lymphoma requires chemotherapy
- GIST is treated with surgical resection; may consider neoadjuvant or adjuvant imatinib if high risk

Prognosis

- Five-year mortality remains high as most patients present with advanced disease at diagnosis.

Acknowledgement The editors would like to acknowledge and thank the following authors for their contributions to the previous edition of the chapter: Sahil B. Gambhir.

Suggested Reading

Abdalla EK, Pisters PW. Staging and preoperative evaluation of upper gastrointestinal malignancies. Semin Oncol. 2004;31(4):513–29.

Ajani JA, Barthel JS, Bekaii-Saab T, et al., NCCN Gastric Cancer Panel. Gastric cancer. J Natl Compr Canc Netw. 2010;8(4):378–409.

Reyes CD, Weber KJ, Gagner M, Divino CM. Laparoscopic vs open gastrectomy. A retrospective review. Surg Endosc. 2001;15:928–31.

Ychou M, Boige V, Pignon J-P, et al. Perioperative chemotherapy compared with surgery alone for resectable gastroesophageal adenocarcinoma: an FNCLCC and FFCCD multicenter phase III trial. J Clin Oncol. 2011;29:1715–21.

Chest Pain After Vomiting

Jordan Shin and Brian R. Smith

Contents

C. de Virgilio, A. Grigorian (eds.), *Surgery*, https://doi.org/10.1007/978-3-032-09799-6_52

Case Study

A 55-year-old man with alcohol use disorder presents to the emergency department after experiencing severe chest pain. He is an obese male with a significant medical history that includes coronary artery disease, sleep apnea, hypercholesterolemia, as well as early liver cirrhosis. The patient states the chest pain started about 18 h ago, after consuming far too much food at a buffet and binge drinking leading to him feeling ill and forcefully vomiting. There was no blood in the vomitus. He states the pain is in his lower chest and radiates to the left side, back, and upper abdomen. The pain is aggravated by swallowing. At initial exam, his blood pressure is 105/90 mmHg, heart rate is 120/min, respiratory rate is 26/min, and temperature is 38.6 °C. He has crepitus with palpation around the sternum. His abdomen is soft and non-tender. A chest X-ray shows a left-sided pleural effusion. Laboratory examination is significant for a white blood count of $17 \times 10^3/\mu L$ (normal 4.1–10.9 × $10^3/\mu L$) with 15% bands (normal <5% bands). Serum troponin-I is 0.1 ng/mL (normal <0.4 ng/mL).

Diagnosis

What Is the Differential Diagnosis? (Table 52.1)

Watch Out

Boerhaave's syndrome has high mortality if not recognized and treated in a timely fashion. The mortality rate is significantly greater in those that have a delay in diagnosis beyond 24 h.

What Is the Most Likely Diagnosis?

In a patient presenting with chest pain after forceful vomiting (retching), accompanied by crepitus with palpation around the sternum, a left-sided pleural effusion, and evidence of a systemic inflammatory response (fever, tachycardia, leukocytosis with a left shift), the most likely diagnosis is Boerhaave's syndrome, a type of spontaneous esophageal rupture.

Table 52.1 Differential diagnosis for case presentation

Diagnosis	Comments
Myocardial infarction	Chest pain, more on the left side, left arm and jaw pain, diaphoresis, ST-segment elevation, and elevated troponins
Pericarditis	Substernal, pleuritic chest pain, worse supine, better leaning forward, fever, tachycardia, friction rub, pulsus paradoxus
Pneumothorax	Chest pain, shortness of breath, tachycardia, decreased/absent breath sounds on the affected side
Pneumonia	Shortness of breath, fever, fatigue, productive cough, and decreased breath sounds on the affected side
Aortic dissection	Shearing or tearing chest pain radiating to upper back, shortness of breath, differences in blood pressure in arms, impending doom, severe hypertension, history of Marfan syndrome
Peptic ulcer disease	Postprandial epigastric abdominal pain, nausea, vomiting, bloating
Acute pancreatitis	Epigastric pain radiating to the back, nausea, vomiting, anorexia, cholelithiasis, alcohol abuse, elevation of amylase/lipase
Mallory-Weiss tear	Forceful vomiting and retching, followed by upper GI bleed, typically in alcoholic or bulimic patients, often resolves spontaneously
Boerhaave's syndrome	Forceful vomiting and retching, followed by chest pain and sepsis typically in patient with alcohol use disorder or bulimia patients, crepitus with palpation around the sternum, left-sided pleural effusion

52

History and Physical

What Are the Risk Factors for Boerhaave's Syndrome?

Patients with alcoholic use disorder have the greatest risk. Binge drinking places patients at risk of forceful vomiting/retching. It can also occur in patients who overeat, which results in aggressive vomiting, those with bulimia, and in those with a hiatal hernia. It most commonly occurs in males 50–70 years old.

Why Is Boerhaave's Syndrome So Often Unrecognized?

Given its mediastinal location, esophageal perforation does not cause peritonitis. Symptoms can be vague. There is a robust differential for a patient who presents with chest pain. Therefore, its manifestations mimic many other diseases.

What Is Mackler's Triad?

Mackler's triad (vomiting, chest pain, and subcutaneous emphysema) is highly suggestive of the diagnosis of Boerhaave's syndrome. The chest pain is usually lower thoracic or retrosternal and is aggravated by swallowing. All three parts of the triad are found in less than one-third of cases, which often lead to a delay in diagnosis. The clinical symptoms most often observed, in decreasing order of frequency, are vomiting (84%), chest pain (79%), dyspnea (53%), epigastric pain (47%), and dysphagia (21%).

What Is the Most Specific Sign of an Esophageal Rupture?

Subcutaneous emphysema after forceful retching is pathognomonic for esophageal rupture. This is identified on physical exam by crepitus with palpation around the sternum. Unfortunately, this finding is not very sensitive, as it is only seen in a minority of patients. Due to the heart beating against air-filled tissues, *Hamman's sign* can be heard over the precordium in mediastinal emphysema. Hamman's sign is a crunching, rasping sound, synchronous with the heartbeat.

What Are the Similarities and Differences Between Boerhaave's Syndrome and Mallory-Weiss Tear? (Table 52.2)

Table 52.2 Comparing boerhaave's syndrome and mallory-weiss tear

	Boerhaave's syndrome	Mallory-Weiss
Population	Alcohol use disorder/bulimia, forceful vomiting	Alcohol use disorder/ bulimia,forceful vomiting
Pathophysiology	*Full-thickness* rupture of the esophagus secondary to increased intragastric pressure	*Partial tear* of mucosal/ submucosa in stomach cardia at gastroesophageal junction, secondary to increased intragastric pressure
Presentation	Thoracic pain radiating to back, left-sided pleural effusion, shortness of breath	Hematemesis
Natural course	Can progress to sepsis and death; may require immediate surgical repair and/or drainage	Most resolve spontaneously; surgery rarely indicated

Pathophysiology

What Are the Most Common Causes of Esophageal Perforation?

The majority of cases of esophageal perforation result from iatrogenic injury, with upper endoscopy being the most frequent cause. Additional causes include traumatic injury (either blunt or penetrating), foreign body ingestion, and malignancy eroding through the esophageal wall. A smaller proportion, approximately 10–20%, are spontaneous perforations, classically referred to as Boerhaave's syndrome. This typically results from a sudden, forceful emesis against a closed cricopharyngeus muscle, leading to a rapid increase in intraesophageal pressure and full-thickness rupture of the esophageal wall.

Why Do Patients with Boerhaave's Syndrome Become So Septic?

The esophageal perforation leads to gross contamination of the mediastinum, predominately with saliva (one of the dirtiest fluids in the body) but also with gastric contents (undigested food particles) and refluxed bile. The perforation often leads to rupture of the pleura as well, which is likely secondary to the gastric and bilious contents eroding through the lining. Once the pleura has been disrupted, gross contamination of the pleural cavity also occurs. It is the mediastinitis and pleuritis that eventually lead to sepsis and multiorgan failure and, if left untreated, will ultimately result in death.

Watch Out

The esophageal tear in Boerhaave's syndrome typically occurs 3–5 cm above the gastroesophageal junction on the *left* side.

Workup

What Is the First Step in Workup for a Patient Suspected of Having Boerhaave's Syndrome?

When a patient presents with chest pain and sepsis, esophageal perforation should be suspected. The initial study should be a chest radiograph. The most common findings are usually left sided and include a pleural effusion and atelectasis. It may also demonstrate pneumomediastinum or a left pneumothorax. It should be noted, however, that a normal chest X-ray will be seen in about 20% of patients. A normal chest X-ray may be due to the fact that the perforation is small, contained within the mediastinum or has sealed, or in the case of iatrogenic perforation, that sufficient time has not passed for air to be present.

Watch Out

Boerhaave's syndrome can easily be confused with pneumonia as both may have a left pleural effusion.

What Is the Role of Oral Contrast Studies in Diagnosing Boerhaave's Syndrome? How About CT?

CT scan with oral contrast is the diagnostic modality of choice for suspected esophageal perforation, including Boerhaave's syndrome. It offers superior sensitivity compared to chest X-ray and traditional contrast esophagography. It may show extraluminal air, provide additional information regarding the location and extent of the perforation, and whether the perforation is contained or freely leaking, as well as the presence of fluid collections. CT also allows for the evaluation of alternative diagnoses such as aortic dissection or pneumonia. While water-soluble contrast esophagography may still be considered in equivocal cases, it is generally reserved as a secondary study when CT findings are nondiagnostic.

What Type of Contrast Should Be Used?

For suspected esophageal perforation, oral contrast-enhanced CT is the preferred initial test, typically using a water-soluble agent such as gastrografin. While gastrografin carries a risk of pneumonitis if aspirated, it is generally well tolerated and preferred over barium due to the latter's potential toxicity if leakage into the peritoneal cavity occurs. Barium is more sensitive for detecting small leaks and may be used following a negative gastrografin study, particularly after esophageal surgery to evaluate for anastomotic dehiscence.

Is There a Role for Endoscopy During Diagnosis?

There is generally no role for endoscopy when perforation is suspected. The concern is that insufflation of air may reopen a sealed perforation or enlarge the perforation.

Management

What Are the Initial Steps in the Management of a Patient with Boerhaave's Syndrome?

As soon as the diagnosis of Boerhaave's syndrome is made, medical management should be initiated in an attempt to treat sepsis. This includes initiating intravenous (IV) fluid resuscitation, placing the patient nothing by mouth (NPO), and starting broad-spectrum antibiotics that cover oral bacteria, as well as an antifungal. An H_2 blocker or proton pump inhibitor should also be initiated to reduce gastric acid secretions.

Watch Out

Remember to start antifungals, in addition to antibiotics in patients with esophageal or gastric perforation.

Does the Time Interval Between Perforation and Intervention Matter?

Yes, time is of the essence. The key to optimal management is the early detection and treatment, ideally within 24 h. Treatment delays greater than 24 h may double the mortality rate.

What Are The Three Main Treatment Options, and How Do You Decide Which One To Choose?

The three treatment options are conservative management, stenting and surgery (Fig. 52.1).

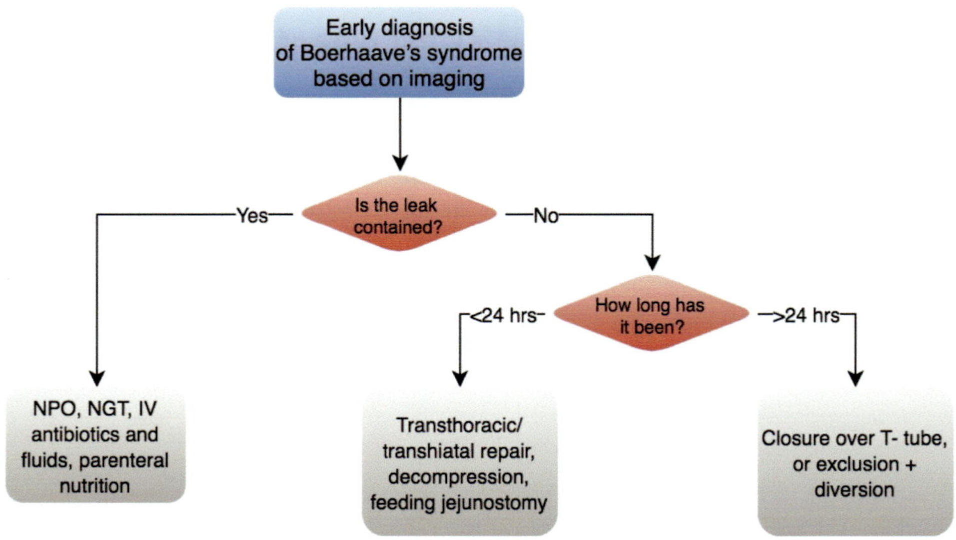

Fig. 52.1 Algorithm for the treatment of a patient with Boerhaave's syndrome

Which Patients Are Appropriate for Conservative Management, and What Does It Constitute?

Conservative (nonoperative) management is an accepted treatment in patients with no signs of sepsis or septic shock, a perforation that has been present for less than 24 h, and a leak that is small and contained or has sealed itself—which happens often. Conservative management consists of continuous nasogastric suction (with careful insertion), intravenous broad-spectrum antibiotics/antifungals, and parenteral nutrition. Repeat imaging should be performed on hospital day 4 or 5 to evaluate for spontaneous closure of the perforation. If there are no signs of extravasation, oral liquid intake may be resumed. Oral antibiotics should be continued for 1–2 weeks, depending on the clinical picture. Currently, there is an approximate 10% failure rate using medical management.

When Is Stenting the Best Option?

Covered stents, placed endoscopically, are considered for patients who fail medical management or for those that have evidence of ongoing esophageal leakage who are either deemed a poor surgical candidates (either due to comorbidities, hemodynamic instability, or presenting very late).

What Are the Surgical Options for a Patient with Boerhaave's Syndrome?

Surgery is indicated if the esophageal perforation has not spontaneously sealed (free leakage into mediastinum or chest), and the patient is a good operative risk, especially if they are exhibiting signs of sepsis (and therefore a need for drainage of the infection). The two main options are primary closure of the perforation and esophageal resection. Primary closure is preferred especially if the perforation is small and recent. All devitalized tissue surrounding the perforation must be debrided in order for surgical treatment to be successful. This includes debridement of the mediastinum as well as the pleura. Following suture closure of the perforation, a reinforcement flap (consisting of a strip of pleura and/or intercostal muscle) should be placed over the suture line to support the closure as well as decrease the chance of a leak, followed by copious irrigation and drainage. With a large hole, or with a prolonged delay, successful primary closure is unlikely, and esophagectomy will be needed. The esophagus is later reconstructed with interposed colon or jejunum.

What Is the Prognosis of a Patient with Boerhaave's Syndrome?

The mortality rates of Boerhaave's syndrome exceed 90% if left untreated and up to 40% after surgical intervention. Death occurs secondary to contamination of the mediastinum and pleura, which eventually leads to sepsis, septic shock, and multiorgan failure. Even with early intervention, mortality is as high as 25%. Delayed time to the operating room is associated with increased mortality. Patients with small, contained leaks without signs of sepsis can be managed nonoperatively with good outcomes.

Area of Controversy

How Effective Are Endoscopic Options for a Patient with Boerhaave's Syndrome?

Endoscopic stent placement is increasingly used in the management of Boerhaave's syndrome, especially in patients with significant comorbidities or those deemed poor surgical candidates. When performed by experienced endoscopists in centers with multidisciplinary expertise, stent therapy can be a viable alternative to surgery. However, observational studies have noted higher rates of reintervention and persistent leak compared to surgical repair. While endoscopic therapy is becoming increasingly used, especially for contained perforations, it is not yet considered the standard of care in all cases. The decision to pursue endoscopic versus surgical management should be individualized and made in consultation with thoracic surgery. Further studies are needed to better define patient selection criteria and long-term outcomes.

Summary of Essentials

History and Physical

- Patients with bulimia and alcohol use disorder are at risk for Boerhaave's syndrome after forceful emesis.
- Iatrogenic injury by upper endoscopy is the most common cause of esophageal perforation.

- Boerhaave's syndrome most commonly presents with thoracic pain radiating to lower back and aggravated by swallowing.
- Mackler's triad (chest pain, vomiting, and subcutaneous emphysema) is suggestive of Boerhaave's syndrome but is found in less than one-third of cases.

Pathophysiology

- Boerhaave's syndrome is a transmural esophageal perforation secondary to increased intragastric pressure induced by vomiting; Mallory-Weiss is from a partial-thickness tear

Workup

- Chest X-ray should be the initial study; look for left-sided pleural effusion, atelectasis, pneumothorax; can be normal in early disease
- Pneumomediastinum after vomiting is pathognomonic
- CT scan of the chest with water-soluble oral contrast should be performed to confirm the diagnosis
- Serum lactate, blood cultures

Management

- Initiate IV fluid resuscitation, NPO, broad-spectrum IV antibiotics and antifungals.
- The time interval between perforation and intervention is critical to the outcome (within 24 h).
- Conservative management with continuous nasogastric suction, intravenous broad-spectrum antibiotics/antifungals, IV fluids, and parenteral nutrition may be considered in healthy patients who have mild sepsis and a sealed perforation or small perforation contained within the mediastinum.
- Gold standard (and with free perforation into chest) is left thoracotomy, with debridement of the necrotic tissue surrounding the perforation, primary suture closure, and coverage with a pedicle flap (pleura, fundoplication, omentum), and wide drainage
- Endoscopic stents are being used more often, but this is not yet considered the standard of care.

Acknowledgements The editors would like to acknowledge and thank the following authors for their contributions to the previous edition of the chapter: Tiffany T. Pham.

Suggested Reading

Griffiths EA, Yap N, Poulter J, Hendrickse MT, Khurshid M. Thirty-four cases of esophageal perforation: the experience of a district general hospital in the UK. Dis Esophagus. 2009;22(7):616–25.

Horwitz B, Krevshy B, Buckman RF Jr, Fisher RS, Dabezies MA. Endoscopic evaluation of penetrating esophageal injuries. Am J Gastroenterol. 1993;88(8):1249–53.

Levy MM, Evans LE, Rhodes A. The surviving sepsis campaign bundle: 2018 update. Intensive Care Med. 2018;44:925–8.

Scheigert M, Beattie R, Solymosi N, Booth K, Dubecz A, Muir A, Moskorz K, Stadhuber RJ, Ofner D, McGuigan J, Stein HJ. Endoscopic stent insertion versus primary operative management for spontaneous rupture of the esophagus (Boerhaave syndrome): an international study comparing the outcome. Am Surg. 2013;79:643.

Upper Gastrointestinal Bleeding

Question Set: Upper Gastrointestinal Bleeding

Questions

1. A 26-year-old man presents with a 6-month history of intermittent difficulty swallowing solid foods. He states that he sometimes has to drink water to help push food down and has had several episodes where food became stuck, requiring him to regurgitate. He denies difficulty swallowing liquids, heartburn, weight loss, or chest pain. His medical history is significant for asthma and seasonal allergies. Upper endoscopy reveals concentric ring-like indentations, longitudinal furrows, and scattered white plaques in the mid-esophagus. What is the most likely diagnosis?
   (A) Achalasia
   (B) Gastroesophageal reflux disease (GERD)
   (C) Eosinophilic esophagitis
   (D) Esophageal adenocarcinoma
   (E) Infectious esophagitis

2. A 70-year-old male with a history of smoking presents with vague upper abdominal and epigastric pain and coffee ground emesis. On esophagogastroduodenoscopy (EGD), a small ulcer is found in the stomach, with evidence of a large submucosal mass underneath the ulcer. Biopsy of the area is negative. CT scan confirms a 4-cm homogeneous, well-circumscribed, submucosal mass in the greater curvature of the stomach. What does this mass most likely represent?
   (A) Gastrointestinal stromal tumor (GIST)
   (B) Gastric adenocarcinoma
   (C) Gastric lipoma
   (D) Metastatic carcinoma
   (E) Solitary fibrous tumor

3. A 65-year-old female presents with recurrent coffee ground emesis. She has had vague upper abdominal pain for the past 2 months, relieved by taking antacids. In addition, she reports an involuntary weight loss of 10 lbs. She denies nonsteroidal anti-inflammatory drug (NSAID) or alcohol use. On physical examination, her blood pressure is 110/70 mmHg and pulse is 80/min. Abdominal examination reveals mild epigastric tenderness with no rebound or guarding. Laboratory values are significant for hemoglobin of 8.3 g/dL (normal 12–15 g/dL) and hematocrit of 24% (36–44%) with a mean corpuscular volume (MCV) of 80 fL (80–100 fL), total bilirubin of 3.0 mg/dL (0.1–1.2 mg/dl), alkaline phosphatase of 250 IU/L (33–131 IU/L), gamma-glutamyl transferase (GGT) of 270 IU/L (6–37 IU/L), alanine transaminase (ALT) of 300 IU/L (<35 IU/L), and aspartate transaminase (AST) of 320 IU/L (<35 IU/L). The most likely diagnosis is:
   (A) Duodenal ulcer
   (B) Gastric ulcer
   (C) Pancreatic cancer
   (D) Ampullary cancer
   (E) Dieulafoy's lesion

4. A 50-year-old Asian female complains of abdominal discomfort and weight loss. She has an esophagogastroduodenoscopy (EGD) performed, and biopsy of a stomach lesion returns as mucosa-associated lymphoid tissue (MALT) lymphoma. Which of the following is the best treatment plan for this patient?
   (A) Chemotherapy
   (B) Radiation therapy
   (C) Combined chemotherapy and radiation
   (D) Clarithromycin, amoxicillin, and a proton pump inhibitor
   (E) Gastric resection

5. Which of the following is the first step in the treatment of a patient with Boerhaave's syndrome?
   (A) Esophagectomy
   (B) Gastric decompression
   (C) Drainage of the mediastinum and pleura
   (D) Primary repair of the perforation with advancement flap coverage
   (E) Fluid resuscitation and intravenous (IV) antibiotics

6. A 65-year-old male presents with iron deficiency anemia. Fecal occult blood testing is positive. Upper endoscopy demonstrates an irregular ulcer in the body of the stomach. Biopsy confirms adenocarcinoma. Which of the following would be the next best step in the management?
   (A) Proceed to gastric resection
   (B) CT scan of the abdomen
   (C) Positron emission tomography (PET) scan
   (D) Endoscopic ultrasound (EUS)
   (E) Chemotherapy

7. A 50-year-old female presents with massive upper GI bleeding. She appears to be lethargic and pale. Blood pressure is 70/50 mmHg, heart rate is 120/min, and respiratory rate is 22/min. The next step in the management is:
   (A) Emergent upper endoscopy
   (B) Transport to the operating room (OR)
   (C) Place bed in Trendelenburg position
   (D) Give two-liter bolus of normal saline
   (E) Insert nasogastric (NG) tube

8. A 48-year-old male presents with vomiting of bright red blood. He states that he has had a 1-month history of epigastric pain that is relieved by eating food. He denies weight loss. He does not take any medications or drink alcohol. He is hemodynamically stable in the emergency department. Following resuscitation, the patient undergoes upper endoscopy which reveals a posterior ulcer in the proximal duodenum which is actively bleeding. Despite numerous attempts at cauterization and injection with epinephrine, the gastroenterologist reports that she cannot stop the bleeding and the blood pressure drops to 70/50 mmHg. The next step in the management is:
   (A) Angiographic embolization
   (B) Transfer to ICU for ongoing transfusion of blood
   (C) Administer vasopressin
   (D) Exploratory laparotomy
   (E) Administer octreotide

9. A 45-year-old male with a history of alcohol use disorder presents to the emergency department with an upper GI bleeding after a night of binge drinking. The patient reports that he repeatedly dry heaved, after which he began to note bright red blood in the vomitus. He is afebrile with normal vital signs. Upper endoscopy reveals a partial

tear in the mucosa and submucosa of the stomach near the gastroesophageal junction. Which of the following is true about this condition?

(A) It is usually related to portal hypertension
(B) It is often associated with a left pleural effusion
(C) It is associated with Helicobacter pylori infection
(D) The bleeding is likely arising from the gastroduodenal artery
(E) The bleeding most often stops spontaneously

10. A 60-year-old male presents with gnawing epigastric pain that has been present for 8 weeks. The pain seems to get worse with eating. He denies nausea, vomiting, or early satiety. He has lost 10 lbs. and he attributes this to a poor appetite. He denies black or bloody stools. Physical examination is unremarkable. What is the next study to be ordered?

(A) Barium swallow
(B) CT scan
(C) Esophagogastroduodenoscopy (EGD)
(D) Six-week trial of proton pump inhibitor
(E) Testing for H. pylori

11. Which of the following is the strongest risk factor for gastric cancer?

(A) Type A blood
(B) H. pylori infection
(C) Smoking
(D) Familial adenomatous polyposis
(E) Family history

12. A 58-year-old man presents to the emergency department with severe chest pain that began after an episode of forceful vomiting. He describes the pain as sharp and radiating to his upper back. He is tachycardic and tachypneic. Physical examination reveals subcutaneous crepitus over the upper chest. Chest X-ray reveals a left pleural effusion and pneumomediastinum. What is the most appropriate next diagnostic step?

(A) Chest CT with oral contrast
(B) Emergent upper endoscopy
(C) Insert left chest tube
(D) Chest X-ray in lateral decubitus position
(E) Serial troponins and ECG monitoring

13. Which of the following is true of Boerhaave's syndrome?

(A) It most often presents with upper GI bleeding
(B) It is most often caused by an iatrogenic injury
(C) It is a partial-thickness tear of the esophagus
(D) It is the most lethal GI perforation
(E) It will require a thoracotomy

14. A young man from Armenia arrives to the emergency department complaining of a progressively bloody cough. He reports night sweats and fevers for the past month. He has been in the United States for 1 week visiting family. As you begin examining him, he coughs up a massive amount (200 mL) of bright red, foamy sputum, and has difficulty speaking. Portable chest X-ray shows multifocal patchy and cavitary opacities in the right upper lobe with mediastinal lymphadenopathy. Given his increased risk for asphyxiation, the patient is intubated and placed in a right lateral decubitus position. What is the next best step in management?

(A) Emergent thoracotomy
(B) Bronchoscopy
(C) Video-assisted thoracic surgery (VATS)
(D) Emergency arteriography
(E) Isoniazid (INH), rifampin, ethambutol, and pyrazinamide

15. A 50-year-old male presents to the emergency department stating that he passed a large amount of maroon stool earlier in the day. He is currently not passing any stool. He has not vomited. He denies abdominal pain or weight loss. He also has a history of nosebleeds. He takes no medications and does not drink alcohol. Physical examination is only significant for small red nodules on his lips. Abdominal examination is unremarkable. Upper endoscopy is negative. Which of the following is most likely to localize the site of the GI bleeding?
    (A) Capsule endoscopy
    (B) CT angiogram
    (C) Lower endoscopy
    (D) Formal angiography
    (E) Technetium-labeled red blood cell scan

16. Successful eradication of *H. pylori* is best documented by:
    (A) EGD with biopsy
    (B) Urea breath test
    (C) Blood antibody test
    (D) Stool antigen
    (E) Documentation is unnecessary provided symptoms have resolved

17. A 65-year-old male presents with melena. He reports no abdominal pain and no vomiting. He denies a prior similar history. In the emergency department, he is tachycardic to 120/min with a blood pressure of 112/80 mmHg. Hemoglobin and hematocrit are 9.2 g/dL (normal 13–16 g/dL) and 28% (40–52%), respectively. Past history is significant for an aortobifemoral bypass 5 years earlier for severe claudication. The patient is admitted to the ICU for resuscitation, the melena ceases, and the hematocrit stabilizes. Upper endoscopy is negative, with no stigmata of bleeding. Following a bowel prep, colonoscopy is also negative. CT scan of the abdomen reveals gas around the proximal aortic graft. Which of the following is true about this condition?
    (A) Formal angiography is likely to demonstrate the source of bleeding
    (B) Gas around the aortic graft is not considered pathologic
    (C) The aortic graft will need to be removed
    (D) Rebleeding is rare
    (E) It will likely resolve with antibiotics

Answers

1. Answer C
   This young man with a history of atopic disease presenting with intermittent solid-food dysphagia without liquid dysphagia and typical endoscopic findings has eosinophilic esophagitis, an allergic inflammatory disorder of the esophagus mediated by a Th2 immune response to food antigens. Endoscopy commonly shows longitudinal furrows, white exudates, and concentric ring-like indentations ("trachealization" of the esophagus). Diagnosis is confirmed via biopsy demonstrating ≥15 eosinophils per high-power field. Treatment includes dietary modification, proton pump inhibitors, and swallowed topical corticosteroids (i.e., budesonide). Achalasia typically causes progressive dysphagia to both solids and liquids and is associated with impaired relaxation of the lower esophageal sphincter (A). GERD can cause dysphagia but does not present with trachealization or eosinophilia on biopsy (B). Esophageal adenocarcinoma usually presents with progressive dysphagia and systemic symptoms like weight loss in older individuals (D). Infectious esophagitis is more common in immunocompromised patients and presents acutely with odynophagia and ulcerations, not concentric rings (E).

2. Answer A
   GISTs are mesenchymal tumors that most often occur in the stomach and small intestine. GISTs often originate from the interstitial cells of Cajal and are typically positive for c-KIT (CD117) on immunohistochemistry. As they grow, they can cause pressure necro-

sis, leading to erosion of the gastric mucosa and GI bleeding. Since the mass is submucosal, attempts at biopsy at the time of upper endoscopy are often negative and may cause bleeding. CT scan typically shows a well-circumscribed homogeneous mass. GISTs are caused by a gain of function mutation (tumorigenesis) in the proto-oncogene c-KIT. Treatment is surgical resection, followed by imatinib mesylate, a selective tyrosine kinase inhibitor with action against mutant c-KIT. Gastric adenocarcinoma starts in the mucosa; it would be unlikely to be biopsy negative (B). A lipoma or a solitary fibrous tumor would not likely erode into the mucosa (C, E). Skin cancer can metastasize to the stomach but does not typically present with a well-circumscribed mass (D).

3. Answer D

The patient is presenting with an unusual combination of an upper GI bleeding (coffee ground emesis) and obstructive jaundice (elevated bilirubin and rise in alkaline phosphatase with proportional rise in ALT and AST). Of the five options, ampullary cancer is the one that would most likely present as such. Pancreatic cancer, though it certainly can cause pain, weight loss, as well as obstructive jaundice, is not associated with iron deficiency anemia or upper GI bleeding (C). Dieulafoy's lesion typically presents with massive upper GI bleeding, due to an abnormally located superficial arteriole that erodes (E). Diagnosis is difficult as it causes a pinpoint bleed that can only be seen when actively bleeding. Duodenal or gastric ulcers would not cause obstructive jaundice (A–B).

4. Answer D

MALT lymphoma is strongly associated with *H. pylori* infection and is unique in that it is potentially curable with antibiotics (i.e., triple therapy). Eradication of *H. pylori* often leads to regression of the lymphoma, particularly in early-stage disease. In addition to biopsy, testing for *H. pylori* should be performed. After triple therapy, cure should be confirmed. If it is determined that triple therapy has failed, other modalities such as chemotherapy, radiation therapy, a combination of both, and/or surgery are utilized (A–C, E).

5. Answer E

All patients presenting with possible esophageal perforation should receive immediate IV fluids and antibiotics for the treatment of sepsis. Gastric decompression, mediastinal and pleural drainage, and primary repair of the esophagus should occur after initial stabilization, ideally within 24 h (B–D). Esophagectomy is reserved for extreme cases with large perforation or wherein primary repair will cause stricture (A).

6. Answer D

EUS is performed as it assists with TNM staging. EUS has been proven to provide more accurate assessment of tumor size, depth, and locoregional lymph node involvement compared to radiographic imaging. Following EUS, the next step would be to perform a CT scan of the abdomen to look for distant metastasis and confirm that the patient is a surgical candidate (B). CT scanning will rule out liver metastasis as well as distant suspicious lymph nodes that were missed on EUS, either of which would preclude a curative resection. Though not the standard of care, PET scan is emerging as an accurate modality for detecting small metastases and lymph node involvement (C). The management of gastric adenocarcinoma is dependent on the staging of the tumor. Surgery with gastric resection is the only potentially curative therapy for resectable gastric cancer (A). Advanced gastric cancer should be considered for a multi-therapeutic approach with chemotherapy (E).

7. Answer D

The patient presented is suffering from a massive UGI bleeding. Management should always begin with the ABCs. Given the large amount of bleeding and hypotension, she needs fluid resuscitation with crystalloid. Trendelenburg helps to improve blood pressure but in this patient may increase risk of aspiration (C). The vast majority of UGI bleeds are controlled endoscopically, so surgery is rarely needed (B). Given the massive bleeding, blood will also likely need to be administered. In a patient with hemodynamic instability from GI bleeding, early transfusion of uncrossmatched O-negative blood should be initiated while awaiting type and cross. There is no value to placing an NG tube (E). Following resuscitation, emergent endoscopy to identify and treat the cause of the bleeding should be performed (A). Additionally, a Foley catheter should be placed to monitor urine output as an indication of the patient's volume status.

8. Answer D
The mainstay of therapy for upper GI bleeding is endoscopic intervention. Techniques utilized include injection of epinephrine, sclerosing agents, clips, and cauterization. On rare occasion, if the bleeding cannot be controlled, then urgent surgical intervention is indicated. In the above case, the appropriate intervention is to surgically open the duodenum and oversew the ulcer in four quadrants to assure the artery has been ligated. The gastroduodenal artery, posterior to the first portion of the duodenum, is the most common source of massive hemorrhage from duodenal ulcers. Continuing blood transfusion alone is not appropriate (B). Although angiographic embolization is occasionally utilized for GI bleeding in poor surgical risk patients, it would not be the first choice in someone who is hemodynamically unstable (A). Vasopressin and octreotide are used in the management of patients suffering from bleeding esophageal varices (C, E).

9. Answer E
The case represents a classic history and endoscopic findings for a Mallory-Weiss tear. The etiology is thought to be a sudden and rapid rise in the transmural pressure gradient at the gastroesophageal (GE) junction, associated with retching. It is most often seen following an alcoholic binge but can also be seen with any forceful vomiting or coughing. It is thought to more likely occur in patients with hiatal hernias. The tear is a longitudinal, partial thickness, in the stomach, near the GE junction. The left gastroduodenal artery is not involved (D). It usually resolves spontaneously. Endoscopic therapy (e.g., cautery or clip) is rarely needed. Though it is seen following an alcohol binge, it is not related to portal hypertension, or *H. pylori*, and does not cause a pleural effusion (A–B). Mallory-Weiss is not to be confused with Boerhaave's syndrome, which can also occur after forceful vomiting. In Boerhaave's syndrome, the rapid rise in intrathoracic pressure can cause a *full-thickness perforation* of the esophagus. The esophageal perforation results in esophageal contents spilling into the mediastinum and sometimes into the left chest, resulting in a left pleural effusion, subcutaneous emphysema, severe chest pain, and, if untreated, sepsis and death. Boerhaave's syndrome requires broad-spectrum antibiotics and emergent surgery to seal the esophageal perforation and drain the mediastinal infection.

10. Answer C
Epigastric pain and symptoms of dyspepsia are extremely common. It is reasonable in most young patients to start with a short trial of proton pump inhibitors (D). Alternatively, clinicians can employ the test-and-treat strategy in which they test for *H. pylori* first (E). Testing should only be done if the clinician plans to offer treatment for a positive test. However, in patients >55 years or in those with ALARM Symptoms (*a*nemia (iron deficiency), *l*oss of weight, *a*norexia, *r*ecent onset of progressive symptoms, *m*elena/hematemesis, *s*wallowing problems), upper endoscopy is required to rule out gastric cancer. CT scan is usually performed after EGD to evaluate for distant metastasis in patients suspected of having gastric cancer (B). Operative resection should not be undertaken until the diagnosis is confirmed and the tumor is staged. Barium swallow may identify gastric ulcers and infiltrating lesions, but it has a high false-negative rate and does not permit biopsy (A). Barium swallow may also be used to evaluate dyspepsia in younger patients.

11. Answer B
H. pylori is the strongest established risk factor for gastric cancer worldwide. *H. pylori* infections lead to gastritis, and without eradication of the infection, inflammatory changes may eventually lead to dysplasia and metaplasia. All the remaining choices increase one's risk of developing gastric cancer but are not considered to be as strong as *H. pylori* (A, C–E).

12. Answer A
This patient has findings concerning for esophageal perforation, which most commonly results from iatrogenic injury during endoscopy. Other causes include trauma, effort rupture (Boerhaave's syndrome), caustic ingestion, or pill esophagitis. Patients typically present with severe retrosternal chest pain radiating to the back, often following episodes of vomiting. Physical exam may reveal subcutaneous emphysema or crepitus, and systemic signs of inflammation such as tachycardia and tachypnea are common. Imaging findings on chest X-ray may include widened mediastinum, pneumomediastinum, pneumothorax, or pleural effusion. However, a CT scan with oral and IV contrast is the preferred next diagnostic study. Chest CT may show indirect signs of perforation such as esophageal wall thickening or mediastinal fluid but may also demonstrate extravasation of the oral contrast into the mediastinum or chest. Another useful study is a water-soluble contrast esophagogram. Emergent upper endoscopy is not typically used to evaluate suspected perforation as insufflation can worsen the injury and the procedure may miss small or contained leaks (B). If a free perforation is confirmed, the patient will likely require surgery to close the hole. A chest tube may eventually be needed, in combination with a thoracotomy, to drain the infection if perforation is confirmed (C). Chest X-ray in lateral decubitus position has minimal diagnostic utility in this context and is not indicated (D). Serial troponins and ECG are appropriate in evaluating cardiac causes of chest pain, but this clinical picture is more consistent with esophageal perforation (E). Once diagnosed, emergent surgical consultation is warranted for operative debridement and repair.

13. Answer D
Boerhaave's syndrome is the term used for a perforation of the esophagus that occurs following forceful emesis (iatrogenic perforation is not called Boerhaave's syndrome) (B). The full-thickness tear causes spillage of GI contents into the mediastinum and even the thorax (C). Since GI contents spill into the mediastinum instead of the peritoneum, the patient does not develop peritonitis. Rather, they often present with fever and chest pain. As such, the diagnosis is often delayed until the patient becomes severely septic. Among GI perforations, it has the highest overall mortality. Boerhaave's syndrome most often occurs in males between the ages of 50 and 70, after excessive intake of food and alcohol. Unlike Mallory-Weiss tears, Boerhaave's syndrome does not typically present with upper GI bleeding (A). Although some patient may require thoracotomy, if the perforation has sealed, treatment is with bowel rest and IV antibiotics. In poor-risk patients, a stent may be placed across the perforation in lieu of surgery (E). Outcomes are dependent on the timeliness of recognition and management.

14. Answer B
Massive hemoptysis with constitutional symptoms as described is likely from tuberculosis (TB). This is further supported by the patient's origin from a TB endemic area (e.g., Armenia, Mexico, Nigeria) and the chest X-ray findings. The most common cause of massive hemoptysis in the world is TB. Immediate intubation is indicated to protect the airway because of the massive amount of foamy sputum preventing him from being able to speak. In addition, any patient with bleeding from a pulmonary source needs to be placed in a dependent position (on the side of the bleeding source) to prevent blood from entering the contralateral lung. This is best done by a right lateral decubitus position in the above patient. The next best step in management involves localizing the source and controlling it with bronchoscopy. Emergent thoracotomy can be considered if initial management options fail to control bleeding (A). VATS offers a minimally

invasive surgical technique to treat certain lung and chest wall diseases but is not currently used much in the emergency setting (C). Angiography with embolization is a therapeutic option for massive hemoptysis, particularly if site of bleeding cannot be localized (D). INH, rifampin, ethambutol, and pyrazinamide are used to treat TB but will not address the patient's acute condition (E).

15. Answer A

Melena can either be from an upper or a lower GI source. The presentation is classic for hereditary hemorrhagic telangiectasia (HHT) (also known as Osler-Weber-Rendu), an autosomal dominant disorder characterized by recurrent epistaxis; telangiectasia/red nodules of the face, lips, and/or GI tract; arteriovenous malformations (AVM); and a family history. GI bleeding most often occurs in the stomach and small bowel. If upper endoscopy is unable to confirm bleeding in the stomach, a capsule endoscopy (gelatin capsule containing a video recorder is swallowed, eventually retrieved in the stool, and permits visualization of the entire bowel) or push enteroscopy is used to assess for small bowel bleeding. Push enteroscopy uses a longer enteroscope or pediatric colonoscope to visualize the proximal jejunum. The subsequent step would be to perform lower endoscopy (after a bowel preparation) (C). However, colonic telangiectasias are very uncommon. Formal angiogram would only be useful if the patient is actively bleeding at a rate of 1 mL/min (the patient is not currently bleeding), is an invasive procedure, and would not permit visualization of the extent of telangiectasias (D). Technetium-labeled red blood cell scan may be useful if the patient is actively bleeding (at a rate of 0.5 ml/min) but is particularly ineffective in localizing the site of bleeding in the small bowel (E). A CT angiogram would not demonstrate telangiectasias of the small bowel (though it would be useful for identifying hepatic AVMs) (B).

16. Answer B

Eradication may be confirmed by a urea breath test, fecal antigen test, or upper endoscopy performed 4 weeks or more after completion of therapy (D). Typically, noninvasive methods should be performed except in cases when a follow-up endoscopy is indicated (e.g., gastric cancer, preneoplastic lesions, MALT lymphoma) (A). Blood antibody test is unable to confirm eradication as immunoglobulin G (IgG) levels will remain elevated after the acute infection is resolved (C). Clinical resolution of symptoms is inappropriate in confirming eradication of *H. pylori*, particularly in the setting of gastric cancer (E).

17. Answer C

GI bleeding, in association with a history of aortobifemoral bypass, is due to an aortoenteric fistula until proven otherwise, a condition where the aortic graft has eroded into the fourth portion of the duodenum. Patients typically have a "herald" bleed, followed later by exsanguinating hemorrhage (D). The first diagnostic test of choice is an upper endoscopy, but in aortoenteric fistulas, it is typically negative as the bleeding results from erosion of the aortic graft into the fourth portion of the duodenum which is usually not well visualized with a standard scope. The negative endoscopy essentially rules out the most common causes of upper GI bleeding which include acute gastritis, as well as gastric and duodenal ulcers. The diagnosis of an aortoenteric fistula is notoriously difficult to make. Angiography is poor at showing any abnormalities with an aortoenteric fistula (A). With an aortoenteric fistula, the aortic graft by definition is infected. Air, fluid, or stranding around the graft on CT scan (beyond 6 weeks after surgery) would be considered pathologic and indicative of a graft infection (B). Delay in diagnosis can lead to catastrophic rebleeding, which has a high mortality rate. Treatment is to remove the graft. This is best done by replacing the infected graft with a human cadaver homograft in situ. Antibiotics alone would not resolve the problem (E).

Urology

Jeremy M. Blumberg

Contents

Scrotal Pain

Areg Grigorian, Fuad F. Elkhoury, and Jeremy M. Blumberg

Contents

C. de Virgilio, A. Grigorian (eds.), *Surgery*, https://doi.org/10.1007/978-3-032-09799-6_53

Case Study

A 14-year-old male presents to the emergency department with nausea, vomiting, and acute onset severe right scrotal pain that started 90 minutes ago while playing soccer. He vomited once soon after pain onset. He denies any trauma. He had a similar past episode 1 year ago that resolved spontaneously 10 minutes after onset. On physical examination, his temperature is 100^F, his right testicle is exquisitely tender to palpation, high riding, and fixed in the scrotum. The left testis is normal lying and non-tender with smooth contours. Right cremasteric reflex is absent.

Diagnosis

What Is the Differential Diagnosis? (▪ Table 53.1)

What Is the Most Likely Diagnosis for This Patient?

A 14-year-old male with acute onset scrotal pain, high riding and tender testicle with horizontal lie, and absent ipsilateral cremasteric reflex has testicular torsion until proven otherwise. Patients may report a similar prior episode.

History and Physical

What Is the Cremasteric Reflex?

The cremasteric reflex is an elevation of the ipsilateral testicle by the cremasteric muscle in response to a stroking motion at the medial aspect of the upper thigh. When the medial thigh is stroked, sensory fibers from the femoral branch of the genitofemoral nerve (L1–L2) are stimulated. The sensory input travels to the spinal cord, where it synapses with the motor nerve from the genital branch of the genitofemoral nerve (L1–L2) to activate the cremasteric muscle and cause ipsilateral elevation of the testis.

▪ **Table 53.1** Differential diagnosis for scrotal pain/mass

Diagnosis	Comments
Testicular torsion	Sudden onset in pubertal child (12–18 years), tender and swollen testicle that is displaced superiorly; mass may be felt in spermatic cord, *absent cremasteric reflex*, nausea, vomiting
Torsion of testicular or epididymal appendage (appendix testis)	Common cause of acute painful hemiscrotum in prepubertal child (7–14 years); the epididymal appendage (appendix testis) is located at the head of the epididymis; *blue-dot sign* is a classic but rare finding; onset of pain is more gradual; *cremasteric reflex is maintained*
Epididymitis and/or orchitis	Scrotal pain in young adult (20–39 years), second peak in men >60, relieved by supporting the scrotum, gradual onset, fever, dysuria, induration; sexually transmitted infections in younger men, *Escherichia coli* in older men; mumps less common; scrotal US showing hyperemia of testis/epididymis
Hydrocele	Fluid in the tunica vaginalis, *transilluminates*, may increase in size with Valsalva if communicating with peritoneum (usually in children), often spontaneously resolves by 1 year of age; idiopathic etiology in adults; may be reactive to inflammation/orchitis
Varicocele	Tortuous dilation of pampiniform plexus, *does not transilluminate;* increases in size with Valsalva, described as a "bag of worms"; may present as scrotal discomfort; may contribute to male infertility
Appendicitis	Anorexia, vague periumbilical abdominal pain, vomiting, localized right lower quadrant pain (McBurney's point)
Fournier's gangrene	Severe necrotizing infection in the perineal and scrotal region occurring most commonly in elderly patients with immunocompromise (diabetes)
Traumatic testicular rupture	History of trauma to scrotum, scrotal pain, hematocele and scrotal hematoma; disruption to the connective tissue enveloping the testicle (tunica albuginea)
Testis tumor	*Painless* testicular mass, does not transilluminate; seminomas (germ cell tumors) are the most common type and are malignant

What Would Cause an Absent Cremasteric Reflex?

The cremasteric reflex is absent with upper and lower motor neuron disorders, spinal cord injury affecting L1–L2 (genitofemoral nerve), accidental transection during hernia surgery, and testicular torsion. Although the cremasteric reflex is usually absent in testicular torsion, its presence does not exclude the diagnosis.

53

What Is the TWIST Score for Testicular Torsion?

The Testicular Workup for Ischemia and Suspected Torsion (TWIST) score is a 7-point tool to evaluate acute scrotal pain. The score includes testicular swelling (2 points), hard testis (2), high-riding testis (1), absent cremasteric reflex (1), and nausea/vomiting (1).

What Is Prehn's Sign? Is It Reliable?

Prehn's sign is positive when patients report pain relief with elevation of scrotal contents and negative when this does not relieve any pain. Classically, patients with epididymitis have a positive Prehn's sign, while testicular torsion patients have a negative sign. However, Prehn's sign is not a reliable distinguishing feature between testicular torsion and epididymitis, as a positive sign does not exclude the diagnosis of testicular torsion.

What Is the Blue-Dot Sign?

This is a pathognomonic sign (Fig. 53.1) for torsion of testicular or epididymal appendage (appendix testis). Palpation reveals a small, firm, tender nodule near the head of the epididymis with a blue discoloration visible through the scrotal skin.

What Are the Four Cardinal Symptoms and Signs of Testicular Torsion?

Nausea/vomiting, testicular pain duration of less than 24 hours, a superiorly displaced testicle, and an absent cremasteric reflex.

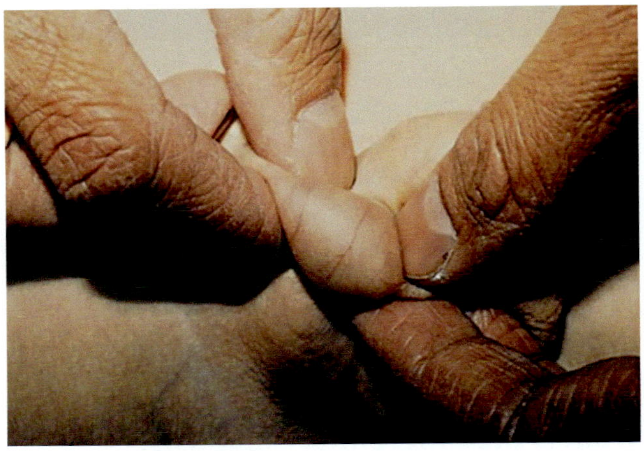

Fig. 53.1 Blue-dot sign. (From Kaplan GW, McAleer IM. Office urology. In: Poppas DP, Retik AB, editors. Pediatric urology. Atlas of clinical urology. London: Current Medicine Group; 2003. Reprinted with permission)

Does a History of Trauma or Presence of Fever Rule Out Testicular Torsion?

No. Some patients report the onset of pain while playing sports or after minor trauma, and they may therefore attribute the pain to a traumatic injury, rather than torsion. Torsion may be accompanied by fever (as well as nausea and vomiting), mimicking a gastrointestinal illness (as in this patient). Thus, it is critical to always examine the scrotum and testicles in adolescents with abdominal complaints.

Pathology/Pathophysiology

What Congenital Defect Predisposes Children to Developing Testicular Torsion?

Congenital defects of the processus vaginalis can lead to failure of the testis to attach to the inner lining of the scrotum (tunica vaginalis), increasing the risk of developing testicular torsion later in life, particularly during adolescence due to rapid testicular growth. In particular, patients with *bell-clapper deformity* are at increased risk of testicular torsion. This occurs when there is a failure of normal posterior anchoring of the gubernaculum, testes, and epididymis, allowing the testes to freely rotate and swing within the tunica vaginalis of the scrotum. This defect is bilateral in about 50% of patients, placing both testes at risk of torsion.

How Does Testicular Torsion Cause Ischemia?

With inadequate fixation of the testis to the tunica vaginalis, the testis twists around the spermatic cord. Typically, torsion initially impedes venous outflow. Arterial flow will subsequently be compromised as venous pressure rises, resulting in ischemia.

How Does One Distinguish Testicular Torsion from Acute Epididymitis?

Acute epididymitis tends to occur in older patients (mean age around 24 years vs. 14 years for torsion) and present with a more gradual onset (>24 hours). Acute epididymitis is associated with testicular swelling (less likely with torsion), dysuria, and worsening pain while standing.

Workup

How Does the TWIST Score Help in Determining What Additional Workup Should Occur?

Time is of the essence with testicular torsion to prevent testicular necrosis. If clinical suspicion is high, such as a TWIST score of 6 or 7, the patient should be taken emergently to the operating room without other tests or imaging. Different authors have used the TWIST score to help define high clinical suspicion as a TWIST score of ≥5 or ≥6.

If Suspicion of Testicular Torsion Is Intermediate, What Additional Workup Should Occur?

Urinalysis should always be ordered to rule out a urinary tract infection or epididymo-orchitis, as these may also present with scrotal pain. Doppler (blood flow) with ultrasound imaging of the scrotum should be obtained (but again only if equivocal clinical findings) provided it does not significantly delay treatment. In the presence of torsion, Doppler interrogation should demonstrate an absence of arterial blood flow in the affected testicle. The ultrasound can demonstrate other etiologies, such as a mass or evidence of trauma. Acute bleeding of testicular parenchyma appears hyperechoic, while older blood will appear hypoechoic (Fig. 53.2).

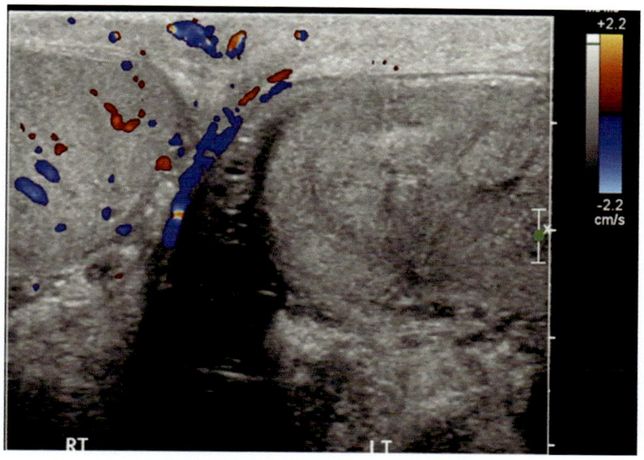

Fig. 53.2 Scrotal Doppler ultrasound showing absent flow in the left testis consistent with testicular torsion. Note: normal color flow in the right testicle (*left side of image*)

In the Trauma Setting, What Are the Most Important Things to Look for on Doppler Ultrasound?

To determine if the tunica albuginea is violated (testicular rupture), as this would warrant surgical repair in the acute setting. One should also confirm adequate blood flow to the testis which ensures that the vascular pedicle is intact. Since torsion often occurs during performance of sporting activities, there may be confusion as to whether the scrotal pain is from trauma or torsion. Absence of arterial flow suggests torsion or severe trauma that has disrupted the blood supply.

Management

In the Setting of Suspected Testicular Torsion, What Is the Optimal Timing from Initial Evaluation to Definitive Management?

The diagnosis of testicular torsion requires immediate surgical consultation. Timing is of the utmost importance because the viability of a torsed testicle depends on how long the testicle remains torsed. Studies suggest nearly 100% viability when detorsion is performed within 6 hours of symptom onset, 50% viability with detorsion after 12 hours, and less than 20% viability with detorsion after 24 hours.

Is There a Role for Manual Detorsion in the Emergency Department?

Manual detorsion may be difficult due to pain and should not replace or delay definitive operative detorsion. However, if immediate surgical intervention is not available, manual detorsion may be attempted with analgesia. In most cases the testes rotates medially during torsion. When facing the patient, manual detorsion involves rotating the right testicle counterclockwise or the left testicle clockwise toward the thigh. Even if manual detorsion is successful, the patient should still undergo surgical exploration.

> **Watch Out**
> While torsion most commonly occurs from medial rotation of the testes, lateral rotation is still possible. If manual detorsion with lateral rotation does not improve symptoms, medial rotation may be attempted.

What Is the Surgical Treatment for Testicular Torsion?

A scrotal exploration is performed and the testicle is untwisted. If the testicle appears ischemic, the surgeon should look for return of pink color and Doppler signals within the testicle and then perform an orchiopexy (testicle sutured to scrotal wall) so as to prevent recurrence. Since patients with torsion of one testicle are at risk of torsion of the contralateral one, bilateral orchiopexy is recommended at the time of surgery.

What If the Testicle Is Necrotic at the Time of Surgical Exploration?

An orchiectomy is performed.

What Is the Recommended Management for Minor Trauma to the Testes?

Minor trauma includes cases where there is no significant swelling, pain, or breaches in the integrity of the skin around the scrotum or the tunica albuginea encasing the testis. These patients can be treated conservatively with scrotal support, ice packs, and nonsteroidal anti-inflammatory drugs.

What Are the Operative Indications for Testicular Trauma?

Operative indications include suspicion of violation of the tunica albuginea, rapidly expanding testicular hematoma, avulsion of the testicular artery, scrotal degloving, and absence of testicular blood flow as evidenced on Doppler ultrasound. With the possible exception of superficial skin lesions, most clinicians elect to explore all penetrating testicular traumas in the operating room. Surgical exploration has proven to increase testicular salvage rates and preserve fertility. Earlier surgical intervention is associated with better outcomes. Delays in management increase the risk of testicular infarction.

What Is the Management of Acute Epididymitis?

Acute epididymitis is the most common cause of scrotal pain in adults. This often presents as unilateral pain and swelling that worsens over the course of several days. Exam may be notable for swelling and tenderness localized to the epididymis on the posterior testis. Pain may be relieved by elevation of the testes (Prehn's sign). Acute epididymitis is most often caused by sexually transmitted infections, particularly *Neisseria gonorrhoeae* and *Chlamydia trachomatis*. Treatment involves supportive care (scrotal elevation, ibuprofen) and antibiotics (ceftriaxone, doxycycline).

Does Loss of a Testicle from Torsion Affect Fertility?

Only one testicle is needed for fertility. In the majority of patients who lose a testicle, fertility is not affected. On occasion, testicular necrosis and loss from torsion can lead to the formation of antisperm antibodies with a subsequent decrease in sperm count and decrease in motility.

Areas Where You Can Get in Trouble

Penile Pain After Sexual Intercourse

An erect penis can fracture during intercourse rupturing the tunica albuginea. Patients may be too embarrassed to report the history leading to the fracture but will often report a "popping" sound heard during the injury. Penile fracture is a surgical emergency and needs to be recognized promptly to undergo corporal repair. Voiding symptoms including dysuria, urinary retention (no urine since the injury), and gross hematuria are rare but need to be worked up with a retrograde urethrogram to rule out a concomitant urethral injury.

Prostatitis

In a patient with a urinary tract infection, bacterial migration from the urethra to the prostate may lead to prostatitis. Typically, infection is caused by *E. coli* or other gram-negative bacteria. Acute prostatitis typically presents with symptoms of a urinary tract infection (dysuria, urgency, frequency) with associated flu-like symptoms (fever, chills, myalgias). It may lead to sepsis requiring hospitalization for intravenous antibiotics and supportive care. Exam is often notable for a tender and swollen prostate. However, vigorous palpation of the prostate in the acute setting may trigger bacteremia and subsequent sepsis. In contrast, chronic bacterial prostatitis may have more subtle symptoms and exam findings. Diagnosis is often made based on a history of chronic or recurrent urogenital symptoms and positive urinalysis, though expressed prostatic secretions may be obtained for confirmation. Typically, at least 6 weeks of antibiotic therapy with a fluoroquinolone or trimethoprim–sulfamethoxazole is required.

Summary of Essentials

Diagnosis

- Four cardinal signs/symptoms of testicular torsion
  - Nausea/vomiting
  - Testicular pain duration of less than 24 hours
  - Superiorly displaced testicle
  - Absent cremasteric reflex
- Apply the TWIST score
- High clinical suspicion is all that is needed to prompt intervention

History and Physical

- Prehn's sign classically negative for testicular torsion; however, this is not reliable
- Blue-dot sign is pathognomonic for appendix testes torsion
- Cremasteric reflex present in appendix testes torsion, absent with testicular torsion

Pathophysiology

- Congenital defects of the processus vaginalis can lead to failure of the testes to attach to the inner lining of the scrotum.
- Adolescent males have rapidly growing testes during puberty, thus predisposing them to testicular torsion.

Workup

- When high clinical suspicion for torsion, no further workup is necessary after history and physical exam.
- If clinical suspicion for torsion is low, urinalysis should always be ordered to rule out a urinary tract infection or epididymo-orchitis.
- If clinical suspicion is intermediate, obtain Doppler ultrasound, an absence of arterial blood flow in the affected testicle confirms diagnosis.
- In trauma setting, look for violation of tunica albuginea on ultrasound.

Management

- Patient should be taken directly to operating room (OR) for surgical detorsion and *bilateral* orchiopexy.
- If immediate surgical intervention is not available, attempt manual detorsion followed by bilateral orchiopexy
- Orchiectomy performed for necrotic testicle.

Suggested Reading

Cummings JM, Boullier JA, Sekhon D, Bose K. Adult testicular torsion. J Urol. 2002;167:2109.

Kapasi Z, Halliday S. Best evidence topic report. Ultrasound in the diagnosis of testicular torsion. Emerg Med J. 2005;22:559.

Mellick LB, Sinex JE, Gibson RW, Mears K. A Systematic Review of Testicle Survival Time After a Torsion Event. Pediatr Emerg Care. 2019;35(12):821–825. https://doi.org/10.1097/PEC.0000000000001287

Qin KR, Qu LG. Diagnosing with a TWIST: Systematic Review and Meta-Analysis of a Testicular Torsion Risk Score. J Urol. 2022 Jul;208(1):62–70. https://doi.org/10.1097/JU.0000000000002496. Epub 2022 Mar 3.

Rabinowitz R. The importance of the cremasteric reflex in acute scrotal swelling in children. J Urol. 1984;132:89.

Wampler SM, Llanes M. Common scrotal and testicular problems. Prim Care. 2010;37:613.

Yecies T, Bandari J, Schneck F, Cannon G. Direction of Rotation in Testicular Torsion and Identification of Predictors of Testicular Salvage. Urology. 2018;114:163–166. https://doi.org/10.1016/j.urology.2017.11.034

Scrotal Mass

Areg Grigorian, Fuad F. Elkhoury, and Jeremy M. Blumberg

Contents

C. de Virgilio, A. Grigorian (eds.), *Surgery*, https://doi.org/10.1007/978-3-032-09799-6_54

Case Study

A 22-year-old male presents with a left scrotal mass. He sustained mild trauma to the left hemiscrotum five weeks ago while playing basketball. The trauma prompted him to palpate his left testicle and he noted a left testicular mass. The patient states that he had mild pain initially that spontaneously resolved and denies any swelling. He says the mass has remained stable in size, like a large almond, and is located "in the middle" of the left testis. He denies subjective fevers, chills, dysuria, gross hematuria, or urethral discharge. Physical examination reveals a firm 2-cm mass within the left testis. There is no pain to palpation. There are no epididymal masses bilaterally, and the right testis is unremarkable. Abdominal exam reveals no masses and no hepatomegaly. There are no supraclavicular nodes and no gynecomastia. Laboratory analysis reveals a normal urinalysis and complete blood count.

Diagnosis

Why Is the Location of a Scrotal Mass Important to Identify?

Identifying the precise location allows for an accurate differential diagnosis based on anatomic origin (i.e., spermatic cord, epididymis, or testes).

Describe the Cause(s) of Scrotal Masses Found Involving the Skin (Table 54.1)

Table 54.1 Scrotal masses involving the skin

Etiology	Features
Epidermoid or pilar cysts	Develop from epidermis or hair follicle and present as painless, slow growing, mobile, fluid-filled nodules; they occur most commonly in areas that have a lot of hair (e.g., scrotum, chest)
Squamous cell carcinoma	Proliferation of squamous cells characterized by formation of keratin pearls; presents as ulcerated, nodular mass with no telangiectasias; occurs in the fifth or sixth decade; associated with human papillomavirus and occupational exposure (soot, oil, and petroleum workers)

What Is the Differential Diagnosis of Scrotal Masses Involving the Spermatic Cord? (Table 54.2)

Table 54.2 Differential diagnosis of scrotal masses involving the spermatic cord

Etiology	Features
Indirect inguinal hernia	Mass increases in size with Valsalva and emerges from internal ring, usually reducible (unless very large); increases in size with standing/Valsalva
Hydrocele	Painless, unilateral scrotal mass, does not extend up spermatic cord, normal testis, transilluminates with light, due to serous fluid accumulation within tunica vaginalis
Varicocele	Feels like a "bag of worms," more common on the left, also increases in size with standing/Valsalva (similar to hernia), does not transilluminate with light, associated with decreased sperm count and infertility

What Is the Differential Diagnosis of Scrotal Masses Involving the Epididymis? (Table 54.3)

Table 54.3 Differential diagnosis of scrotal masses involving the epididymis

Etiology	Features
Epididymitis	Painful, tender epididymis, associated with urinary tract infection or sexually transmitted infection; scrotal erythema/cellulitis, positive "Prehn's sign" (relief of pain with elevation)
Spermatocele	Also called epididymal cyst, benign, typically painless, fluid-filled mass, cephalad and distinct from the testis, may transilluminate with light
Torsion of testicular epididymal appendage (appendix testes)	Most common cause of acute painful hemiscrotum in a child; the epididymal appendage (appendix testis) is located at the head of the epididymis; blue-dot sign is a classic finding; onset of pain is more gradual; cremasteric reflex is maintained

What Is the Differential Diagnosis of Scrotal Masses Found Involving the Testes? (Table 54.4)

Table 54.4 Differential diagnosis of scrotal masses involving the testes

Etiology	Features
Orchitis	Painful, tender testicle, most often viral (mumps) but also bacterial, associated with sexually transmitted infection (in which case epididymis is also affected)
Testicular torsion	Sudden, severe onset of pain, testis high-riding, negative Prehn's sign (pain not alleviated with elevation), most common in pubescent males, also seen in neonates, loss of cremasteric reflex, *surgical emergency*
Testicular cancer	Presents as firm, painless testicular mass that does not transilluminate; seminoma (germ cell tumor) is the most common type

What Is the Most Likely Diagnosis for This Patient?

In a 22-year-old male with a painless, firm, non-tender testicular mass, testicular cancer is the most likely diagnosis. Despite a history of trauma, a young man (20–40 years old) with a testicular mass should be presumed to have testicular cancer until proven otherwise. Trauma to the scrotum or groin may prompt men to examine their testes leading to the discovery of an otherwise painless mass.

History and Physical

What Features on History and Physical Examination Favor the Diagnosis of Testicular Cancer?

Any painless mass within the testicle is cancer until proven otherwise. Most patients with testicular cancer present without symptoms and most are young adults (average age between 20 and 35 years). On physical exam, the mass is within the testicle (as opposed to separate from it). Rarely, patients with testicular cancer may also have gynecomastia secondary to hormonally active tumors (secreting human chorionic gonadotropin).

What Is the Implication of Constitutional Symptoms in Association with a Painless Testicular Mass?

The presence of constitutional symptoms in association with a painless testicular mass is highly suggestive of metastatic testicular cancer. Symptoms such as back or abdominal pain, weight loss, and nausea suggest retroperitoneal lymph node metastasis, whereas cough and shortness of breath suggest pulmonary metastasis.

What Risk Factors for Testicular Cancer Should Be Obtained on History?

The vast majority of patients have no risk factors. The main risk factor is cryptorchidism (undescended testicle). Other risk factors include personal history of testicular cancer (contralateral testicle), family history of testicular cancer, Klinefelter's syndrome, and white race.

What Features on Physical Examination Favor a Nonmalignant Etiology?

Masses that are bilateral, painful, mobile, and fluid-filled and that transilluminate are less likely to be cancerous.

What Are the Main Diagnoses to Consider in the Presence of a Very Painful Scrotal Mass?

Epididymitis and/or orchitis would be highest on the differential. During pubescence, testicular torsion and torsion of the appendix testis should be considered. An incarcerated hernia can be extremely painful but is separated from the testicle and epididymis.

What Benign Processes Are Typically Painless?

Spermatocele, varicocele, and hydrocele are usually painless. Careful examination will demonstrate that these masses are separated from the testicle itself.

What Physical Exam Maneuver Can Help Identify a Varicocele?

A varicocele typically disappears when the patient is supine and reappears upon standing due to gravitational pooling of blood in the pampiniform plexus. It enlarges with Valsalva and feels like a soft, compressible "bag of worms" above the testicle, most often on the left side. In contrast, an inguinal hernia may also enlarge with Valsalva and reduce when supine, but it often presents as a firmer, more discrete mass that may extend through the inguinal canal and into the scrotum. Hernias are usually palpable at the external inguinal ring and may produce a cough impulse or bowel sounds if they contain intestine. Careful examination in both standing and supine positions, with and without Valsalva, helps distinguish a varicocele from an inguinal hernia. When the diagnosis remains uncertain, scrotal ultrasound with Doppler can aid differentiation.

Watch Out
Varicocele is associated with infertility.

Pathology/Pathophysiology

Does Cryptorchidism Increase the Risk of Developing Testicular Cancer in the Undescended Testicle, the Contralateral Descended Testicle, or Both?

Both. Testicular cancer is more likely to occur in the undescended testicle. However, in nearly 25% of patients with cryptorchidism that have testicular cancer, the contralateral descended testicle also develops testicular cancer. This suggests that an undescended testicle may not play a direct role in the development of testicular cancer, but rather, there is some other phenomenon that leads to both testicular cancer and abnormal descent of the testicles during embryologic development.

What Is the Most Common Subtype of Testicular Tumor? Is It Malignant?

Seminoma, a germ cell tumor, is the most common subtype and is considered malignant.

What Are the Major Pathologic Subtypes of Testicular Cancers? (Table 54.5)

Table 54.5 Major subtypes of testicular cancer

Seminomatous germ cell tumors (65%)	
Seminoma	Most common type in adults, highly responsive to radiotherapy and chemotherapy, metastasize late, excellent prognosis, normal AFP, possibly elevated β-hCG
Nonseminomatous germ cell tumors (35%)	
Embryonal carcinoma	Malignant, necrosis common, aggressive with early hematogenous spread, elevated AFP and/or β-hCG
Yolk sac	Most common type in children, malignant, elevated AFP
Choriocarcinoma	Malignant, early hematogenous spread, elevated β-hCG
Teratoma	Benign and malignant types, derived from ≥2 embryonic layers, elevated AFP and/or β-hCG; resistant to chemotherapy and radiation
Mixed germ cell	Benign and malignant types, multiple nonseminomatous components
Sex-cord stromal tumors	
Leydig cell	Most are benign, associated with androgen (precocious puberty) and estrogen (gynecomastia) production
Sertoli cell	Most are benign often clinically silent
Other	
Lymphoma	Malignant, commonly bilateral, occurs in older males, typically diffuse large B-cell type; treat with chemotherapy

AFP alpha-fetoprotein, *β-hCG* human chorionic gonadotropin.

What Causes Gynecomastia in Patients with Testicular Cancers?

Choriocarcinoma, a germ cell tumor, is associated with ectopic human chorionic gonadotropin (hCG) production. Elevated hCG can stimulate breast tissue, resulting in gynecomastia. It may also cause symptoms of hyperthyroidism without goiter, as the alpha subunit of hCG mimics thyroid-stimulating hormone. In contrast, Leydig cell tumors, which are non-germ cell testicular neoplasms, can also cause gynecomastia through direct estrogen production. This leads to suppression of luteinizing hormone and follicle-stimulating hormone, but serum tumor markers such as hCG and alpha-fetoprotein (AFP) are typically not elevated in these cases.

What Are the Differences Between Epididymitis and a Spermatocele?

Epididymitis involves an infection of the epididymis (Table 54.6) and is an acute process that is often confused with torsion. Patients will often complain of dysuria and a tender epididymis. Spermatoceles develop as a result of a retention cyst, often at the head of the epididymis. They are often asymptomatic but can present clinically as painless masses distinct from the testes that will transilluminate with light. In young adults, the etiology is usually related to a sexually transmitted infection. In older adults, the etiology is related to a urinary tract infection.

Table 54.6 Organisms causing epididymitis

Organism	Age
Chlamydia trachomatis (serotypes D–K), Neisseria gonorrhoeae	Young adult (<35)
Escherichia coli, Pseudomonas	Older adult (>35)

Why Does a Varicocele Form? Why Is It More Often on the Left? Why Does It Affect Fertility?

The pathophysiology of a varicocele relates to impaired venous drainage. Veins in the pampiniform plexus slowly and progressively dilate and enlarge over time as a result of impaired drainage. It occurs more commonly on the left as venous drainage is less optimal. The left testicular vein enters the left renal vein at a right angle and can get compressed between the superior mesenteric artery and aorta (nutcracker phenomenon). The right testicular vein drains directly into the inferior vena cava (IVC) at a more favorable angle. Stasis of venous blood appears to increase testicular temperature, increase seminal oxidative stress, and damage sperm DNA.

Watch Out

Sudden, new-onset varicocele in an adult, particularly if right-sided or persistent when supine, may indicate obstruction of the gonadal vein by a retroperitoneal mass such as renal cell carcinoma. Compression of the left renal vein (e.g., by a left-sided renal tumor) can also cause a sudden left-sided varicocele. In adults with sudden onset varicocele, order a CT scan of the abdomen and pelvis to evaluate for an underlying malignancy. In children, a sudden or atypical varicocele warrants abdominal ultrasound to assess for secondary causes.

What Is the Pathophysiology of a Hydrocele?

During fetal development, the peritoneum extends into the scrotum through the inguinal canal, and the testes descend into the scrotum through this channel, called the processus vaginalis. The processus vaginalis normally closes during development, with the remaining peritoneal layer around the testes now called the tunica vaginalis. Occasionally, the processus vaginalis remains patent, resulting in peritoneal fluid flowing into the tunica vaginalis to create a *communicating* hydrocele. Hydroceles in newborns tend to resolve within the first year of life as the patent processus vaginalis closes. Unresolving communicating hydroceles require a high ligation of the patent processus vaginalis (essentially the same operation as an indirect hernia repair in an infant). In older men, hydroceles tend to be *non-communicating*, due to secretion of serous fluid from the tunica vaginalis. The size of the opening of the processus vaginalis determines whether only fluid enters (hydrocele) or bowel (hernia).

Workup

What Is the Key Imaging Modality for a Patient with a Painless Testicular Mass?

Ultrasound is the best imaging. The demonstration on ultrasound of a solid mass (Fig. 54.1) within the testicle makes the likelihood of cancer very high, whereas a purely cystic, fluid-filled mass has a very low likelihood

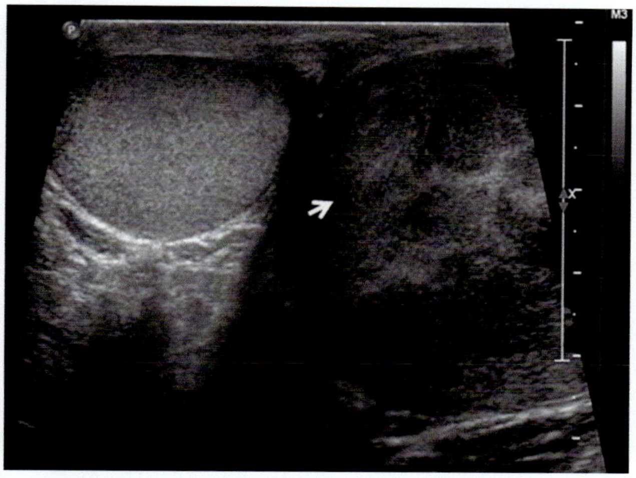

Fig. 54.1 Scrotal ultrasound showing an enlarged testicle with heterogeneous echotexture suggestive of infiltrative cancer. Compare with normal testis on the left of the image. *White arrow: abnormal testicle*

of being malignant. Seminomas tend to be well circumscribed and hypoechoic, whereas nonseminomas are hyperechoic with indistinct borders.

Once a Solid Testicular Mass Is Identified, What Additional Imaging Is Recommended?

Staging should then be performed with a CT scan of the abdomen and pelvis (to look for retroperitoneal lymph node metastasis) and a chest X-ray (to look for pulmonary metastasis). If retroperitoneal lymph node metastases or a pulmonary nodule is discovered, a CT of the chest should be considered. Patients with neurologic symptoms should also have a CT or MRI of the brain.

Watch Out

In rare cases, a patient may present with metastatic testicular cancer but no palpable testicular mass. These cases may represent a "burned-out" testicular tumor in which the tumor outstrips its blood supply and regresses. Ultrasound may show testicular atrophy or microcalcifications.

What Relevant Blood Tests Should Be Obtained in a Patient with Testicular Cancer?

There are three blood tests: AFP, β-hCG, and lactate dehydrogenase (LDH). These should be ordered when one suspects testicular cancer, as they are used for diagnosis, staging, and prognostication. β-hCG is elevated in some seminomatous cancers and in most nonseminomatous ones, whereas AFP is *only* elevated in nonseminomatous cancer. LDH levels are useful for prognostic purposes (high levels suggest a large tumor bulk), and very high levels (along with high levels of hCG and AFP) are associated with a poor prognosis.

Is Percutaneous Biopsy for a Testicular Tumor Recommended?

No. There is a high risk of seeding or spreading the cancer with a biopsy.

What Are the Key Differences Between a Seminoma and Nonseminoma? (Table 54.7)

Table 54.7 Comparison of seminoma and nonseminoma

	Seminoma	Nonseminoma
Incidence	Most common	Less common
Elevated AFP levels	No	Common
Elevated β-hCG levels	Rare	Common
Radical inguinal orchiectomy	Yes	Yes
Radiation therapy	Radiosensitive	Not radiosensitive
Chemotherapy	Yes	Yes
Retroperitoneal lymph node dissection	No	Yes (many patients)

AFP alpha-fetoprotein, *β-hCG* human chorionic gonadotropin.

Management

How Is Pathologic Confirmation of Testicular Cancer Determined?

In patients with a testicular mass that is highly suspicious for malignancy (based on physical exam and ultrasound), radical inguinal orchiectomy is performed. The procedure is performed via an inguinal incision and consists of the removal of the testicle and spermatic cord up to the point where it exits from the internal ring. In rare cases of bilateral testicular cancer or planned bilateral orchiectomy, testosterone replacement and fertility counseling are required.

Why Is an Inguinal Incision Preferred Over a Scrotal One?

Orchiectomy via a trans-scrotal incision is associated with a higher rate of local recurrence and scrotal seeding. The inguinal incision also allows a longer portion of the spermatic cord to be removed.

What Other Treatment Modalities Are Utilized After Initial Surgery for Testicular Cancer?

Radiation, chemotherapy, and retroperitoneal lymph node dissection (RPLND) are additional treatment strategies utilized. The decision as to which of these modalities to use depends on the type and stage of the cancer. For instance, seminomas are highly radiosensitive and chemosensitive, so the majority of patients receive chemotherapy or radiation therapy postoperatively. Most nonseminomas respond well to chemotherapy. RPLND is primarily recommended for nonseminomas. Testicular cancers metastasize first to the retroperitoneal (para-aortic) lymph nodes due to embryologic descent, whereas scrotal lesions drain to superficial inguinal nodes.

What Should Be Recommended for Patients About to Undergo Orchiectomy and/or Chemotherapy?

Patients who will undergo chemotherapy may have infertility issues as a result of their treatment. Although removing one testicle should not significantly affect fertility, patients should be offered sperm banking preoperatively to afford them a better chance to have children in the future.

Does Unilateral Orchiectomy Lead to Impotence?

No. Unilateral orchiectomy does not affect erectile function. However, RPLND can injure nerves that affect ejaculatory function.

Areas Where You Can Get in Trouble

Rapidly Expanding Scrotal Mass Following Blunt Trauma

A rapidly enlarging scrotal mass after blunt trauma should raise concern for a significant hematoma, which in rare cases can lead to testicular compartment syndrome. This occurs when increasing pressure within the tunica albuginea impairs testicular perfusion, risking ischemia. While scrotal ultrasound is useful to assess for hematoma and rule out testicular rupture, preserved flow on Doppler does not exclude evolving compartment syndrome. If the scrotum becomes tense, exquisitely tender, or continues to expand rapidly, urgent surgical exploration with hematoma evacuation is indicated to prevent irreversible testicular damage. Delay in intervention can lead to testicular infarction and loss.

Summary of Essentials

History and Physical

- Male patients aged 20–40 with a non-tender testicular mass should raise suspicion for testicular cancer.
- History of cryptorchidism increases lifetime risk, even in the contralateral descended testis.
- Gynecomastia may result from elevated hCG (choriocarcinoma) or estrogen-producing Leydig cell tumors.

Pathology/Pathophysiology

- Seminomas are the most common testicular cancer and are highly radiosensitive.
- Nonseminomas (embryonal carcinoma, yolk sac, choriocarcinoma, teratoma) are more aggressive and more likely to have elevated tumor markers.
- Varicocele is more common on the left due to drainage into the left renal vein; right-sided, acute onset, or non-decompressing varicocele warrant abdominal imaging to rule out malignancy.
- Testicular tumors metastasize to retroperitoneal (para-aortic) lymph nodes, not superficial inguinal nodes.

Workup

- Ultrasound will show a solid mass within the testicle in testicular cancer.
- Tumor markers (AFP, β-hCG, LDH) aid in diagnosis, staging, and monitoring
- CT of abdomen and pelvis should be used for staging.
- Biopsy is contraindicated as it may seed cancerous cells.

Management

- Radical inguinal orchiectomy is both diagnostic and therapeutic for testicular cancer.
- Seminomas are treated with radiation or chemotherapy; nonseminomas usually require chemotherapy and possibly RPLND.
- Sperm banking should be offered preoperatively in patients undergoing orchiectomy or chemotherapy.
- Unilateral orchiectomy does not cause impotence, but RPLND may affect ejaculatory function.

Suggested Reading

Bosl GJ, Motzer RJ. Testicular germ-cell cancer. N Engl J Med. 1997;337:242.

Kurklinsky AK, Rooke TW. Nutcracker phenomenon and nutcracker syndrome. Mayo Clin Proc. 2010;85(6):552–9.

Marth D, Scheidegger J, Studer UE. Ultrasonography of testicular tumors. Urol Int. 1990;45:237.

Powell TM, Tarter TH. Management of nonpalpable incidental testicular masses. J Urol. 2006;176:96.

Blood in Urine

Jeremy M. Blumberg, Fuad F. Elkhoury, and Kiran Gollapudi

Contents

C. de Virgilio, A. Grigorian (eds.), *Surgery*, https://doi.org/10.1007/978-3-032-09799-6_55

Case Study

A 68-year-old man presents to the emergency department complaining of blood in his urine as well as small blood clots for 3 days. He denies dysuria, nocturia, urinary frequency or hesitancy, or a decreased urinary stream. He denies any fevers, chills, or weight loss. He has had similar episodes of visible blood in his urine in the last several months and has been treated twice with antibiotics for a possible urinary tract infection without improvement. He has a history of hypertension for which he takes a beta-blocker; otherwise he has had no surgeries and takes no other medications. He denies any family history of malignancy or renal disease. He denies any history of trauma and does not vigorously exercise. He has a 40-pack-year history of smoking and worked as a painter. On physical exam, he is afebrile with normal vital signs. His abdomen is soft, without any palpable masses. His genitourinary exam reveals a normal circumcised phallus without lesions and normal bilateral descended testicles. On digital rectal exam, his prostate is small without any nodularity, induration, or tenderness. On laboratory exam, his hematocrit is 42%, creatinine is 1.0 mg/dL, international normalized ratio (INR) and partial thromboplastin time (PTT) are normal, and prostate-specific antigen (PSA) is within normal limits. His urinalysis shows a large number of red cells, no white cells, no casts, and no bacteria.

Diagnosis

What Is the Differential Diagnosis for Gross Hematuria? (Table 55.1)

What Are the Most Likely Diagnoses for This Patient?

This patient presents with several concerning features for a urologic malignancy, including advanced age, persistent macroscopic hematuria with clots, absence of

Table 55.1 Differential diagnosis for gross hematuria

Condition	Comments
Acute cystitis	Bladder infection most commonly caused by enteric bacteria such as *Escherichia coli*; frequency, urgency, burning; pyuria, bacteriuria
Bladder cancer	Mainly urothelial carcinoma (formerly known as transitional cell carcinoma); painless hematuria; risk factors include tobacco and exposure to automobile exhaust or industrial solvents
Benign prostatic hyperplasia (BPH)	Obstruction of the urethra by an enlarged prostate; frequency, urgency, hesitancy, slow stream, nocturia
Nephrolithiasis (kidney stones)	Calcium, uric acid, cysteine, or struvite; severe pain often in the flank
Hemolytic transfusion reaction	Immune-mediated (i.e., ABO antibodies) or non-immune mediated (pre-existing damage to blood products from heat, mechanical damage, etc.); presents with triad of fever, flank pain, hemoglobinuria
Pyelonephritis	Mainly ascending infection of the kidney from a lower urinary tract infection; may cause systemic symptoms; costovertebral angle tenderness on percussion
Prostate cancer	Most common non-skin malignancy in males; diagnosed via digital rectal exam, PSA, and/or biopsy; gross hematuria is rare
Urethral stricture	Similar symptoms to BPH; usually benign, caused by scarring from infection, instrumentation, trauma, or rarely cancer
Trauma	Injury to genitourinary tract such as traumatic Foley placement, pelvic fracture can injure bladder
Polycystic kidney disease	Flank pain, enlarged liver, kidney stones, hypertension; risk of subarachnoid hemorrhage (intracranial aneurysms); often positive family history, autosomal dominant
Exercise induced	Most commonly with running, resolves in a few days

pain, history of smoking, and occupational exposure to carcinogens as a painter. The lack of lower urinary tract symptoms such as hesitancy or nocturia, a normal prostate exam, and no history of trauma or vigorous exercise reduce the likelihood of benign causes such as BPH, prostatitis, or exercise-induced hematuria. Additionally, the absence of infection on urinalysis, normal renal function, and no proteinuria or casts makes glomerular disease unlikely. These findings increase the likelihood of a urologic malignancy, most likely bladder cancer, which requires further evaluation.

History and Physical

What Are the Differences Between Gross and Microscopic Hematuria?

Gross or macroscopic hematuria is suspected when urine is visibly pink, red, or brown or when blood clots are voided. Microscopic hematuria is discovered by the presence of red blood cells (RBCs) or heme on urinalysis. Urologic malignancy is six to seven times more common in patients with gross hematuria. A single urinalysis with ≥3 RBCs/HPF is sufficient to warrant a complete workup in patients with significant risk factors.

Why Is the Color and Consistency of the Urine Important? (◘ Table 55.2)

Other than Blood, What Can Make Urine Appear Red?

Certain foods (beets, rhubarb) and drugs (rifampin, sulfonamides, phenazopyridine, nitrofurantoin, phenytoin, levodopa, methyldopa, quinine, chloroquine, adriamycin, metronidazole) can have this effect (called pseudohematuria). Additionally, rhabdomyolysis—the destruction of muscle tissue, as in crush injuries or following vigorous exercise—may release sufficient myoglobin into the bloodstream, and subsequently into the urine, to make the urine appear red or brown. Dark urine may also be seen in patients with elevated levels of conjugated bilirubin, as in biliary obstruction or certain metabolic diseases of the liver.

◘ Table 55.2 Implications of abnormal color/consistency of urine

Color/consistency	Implication
Bright red, thick consistency	*Moderate or severe active bleeding*
Pink	*Mild active bleeding*
Brown	*Old blood; glomerular bleeding*

Does It Matter if Hematuria Is at the Beginning of the Urine Stream or at the End?

Yes. Hematuria present during the beginning of urine stream (*initial hematuria*) but then quickly fades away is suggestive of a urethral disease. Hematuria that appears near the end of the urine stream (*terminal hematuria*) is suggestive of bladder or prostate pathology. If the hematuria is present from beginning to end (*total hematuria*), then the kidneys, ureters, or bladder can be involved.

What Is the Importance of Pain in Association with Hematuria?

Pain in association with hematuria strongly suggests infection or urinary obstruction. As such, urinary tract infection, prostatitis, pyelonephritis, and nephrolithiasis would be higher on the differential.

What Is the Classic Presentation for Nephrolithiasis?

Ureteral stones present with acute colicky flank pain that may extend into the groin area if the stone is close to the bladder. The pain is described as colicky, with periods of severe pain during which the patient will not be able to stay still and will shift positions in an attempt to relieve their pain, followed by temporary resolution of the pain. This tendency to move around can help differentiate these patients from those with peritonitis as the latter prefer to remain rigid. Patients with nephrolithiasis may also complain of nausea, vomiting, and dysuria.

What Are the Risk Factors for Nephrolithiasis?

Prior episodes of nephrolithiasis, family history, high protein diet, males > females, low fluid intake, dehydration, recurrent urinary tract infections, diabetes, gout, renal tubular acidosis, electrolyte abnormalities (e.g., hypercalcemia), and certain medications (e.g., acetazolamide, furosemide, allopurinol).

How Does Autosomal Dominant Polycystic Kidney Disease Present?

Autosomal dominant polycystic kidney disease results from a mutation in the *PDK1* or *PDK2* gene, leading to the growth of renal cysts early in life. Clinical symptoms typically manifest between the ages of 30 and 50. Hypertension is a common presenting sign. Cyst rupture may present with recurrent flank pain and hematuria. Patients will experience progressive renal dysfunction; the majority will advance to end stage renal disease. Other associated conditions include mitral valve prolapse, aortic regurgitation, diverticulosis, brain aneurysms, liver cysts, and nephrolithiasis.

What Are the Most Common Symptoms/ Presentation for Renal Cancer?

In most patients, renal cancer is discovered incidentally as a mass on imaging for other complaints. The classic triad includes flank pain, abdominal mass, and hematuria, but this is seen in only 10–15% of patients. Rarely, a sudden onset of a varicocele suggestive of tumor infiltrating into the inferior vena cava or left renal vein may be the only clue. It is important to differentiate renal cancer from polycystic kidney disease, which is typically bilateral and is associated with progressive renal failure.

What Are the Main Risk Factors for Renal Cancer?

Smoking, male gender, older age, obesity, family history, and exposure to certain heavy metals and chemicals.

What Is the Most Common Presentation for Bladder Cancer? What Are the Risk Factors?

Painless gross hematuria. A minority of patients will have urinary symptoms. Similar to renal cancer, risk factors include smoking, male gender, older age, family history, and exposure to heavy metals and chemicals. In addition, chronic bladder irritation and inflammation (from recurrent urinary tract infections, indwelling Foley, pelvic irradiation) increase the risk.

What Is the Most Common Presentation for Prostate Cancer? What Are the Risk Factors?

Most prostate cancers are discovered incidentally because of PSA screening. On occasion, patients may present with urinary symptoms similar to BPH. With metastatic disease, the patient may present with bone pain, obstructive renal failure, or weight loss. The main risk factors are age > 50 years, black race, high fat diet, and family history.

What Comprises the Urinary Tract and Where Along the Tract Can Bleeding Arise?

The kidneys, ureters, bladder, and urethra make up the urinary tract. The kidneys and ureters make up the *upper* urinary tract, while the bladder and urethra comprise the *lower* urinary tract. Bleeding can arise from anywhere along the tract, from the glomerulus to the distal urethra.

Pathology/Pathophysiology

Where Do Renal Stones Develop and in What Circumstances Do They Lead to Symptoms?

Stones can develop anywhere in the urinary tract but typically originate from the kidney or the renal pelvis. Many of these stones (<5 mm) will pass freely into the bladder and eventually exit the body during micturition. Stones do not cause symptoms unless they get lodged somewhere in the urinary tract and cause obstruction. The most common locations for a stone to get stuck are at points of narrowing in the genitourinary tract: (1) the ureteropelvic junction, (2) where the ureter crosses the iliac vessels, and (3) the ureterovesical junction.

Why Do High Protein Diets Increase the Risk of Developing Renal Stones?

Breakdown of protein (e.g., fish, red meat, chicken) lowers the urinary pH and increases excretion of uric acid which can contribute to the formation of stones. Decreasing dietary protein, oxalate, and sodium intake decreases the risk of developing renal calculi.

What Is the Most Common Type of Renal Stone and What Is the Leading Cause of This Type of Stone?

The most common renal stone (◘ Table 55.3) is calcium oxalate. The leading cause of calcium oxalate renal stones is hypercalciuria (◘ Fig. 55.1).

What Is the Most Common Type of Renal Cancer?

Renal cell carcinoma (RCC) is the most common primary tumor of the kidney. RCC arises from the renal tubule cells, and nearly one-third of patients have metastatic disease at the time of presentation. The most common histologic subtypes include clear cell (70%), papillary (15%), and chromophobe (5%).

Where Is the Most Common Location for RCC Metastasis?

The lung, though RCC, is known to metastasize to many different organs. The most common tumor to metastasize to the thyroid is RCC.

What Genetic Syndromes Are Associated with RCC?

Most cases of RCC are sporadic, but several familial syndromes are associated with RCC. These syndromes include von Hippel-Lindau (autosomal dominant, mutation of chromosome 3p), tuberous sclerosis (autosomal dominant, mutation of chromosome 9), and Birt-Hogg-Dube (autosomal dominant, mutation of chromosome 17).

What Paraneoplastic Syndromes Are Associated with RCC? (◘ Table 55.4)

What Is the Most Common Type of Bladder Cancer?

The most common type of bladder cancer is urothelial cell carcinoma (UCC), formerly referred to as transitional cell carcinoma. UCC can arise from the renal collecting system, ureters, bladder, or urethra. UCCs are

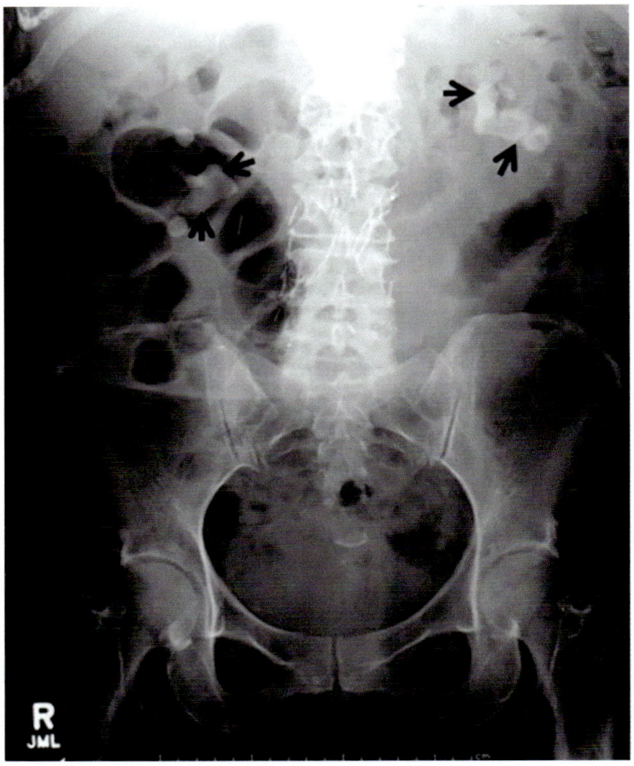

◘ **Fig. 55.1** Abdominal X-ray showing branching radiopaque stones outlining the renal collecting system, consistent with staghorn calculi

◘ **Table 55.3** Renal stones

Type	Etiology	Radiology	Features
Calcium oxalate	Hypercalciuria, Crohn's disease	Radiopaque	Most common type
Struvite	Urinary tract infection secondary to urease + organism (e.g., *Proteus*, *Klebsiella*)	Radiopaque	Women are affected more often; can form staghorn calculi (outlining renal pelvis)
Calcium phosphate	Renal tubular acidosis, hyperparathyroidism	Radiopaque	Form more readily in alkalinized urine
Uric acid	Low urinary pH, gout, chemotherapy, patients with ileostomy	*Radiolucent*	Treated by increasing urinary pH (e.g., alkalinizing agents)

Table 55.4 Paraneoplastic syndromes associated with renal cell carcinoma

Paraneoplastic syndromes	Mediator
Polycythemia	Increased erythropoietin production
Hypercalcemia	PTH-related peptide hormone production
Hypertension	Increased renin production
Cushing's syndrome	Ectopic cortisol production
Stauffer's syndrome	Reversible liver dysfunction; ↑ALP, ↑GGT, ↑ESR; hepatosplenomegaly; unknown mechanism

PTH parathyroid hormone, *ALP* alkaline phosphatase, *GGT* gamma-glutamyl transferase, *ESR* erythrocyte sedimentation rate

graded as either low grade or high grade. They are staged based on the depth of their invasion.

What Is the Most Common Type of Prostate Cancer?

Prostatic adenocarcinoma.

> **Watch Out**
> History of cancer plus new focal vertebral tenderness suggests vertebral metastasis. Pain is typically focal, worse at night, and not relieved by rest. Look for red flags like hypercalcemia, neurologic deficits, weight loss, or B symptoms.

Workup

What Is the Next Step in the Workup after a Positive Urine Dipstick for Blood?

A positive dipstick analysis should be confirmed with a microscopic urinalysis. This analysis will provide the number of RBCs/HPF, the number of white blood cells (WBCs), and the presence of bacteria. In addition, the presence of crystals can be determined. Furthermore, the presence of dysmorphic RBCs and red blood cell casts suggests a glomerular source of bleeding.

Table 55.5 Recommended studies for hematuria work-up

Lab tests	Why order?
Complete blood count	White blood cell count if concerned about infection
	Hemoglobin to determine if anemic from hematuria
	Platelet count may reveal thrombocytopenia
Metabolic panel	BUN and creatinine to evaluate renal function
PT/PTT/INR	Rule out coagulopathy
PSA	Screen for prostate cancer in appropriate patients, can also be elevated in setting of urinary tract infection or recent instrumentation
Urine culture	Rule out infection
Urine cytology	Rule out urothelial malignancy

What Additional Laboratory Tests Should Be Ordered During the Hematuria Workup? (Table 55.5)

What Is the Best Diagnostic Test for Nephrolithiasis?

The best diagnostic test is a renal protocol (non-contrast) CT, which is highly sensitive for detecting stones and more accurate than X-ray or ultrasound. In pregnant patients and women of childbearing age, ultrasound is preferred despite its lower sensitivity.

What Further Workup Is Recommended in the Presence of Gross Hematuria?

The strongest predictors for cancer are age over 50 and a history of gross (macroscopic) hematuria. As such, the majority of patients who present with gross hematuria should undergo a workup for malignancy. The workup consists of a CT urogram, urine cytology, and cystourethroscopy (for bladder and urethral pathology). CT urogram consists of a non-contrast study (for urolithiasis), along with nephrographic (for renal masses), and excretory phases (for urothelial lesions). Further workup is dictated based on the findings from these studies.

Does Negative Urine Cytology Rule Out a Malignancy?

No. A urine cytology detects abnormal-appearing urothelial cells that are concerning for a urothelial carcinoma of the bladder. The higher the tumor grade, the more likely urine cytology will be positive. The sensitivity of urine cytology for low-grade tumors is less than 50%. Also, in the presence of significant hematuria, cytopathologic analysis may not be able to pick up abnormal cells in the background of a significant number of RBCs.

Management

Renal Stones

What Is the Best Management for Nephrolithiasis? How Does the Size of the Stone Change Management?

Renal stones that are <5 mm are likely to pass on their own and should be managed with supportive therapy unless the patient is septic, has a solitary kidney, or has uncontrolled pain. Alpha-blockers such as tamsulosin can also be given to relax the ureteral wall. Stones between 5 and 9 mm should be managed using clinical judgment. Stones larger than 9 mm are unlikely to pass spontaneously and will therefore require more invasive treatment.

What Are the Emergent Surgical Indications for Renal Stones?

Obstructive stones that lead to urosepsis, intractable pain, progressive renal damage, or a solitary kidney (i.e., the patient only has one functional kidney) require ureteral stent placement or percutaneous nephrostomy tube placement.

Renal Masses

What Are the Treatment Options for Renal Masses Concerning for RCC?

Renal masses that are concerning for RCC are treated either with radical or partial nephrectomy depending on the size and location of the mass. In patients with small masses, or who are poor surgical candidates, surveillance and thermal or cryoablation are also options.

What Is a Radical Nephrectomy?

A radical nephrectomy is the removal of the kidney, perinephric fat, Gerota's fascia, ureter, lymph nodes, and, possibly, ipsilateral adrenal gland. However, in most cases, the ipsilateral adrenal gland can be preserved.

Bladder Cancer

How Is Urothelial Cell Carcinoma of the Bladder Treated?

UCC involves transurethral resection for both diagnosis and staging. Superficial, non-muscle-invasive tumors are treated with complete transurethral (endoscopic) resection and may also receive intravesical therapy such as mitomycin or bacillus Calmette-Guérin (BCG). Due to a high recurrence rate, patients require close surveillance with regular cystoscopy. For muscle-invasive disease, treatment depends on the extent of involvement. Tumors limited to a small area may be managed with partial cystectomy. However, larger tumors or those involving multiple bladder regions require radical (total) cystectomy with urinary diversion.

> **Watch Out**
> BCG is also used as a vaccine against tuberculosis in other countries but not the United States.

Prostate Cancer

What Is a Radical Prostatectomy? Which Patients Are Appropriate Candidates for This Procedure?

Removal of the prostate and seminal vesicles. Patients with disease contained to the prostate and a life expectancy of at least 10 years are good candidates. Patients should undergo imaging with bone scans, CT, or MRI to evaluate for metastasis. Metastatic prostate cancer leads to excessive bone formation; these osteoblastic metastases will appear as very dense, sclerotic lesions in the bone.

What Are Nonsurgical Treatments for Prostate Cancer?

External beam radiation, brachytherapy (placement of radioactive beads within the prostate), and androgen deprivation therapy. Patients who are poor surgical candidates or who have reduced life expectancy due to some other cause may receive nonsurgical therapy or active surveillance.

Special Circumstances

What Are the Next Steps in Management if Significant Hematuria Persists Despite Foley Catheter Placement and Manual Irrigation?

If the patient continues to have significant hematuria after manual irrigation, a three-way Foley catheter can be placed, and continuous bladder irrigation can be initiated. Continuous irrigation helps prevent the formation of new blood clots and also decreases exposure of potential bleeding sites in the lower urinary tract to urokinase. Urokinase is a serine protease that is present in urine that activates plasmin and the thrombolytic cascade. If hematuria does not improve or resolve with bladder irrigation, the patient may be taken to the operating room for cystoscopy. Cystoscopy allows for adequate clot evacuation, diagnosis of lower urinary tract pathology, and fulguration (i.e., electrical cauterization) of bleeding sites.

Areas You Can Get into Trouble

Not Placing a Foley Catheter in the Setting of Significant Gross Hematuria

A Foley catheter should be placed if the patient has significant gross hematuria or blood clots. Failure to do so may result in urinary retention due to obstruction from the blood clots. All of the blood clots should be manually irrigated out of the bladder with a catheter tip syringe with either sterile saline or water. When hematuria is secondary to urethral or prostatic trauma following instrumentation or Foley catheter placement, the Foley catheter itself can act to tamponade bleeding sites.

Placing a Foley Catheter in the Setting of Trauma and Blood at the Urethral Meatus

Conversely, a Foley catheter should not be placed if there is blood at the urethral meatus following major trauma, as this may indicate a urethral injury. Blind catheterization risks converting a partial tear into a complete transection. The next best step is retrograde urethrography (RUG) to assess for injury. If a posterior urethral injury is identified, typically associated with pelvic fractures, bladder decompression should be achieved with a suprapubic catheter. Anterior urethral injuries, such as those from blunt trauma to the erect penis resulting in penile fracture, require emergent urethral repair with intraoperative catheter placement.

Bladder Rupture After Blunt Trauma

Bladder rupture should be suspected in a patient with gross hematuria following blunt trauma and are divided into intraperitoneal and extraperitoneal injuries. Intraperitoneal injuries tend to occur in patients with a full bladder who suffer lower abdominal trauma. The dome of the bladder (weakest part of the bladder) blows out, and urine leaks into the peritoneum. There may not necessarily be a pelvic fracture. Extraperitoneal injuries are associated with pelvic fractures that typically lead to injury to the lateral or posterior surface of the bladder. A bone fragment may puncture the bladder, with urine leakage into the extraperitoneal space. Diagnosis is made with a CT-retrograde cystogram. With intraperitoneal injuries, the CT scan may show a large amount of free fluid (without injury to a solid organ), suggesting that the fluid may be urine and not blood. Since intraperitoneal injuries cause leakage of urine into the peritoneal cavity, the patient may develop urinary ascites, sepsis, and the peritoneum may reabsorb the urine leading to a pseudo renal failure as the blood urea nitrogen (BUN) and creatinine increase. As such, surgical repair is indicated in intraperitoneal injuries. Extraperitoneal injuries on the other hand are small, localized, and often heal on their own. Therefore, management is typically conservative and includes 2 weeks of catheter decompression.

Can Gross Hematuria Be Associated with an Abdominal Aortic Aneurysm (AAA)?

Yes, an AAA can rupture into the inferior vena cava forming an aortocaval fistula or into the iliac veins leading to venous congestion of retroperitoneal organs, including the kidneys and bladder, and present with gross hematuria. The patient would present with sudden onset of back pain, hypotension, tachycardia, as well as swelling of the lower extremities and high-output congestive heart failure.

Fever, Flank Pain, and Gross Hematuria Following a Blood Transfusion

Acute hemolytic transfusion reaction is a rare, though life-threatening, immune-mediated response that occurs within 24 hours of transfusion. This results from an antibody response to mismatched blood, typically in the setting of ABO incompatibility. Most often, immunoglobulin M (IgM) antibodies against donor antigens lead to intravascular hemolysis. Patients will present with hemoglobinuria, flank pain, and fever. The complement-mediated reaction will result in a positive direct antiglobulin (Coombs) test. Treatment includes immediate discontinuation of the transfusion and supportive care. The most common cause of acute hemolytic transfusion reactions is preventable error, such as unidentified incompatibility, mislabeling of blood products, or misidentified patients.

Summary of Essentials

History and Physical

- Pain with hematuria suggests urinary tract infection or urinary obstruction.
- Painless gross hematuria raises suspicion for malignancy (especially in the elderly).
- Inquire about risk factors for malignancy.

Pathology/Pathophysiology

- Gross hematuria: urine that is visibly red, pink, or brown.
- Microscopic hematuria: urine appears normal but RBCs are detected on urinalysis.
- Pseudohematuria: red urine (without RBCs) due to certain foods, drugs, or metabolic disorders.
- RCC is usually asymptomatic and discovered incidentally.
- Bladder cancer usually presents as painless gross hematuria.
- Prostate cancer is usually discovered by PSA screening and prostate biopsy.
- Adenocarcinoma is the most common.
- Kidney stone: calcium oxalate is the most common.

Workup

- Urine dipstick (for blood, protein), microscopic urinalysis.
- Suspected kidney stone: non-contrast CT; in women of childbearing age and children, ultrasonography should be used instead
- Most kidney stones are radiopaque (visible on X-ray)
- Gross hematuria (especially if >50 years old)—malignancy workup:
- CT urogram
- Urine cytology
- Cystourethroscopy

Management

- Kidney stones
- <5 mm: will likely pass spontaneously, alpha-blockers such as tamsulosin
- 5–9 mm: management individualized
- >10 mm: extracorporeal shock wave lithotripsy, percutaneous nephrostomy, ureteroscopy, or rarely nephrolithotomy
- Renal cancer
- Partial or radical nephrectomy
- Bladder cancer
- Transurethral resection, infusion of mitomycin or BCG, or radical cystectomy
- Prostate cancer
- External beam radiation, brachytherapy, androgen deprivation therapy, radical prostatectomy, or active surveillance

Suggested Reading

Cohen RA, Brown RS. Clinical practice. Microscopic hematuria. N Engl J Med. 2003;348:2330.

Holzbeierlein JM, Bixler BR, Buckley DI, et al. Diagnosis and Treatment of Non-Muscle Invasive Bladder Cancer: AUA/SUO Guideline: 2024 Amendment [published correction appears in J Urol. 2024 Dec;212(6):936. https://doi.org/10.1097/JU.0000000000004251.]. J Urol. 2024;211(4):533–538. https://doi.org/10.1097/JU.0000000000003846

Khadra MH, Pickard RS, Charlton M, et al. A prospective analysis of 1,930 patients with hematuria to evaluate current diagnostic practice. J Urol. 2000;163:524.

Nakamura K, Kasraeian A, Iczkowski KA, et al. Utility of serial urinary cytology in the initial evaluation of the patient with microscopic hematuria. BMC Urol. 2009;9:12.

Salo JA, Verkkala KA, Ala-Kulju KV, Heikkinen LO, Luosto RV. Hematuria is an indication of rupture of an abdominal aortic aneurysm into the vena cava. J Vasc Surg. 1990;12(1):41–4.

Urology

Question Set: Urology

Questions

1. A 17-year-old male with a history of sickle cell disease presents to the emergency department with painful penile erection for the past 6 h. He denies trauma. He reports that the erection began shortly after using alcohol and spending time in a cold swimming pool. On physical examination, the penis is rigid and tender. The glans is soft. There are no signs of trauma or infection. Vital signs are within normal limits. Cavernosal blood gas is obtained and reveals pH 7.02, partial pressure of oxygen (pO_2) 26 mmHg, and partial pressure of carbon dioxide (pCO_2) 65 mmHg. What is the most appropriate next step in management?
   (A) Administer oral pseudoephedrine
   (B) Irrigation and aspiration of the corpora cavernosa
   (C) Trial of warm compresses and observation
   (D) Intramuscular corticosteroids
   (E) Intravenous (IV) antibiotics and penile ultrasound

2. A 10-year-old boy presents to his doctor for follow-up 2 weeks after having an upper respiratory tract infection (URI). He complains of pain in his scrotum. It has been bothering him for the past 3 days but is more painful today. A scrotal ultrasound demonstrates an enlarged and rounded epididymis. His scrotal skin appears thickened. What other finding(s) would you suspect in this patient's history and physical?
   (A) Skin lesions and abdominal pain
   (B) Recent weight loss, night sweats, and fevers
   (C) Recent epididymitis
   (D) Sores in the mouth and swelling of the eyes
   (E) Painful urination

3. A male infant presents with a mass in his scrotum that has been present since birth. His mother states that the mass changes in size when the infant cries and does not seem to be painful. On exam, the mass appears to be adjacent to his testicle which is palpated posteriorly. The mass is soft and non-tender and transilluminates. There is no bulge or mass at the internal ring. What is the most appropriate next step in the management?
   (A) Surgical management
   (B) Medical management
   (C) Ultrasound
   (D) Needle aspiration
   (E) Reassurance

4. A 50-year-old man arrives to the emergency department with severe acute colicky flank pain and hematuria. The patient has a long-standing history of gout. Which of the following is true regarding the type of kidney stone the patient likely has?
   (A) Most are radiopaque
   (B) They are often seen in patients with hyperparathyroidism
   (C) Shock wave lithotripsy is not helpful
   (D) Sodium bicarbonate administration is beneficial
   (E) Suppressive antibiotics are helpful in prevention

5. A 20-year-old male presents with a right testicular mass. He noticed the mass after getting kneed in the groin during a basketball game 3 weeks earlier. He states that the mass is not tender. He denies any other symptoms. On physical examination, there is a firm 2-cm mass within the right testicle. Ultrasound confirms a 2-cm homogeneous mass within the right testicle. CT scan of the abdomen and pelvis is negative. Chest X-ray is negative. Which of the following is the most appropriate next step in management?
   (A) Radical inguinal orchiectomy
   (B) Scrotal orchiectomy
   (C) Fine needle aspiration
   (D) Open testicular biopsy
   (E) Percutaneous biopsy

6. A 78-year-old man arrives to the emergency department with colicky flank pain for the past 4 days that is now accompanied by nausea, vomiting, fever, and hematuria. Past medical history is significant for congestive heart failure and prior myocardial infarction. On physical examination, the patient has a blood pressure of 100/60 mmHg, temperature of 38.0 °C, and a heart rate of 110/min. Urinalysis reveals 150 red blood cell (RBC)/hpf and 20 white blood cell (WBC)/hpf. Laboratory tests demonstrate a WBC of $15 \times 10^3/\mu L$ (normal $4.1–10.9 \times 10^3/\mu L$) with 10% bands. Imaging demonstrates a 10-millimeter stone lodged in the ureterovesical junction with dilation of the right renal calyx. Broad-spectrum antibiotics are administered intravenously. What is the best next step in management?
   (A) Percutaneous nephrostomy tube
   (B) Open nephrostomy
   (C) Shock wave lithotripsy
   (D) Placement of a ureteral stent
   (E) Admit to intensive care unit (ICU) for close monitoring

7. A 45-year-old male presents with a new scrotal mass on the right side that developed abruptly a week earlier. It is non-tender. He reports no history of trauma. When the patient is standing, the scrotal mass is separate from the testicle and epididymis, feels like a "bag of worms," and is soft, compressible, and non-tender. With the patient supine, the mass is unchanged. The left side is normal. What is the most appropriate next step in the management?
   (A) Scrotal support and nonsteroidal anti-inflammatory drugs (NSAIDs)
   (B) Surgical intervention
   (C) CT of the abdomen
   (D) Reassurance and observation
   (E) Ultrasound-guided biopsy of the mass

8. A 15-year-old boy arrives to the emergency department 4 h after experiencing a sudden onset of right testicular pain while playing soccer. He does not recall any specific trauma to his testicle during the game. He also reports nausea and vomiting. Physical examination reveals a tender and swollen right testicle that is displaced superiorly. The testicle appears to be lying transversely. He has an absent cremasteric reflex on the right. The left testicle is normal in location and is non-tender. What is the next step in management?
   (A) Ultrasound
   (B) Color Doppler ultrasound
   (C) Right orchiopexy
   (D) Bilateral orchiopexy
   (E) Scrotal support and nonsteroidal anti-inflammatory drugs

9. A 26-year-old man that recently emigrated from Sudan to the United States arrives to your office complaining of red urine. He does not experience any pain but says that for the last week his urine has appeared red. He also reports night sweats, fevers, and losing 10 lbs. over the last 2 months without a change in his appetite. Cystoscopy is

performed, and biopsies are taken of a tumor that appears nodular with a plaque-like and irregular surface. What is most likely to be seen on microscopic analysis?

(A) Urothelial carcinoma (transitional cell carcinoma)
(B) Squamous cell carcinoma
(C) Adenocarcinoma
(D) Mucinous (colloid) carcinoma
(E) Small cell carcinoma

10. A 7-year-old boy presents to the doctor with a non-tender scrotal mass. His vitals are normal, and he has no complaints. His mother reports that he has been behaving more aggressively at home and has gotten into two fights at school over the past month. Physical examination reveals a firm 2.5-cm mass within the right testicle. There are no epididymal masses bilaterally, although both testicles appear to be enlarged. He also has axillary hair. Laboratory analysis reveals a normal urinalysis. What is the most likely etiology of the testicular mass?

(A) Leydig cell tumor
(B) Sertoli cell tumor
(C) Seminoma
(D) Teratoma
(E) Juvenile granulosa cell tumor

11. An infant is found to have an undescended left testicle shortly after birth. During his 6-month checkup, the left testicle remains undescended. Which of the following statements is most accurate regarding the management and long-term risks of this condition?

(A) Immediate orchiopexy eliminates the risk of testicular cancer
(B) Orchiopexy within the next 6 months reduces cancer risk to normal levels
(C) Hormonal therapy is the preferred first-line approach
(D) Observation until age 2 is recommended before intervening
(E) Even after orchiopexy, testicular cancer risk remains higher than in boys without cryptorchidism

12. A 52-year-old male is brought to the hospital by his wife with complaints of intense pain that started around his right flank and now radiates to his right groin. He said that his urine appears pink. He appears to be in severe pain and is unable to remain still during examination. His abdominal exam is unremarkable. Urinalysis reveals 100 RBC/hpf. IV fluids and analgesics are administered. Which of the following is the most appropriate imaging?

(A) Helical CT scan of the abdomen and pelvis without contrast
(B) Helical CT scan of the abdomen and pelvis with contrast
(C) Upright abdominal X-ray
(D) Intravenous pyelogram (IVP)
(E) Renal ultrasound

13. A 30-year-old male restrained driver is involved in a high-speed motor vehicle accident. In the emergency department, he has a strong odor of alcohol. Blood pressure is 120/70 mmHg and heart rate is 80/min. His abdomen appears distended and mildly tender diffusely. The pelvis is stable. On rectal exam, the prostate feels normal. There is no blood at the urethral meatus. On insertion of a Foley catheter, there is gross hematuria. CT scan of the abdomen and pelvis with oral and IV contrast reveals a large amount of free fluid and contrast in the peritoneum. The liver and spleen appear to be normal as does the pelvis. What part of the genitourinary tract is most likely injured?

(A) Ureter
(B) Base of the bladder
(C) Bladder dome
(D) Renal hilum
(E) Urethra

neal injuries will demonstrate a large amount of intraperitoneal free fluid (and contrast) on CT scan. Although the free fluid might initially be thought of as being blood, the absence of liver or spleen injury raises suspicion that the fluid is urine. Intraperitoneal injuries require laparotomy and repair. The bladder dome is the only region covered by the peritoneum and is considered the weakest portion. Thus, it is the only portion prone to rupture in the peritoneum and lead to chemical peritonitis. However, the most common overall location of bladder rupture is at the base of the bladder, which is located in the retroperitoneum and will not present with peritonitis (B). Retroperitoneal bladder injuries are most often associated with pelvic fractures and can be managed nonoperatively with a Foley catheter. The ureter and renal hilum are also located in the retroperitoneum (A, D). Urethral injury is associated with blood at the urethral meatus and would not be expected to cause free fluid in the peritoneum (E).

14. Answer D

Varicocele is often an asymptomatic condition, but patients may complain of a vague discomfort and/or pain in the scrotum. The affected side will have a mass that feels similar to a "bag of worms" and will disappear upon lying down and reappear when the patient stands up. Varicoceles develop as a result of tortuous dilation of the pampiniform plexus of the veins surrounding the spermatic cord and testis. About 80% occur on the left side (A). Since it is a venous drainage problem, varicoceles increase in size with Valsalva. Unlike a hydrocele that transilluminates (as it contains clear fluid), a varicocele does not (C). In adolescents with varicoceles, surgical repair is indicated when there is ipsilateral testicular atrophy or evidence of impaired fertility. A testicle that is high in the scrotum would raise concern for testicular torsion (if associated with sudden pain) or a partially undescended testicle (B). An absent cremasteric reflex is seen with testicular torsion (E).

15. Answer D

The history of sudden penile pain following trauma combined with the physical examination is consistent with a penile fracture, which requires urgent surgical repair. It is due to a tear in the tunica albuginea with subsequent rupture of one or both of the corpus cavernosum. Failure to recognize and surgically manage the injury often results in permanent erectile dysfunction. Men are often embarrassed to describe the true nature of the injury, so they fabricate stories that don't fit the clinical picture. Penile fractures most often occur during vigorous sexual activity. Most patients describe a "snapping" sound preceding the fracture. A hematoma rapidly develops within the corpus cavernosum and presents as a blue discoloration at the base of the penis, which is deviated at the fracture site. Prior to surgical exploration, a urethral injury should be ruled out with a retrograde urethrogram. CT scan and cystoscopy play no role in the evaluation of penile fractures (A–B). Analgesics and best rest are not acceptable options for a patient suspected of having a penile fracture (C). Temporary suprapubic catheter would not help address the underlying problem (E).

16. Answer C

Patients with Crohn's disease that present with flank pain and hematuria should raise suspicion for nephrolithiasis secondary to hyperoxaluria. Her laparotomy scar suggests that she had an ileocolic resection, which would predispose her to fat malabsorption as the terminal ileum is the principal site for fat absorption. In healthy patients, intraluminal calcium binds to oxalate to prevent its reabsorption from the gastrointestinal (GI) tract. In patients with increased amounts of fat in the GI lumen (e.g., Crohn's disease status-post ileocolic resection), the calcium preferentially binds to fat leaving the unbound oxalate available for reabsorption and, thus, increases the risk of developing calcium oxalate renal stones. Hypercalciuria would have been the most likely etiology had she not had Crohn's disease (B). Urease-producing bacteria are associated with struvite stones and recurrent urinary tract infections (D). Gallstones do not cause flank pain or hematuria, and mesalamine is not a known risk factor for the development of renal stones (A, E).

Vascular

Christian de Virgilio

Contents

Transient Loss of Vision in the Right Eye

Areg Grigorian, Jessica Beth O'Connell, and Christian de Virgilio

Contents

C. de Virgilio, A. Grigorian (eds.), *Surgery*, https://doi.org/10.1007/978-3-032-09799-6_56

Case Study

A 60-year-old male presents with an episode of vision loss in his right eye. The event occurred a week ago, while he was watching television, and resolved spontaneously after about 20 minutes. He described it as a curtain or shade that descended over his eye from top to bottom. He denied having any pain in the eye. He also denied any headaches, tiredness in his jaw while chewing, or any generalized fatigue. He denied any episodes of weakness or numbness on one side of his body or changes in his speech. He has a 30-pack-year history of smoking. He also has a history of hypertension and hypercholesterolemia. He denied a history of coronary artery disease or diabetes. He takes a beta-blocker and a statin. Physical examination reveals a systolic blood pressure of 140/70 mmHg. He has normal carotid pulses with a right carotid bruit. Neurologic examination is normal.

Diagnosis

What Is the Differential Diagnosis for Transient Monocular Vision Loss? (Table 56.1)

What Is the Most Likely Diagnosis for This Patient?

Transient loss of vision, without other associated symptoms (such as headache, eye pain, floaters, and jaw tiredness when chewing), in a smoker with a carotid bruit is most likely due to atherosclerotic plaque from the internal carotid artery (ICA).

History and Physical Examination

What Is the Term for the Eye Symptom the Patient Describes?

Amaurosis fugax is derived from Greek (amaurosis meaning darkness) and Latin (fugax meaning fleeting). The term describes transient vision loss and is described as a "curtain" or "shade" descending the field of vision in one eye. It is often the result of atherosclerotic debris from a plaque in the ICA that embolizes to the ophthalmic artery (the first branch of the ICA in the brain), leading to temporary ipsilateral retinal ischemia that typically lasts for minutes.

Table 56.1 Differential diagnosis for transident monocular vision loss

Category	Conditions
Circulatory	*Embolus* from the carotid artery
	Central retinal artery occlusion with *cherry red spot* on fundoscopy
	Severe orthostatic hypotension; seen in diabetics
	Giant cell arteritis; jaw claudication, headaches, and increased erythrocyte sedimentation rate (ESR)
	Retinal vein occlusion; associated with chronic glaucoma, diabetes, and coagulopathy; patients report painless, monocular "cloudy vision," and fundoscopy shows cotton wool spots, edema, and retinal hemorrhages
Ocular	*Retinal detachment*; floaters
	Open-angle glaucoma; gradual loss of vision (from peripheral to central)
Neurologic	*Papilledema*; associated with increased cerebral pressure (e.g., malignant hypertension, pseudotumor cerebri), headache, and bilateral disk swelling
	Optic neuritis; associated with multiple sclerosis, inflammation of the optic nerve, painful visual loss
	Retinal migraine or aura; result of vasospasm; painful vision loss

In a Patient with This Eye Symptom, What Finding on Fundoscopic Ophthalmologic Examination Would Support a Carotid Artery Source of the Symptom?

Hollenhorst plaques may be seen. These are cholesterol microemboli seen within the retinal arterioles that have a bright, yellow, and refractile appearance. They are considered highly suggestive of embolization from a plaque at the carotid bifurcation.

What If the Patient Instead Described Transient Motor and Sensory Loss of the Left Arm and Leg, What Term Would Be Used for Such a Symptom?

This is another symptom of carotid embolization. It is called a hemispheric TIA (transient ischemic attack). This is a focal neurologic deficit that lasts <24 hours; however, the vast majority lasts 30 minutes or less.

How Does One Distinguish a TIA from a Stroke?

The symptoms of a stroke persist >24 hours. Since most TIAs last less than an hour, symptoms lasting beyond that time are highly suggestive of a stroke.

What Does a Carotid Bruit Signify?

It is indicative of turbulent flow, most often due to a hemodynamically significant stenosis of the internal carotid artery due to atherosclerosis. The turbulent flow causes the artery distal to the stenosis to vibrate.

What Else Can Cause a Bruit in the Neck?

Other causes include a murmur transmitted from the heart to the neck, such as from aortic stenosis (such a murmur will typically be louder when auscultated at the left sternal border as compared to the neck, and intensity will decrease with Valsalva), stenosis of the external carotid artery (ECA; considered a benign problem), and stenosis of the subclavian artery (can cause subclavian steal syndrome).

What Is Subclavian Steal Syndrome?

Subclavian steal syndrome is classically associated with stenosis of the left subclavian artery proximal to the vertebral artery branch point. With arm exercise demand increases and resistance decreases. The left arm becomes tired. To compensate, blood flows in a retrograde fashion down that the vertebral artery into the arm, stealing blood from the posterior brain. Patients report transient vertigo, dizziness, and less commonly syncope, during arm exercise.

Are Dizziness, Syncope, and Headaches Considered Symptoms of Carotid Stenosis?

No. Rarely, bilateral carotid stenosis can lead to syncope secondary to cerebral hypoperfusion. Dizziness and syncope may be symptoms of disease in the posterior circulation of the brain.

What Are the Risk Factors for Carotid Stenosis?

The risk factors for carotid stenosis are older age, male gender, hypertension, smoking, hypercholesterolemia, diabetes, and obesity.

Anatomy

What Are the Branches of the ECA?

The branches of the external carotid artery can be remembered with "some attendings like freaking out potential medical students": *s*uperior thyroid, *a*scending pharyngeal, *l*ingual, *f*acial, *o*ccipital, *p*osterior auricular, and *m*axillary arteries.

What Is the First Branch of the ICA?

The first branch is the ophthalmic artery which occurs intracranially. The ICA has no branches in the neck.

What Is the Classic Anterior Circulation Ischemic Stroke in Terms of Arterial Distribution and Symptoms?

An anterior circulation ischemic stroke (◘ Table 56.2) is the most common type (70% of cases) of stroke. The cortex is supplied by branches of the two internal carotid arteries and two vertebral arteries. The anterior cerebral artery (ACA) and the middle cerebral artery (MCA), both of which branch from the internal carotid, connect with the posterior cerebral artery (derived from the basilar artery) to form the circle of Willis. The MCA primarily supplies the lateral surface of the frontal, parietal, and superior temporal lobes. The deeper branches supply the basal ganglia and internal capsule. An occlusion of the MCA is the most common location for an anterior circulation stroke, resulting in contralateral spastic paralysis/weakness, gaze palsy, and aphasia.

Why Is It Important to Distinguish Between Anterior and Posterior Circulation Symptoms?

Carotid plaques embolize to the anterior circulation, most often to the middle cerebral and less commonly into the anterior cerebral artery, thus causing anterior circulation symptoms. If the patient's symptoms are related to posterior circulation ischemia, then a carotid plaque should not be implicated as the source of the ischemia, and, therefore, carotid endarterectomy would not be beneficial.

Pathophysiology

What Are the Two Main Causes of Stroke?

Strokes are broadly categorized into ischemic and hemorrhagic types. Ischemic stroke (most common, about 85%) occurs when there is a blockage to the blood supply to the brain, whereas hemorrhagic stroke occurs when an artery ruptures and bleeds. The main causes of ischemic strokes are emboli (clot from somewhere else) and thrombosis (clot forming within the intracranial arteries). Causes of hemorrhagic stroke include *intracerebral* hemorrhage due to poorly controlled hypertension, trauma, congenital arteriovenous malformations, and *subarachnoid* hemorrhage due to a ruptured intracranial aneurysm.

Watch Out
Uncontrolled hypertension is a strong risk factor for both ischemic and hemorrhagic strokes.

What Are the Main Sources of Cerebral Emboli?

Emboli arise from the rupture of plaque in the ICA at the carotid bifurcation and from the heart (left atrial thrombus in association with atrial fibrillation, mural thrombus in association with acute myocardial infarction [MI], endocarditis). Less commonly, plaque from the aortic arch can embolize.

◘ **Table 56.2** Anterior circulation

Artery	Branches from	Supplies	Presentation with ischemia
Ophthalmic artery	Internal carotid artery	Retina	Ipsilateral amaurosis fugax; patients report sudden onset of painless loss of vision
Anterior cerebral artery	Internal carotid artery	Medial surfaces of the frontal and parietal lobes, corpus callosum, anterior portions of the basal ganglia, and internal capsule	Contralateral and greater motor and sensory loss in the lower extremities than upper extremities, gait apraxia
Middle cerebral artery	Internal carotid artery	Lateral frontal, parietal, and superior temporal lobes, insula, claustrum, internal capsule	Contralateral and greater motor and sensory loss of the upper extremities than the lower extremities, gaze palsy, aphasia, the *most common form* of anterior circulation ischemic stroke

Watch Out

If a patient presents with a TIA or stroke in association with a deep vein thrombosis, consider *paradoxical embolus*, which travels from the vein to the right heart, across a patent foramen ovale to the left heart, and then to the carotid artery.

What Is a Lacunar Stroke?

A lacunar stroke is an ischemic stroke that is caused by an occlusion of the deep penetrating arteries. The main risks are severe hypertension and diabetes. Lacunar infarcts are not generally thought to be due to large vessel (carotid) or cardiac embolization. Lacunar strokes involve deep brain structures such as the basal ganglia, internal capsule, and thalamus.

How Is an Atherosclerotic Plaque Formed?

The initiating event leading to plaque formation is believed to be endothelial damage. Damaged vessel walls release thrombin, adenosine diphosphate, and cytokines stimulating platelet migration. This initiates a cascade of events ultimately leading to smooth muscle proliferation and fibroplasia resulting in a narrowed vessel.

Why Does Atherosclerotic Plaque Localize at the Bifurcation of the Carotid Artery?

Atherosclerotic plaque has a predilection for developing at arterial bifurcations. Bifurcations cause alterations in blood flow. Specifically, it alters the shear stress (forces) applied to the arterial intima. High shear stress (seen at the *inner* wall or flow divider of bifurcations) is healthy for the intima, whereas low shear stress (seen in *outer* walls) promotes plaque buildup. Additionally, blood flow in the outer wall of a bifurcation has areas of transient reversal of flow with stasis of blood. This transient reversal of blood flow coupled with the low shear stress within the region promotes conditions favorable for additional plaque buildup at the outer walls.

Watch Out

Low shear stress promotes atherosclerotic plaque buildup.

How Does a Carotid Stenosis Typically Cause Symptoms?

Symptoms of carotid stenosis are most often caused by embolization of atherosclerotic debris from the ICA at the carotid bifurcation, which subsequently travels distally to the cerebral circulation. This embolic phenomenon can lead to transient ischemic attacks or strokes. Hemodynamically significant stenosis, by itself, rarely causes symptoms because collateral circulation from the contralateral carotid and vertebral arteries, via the circle of Willis, typically maintains adequate cerebral blood flow. Therefore, it is the embolic, rather than the flow-limiting, effect of carotid disease that is responsible for most clinical manifestations.

Is the Degree of ICA Stenosis Related to the Risk of Symptoms Developing?

As the atherosclerotic burden increases, the risk of developing symptoms increases. Larger plaques are more unstable and prone to rupture leading to a greater chance of distal embolization.

If a Patient Had Multiple TIAs with the Same Symptom Each Time, What Is the Most Likely Source of the TIA?

The most likely source would be the carotid artery. Blood flows in concentric laminar rings, and emboli originating from a carotid plaque tend to follow the same vascular path, lodging at the same distal branch point. This results in recurrent, stereotyped neurologic deficits. In contrast, emboli from a cardiac source such as atrial fibrillation can travel unpredictably throughout the systemic circulation, potentially causing a range of symptoms including stroke, limb ischemia, or mesenteric ischemia.

What Happens When the ICA Occludes?

The ICA typically occludes at its origin at the bifurcation in the neck. Since there are no branches in the neck, clot often propagates up into the brain. Depending on collateral blood flow, the clot may stop just before the ophthalmic artery or progress into the ACA or MCA. Thus, the occlusion may cause no symptoms, a TIA, or a stroke. Collateral blood flow is supplied by the circle of Willis.

What Is a Symptomatic Carotid Artery Stenosis?

A symptomatic carotid artery stenosis is one in which plaque from the carotid bifurcation is thought to be the source of emboli to the brain resulting in a TIA or a stroke within the anterior circulation. So classically, a carotid stenosis would be considered symptomatic if it results in ipsilateral amaurosis fugax with contralateral weakness/paralysis/numbness (transient, TIA or permanent, stroke).

What Additional Symptom Can Help Differentiate Left from Right Carotid Artery Stenosis?

Since Broca's area is in the left cerebral hemisphere, a stenosis of the left ICA can result in aphasia.

Workup

How Useful Is the Presence of a Bruit for Detecting Carotid Artery Stenosis?

The sensitivity and specificity of auscultation in detecting carotid artery stenosis are about 60% and 98%, respectively. Because of the low sensitivity, physical examination is not sufficient in ruling out the carotid artery as the source of stroke.

What Is the Diagnostic Test of Choice for the Workup of Possible Carotid Stenosis?

Carotid duplex scan is the first step in working up carotid stenosis. This noninvasive tool uses ultrasonography to visualize the plaque and Doppler to measure the rise in velocity of blood flow at the narrowed segment, which is proportional to the degree of stenosis.

Are Additional Diagnostic Studies Warranted?

Carotid duplex is somewhat operator dependent and provides a range of % stenosis (0–49%, 50–69%, 70–99%, occluded). Though additional studies are not needed,

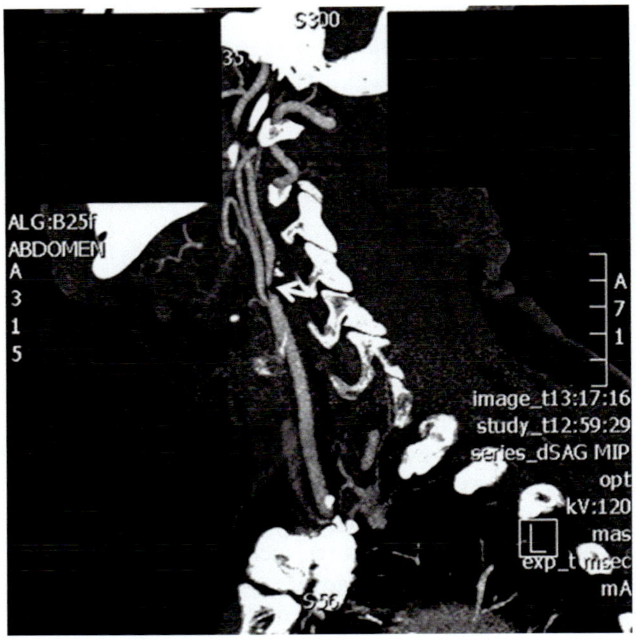

Fig. 56.1 Lateral CT angiogram showing high-grade stenosis at the origin of the internal carotid artery (*white arrow*)

many surgeons obtain a second study to confirm the exact percent of the ICA stenosis, either via CTA or MRA (Fig. 56.1). Formal angiogram is rarely used due to cost, invasiveness, and its risk of causing a stroke (the catheter that is inserted into the carotid artery may break off plaque).

Management

What Are the Three Management Options for Symptomatic Carotid Stenosis?

The three management options for symptomatic carotid stenosis are medical management alone, carotid endarterectomy (CEA), and carotid artery stenting (CAS). CAS includes transfemoral stenting and transcarotid (TCAR: transcarotid artery revascularization). All patients should receive medical therapy, including antiplatelet agents and a statin, regardless of whether they undergo a procedure. CEA is preferred in patients with significant stenosis who are good surgical candidates. CAS is generally reserved for patients at high surgical risk or with anatomy not amenable to open surgery, although with the advent of TCAR this is changing (see below). The choice between options depends on stenosis severity, surgical risk, and anatomic accessibility.

At What Percent of ICA Stenosis Should CEA Be Considered in Symptomatic Patients?

Benefit is greatest in symptomatic patients with high-grade (70–99%) stenosis. Benefit is greater (a) with hemispheric symptoms than amaurosis fugax, (b) in men than women, and (c) with increasing degree of stenosis. Refer to ◻ Table 56.3.

Following a Stroke or TIA, What Is the Optimal Timing of CEA?

CEA should optimally be performed within 2 weeks. The greatest risk of another embolic event is within that time frame. As such, the benefit of CEA is greatest within this time period. The longer one waits, the greater the risk of another embolic stroke, thus obviating the benefit of CEA.

Why Is CEA Not Recommended for a Symptomatic Patient with an Occluded (100% Stenosis) ICA?

CEA is not performed in cases of complete ICA occlusion because there is no antegrade flow, and therefore no ongoing risk of embolization from the occluded segment. Surgical intervention in this setting offers no benefit and carries significant risk, as the artery is thrombosed and the clot often extends intracranially, making revascularization technically unfeasible and potentially harmful.

◻ **Table 56.3** Management of carotid stenosis in a symptomatic patient

Degree of stenosis	Management
100%	Aspirin, statin, and/or clopidogrel
70–99%	CEA
50–69%	CEA is of less benefit (more benefit in men and if symptoms are hemispheric; no benefit in women and if symptom is amaurosis fugax)
<49%	Aspirin, statin, and/or clopidogrel

What Is the Role of CEA in a Patient with Symptomatic ICA Stenosis that Resulted in Complete Paralysis of the Arm and Leg As Well As Aphasia?

There is no role for CEA in a patient following a stroke that causes severe neurologic deficits (complete hemiplegia). The goal of CEA is to protect the remaining viable motor and language regions, so as to prevent further damage. With complete hemiplegia and aphasia, there is essentially no further viable motor cortex to protect, and thus the risks of surgery outweigh the benefits.

What Is the Anticipated Stroke Risk Reduction for CEA for a Symptomatic 70–99% ICA Stenosis?

For a 70–99% stenosis, CEA plus ASA (as compared with ASA alone) lowers the stroke rate at *2 years* from 26% to 9%.

What Is the Management of Carotid Stenosis in an Asymptomatic Patient? (◻ Table 56.4)

At What Percent of ICA Stenosis Should CEA Be Considered in *Asymptomatic* Patients?

Benefit is greatest in asymptomatic patients with 80–99% stenosis. Benefit is greater in men versus women and with increasing degree of stenosis. However the benefit

◻ **Table 56.4** Management of carotid stenosis in asymptomatic patient

Degree of stenosis	Management
100%	Aspirin, statin, and/or clopidogrel
60–99%	CEA for men, medical management for women
<59%	Aspirin, statin, and/or clopidogrel

CEA carotid endarterectomy, *ASA* aspirin

of CEA for asymptomatic patients is controversial, and recent studies suggest there may be no benefit.

What Is the Anticipated Stroke Risk Reduction for CEA for an Asymptomatic 60–99% ICA Stenosis?

CEA reduces stroke at *5 years* from 11% to 5% (or annually from about 2% to 1%).

Why Is There Less Benefit from CEA in Women?

The data suggests that women are more likely to have unfavorable outcomes, such as surgical mortality, neurologic morbidity, and recurrent stenosis. This is likely a reflection of the fact that women have smaller caliber vessels putting them at risk for developing recurrent stenosis and perioperative carotid thrombosis.

What Medications Have Been Shown to Reduce the Risk of Perioperative Stroke After CEA?

Aspirin, statins, clopidogrel, and antihypertensive agents to control blood pressure have been shown to reduce the risk of perioperative stroke after CEA. Aspirin should be continued before and after surgery, and statins are associated with improved perioperative and long-term outcomes. Clopidogrel is not routinely used and is sometimes indicated for dual antiplatelet therapy.

> **Watch Out**
> Statins not only lower serum cholesterol level, they also stabilize atherosclerotic plaque to prevent rupture and embolus (pleiotropic effect).

Why Is Blood Pressure Control Important Prior to CEA?

Poorly controlled blood pressure has been shown to increase the risk of perioperative stroke. In addition, the manipulation of the carotid artery (and carotid sinus) during CEA is associated with baroreceptor dysfunction.

What Complication Likely Occurred in a Patient Complaining of a Severe Headache Days After CEA?

This is concerning for *cerebral hyperperfusion syndrome* and occurs in 1% of CEA patients about 2–7 days after surgery. It is thought to occur as a result of impaired autoregulation of cerebral blood flow from long-standing stenosis of the carotid artery resulting in a compensatory dilation of distal cerebral vessels to maintain adequate cerebral blood flow. Once the carotid stenosis is repaired, autoregulation is not able to immediately adjust to the sudden increase in blood flow. Patients complain of a severe frontal headache, possibly followed by seizures and, rarely, intracerebral hemorrhage.

What Cranial Nerves Are at Risk of Injury During CEA? (Table 56.5)

> **Watch Out**
> The most common cranial nerve injury following CEA is to the hypoglossal nerve (tongue deviation to side of injury), followed by injury to the recurrent laryngeal nerve (hoarseness).

What Is an Acceptable Risk of Stroke/Death Following CEA?

The acceptable risk of stroke/death following CEA is <3% for asymptomatic CEA and <6% for symptomatic CEA.

Table 56.5 Cranial nerves at risk during CEA

Cranial nerve	Presentation
VII (marginal mandibular branch)	Droop in the corner of the mouth
IX (glossopharyngeal nerve)	Difficulty in swallowing
X (vagus nerve)	Hoarseness due to recurrent laryngeal nerve coming off distal to injury
XI (spinal accessory nerve)	Diminished or absent function of the sternocleidomastoid or trapezius muscles
XII (hypoglossal nerve)	Tongue deviation to the side of injury

What Is the Role of Mechanical Thrombectomy in the Management of Ischemic Stroke?

Mechanical thrombectomy is indicated in patients with acute ischemic stroke due to large vessel occlusion, most commonly in the MCA. It is performed by interventional radiologists and is most effective when initiated within 6 hours of symptom onset, though select patients with favorable imaging may benefit up to 24 hours out. It is used in conjunction with, or following intravenous thrombolytics if the patient is eligible. Thrombectomy is not a treatment for carotid stenosis itself but may be performed in patients with carotid-origin emboli who develop a large vessel stroke.

What Imaging Is Required Before Performing Mechanical Thrombectomy?

Non-contrast head CT is performed first to rule out hemorrhage. If no hemorrhage is seen, CT angiography is used to identify large vessel occlusion, and CT perfusion may be used to assess the extent of salvageable brain tissue (penumbra). Patients with small core infarct volume and significant penumbra may be eligible for thrombectomy even beyond the traditional 6-hour window.

Area Where You Can Get in Trouble

New Neurologic Deficit in the Postoperative Recovery Room After CEA

New neurologic deficits (weakness of extremity, loss of speech) occurring immediately after CEA (in the recovery room) are concerning for thromboembolic phenomena or a residual intimal flap at the repair site. The patient should immediately be given systemic heparin and taken back to the operating room for exploration (do not waste time with imaging).

Area of Controversy

Carotid Stenting Versus CEA for Symptomatic High-Grade (>70%) ICA Stenosis

CEA remains the standard treatment for symptomatic high-grade ICA stenosis and is associated with a lower risk of perioperative stroke compared to transfemoral CAS. Transfemoral CAS was developed as a less invasive alternative for patients at high surgical risk. Advantages of transfemoral CAS include avoidance of general anesthesia, no neck incision, and a lower risk of cranial nerve injury and myocardial infarction. However, CAS carries a higher risk of perioperative stroke (wires are passed through the aortic arch and carotid) and is generally not recommended for asymptomatic disease. CAS is best reserved for symptomatic patients with a hostile neck (e.g., prior surgery, radiation, or high lesion location) or those who are poor candidates for open surgery. TCAR involves placing the stent directly into the carotid though a small neck incision and using flow reversal to prevent embolization. It appears to have the same low risk of stroke as CEA, but less risk of cranial nerve injury. It is becoming more widely adopted.

Carotid Artery Disease (◘ Fig. 56.2)

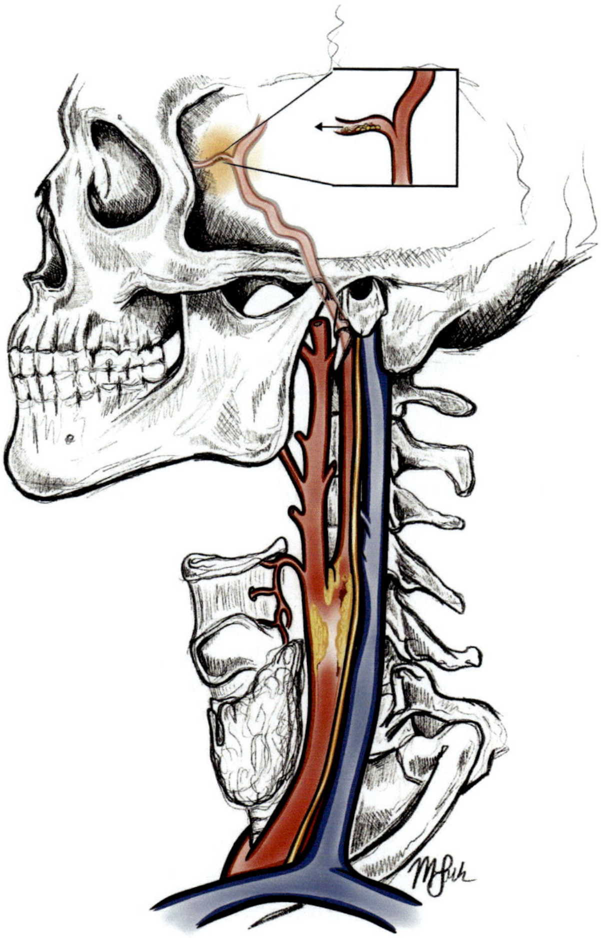

◘ **Fig 56.2** **Carotid artery embolism:** An atherosclerotic plaque within the common carotid artery can serve as a source of emboli, which can travel to arteries like the ophthalmic artery

Summary of Essentials

Differential Diagnosis

- Transient monocular vision loss (amaurosis fugax) differential includes carotid embolus, central retinal artery occlusion, giant cell arteritis, retinal vein occlusion, retinal detachment, papilledema, and optic neuritis

History

- TIA <24 hours, stroke >24 hours.
- Classic carotid symptoms: ipsilateral amaurosis fugax and contralateral arm/leg weakness or numbness ± aphasia (if left-sided).
- Carotid stenosis is more common in men, smokers, and those with hypertension and hyperlipidemia.
- Dizziness, syncope, and headaches are not typical symptoms of carotid stenosis.
- Stroke: the fourth leading cause of death in the United States.

Physical Exam

- Hollenhorst plaques (emboli to the retina on fundoscopic exam).
- Carotid bruit is specific but not sensitive.

Pathology/Pathophysiology

- Symptoms of carotid disease are most often due to embolization, not flow limitation.
- Low shear stress promotes atherosclerotic plaque formation.
- ICA stenosis affects anterior circulation; most commonly causes MCA infarcts.
- Posterior circulation ischemic stroke not from carotid disease (most often from cardiac embolus).
- Carotid stenosis is a marker for systemic atherosclerosis; MI is the most common cause of death in these patients.

Workup

- Carotid duplex to determine % ICA stenosis.
- Confirmatory imaging recommended (CTA or MRA).
- Mechanical thrombectomy may be indicated in acute ischemic stroke due to large vessel occlusion, particularly MCA territory strokes, typically within 6 hours (up to 24 in select cases).

Management

- All patients should receive medical therapy (aspirin, statin, blood pressure control)
- CEA
  - Greatest benefit for symptomatic 70–99% ICA stenosis
  - Less benefit for symptomatic 50–69% ICA stenosis
  - Questionable benefit for asymptomatic stenosis
  - No benefit for <50% ICA stenosis
- Transfemoral carotid stenting
  - Higher risk of stroke than CEA (less risk of perioperative MI)
  - Best used for symptomatic ICA stenosis with high cardiac risk or hostile neck (radiated, prior surgery)
  - Not indicated for asymptomatic ICA stenosis
- TCAR: Similar risk of stroke as CEA, less risk of cranial nerve injury

Suggested Reading

Barnett HJ, Taylor DW, Eliasziw M, et al. Benefit of carotid endarterectomy in patients with symptomatic moderate or severe stenosis. North American Symptomatic Carotid Endarterectomy Trial Collaborators. N Engl J Med. 1998;339(20):1415–25.

Brott TG, Hobson RW 2nd, Howard G, et al. Stenting versus endarterectomy for treatment of carotid-artery stenosis. N Engl J Med. 2010;363:11–23.

Executive Committee for the Asymptomatic Carotid Atherosclerosis Study. Endarterectomy for asymptomatic carotid artery stenosis. JAMA. 1995;273:1421–8.

Kashyap, Vikram S., Alexander H. King, Mazin I. Foteh, Matthew Janko, Jeffrey Jim, Raghu L. Motaganahalli, Jeffrey M. Apple, Saideep Bose, and Norman H. Kumins. "A multi-institutional analysis of transcarotid artery revascularization compared to carotid endarterectomy." Journal of vascular surgery 70, no. 1 (2019): 123–129.

North American Symptomatic Carotid Artery Trial Collaborators. Beneficial effect of carotid endarterectomy in symptomatic patients with high-grade carotid stenosis. N Engl J Med. 1991;325:445–53.

Right Calf Pain with Walking

Cooper Nagaki and Christian de Virgilio

Contents

C. de Virgilio, A. Grigorian (eds.), *Surgery*, https://doi.org/10.1007/978-3-032-09799-6_57

Case Study

A 65-year-old male presents with a 5-month history of progressively worsening right calf pain upon walking. He describes the pain as a tightening or cramping, and it comes on after walking two blocks. The pain forces him to stop walking and is relieved after he sits down for 5 minutes. The pain comes on consistently at the same two-block walking distance each time, unless he walks fast or uphill, in which case he can walk much less. He denies waking up at night with pain in his foot. He reports a 40-pack-year smoking history and is taking antihypertensives. He has normal 2+ femoral pulses bilaterally; nonpalpable (0) popliteal, dorsalis pedis, and posterior tibial pulses on the right side; and diminished (1+) popliteal, dorsalis pedis, and posterior tibial pulses on the left. He is moderately obese, yet both legs appear to be thin. The skin on his lower legs appears thin and shiny, flaky, and dry, with no hair. His toenails are thickened. There are no ulcers on his feet. Capillary refill is diminished in his right foot at 4 seconds (normal ≤2 seconds). Laboratory values reveal a total cholesterol of 280 mg/dL (normal <200 mg/dL), low-density lipoprotein (LDL) of 160 mg/dL (65–180 mg/dL), and a high-density lipoprotein (HDL) of 35 mg/dL (>35 mg/dL).

Diagnosis

What Is the Differential Diagnosis? (Table 57.1)

Table 57.1 Differential diagnosis for case presentation

Disease	Pathophysiology	Symptoms
Peripheral arterial disease	Atherosclerotic plaque obstructing blood flow	Pain with walking
		Relieved with a few minutes of rest
		Reproducible at the same walking distance
Osteoarthritis of the hip or knee	Mechanical degeneration of joint structures	Not relieved with a few minutes of rest
		Not reproducible at the same walking distance
Spinal stenosis	Narrowing of the spaces of the vertebral column causing nerve root compression (neurogenic claudication)	Generalized weakness of both legs that worsens with walking
		Relieved by leaning forward
Sciatica	Irritation or compression of the sciatic nerve	Buttock pain, leg pain "shooting" down the posterior thigh
Chronic venous stasis	Incompetence of vein valves, pooling of blood in the legs	Worse after prolonged standing (end of the day)
		Leg swelling
		Relieved by elevating legs and wearing compression stockings

What Is the Most Likely Diagnosis?

In an elderly patient with a long-standing smoking history, hypertension, hypercholesterolemia, and a 5-month history of progressively worsening and reproducible right calf pain with exercise, the most likely diagnosis is claudication secondary to peripheral arterial disease (PAD). In addition, his physical exam (thin, flaky, dry, hairless legs) and diminished pulses are consistent with the diagnosis.

History and Physical

What Is Claudication, and What Is the Three-Part Definition that Should Be Obtained by History?

Claudication derives from the Latin word *claudicare* which means "to limp." It is caused by a reduction in blood flow to the leg muscles, most commonly by an atherosclerotic plaque. It is not typically due to a blood clot or embolization. The reduced arterial blood supply cannot meet the metabolic demand of the muscles utilized during walking. The diagnosis can readily be suspected based on the three-part definition obtained by history: (1) pain in the leg with walking, (2) relieved within a few minutes of rest, and (3) reproducible at the same walking distance each time.

Claudication Is a Symptom of What Underlying Disease?

Claudication is a symptom of PAD, commonly caused by atherosclerosis. PAD primarily affects the lower extremities, though it can also involve the upper extremities, intestinal, and renal arteries.

What Are the Main Risk Factors for PAD?

Modifiable risk factors for PAD include smoking, obesity, sedentary lifestyle, hypertension, diabetes, and hypercholesterolemia. Non-modifiable risk factors for PAD include advanced age, male gender, and family history of cardiovascular disease.

What Is the Spectrum of Severity in PAD?

The spectrum of severity is categorized by the Rutherford classification of chronic limb ischemia (◘ Table 57.2).

◘ **Table 57.2** The Rutherford classification system of chronic limb ischemia

Category	Patient presentation
0	Asymptomatic
1	Mild claudication
2	Moderate claudication
3	Severe claudication
4	Ischemic rest pain
5	Minor tissue loss
6	Major tissue loss

What Is Critical Limb-Threatening Ischemia (CLTI)?

CLTI is a term used for severe, advanced PAD that places the limb at significant risk of amputation. It includes Rutherford categories 4, 5, and 6.

What Is Ischemic Rest Pain, and How Does It Present?

Ischemic rest pain is a sign of advanced PAD (Rutherford class 4). It typically occurs in the toes, where blood flow is most limited. This pain usually presents at night when the patient is lying flat, as the patient's arterial blood flow is so severe that gravity is needed to aid blood flow to the foot. Patients with ischemic rest pain wake up due to aching or numb toes, prompting them to walk around or dangle the leg over the bed. In severe cases, they may need to sleep with the leg in a dependent position, such as in an inclined bed or chair, to alleviate the pain.

Watch Out

Always ask about rest pain, as the presence of rest pain identifies a patient as having CLTI. Ask the patient specifically if they ever wake up at night with pain in their foot and what they do to relieve it (such as dangle the foot over the edge of the bed or get out of bed). Rest pain can be confused with diabetic neuropathy. Neuropathic pain tends to be burning in nature, involves the whole foot (both feet usually), and is not relieved by dependency.

What Is Buerger's Sign?

It is a physical examination sign of CLTI. The affected foot turns pale after it is elevated (usually for 2 minutes). Once the patient sits up and dangles the foot down, it becomes ruborous (like a cooked lobster) due to marked arteriolar dilation from chronic severe ischemia that causes a reactive hyperemia. Patients with ischemic rest pain typically will manifest Buerger's sign. Such patients will also have multiple levels of arterial obstruction and an accompanying low ankle–brachial index (ABI) of <0.4. The absence of Buerger's sign makes ischemic rest pain less likely.

Watch Out
Do not confuse Buerger's sign with Buerger's disease (thromboangiitis obliterans), which presents with cyanotic and blue digits, typically in young male smokers.

How Is the ABI Measured?

It is measured with the patient in a supine position. A handheld Doppler and a blood pressure (BP) cuff are needed to measure ABI. The BP cuff is inflated, while the Doppler is held on the dorsalis pedis artery. The cuff is inflated until the Doppler signal disappears. The cuff is slowly deflated until the signal returns. The systolic pressure at which the signal returns is recorded. The process is repeated with the posterior tibial and bilateral brachial arteries. The ABI is the ratio of the highest systolic pressure at the ankle *or* foot (of the side in question) over the highest brachial systolic pressure (of the right *or* left side).

How Many Pulses Should Be Examined?

Seventeen pulses should be examined: superficial temporal, carotid, brachial, radial, femoral, popliteal, posterior tibial, dorsalis pedis bilaterally, and aortic.

In Addition to a Pulse Deficit, What Other Findings on Leg Examination Would Support PAD?

PAD leads to reduced blood supply, resulting in muscle atrophy, hair loss, dry and scaly skin, and thin, shiny skin. Ulcers may develop, and capillary refill time is prolonged (normally ≤2 seconds).

Watch Out
Ulcers at the most distal aspects of the extremities (e.g., toes) are generally arterial in etiology, whereas more proximal ulcers (e.g., malleoli) are generally venous in etiology.

Anatomy

What Muscle Groups Are Affected by Claudication?

Claudication may affect all the major muscle groups associated with walking, including the buttock, anterior thigh, calf, and rarely the foot muscles. The calf muscles are supplied by the superficial femoral artery (SFA). The SFA, which travels through the Hunter/adductor canal, is the most common site for atherosclerosis in the lower extremities; therefore, calf claudication is the most common location of pain. The internal iliac arteries supply the buttocks. Thus, stenosis above the internal iliac arteries (aorta, common iliac arteries) would cause buttock claudication. The hamstrings are not primarily utilized for walking. Thus, pain in the back of the thigh is not characteristic of claudication. Foot claudication is extremely rare and is most often seen in Buerger's disease, as they typically have isolated tibial artery disease.

Where Is the Hunter/Adductor Canal Located?

This aponeurotic tunnel extends from the apex of the femoral triangle to the opening of adductor magnus (adductor hiatus). The SFA runs through this canal and becomes the above-knee popliteal artery just distal to it. The adductor canal is bordered anteriorly by the sartorius muscle, laterally by the vastus medialis, and posteriorly by the adductor longus and adductor magnus.

Watch Out
The common femoral artery is the most common location of arterial emboli, while the more distal SFA is the most common location of atherosclerotic plaque.

Pathophysiology

What Is Dependent Rubor?

Dependent rubor is a sign of advanced chronic ischemia. It occurs when the arterioles in the foot remain vasodilated, causing blood to pool in a dependent (lowered) position. This vasodilation compensates for poor blood and oxygen delivery. Dependent rubor confers a higher risk of CLTI (ischemic rest pain or nonhealing ulcers) compared to claudication alone.

Why Is the Onset of Claudication Consistently at the Same Walking Distance?

Claudication is typically due to an atherosclerotic plaque, a fixed lesion that restricts blood flow by a consistent amount. Thus, patients often experience pain after walking a predictable distance, helping differentiate claudication from other leg pain causes. If a patient describes significant variability in walking ability (e.g., one day walking only a few steps, another day walking a mile), this is less consistent with claudication. Slight variations in pain onset can occur with changes in effort, such as walking faster, slower, uphill, or downhill, as these alter oxygen demand.

What Other Disease Processes Can Cause Claudication?

Buerger's disease, vasculitis, and entrapment of the popliteal artery can also cause claudication.

What Condition Is Classically Associated with Claudication in the Upper Extremities?

Subclavian steal syndrome is classically associated with upper extremity claudication. In this condition, an atherosclerotic plaque narrows the proximal subclavian artery, most often on the left. During arm activity (such as combing or brushing hair), blood is diverted in a retrograde fashion from the vertebral artery into the subclavian artery to supply the working limb. This "steals" blood from the vertebrobasilar system, potentially leading to symptoms such as vertigo, dizziness, or presyncope during arm exertion, in addition to arm fatigue or claudication. A significant difference in systolic blood pressure between the arms supports the diagnosis.

What Is Buerger's Disease?

It is also known as thromboangiitis obliterans and is seen in young (<40 years), predominantly male, smokers. It is an inflammatory and thrombotic process that causes occlusion of small- to medium-sized arteries, veins, and nerves of the upper and lower extremities. Patients present with claudication of the leg, foot, arm, or hand, which can progress to ischemic rest pain and ulcerations of the toes, feet, and fingers. It is associated with a high rate of amputation and a lack of response to angioplasty or bypass. The only effective treatment is smoking cessation.

What Is Leriche's Syndrome (Aortoiliac Occlusive Disease)?

It is a chronic, slowly developing occlusion of the infrarenal aorta most often seen in smokers, characterized by a triad: (1) bilateral buttock and thigh claudication, (2) absent femoral pulses, and (3) impotence. Since the aorta is occluded, the blood flow to the internal iliac arteries is compromised, which in turn decreases blood supply to internal pudendal arteries causing erectile dysfunction. Because of the slow progressive nature, collaterals have time to enlarge and compensate, such that most patients only have claudication and not ischemic rest pain.

Workup

What Is the Next Step in the Diagnostic Workup?

The ABI and arterial duplex scan are the next steps in the diagnostic workup. The ABI measures the ratio of the systolic pressure in the foot (ankle) to the systolic pressure in the arm (brachial artery). The normal ABI ranges from 1 to 1.2 because the ankle pressure in the supine position can be as much as 20% higher than in the arm. The arterial duplex scan uses a combination of ultrasound to detect plaques in the arteries and Doppler to detect areas of elevated velocity of blood flow, indicating that the plaque is causing a hemodynamically significant stenosis. The diagnosis of PAD can be established based on these two studies.

Watch Out

The API (arterial pressure index) is used in trauma and compares the systolic pressure in the injured extremity with the contralateral uninjured extremity. A ratio <0.9 is considered abnormal.

How Is PAD Defined? (Table 57.3)

Table 57.3 Relationship of ABI to presence/severity of PAD

Normal ABI	1.2–1.0
Mild disease	0.9–0.7
Moderate disease	0.7–0.4
Severe disease/rest pain	<0.4

Watch Out

PAD is defined as ABI < 0.9.

What Is the Typical ABI of a Patient with Claudication? Rest Pain?

Patients with claudication usually have an ABI in the 0.6–0.8 range. Patients with ischemic rest pain or tissue loss usually have an ABI < 0.4.

Once the Diagnosis of PAD Is Established with ABI and Duplex, Are Further Studies Needed? If So, What Study?

It depends. If the patient only has claudication, since the initial management is medical, additional studies are not needed. On the other hand, if the patient has CLTI, a computed tomography angiography (CTA) is recommended as it will help plan intervention (Figs. 57.1 and 57.2).

What is a Formal Angiogram?

A formal angiogram is typically performed via a femoral arterial puncture. The angiogram can be diagnostic (to plan a bypass) and/or therapeutic (when an artery undergoes balloon angioplasty and/or stenting).

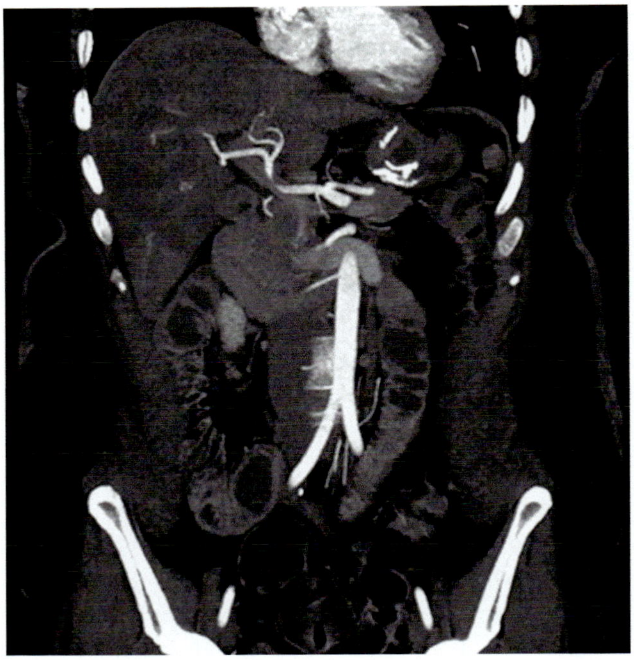

Fig. 57.1 Coronal CT angiogram showing a normal aorta and common iliac arteries

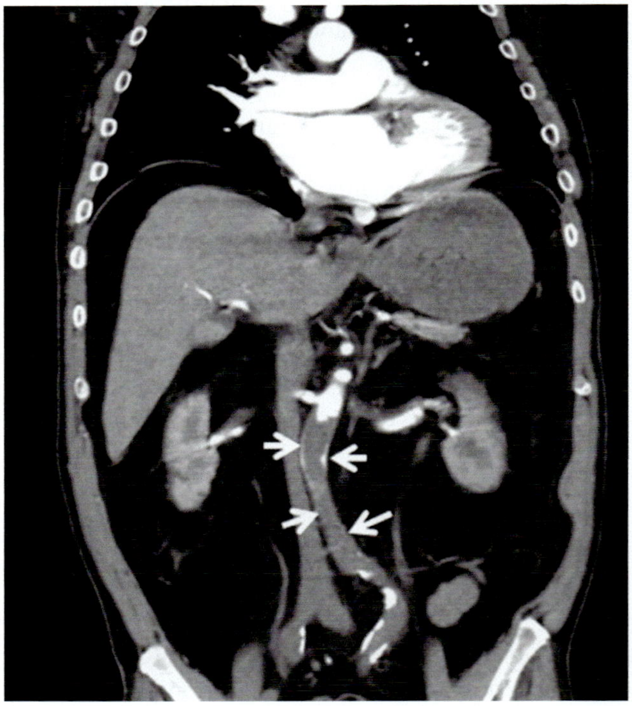

Fig. 57.2 Coronal CT angiogram showing occlusion of the abdominal aorta just below the renal arteries

Prognosis

What Is the Risk of Limb Loss for Patients with Claudication?

Provided the patient does not have ischemic rest pain or tissue loss, the 5-year risk of limb loss for all comers with claudication is surprisingly low at < 5%. The 10-year risk of limb loss is 10%.

What Is the Risk of Limb Loss for Patients with Ischemic Rest Pain in the Foot?

Rest pain makes it highly likely (50%) that the patient will have limb loss at 1 year if no intervention is performed.

What Symptoms/Signs Are Considered an Indication for More Aggressive Management?

CLTI (ischemic rest pain, nonhealing ulcer, and gangrene) are indications for more aggressive intervention.

Management

What Is the Initial Management of Claudication?

Given the low risk of limb loss, initial management of claudication is primarily medical, targeting modifiable risk factors. The most effective treatment for claudication is a supervised walking program (walking 45 minutes daily for at least a month). Smoking cessation is also important. Additional management involves controlling hypertension, coronary artery disease, hypercholesterolemia, diabetes, and obesity through antihypertensives, aspirin, statins, glucose control, and dietary changes. While these latter measures can slow atherosclerosis progression, they may not directly improve walking distance.

Are There Any Drugs Specifically Approved by the Food and Drug Administration (FDA) for Claudication?

Two drugs are FDA-approved for claudication, with only one considered effective. *Cilostazol* is the preferred choice, improving symptoms in about 50% of patients within a month. It works by inhibiting platelet aggregation, promoting vasodilation, and lowering triglycerides but is contraindicated in heart failure. *Pentoxifylline*, also FDA-approved, is less effective (comparable to placebo) and acts by reducing blood viscosity and increasing red blood cell flexibility.

What About a Statin? Does It Improve Claudication?

Statins are recommended for all patients with PAD, regardless of cholesterol levels, due to their plaque-stabilizing and anti-inflammatory effects, which significantly reduce the risk of myocardial infarction (MI) and stroke. For patients with elevated cholesterol, the goal is to achieve a low-density lipoprotein (LDL) level of <70 mg/dL. Their primary role in PAD is cardiovascular risk reduction, not direct symptom relief.

What About Aspirin? Does It Improve Claudication?

Aspirin does not directly improve claudication. However, since there is a strong association between PAD and coronary and carotid atherosclerosis, aspirin is thought to reduce the risk of cardiovascular events such as stroke and myocardial infarction. Aspirin inhibits platelet aggregation by suppressing the platelet's ability to produce thromboxane A2 due to its irreversible inactivation of the cyclooxygenase enzyme.

What About Clopidogrel?

Clopidogrel irreversibly inhibits platelet aggregation by selectively inhibiting the binding of adenosine diphosphate to the platelet P2Y12 receptor. It does not directly lead to an improvement in claudication or walking distance. However, in patients with PAD it has been shown to reduce the composite endpoint of stroke, myocardial infarction, or other vascular deaths. However, it has a higher risk of bleeding; thus, it is not routinely used in all patients with PAD, and there is debatable benefit to its routine use in combination with aspirin.

What About Anticoagulants Such as Heparin or Warfarin?

Claudication is due to an atherosclerotic plaque obstructing the blood flow and *not* a blood clot or embolization. As such, there is no role for anticoagulants.

What Are the Invasive Therapeutic Options?

Invasive therapeutic options are endovascular angioplasty/stenting (preferable in most patients) and open surgical techniques (endarterectomy or bypass).

If Medical Management Fails, Which Patients with Claudication Are Candidates for an Invasive Therapeutic Approach?

Patients with disabling claudication (Rutherford class 2 or 3) may be considered for invasive treatment provided (1) they are good-risk candidates for an intervention and (2) the symptoms are significantly affecting their lifestyle. For example, an elderly frail patient on home oxygen for pulmonary disease would not be a good-risk candidate, and their walking distance is more likely limited by their pulmonary disease than by the PAD. A security guard or a mail carrier would much more likely be limited by the PAD (and benefit from intervention). There is no role for invasive intervention in asymptomatic PAD.

Which Patients with PAD Should Go Directly to an Invasive Therapeutic Approach Rather Than an Initial Attempt at Medical Management?

Patients with CLTI (Rutherford classes 4–6) should go directly to an invasive therapeutic approach as their risk of limb loss is significantly higher.

What Is the 5-Year Mortality for Patients with PAD?

Mortality for patients with moderate PAD is 30% at 5 years and is 60% for patients with severe disease. This is due to myocardial infarction, primarily, and stroke. Mortality is even higher for patients who continue to smoke.

Key Areas Where You Can Get in Trouble

Confusing the Dependent Rubor of Rest Pain with Cellulitis (or Confusing Dependent Rubor with a Well-Perfused Foot)

In patients with advanced PAD, ischemic rest pain is constant, requiring the patient to even sleep with their feet dangling or to sleep in a chair. This may lead to some dependent edema in the leg, as well as to dependent rubor. The combination of redness and edema may confuse the diagnosis, and the clinician can mistake ischemia with cellulitis. The two can be distinguished by raising the foot. In ischemia, the red skin will be cool to touch, and upon elevation for 1–2 minutes, the rubor will disappear, and the foot will turn pale. With cellulitis, the red skin will feel warm, and the red color will *persist* with elevation.

Assuming an ABI of >1.0 Is a Sign of Normal Circulation in a Diabetic Patient

Diabetic patients may develop falsely elevated (>1.2) or falsely normal ABIs. Diabetic patients develop a unique form of arteriosclerosis known as *Monckeberg's arteriosclerosis* or *medial calcinosis*. It involves intense calcification of the medial layer of the artery (typically the tibial vessels below the knee), which causes them to become rigid like a lead pipe. The result is that when one attempts to obtain an ABI, the blood pressure cuff is either unable to compress the artery or the pressure required to compress the artery is falsely elevated. This typically affects the tibial vessels, sparing digital vessels in the toes. As such, toe pressures in diabetics are more reliable, as are other measures of distal perfusion, including transcutaneous oximetry.

Areas of Controversy

Should a Patient with Claudication Who Is Still Smoking Undergo an Invasive Procedure?

As explained above, claudication (in the absence of CLTI) is not considered limb threatening. The primary treatment modality is lifestyle and risk factor modification. Studies have shown that if patients continue to smoke, the disease will progress. Smoking is associated with worse outcomes after angioplasty, stenting, and bypass. Thus, many surgeons do not advocate pursuing aggressive intervention in patients with claudication until they have quit smoking. The counterargument is that the patient may need to see an immediate improvement in walking in order to embrace a healthier lifestyle.

Should a Patient with Claudication Ever Undergo an Invasive Procedure?

Some recent studies suggest that a patient with claudication who undergoes endovascular procedures such as balloon angioplasty or stenting may be at higher long-term risk of limb loss than those who are managed medically. This may be due to the fact that endovascular procedures tend with time to re-stenose or occlude. When a stent occludes, the patient may present with sudden acute limb ischemia. This in turn leads to multiple repeat interventions, each of which carry a risk of causing embolization and limb loss.

In a Patient with CLTI (Rutherford Class 4, 5, or 6), Is It Better to Attempt an Endovascular Approach (Angioplasty/Stenting) or to Perform an Open Surgical Bypass (Using Reverse Saphenous Vein)?

A recent randomized study demonstrated that in patients with CLTI who had an adequate great saphenous vein for surgical bypass, the incidence of a major adverse limb event or death was significantly lower in the surgical bypass group as compared to the endovascular group. In the absence of an adequate saphenous vein, surgical bypass (using spliced vein, arm vein or synthetic grafts) has similar outcome to endovascular procedures.

Summary of Essentials

History

- Calf, thigh, or buttock pain with walking, relieved by rest, reproducible at the same distance is suggestive of claudication.

Physical Exam

- Absent pulses, muscle atrophy, hair loss, dry and atrophic skin, toe ulcers, and thickened toenails suggest PAD

Pathology/Pathophysiology

- SFA is the most common site of atherosclerotic disease in the lower extremities (Hunter canal).

Differential Diagnosis

- Neurogenic claudication (spinal stenosis), arthritis, sciatica, and chronic venous stasis.

Diagnosis

- By history and physical exam supplemented by ABI with Doppler and duplex ultrasound.
- Reserve CT or MR angiogram only if intervention is planned.

Management

- Conservative for claudication (Rutherford classes 1–3): smoking cessation, walking program, statin, and aspirin
- Best drug for claudication is cilostazol (improves walking distance).
- Interventional if with ischemic rest pain or tissue loss (Rutherford classes 4–6).
- Invasive treatment options include angioplasty/stenting (for stenosis and short occlusions), endarterectomy, and surgical bypass (long occlusions).
- Surgical bypass better than endovascular if adequate saphenous vein.

Prognosis

- Five-year risk of limb loss less than 5% with claudication.
- Five-year mortality 30% (due mainly to MI).

Special Situations

- Subclavian steal syndrome: arm claudication and dizziness.
- Leriche's syndrome: buttock claudication, absent femoral pulses, and impotence.
- Buerger's disease: young male smokers with distal artery and vein occlusions.

Watch Out

- Falsely normal ABI in diabetics with medial calcinosis.

Acknowledgments The editors would like to acknowledge and thank the following authors for their contributions to the previous edition of the chapter: Divya Ramakrishnan.

Suggested Reading

Farber A, Menard MT, Conte MS, et al. BEST-CLI Investigators. Surgery or Endovascular Therapy for Chronic Limb-Threatening Ischemia. N Engl J Med. 2022 Dec 22;387(25):2305–2316. https://doi.org/10.1056/NEJMoa2207899. Epub 2022 Nov 7. PMID: 36342173.

Hirsch AT, Criqui MH, Treat-Jacobson D, et al. Peripheral arterial disease detection, awareness, and treatment in primary care. JAMA. 2001;286:1317.

Layden J, Michaels J, Bermingham S, et al. Diagnosis and management of lower limb peripheral arterial disease: summary of NICE guidance. BMJ. 2012;345:e4947.

McDermott MM, Greenland P, Liu K, et al. Leg symptoms in peripheral arterial disease: associated clinical characteristics and functional impairment. JAMA. 2001;286:1599.

Rooke TW, Hirsch AT, Misra S, et al. Management of patients with peripheral artery disease (compilation of 2005 and 2011 ACCF/AHA Guideline Recommendations): a report of the American College of Cardiology Foundation/American Heart Association Task Force on Practice Guidelines. J Am Coll Cardiol. 2013;61:1555.

Sudden Onset of Severe Left-Sided Abdominal Pain

Cooper Nagaki, Michael de Virgilio, and Nina M. Bowens

Contents

C. de Virgilio, A. Grigorian (eds.), *Surgery*, https://doi.org/10.1007/978-3-032-09799-6_58

Case Study

A 67-year-old obese male presents to the emergency department with sudden onset of severe left-sided abdominal pain that radiates to the left flank and back. The pain began 2 h ago while he was watching television. He has never had the pain before. He denies any nausea or vomiting, changes in bowel habits, or bloody/black stools. His history is significant for chronic obstructive pulmonary disease (COPD) and well-controlled hypertension. He does not drink alcohol but has a 35 pack-year smoking history. On physical exam, blood pressure is 90/60 mmHg, heart rate is 120/min, respiratory rate is 24/min, and he is afebrile. He appears to be in moderate distress secondary to pain and is diaphoretic. Lungs are clear bilaterally to auscultation without rales or rhonchi. Cardiac exam reveals a regular rhythm without murmurs, rubs, or gallops. His abdomen is moderately tender to palpation diffusely but worse in the mid-abdomen and in the left lower quadrant. He has no rebound or guarding. A palpable, tender pulsatile mass is felt in the midline just above the umbilicus. Rectal exam reveals no blood, stool, or masses. Femoral, popliteal, and pedal pulses are 1+ bilaterally. Laboratory examination reveals a hemoglobin of 10.1 g/dL (normal 12.3–15.7 g/dL), hematocrit of 30.3% (37–46%), and white blood cell count of 11 × 10^3/μL (4.1–10.9 × 10^3/μL), aminotransferase (AST) of 44 μ/L (5–35 μ/L), alanine aminotransferase (ALT) of 65 μ/L (7–56 μ/L), lipase of 50 μ/L (7–60 μ/L), and amylase of 62 μ/L (30–110 μ/L).

Diagnosis

What Is the Differential Diagnosis? (Table 58.1)

What Is the Most Likely Diagnosis?

In an elderly patient with a history of smoking, hypertension, and chronic obstructive pulmonary disease who presents with a pulsatile abdominal mass, sudden onset of abdominal and left flank pain, hypotension, tachycardia, pallor, and diaphoresis, the most likely diagnosis is a ruptured abdominal aortic aneurysm (AAA). The presence of anemia without an identifiable external source of bleeding further supports this diagnosis, as the rupture of an aneurysm into the retroperitoneum can lead to significant blood loss without external signs.

History and Physical Examination

What Is the Typical Presentation for an Unruptured AAA?

Most unruptured AAAs are asymptomatic and therefore go undetected. In most patients, the first symptom of an AAA is rupture, which is often fatal. For this reason, AAA is referred to as a silent killer. Most AAAs are discovered incidentally (CT, ultrasound) during the

Table 58.1 Differential diagnosis for the case presentation

Diagnosis	History and physical examination
Ruptured AAA	Caucasian, elderly, male, smoker with sudden onset of severe abdominal, left flank, left groin, and/or lower back pain; pulsatile abdominal mass; tachycardia; and hypotension
Perforated gastric or duodenal ulcer	Sudden onset of epigastric pain which then becomes diffuse, history of steroid or chronic NSAID use, abdominal guarding, rigidity, and rebound tenderness
Aortic dissection	Sharp, tearing chest pain radiating to the back; history of hypertension
Pancreatitis	Epigastric pain radiating to the back, nausea, vomiting, anorexia, fever, and tachycardia, associated with cholelithiasis and alcohol abuse
Diverticulitis	Pain begins in left lower quadrant and may become diffuse; fever, nausea, diarrhea, constipation, common in elderly
Renal Colic	Flank pain radiating to groin, hematuria

AAA abdominal aortic aneurysm, *NSAID* nonsteroidal anti-inflammatory drug

workup for other medical problems. Rarely, as an AAA enlarges, patients can experience chronic lower back pain from compression of the spine. Thrombus commonly forms within the outer walls of an AAA. Rarely, the thrombus may embolize to the lower extremities, resulting in acute limb ischemia.

What Are the Risk Factors for AAA?

Risk factors include smoking, age ≥ 65, Caucasian race, male, coronary artery disease, a history of extra-abdominal aneurysm such as femoral or popliteal aneurysms, peripheral arterial disease, family history of AAA, COPD, and hypertension.

Watch Out
Smoking is by far the strongest risk factor for AAA, while hypertension is the strongest risk factor for aortic dissection. Smoking one or more packs of cigarettes a day is associated with a 12-fold increased risk for developing an AAA.

Is Diabetes a Risk Factor for AAA?

No. While diabetes is an important risk factor for intimal atheroma formation, myocardial infarction, stroke, and peripheral arterial disease, it is actually *protective* against AAA. While the protective mechanism of diabetes is not fully understood, one hypothesis is that glycation of matrix metalloproteinases (MMPs; discussed in *Pathophysiology*) leads to their deactivation and thus decreases aortic remodeling.

Is There a Role for Physical Examination in the Detection of AAA? What Are the Limitations?

AAA can be detected on physical examination but should not be used as the sole modality for screening. The sensitivity and specificity of physical examination improve with increasing AAA size but decrease with higher body mass index, making obesity the most significant limiting factor in detecting an AAA on physical exam. In addition, the value of physical examination varies by practitioner and is limited in detecting smaller aneurysms.

Is There a Role for AAA Screening? If So, Who Should Be Screened and How Often?

The American College of Cardiology, American Heart Association, and the US Preventive Services Task Force recommend screening with physical exam and one-time abdominal ultrasound for men between ages 65 and 75 who have had *any* smoking history. First-degree relatives of a patient with an AAA should be screened at age 65. If an AAA is found, it should be followed by annual ultrasonography if it is between 4.0 and 4.9 cm and biannually if between 5.0 and 5.4 cm. Screening has been shown to reduce aneurysm-related mortality by approximately 50%.

Watch Out
Screening for AAAs with a one-time ultrasound is recommended for *male* smokers between ages 65 and 75.

Shouldn't Women Who Have Smoked Also Be Screened for AAA?

There is insufficient evidence to recommend screening in women who smoke, as women are about four times less likely to develop AAA than men. However, women with AAA tend to rupture at smaller diameters and have greater mortality than men.

In a Patient with an AAA, What Other Arteries Might Have Aneurysms? How Would You Screen for Them? What Is the Main Risk Associated with Those Aneurysms?

Femoral and popliteal artery aneurysms are associated with an AAA, with popliteal artery aneurysms being more common. These aneurysms are bilateral in 50% of patients and may sometimes be detected during a physical exam. However, the recommended screening modality for detecting these peripheral aneurysms is a duplex ultrasonography in patients known to have an AAA. Rupture of femoral and popliteal aneurysms is extremely rare. The main risk of these aneurysms is limb ischemia, from either arterial thrombosis or distal embolization.

> **Watch Out**
> A thrombosed popliteal aneurysm should be on the differential of acute limb ischemia. It is associated with a high risk of limb loss.

> **Watch Out**
> Thoracic aneurysms can present with dysphagia, hoarseness, dyspnea, and upper extremity edema due to mass effect and compression of the esophagus, recurrent laryngeal nerve, and central veins.

> **Watch Out**
> The most common *visceral* artery aneurysm is splenic.

Pathophysiology

What Is the Normal Diameter of the Infrarenal Aorta in Men? Women?

The normal size of the infrarenal aorta is 2.0 cm in men and 1.8 cm in women.

What Is the Primary Defect in AAA?

Although AAA is a multifactorial disease process, it ultimately results from the degeneration of the medial layer through degradation of elastin and collagen.

At What Diameter Is the Infrarenal Aorta Considered to Be Aneurysmal?

For an artery to be considered an aneurysm, there must be a focal area that is 1.5 times larger than the diameter of the non-aneurysmal artery above. In the case of the infrarenal aorta, this would mean a diameter of about 3 cm or more.

What Is the Average Annual Growth Rate of AAA?

Studies examining the annual growth rate of small AAAs estimate a rate of 2–4 mm/year. Patients with rapid expansion (>5 mm/6 months) should be referred for elective repair. In addition, routine monitoring is important as expansion tends to be in stepwise growth spurts rather than linear.

What Factors Influence Growth Rate?

Ongoing smoking has been found to increase the growth rates of AAA, whereas patients with diabetes have slower growth rates. Diastolic hypertension appears to increase growth rate as well. However, the use of blood pressure medications has not been shown to consistently slow the growth rates of AAA.

What Are Matrix Metalloproteinases (MMPs), and What Is Their Role in AAA Formation?

MMPs are important for collagen turnover, which is vital to inflammation and wound healing. Patients with AAA have abnormally high levels of MMP activity in the aortic wall, which weaken the arterial wall and contribute to the dilation of the aneurysm over time.

> **Watch Out**
> The antidiabetic drug metformin is associated with reduced AAA growth in clinical studies and may be the reason why diabetes is protective against AAA.

Is There a Genetic Component to AAA Formation?

Family history is a risk factor for AAA. First-degree relatives of patients with AAAs have up to a 12-fold higher risk of developing the disease, and the risk is even higher in siblings of patients with AAAs. Interestingly, while male sex is an independent risk factor for AAA, familial clustering appears more common in females.

If an AAA Ruptures, Where Does It Typically Do So?

AAAs most commonly rupture into the retroperitoneum (the aorta is a retroperitoneal structure) and most often to the left (the vena cava is on the right and may prevent rupture to that side). Free rupture into the peritoneum is rare and would likely lead to immediate death as there is no ability to tamponade the bleeding.

Watch Out

Rarely, an AAA can erode into the inferior vena cava or iliac veins, creating an aortocaval fistula. These patients classically present with high output congestive heart failure, bilateral leg edema, and an abdominal bruit or thrill. Rarely, patients may have hematuria with retroperitoneal congestion.

What Is the Relationship Between AAA Rupture and Size?

As the aneurysm enlarges, the risk of rupture also increases. AAAs with a 4–5 cm diameter have a <1% annual chance of rupturing versus 30–50% in an AAA >8 cm diameter.

Other Than AAA Size, What Are Other Risk Factors for AAA Rupture?

Poorly controlled blood pressure, active smoking, and female gender have been associated with an increased risk of AAA rupture.

What Are the Primary Differences Between an Aortic Dissection and an AAA? (◘ Table 58.2)

Workup

What Is the First Step in the Evaluation of a Patient with a Suspected Ruptured AAA?

Although the ABCs of resuscitation should be followed, there are special considerations for intubation and fluid management. If the patient is not in respiratory failure, intubation should be *delayed* until the patient is in the operating room (OR) and prepped and draped, and ready for immediate surgical intervention. This is because the medications used for induction and intubation can exacerbate hypotension and may precipitate cardiac arrest. The surgical team must be prepared to make a skin incision immediately after induction if necessary. Two large-bore intravenous (IVs) should be established to facilitate resuscitation or blood transfusion as needed.

In a Patient with Suspected Ruptured AAA, What Is the Goal of Fluid Resuscitation?

In a patient with suspected ruptured AAA, the goal of fluid resuscitation is to achieve permissive hypotension rather than aggressive normalization of blood pressure. The primary objective is to maintain sufficient perfusion to ensure normal mentation, without aiming to restore a normal systolic blood pressure. This strategy minimizes the risk of exacerbating hemorrhage, as the rupture in

◘ Table 58.2 Comparison of aortic dissection and abdominal aortic aneurysm

	Aortic dissection	AAA
Population	White male 40–70 years old or young patients with connective tissue disease (e.g., Marfan, Ehlers-Danlos)	White male ≥ age 65
Strongest risk factor	Hypertension	Smoking
Presentation	Sharp, tearing chest pain radiating to the upper back	Usually asymptomatic; if ruptured, will present with severe abdominal pain, pulsatile abdominal mass, and shock
Pathophysiology	Intimal tear with dissection of blood through the medial layer forming a true and false lumen	Multifactorial processes leading to weakened medial layer
Location	Ascending aorta/aortic arch (Stanford A) or descending thoracic aorta (Stanford B) (distal to left subclavian); high stress regions	Usually arises below renal arteries but above the iliac arteries

the aorta is often temporarily contained by vasoconstriction and clot formation. Excessive fluid resuscitation before surgical control of the bleeding can disrupt these clots, raise systolic blood pressure, and dilute coagulation factors, all of which can worsen bleeding and reduce the chances of survival.

What Imaging Is Recommended for Suspected Ruptured AAA in a Hemodynamically Stable Patient?

In a stable patient, the recommended imaging modality for suspected ruptured AAA is a computed tomography angiography (CTA). This offers the benefits of (1) confirming whether there is a ruptured AAA versus another diagnosis and (2), if it is a ruptured AAA, determining whether an endovascular approach is feasible (◘ Figs. 58.1 and 58.2).

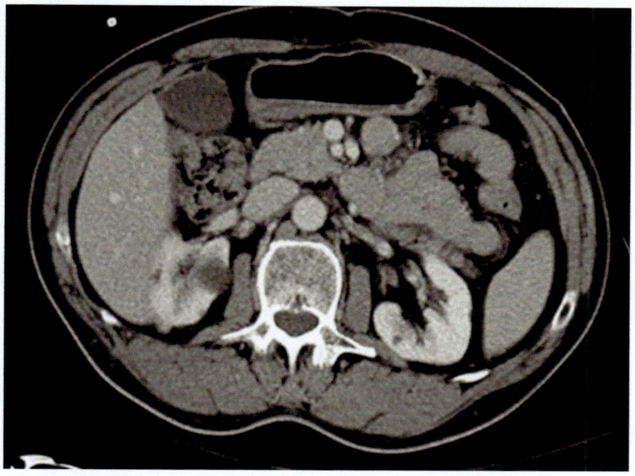

◘ **Fig. 58.1** Axial CT showing a normal aorta

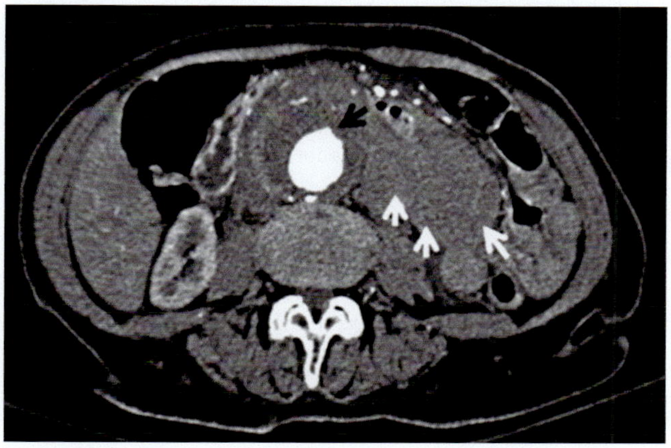

◘ **Fig. 58.2** Axial CT showing a ruptured abdominal aortic aneurysm with thrombus and large left-sided fluid collection consistent with rupture. *Black arrow: thrombus. White arrows: fluid collection*

How Does the Imaging of Choice Differ in a Hemodynamically Unstable Patient?

In the hemodynamically unstable patient, there is no role for CT scan. A bedside abdominal ultrasonography is used to confirm the presence of a large AAA. Since the rupture is usually retroperitoneal, the ultrasound may not demonstrate the rupture, as it cannot reliably detect bleeding in the retroperitoneum. As such, a presumptive diagnosis of a ruptured AAA is made by combining the clinical presentation, physical exam, and the finding of a large AAA on ultrasound. The patient should then be taken directly to the operating room for an exploratory laparotomy.

Management

How Does AAA Size and Growth Rate Influence Management for an Asymptomatic AAA in Males? (◘ Table 58.3)

Non-ruptured Asymptomatic AAA

Why Wait for the AAA to Reach this Size? Why Not Repair a Smaller AAA Since the Patient Is Theoretically Healthier and Is Younger?

The annual risk of rupture for an aneurysm <5.5 cm is very low, and morbidity and mortality of repair are greater than the risk of death from rupture. Two large studies have demonstrated no survival benefit for early intervention for AAA <5.5 cm. Since the diameter of aortas is smaller in women, and women with AAA have a higher risk of rupture, most surgeons recommend a lower threshold for repair (> 5.0 cm).

◘ **Table 58.3** Recommendations for management of AAA based on size

AAA measurement	Management
3.0–3.9 cm	Ultrasound every 3 years
4.0–4.9 cm	Annual ultrasound
5.0–5.4 cm	Ultrasound every 6 months
>5.5 cm	Elective repair
Enlarging >1 cm/year or symptomatic	Elective repair

What Surgical Options Are Available for Asymptomatic AAA?

The two available options are open repair and endovascular aneurysm repair (EVAR) with EVAR being the preferred approach in the US.

> **Watch Out**
> The main source of perioperative morbidity and mortality following both open repair and endovascular AAA repair is myocardial infarction.

How Do the Two Surgical Approaches Compare in Terms of Perioperative Morbidity and Mortality? What About Long-Term Mortality?

EVAR has a lower perioperative mortality rate compared to open repair. However, long-term survival is *equivalent* for open repair and EVAR. This is likely related to the fact that EVAR reduces but does not eliminate the risk of AAA, and EVAR is associated with higher rates of re-intervention and re-intervention-associated complications.

Ruptured AAA

What Are the Surgical Options for a Patient with a Ruptured AAA?

For patients with a ruptured AAA most surgeons prefer EVAR over open repair. If the patient is hemodynamically unstable, and there is no time to obtain a CT scan, open repair may be necessary. Recent studies show that outcomes are the same for both approaches in terms of long-term mortality.

What Anatomical Factors Make an AAA Unsuitable for EVAR?

An AAA may be unsuitable for EVAR if there is insufficient length of normal aorta between the renal artery orifices and the start of the infrarenal aneurysm (known as the neck). A short or inadequate aortic neck makes it difficult to securely deploy the stent without risking occlusion of the renal arteries or the development of an endoleak. Other contraindications are access vessels that are too small, and severe atherosclerosis in the iliac arteries.

What Is the Mortality Risk if an AAA Ruptures?

Overall mortality from AAA rupture is estimated at 80–90%. Approximately half of all patients with ruptured AAA die before reaching a hospital, and of those who do arrive to the hospital alive, about 50% will die.

What Is the Main Achilles Heel of Endovascular Repair?

The main concern of EVAR is failure to fully exclude the aortic aneurysm. Persistent arterial flow into the aneurysm sac is known as an endoleak (Table 58.4). The concern of a persistent endoleak, particularly one at a high systolic pressure, is that the aneurysm will continue to grow and may eventually rupture despite treatment with EVAR. At the end of EVAR, a completion angiogram should be performed to identify an endoleak before leaving the operating room. After successful EVAR, patients require annual surveillance for life to determine if an endoleak develops later.

How Should Patients Be Monitored After an Endovascular AAA Repair?

Following EVAR, the gold standard for monitoring is CTA. Patients undergo CTA at 1 month and 1 year following EVAR and then yearly to evaluate for late endoleak. Duplex ultrasonography is an adjunctive tool for EVAR surveillance, although it has diminished specificity when compared to CTA.

Are There Any Consequences To Annual CT Scans?

Some studies suggest that there is an increased risk of abdominal cancer after EVAR. This may be related to the numerous CT scans that patients undergo.

Table 58.4 Five types of endoleaks

Type	Features
I	Anterograde or retrograde flow from inadequate proximal or distal seal of the stent graft against the arterial wall; most worrisome and *requires repair* before leaving the operating room
II	Retrograde flow from patent branches within the aneurysm sac (i.e., lumbar, inferior mesenteric); *most common*, usually benign, and does not lead to sac growth
III	Flow between junctional areas of overlapping stents within the aortic and iliac vessels
IV	Flow through the graft due to overly porous stent material or fabric tear
V	Also referred to as *endotension*; considered idiopathic as sac enlarges without evidence of a leak site

Areas Where You Can Get in Trouble

Assuming That an AAA Is Not Ruptured Because No Contrast Extravasation Is Seen on CT

A patient with a ruptured AAA may present with reasonable vital signs, implying that the site of rupture is temporarily contained without current bleeding. CT imaging of this patient may not show contrast extravasation outside the lumen of the aorta but will have fluid or stranding in the retroperitoneum around the aorta, representing clotted blood. In the setting of acute abdominal pain, retroperitoneal fluid and fat stranding adjacent to the aorta represents an emergent ruptured AAA until proven otherwise.

Early-Onset Diarrhea After AAA Repair

Ischemic colitis is a significant early complication of infrarenal AAA repair, caused by inadequate perfusion of the descending and sigmoid colon following ligation or exclusion of the inferior mesenteric artery (IMA). It typically presents within days (or hours) postoperatively with left-sided abdominal pain, bloody diarrhea (though not always bloody), fever, and leukocytosis. Workup involves flexible sigmoidoscopy which may reveal edema, ulceration, and friability in the sigmoid colon. Management includes fluid resuscitation, bowel rest, and broad-spectrum IV antibiotics. Surgery (e.g. sigmoid resection with colostomy) is reserved for patients with clinical deterioration, peritonitis, or full-thickness necrosis.

> **Watch Out**
> The *greatest* risk factor for ischemic colitis following AAA repair is hypotension and hypoperfusion in the setting of a ruptured AAA.

GI Bleed After AAA Repair

An aortoenteric fistula is a rare but life-threatening complication of AAA repair, involving erosion between the aortic graft and the duodenum. This condition can occur months to years postoperatively and often presents with a "sentinel bleed," a self-limited episode of upper gastrointestinal (GI) bleeding or melena that precedes a catastrophic hemorrhage. The fistula commonly forms between the aortic graft and the fourth portion of the duodenum. Diagnosis is challenging, as upper endoscopy is often negative. Often the only clue is air or fluid around the aortic graft on CT scan, indicating infection. Since the aortic graft is infected from duodenal bacteria, management requires excision of the aortic graft with placement of an aortic homograft (cadaver aorta) and long-term antibiotic therapy.

Area of Controversy

Since EVAR Has a Lower Risk of Perioperative Mortality Than Open Repair, Should We Lower Our Threshold for AAA Repair (i.e., <5.5 cm) If the Patient Is an EVAR Candidate?

Although EVAR has a lower risk of perioperative complications and death than open repair, it is still associated with significant potential complications. In addition, patients with small AAA often have significant coexisting medical problems, so they are more likely to die in the long term from a cardiac event or from cancer than from a ruptured aneurysm. To date, there is no evidence that male patients who are EVAR candidates would benefit from AAA repair at less than 5.5 cm.

Which Is the Best Option for Elective AAA Repair, Open or EVAR?

While EVAR has better short-term morbidity and mortality, long-term mortality has been reported to be the same. More recently, however, some studies suggest that open repair may have better long-term survival beyond 8 years. EVAR requires yearly monitoring with CT scan, more reinterventions, and does not completely eliminate the risk of rupture due to endoleaks. Thus, in younger, good operative risk patients, open repair may now be preferrable.

Abdominal Aortic Aneurysm (AAA) (Fig. 58.3)

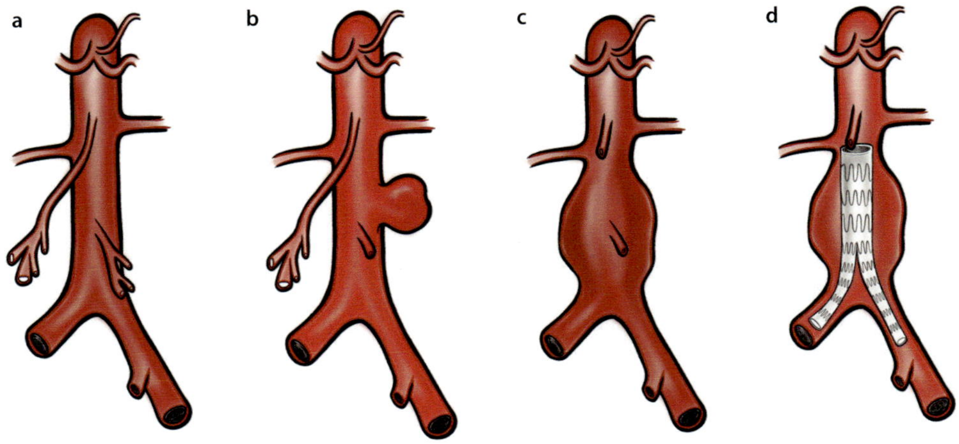

Fig. 58.3 A normal aorta. **a** can progress to a saccular **b** abdominal aortic aneurysm or a fusiform abdominal aortic aneurysm **c**. Endovascular aortic repair (EVAR) is a procedure that endovascularly inserts a stent graft to reinforce the aortic wall and reduce risk of aneurysm rupture **d**

Summary of Essentials

History and Physical Examination

58

- AAA is a silent killer; most are asymptomatic until rupture.
- Ruptured AAA should be suspected in elderly, male smokers who present with acute abdominal pain radiating to the back or left flank, a pulsatile abdominal mass, hypotension, tachycardia, pallor, and diaphoresis.
- Many patients are obese, so a pulsatile abdominal mass may not be palpable.

Diagnosis

- In unstable patients, there is no time for a diagnostic workup, so diagnosis is based on history and physical exam.
- In stable patients, CTA will elucidate the anatomy and determine whether the patient is a candidate for endovascular repair.
- Abdominal ultrasound can diagnose the presence of an AAA and its size but is not accurate for determining rupture.

Screening

- Ultrasound screening
  - Men (not women) aged 65–75 with any smoking history or beginning at age 65 if they have a first-degree relative with AAA.
  - Patients with femoral or popliteal artery aneurysm.
  - An aortic diameter >3 cm is considered aneurysmal.

Management

- Ruptured AAA
  - Obtain IV access but limit fluids
  - Permissive hypotension (as low as 70 mmHg), maintain mentation
  - Avoid intubation until in the operating room
- Repair via open or EVAR
- Non-ruptured AAA
  - Men
  - <5.5 cm, observe
  - >5.5 cm, repair
  - Women
  - Consider repair if > 5.0 cm
  - Open or EVAR

Complications

- Myocardial infarction is the most common cause of death.
- Colonic ischemia: postoperative bloody diarrhea (early, days after surgery).
- Aortoenteric fistula: GI bleed (late, months to years later).

Suggested Reading

Bhak RH, Wininger M, et al.; Aneurysm Detection and Management (ADAM) Study Group. Factors associated with small abdominal aortic aneurysm expansion rate. JAMA Surg. 2015 Jan;150(1):44–50. https://doi.org/10.1001/jamasurg.2014.2025. PMID: 25389641.

Chaikof EL, Dalman RL, Eskandari MK, et al. The Society for Vascular Surgery practice guidelines on the care of patients with abdominal aortic aneurysm. J Vasc Surg. 2018;67(1):2–77.

Fink HA, Lederle FA, Roth CS, Bowles CA, Nelson DB, Haas MA. The accuracy of physical examination to detect abdominal aortic aneurysm. Arch Intern Med. 2000;160(6):833–6.

Golledge J, Karan M, Moran CS, et al. Reduced expansion rate of abdominal aortic aneurysms in patients with diabetes may be related to aberrant monocyte-matrix interactions. Eur Heart J. 2008;29(5):665–72.

Kent KC, Moscucci M, Mansour KA, DiMattia S, et al. Retroperitoneal hematoma after cardiac catheterization: prevalence, risk factors, and optimal management. J Vasc Surg. 1994;20(6):905–13.

Kessler V, Klopf J, et al. AAA Revisited: A Comprehensive Review of Risk Factors, Management, and Hallmarks of Pathogenesis. Biomedicines. 2022 Jan 2;10(1):94. https://doi.org/10.3390/biomedicines10010094. PMID: 35052774; PMCID: PMC8773452.

Takayama T, Yamanouchi D. Aneurysmal disease: the abdominal aorta. Surg Clin N Am. 2013;93(4):877–91, viii.

Yei K, Mathlouthi A, et al. Long-term Outcomes Associated With Open vs Endovascular Abdominal Aortic Aneurysm Repair in a Medicare-Matched Database. JAMA Netw Open. 2022 May 2;5(5):e2212081. https://doi.org/10.1001/jamanetworkopen.2022.12081. PMID: 35560049; PMCID: PMC9107027.

Cold, Painful Right Lower Extremity

Manan P. Shah, Nina M. Bowens, and Christian de Virgilio

Contents

C. de Virgilio, A. Grigorian (eds.), *Surgery*, https://doi.org/10.1007/978-3-032-09799-6_59

Case Study

A 65-year-old female presents to the emergency department with a 4-h history of sudden onset of right leg pain, coolness, weakness, and numbness. She has no prior similar history. The pain began while she was sitting watching television. She has a history of hypertension and hypercholesterolemia and takes medication for both. She denies smoking. On review of systems, she has no prior history of pain in her right leg with walking. On physical examination, her lungs are clear to auscultation. Her heart rate is irregularly irregular without murmurs, rubs, or gallops. Her abdomen is soft and non-tender without a pulsatile mass. On the left side, the femoral, popliteal, dorsalis pedis, and posterior tibial pulses are 2+, with biphasic signals on Doppler. On the right side, the femoral, popliteal, dorsalis pedis, and posterior tibial pulses are absent, with faint monophasic signals on Doppler. Her right calf is tender to palpation but is not edematous. She has normal appearing, supple skin in her legs with a normal hair pattern. The left foot is pink and warm with a two-second capillary refill and normal motor and sensory function. Her right foot is pale and feels much colder than the left; capillary refill time is six seconds. The toes have decreased sensation to touch. Her strength is diminished in both plantar flexion and dorsiflexion of the ankle at 4+/5.

Diagnosis

What Is the Differential Diagnosis? (▫ Table 59.1)

What Is the Most Likely Diagnosis?

This patient's presentation is most consistent with acute limb ischemia (ALI). The presence of motor weakness often creates confusion and may inappropriately steer the clinician toward a neurologic diagnosis. However,

▫ **Table 59.1** Differential diagnosis for case presentation

Differential diagnosis	**Key features/findings**
Acute limb ischemia	Pain, pallor, pulselessness, paresthesias, paralysis, and poikilothermia; history of PAD, atrial fibrillation
Compartment syndrome	Severe pain in calf with passive motion of ankle, tense leg, elevated CPK level
Deep vein thrombosis	Prolonged stasis, hypercoagulable state, endothelial injury (*Virchow's triad*)
Cerebrovascular accident	May cause numbness and weakness but not pain or pulselessness; other neurological signs may be present
Disk herniation	History of back pain, DJD; paresthesias in dermatomal distribution (e.g., sciatica), possible weakness and sensory changes, but pulses present
Spinal cord tumor	Presents similarly to disk herniation; consider in patients with history of metastatic malignancy, normal pulses

PAD peripheral arterial disease, *DJD* degenerative joint disease

the pale, cold foot, combined with the absence of palpable pulses, as supported by monophasic Doppler signal, rules out the majority of the diagnoses in the differential. The presence of an irregularly irregular heartbeat (e.g., atrial fibrillation) points toward a cardioembolic etiology of the ALI.

History and Physical

What Is the Difference in Timing Between Acute and Chronic Limb-Threatening Ischemia (CLTI)?

ALI refers to a sudden decrease in limb perfusion that threatens limb viability and typically presents with symptoms for less than 2 weeks. In contrast, CLTI is defined as ischemia of longer than 2 weeks' duration, usually in the setting of progressive peripheral arterial disease (PAD), and is characterized by three conditions: rest pain, non-healing ulcers, or gangrene.

What Are the "Ps" of Acute Limb Ischemia?

Various references use either 5 or 6 Ps, and differ slightly. The Ps of compartment syndrome are pain (often described as out of proportion to the injury and pain on passive motion), paresthesia (tingling or numbness), pallor (paleness of the skin), paralysis (weakness or inability to move the affected limb), pulselessness (absent pulses, a late finding), and pressure (a swollen or tense extremity or compartment). Others add another P, poikilothermia, defined as a change in temperature or coolness. Pulselessness is considered the defining feature of ALI, but pain is often the presenting symptom. Pain associated with ALI is frequently located in the foot and calf and occurs at rest. Numbness is present in more than half of the patients with ALI. Paralysis is the most ominous sign of the "Ps" and is a sign of severe ischemia that may be irreversible.

Why Is the Cardiac History Important in Determining the Etiology of ALI?

An embolus is the most common etiology (▫ Table 59.2) for ALI with 80% of emboli coming from the heart. ALI after a myocardial infarction is oftentimes due to embolization of a left ventricular thrombus.

Watch Out

Abrupt cessation of warfarin (e.g., patient runs out of medication) in a patient with atrial fibrillation can lead to rebound hypercoagulability and higher risk of embolic events.

▫ **Table 59.2** Common causes of acute limb ischemia

	Etiology	Key features/findings
Thrombosis	Thrombosis of stenosed artery	Vascular risk factors, history of claudication, signs of chronic ischemia in contralateral limb
	Thrombosis of previous graft	Vascular risk factors, known previous graft, surgical scars
	Hypercoagulable disorder	Known coagulopathy, history of prior de novo thrombosis, no prior history of atherosclerotic PAD
	Arterial trauma	Recent trauma, recent vascular intervention
Embolus	Cardioembolic	Atrial fibrillation, valvular disease, CHF, recent MI, ventricular aneurysm, left atrial myxoma
	Embolism from popliteal/aortic aneurysm	Palpable pulsatile abdominal or popliteal mass
	Paradoxical embolism	DVT sends clot to the heart, crosses cardiac septal defect with embolization to the arterial tree
Others	Acute aortic dissection	Type A (involves aortic arch), type B (descending aorta), tearing back pain, Marfan's syndrome, hypertension
	Systemic shock	Limb ischemia may be a late manifestation of severe shock, particularly with underlying chronic occlusive disease or high doses of vasopressors

PAD peripheral arterial disease, *CHF* congestive heart failure, *MI* myocardial infarction, *DVT* deep vein thrombosis

> **Watch Out**
> A ruptured popliteal cyst can closely mimic DVT with calf pain, swelling, and tenderness. Ecchymosis may track to the medial malleolus, known as the crescent sign. Symptoms often follow minor trauma or strain. Systemic signs such as fever are typically absent. Ultrasound is necessary to rule out DVT. Management is conservative with rest, non-steroidal anti-inflammatory drugs (NSAIDs), and leg elevation.

What Are the Key Findings That Point Toward an Embolic Etiology Rather Than a Thrombotic Event?

An embolic etiology is more likely when symptoms present suddenly and asymmetrically, without prior claudication or CLTI. Key features include acute onset in a previously asymptomatic limb and the presence of a known embolic source, such as atrial fibrillation (as seen in the irregularly irregular rhythm in the patient above) or a recent myocardial infarction. In contrast, thrombotic events typically occur over time in the setting of underlying peripheral artery disease, which is often bilateral and symmetric due to chronic atherosclerosis. A more gradual presentation suggests an acute-on-chronic picture, rather than a true embolic event.

Why Is It Important to Examine the Contralateral, Nonischemic Limb?

Examining the contralateral leg allows the provider to compare each leg when assessing the subjective findings of pallor and poikilothermia. It also provides important clues regarding the etiology of ischemia. If the nonischemic limb has evidence of chronic decreased perfusion, such as diminished pulses, hair loss, or atrophic skin changes, this suggests that the patient has PAD, which raises suspicion for a thrombotic etiology of ALI. Since PAD is a diffuse disease process in the peripheral vasculature, the lack of any chronic ischemic changes in the contralateral leg makes an embolic cause more likely.

How Would You Best Assess This Patient's Atherosclerotic Disease History?

The patient should be asked about a history of intermittent claudication and risk factors such as smoking, diabetes, hypertension, hypercholesterolemia, and history of coronary artery disease.

Why Is It Important to Ask About Past Interventions for PAD?

It is important to determine if the patient has had previous interventions for PAD, as thrombosis of a previous bypass or stent is a frequent cause of ALI. Iatrogenic trauma such as that caused by recent arterial catheterization (e.g., for coronary stenting) may also cause arterial thrombosis.

How Do Peripheral Artery Aneurysms Typically Present, and What Are Their Common Associations?

Peripheral artery aneurysms are most common in the popliteal artery. They are often bilateral and most are asymptomatic. Since they may contain thrombus, the most common presentation is ALI, due to thrombosis of the artery or distal embolization. Very rarely, they may compress adjacent structures, nerves, and veins. This can result in neuropathy or venous thrombosis. These aneurysms are frequently associated with abdominal aortic aneurysms, so patients diagnosed with a popliteal artery aneurysm should undergo ultrasound screening for concurrent aortic aneurysms.

Pathophysiology

Where in the Arterial Tree Do Cardiac Emboli Tend to Lodge?

Generally, emboli lodge at arterial bifurcations (■ Table 59.3) due to the sudden reduction in arterial diameter as the artery branches. The bifurcation of

Table 59.3 Common locations of lower extremity embolic occlusion and their presentations

Location	Pulses	Symptoms
Aortic bifurcation	Absent bilaterally	Bilateral pain/weakness of thighs/calves, mottling of skin distal to umbilicus
Common femoral bifurcation	Absent throughout affected limb	Unilateral calf and foot pain
Popliteal bifurcation	Femoral pulse present, pedal pulses absent; popliteal pulse may be present as well	Unilateral foot pain; calf pain may be present as well

the common femoral artery is the most common location for an embolus to lodge in the lower extremity.

Why Do Aneurysms Cause Thrombus Formation?

An aneurysm is a focal area of arterial dilation. At its widest points, blood flow becomes static, with eddy currents (much like where a river suddenly widens), leading to thrombus formation.

How Does Peripheral Arterial Disease Lead to Acute Limb Ischemia?

Thrombotic causes of ALI (approximately 50–60% of cases) are usually associated with underlying atherosclerotic disease. There are two primary mechanisms believed to be responsible for atherosclerosis-related limb ischemia. Plaque buildup can lead to a progressive narrowing of the artery with subsequent low-flow states and stasis that can lead to sudden thrombosis of the artery. The second mechanism involves intraplaque rupture with local hypercoagulability and hemorrhage, which can also suddenly occlude the artery, leading to thrombus formation.

How Long Can Muscle Tissue Withstand Ischemia Before Irreversible Damage Occurs?

Physiologic studies show that after an acute ischemic event, skeletal muscle tissue begins to show signs of irreversible cell damage after three hours and progresses to complete cell damage at six hours. Thus, rapid diagnosis and treatment within six hours are essential in suspected ALI. Every hour counts.

Workup

What Is the First Step After Suspecting ALI?

It is critically important to start therapeutic anticoagulation (often with initiation of heparin infusion) even prior to confirming the diagnosis with imaging. This prevents thrombus propagation while the patient undergoes further workup.

What Does a Doppler Probe Detect and What Are the Three Signals?

Blood flow is detected by a handheld Doppler probe and converted to an audible acoustic signal. Doppler assessment is frequently more sensitive than the ability to palpate a pulse. The signal should be reported as triphasic, biphasic, monophasic, or absent. A healthy peripheral artery produces a triphasic signal (three sounds). This reflects initial forward systolic flow, followed by early-diastolic retrograde flow attributable to high resistance, and finally forward diastolic flow. Biphasic signals are often normal but may represent an early disease state. Monophasic signals workup are clearly abnormal and signify a severe reduction in blood flow. Most patients with ALI have absent Doppler signals or, at best, faintly monophasic signals.

Is the Ankle–Brachial Index Useful for ALI?

The ankle–brachial index (ABI) is useful in patients with claudication or CLTI. An ABI <0.9 confirms the diagnosis of PAD. With ALI, however, the blood flow in the foot is severely reduced such that a blood pressure, and therefore an ABI, is typically not measurable; therefore, the ABI has limited utility.

How Is the Severity of ALI Determined?

The severity of ALI is determined clinically, not radiographically. Severity is based on the motor and sensory exam. Patients are placed in four categories of severity: (1) normal motor and sensory exam, (2a) diminished sensation but normal motor exam, (2b) diminished motor and sensory exam, and (3) complete absence of sensation and movement. Doppler signal is also important as a measure of whether any arterial blood flow is present.

What Imaging Is Recommended?

The diagnosis of ALI is extremely time sensitive. Duplex ultrasound scanning is a simple and convenient imaging modality to use for initial evaluation of ALI. A normal duplex scan is an inexpensive way to effectively rule out ALI. Though it is useful for examining the affected limb, it does not provide information about the proximal arterial tree (aorta and iliac arteries). Thus, a computed tomography angiography (CTA) of the abdomen, pelvis, and both lower extremities is the gold standard as it can be performed quickly. Not only does it demonstrate the site of the occluded artery, it can often provide clues as to the etiology by demonstrating atherosclerotic plaques, aneurysms, or arterial dissection.

What Additional Imaging Should Be Done If an Embolus Is Suspected as the Cause for ALI? If a Paradoxical Embolus Is Suspected?

If an embolus is suspected, a cardiac workup with transthoracic echocardiography should be obtained to evaluate for intracardiac thrombus. If there are clinical clues suggestive of a paradoxical embolus, such as recent air travel, surgery, or signs of DVT like unilateral leg swelling, a venous duplex scan of the lower extremities should be performed to assess for DVT. In such cases, a transthoracic echocardiogram with a bubble study should be performed to evaluate for a right-to-left shunt, such as a patent foramen ovale, that could allow venous thrombi to enter the arterial circulation.

Management

What Are the Three Most Important Initial Management Steps?

Anticoagulation with heparin should be started immediately (provided there is no contraindication such as bleeding) once the diagnosis of ALI is suspected. Do not wait for imaging in someone with a cold, pulseless foot. While heparin will not dissolve the clot, it is essential in *preventing* clot propagation into unaffected vascular beds, while the patient's endogenous fibrinolytic system dissolves the clot. In addition to anticoagulation, the affected limb should be placed in a dependent position to improve flow. Finally, intravenous (IV) fluids should be started as volume expansion helps optimize perfusion through collateral vessels.

What Are the Main Therapeutic Options for ALI?

The two mainstay treatment options for ALI are endovascular and open surgical revascularization. Endovascular treatment relies on catheter-based methods to achieve clot dissolution; these include catheter-directed tissue plasminogen activator (tPA) thrombolysis, percutaneous aspiration thrombectomy, or percutaneous mechanical thrombectomy. Surgical options include surgical (Fogarty balloon) embolectomy, endarterectomy, and distal bypass. In some cases, heparin alone may be the best treatment option, particularly in patients with mild ischemia who are at high risk of complications from thrombolysis or surgery.

> **Watch Out**
> Unlike the trauma population where the contralateral vein is typically used, in patients with ALI undergoing bypass surgery, the *ipsilateral* greater saphenous vein is the conduit of choice.

What Are the Absolute Contraindications to Thrombolytic Therapy? Relative Contraindications?

The absolute contraindications are recent stroke or transient ischemic attack, active or recent bleeding, and significant coagulopathy. Relative contraindications include recent (<2 weeks) major surgery, recent trauma, uncontrolled hypertension, intracranial pathology, and pregnancy. tPA should only be used for a maximum for 48 h, at which point the risk of bleeding increases significantly.

How Does One Choose Between Open Surgery and Endovascular Therapy?

Endovascular therapy, though less invasive, may take 24–48 h to be completely effective. Thus, it is appropriate and preferred for most patients with less severe ischemia (those with a normal motor/sensory exam) or with only a sensory deficit. Open surgical intervention is preferred for patients with severe ALI (those with a motor deficit) when immediate revascularization is indicated.

Who Is the Best Candidate for Surgical Balloon Embolectomy?

Surgical embolectomy (with a Fogarty balloon) is best used for emboli from the heart. In the setting thrombosis due to underlying atherosclerosis, an embolectomy will not work as it cannot remove underlying plaque.

What Is the Treatment for Irreversible Limb Ischemia?

When ALI presents with complete motor and sensory loss, the tissue damage is irreversible, so primary amputation should be performed. Attempting revascularization in this setting is contraindicated, as the risk of reperfusion injury is extremely high.

What Are the Potential Dangerous Sequelae of Reperfusion Following ALI?

Reperfusion of ischemic muscle can lead to a constellation of serious complications collectively known as *ischemia–reperfusion syndrome*. These complications are caused by toxic products that are released from the damaged tissue into the general circulation. Rhabdomyolysis is the primary concern and can lead to acute renal failure in severe cases. Thus, it is important to monitor for elevated serum creatine phosphokinase (CPK) and myoglobinuria when revascularization is performed. Hyperkalemia and acidosis may also occur as part of reperfusion syndrome as large amounts of potassium and acid are released from the ischemic muscle, leading to cardiac arrest. Reperfusion syndrome can occur even with less severe ALI. Compartment syndrome is also a complication of reperfusion injury, as the reperfused muscle swells.

Areas Where You Can Get into Trouble

Failing to Monitor for Elevated CPK and Myoglobinuria

Rhabdomyolysis is a potentially serious complication of reperfusion of a limb, with up to 20% of patients showing laboratory evidence of myoglobinuria. Of patients with CPK >5000 units/L, approximately half will develop acute kidney injury (AKI) caused by heme pigment, which precipitates in tubules leading to cast formation and direct toxic injury to proximal tubular cells. If rhabdomyolysis is suspected, prompt therapy with IV fluids (normal saline) should be started. IV fluids enhance renal perfusion and prevent ischemic injury while simultaneously increasing urine flow in order to limit intratubular cast formation and increase heme excretion. The prognosis for heme pigment-induced AKI is favorable with many patients returning to normal renal function.

Following Revascularization, the Patient Develops Peaked T Waves on the EKG

Peaked T waves are an early sign of hyperkalemia. It should be treated promptly with IV calcium gluconate which counteracts the effects of potassium on resting membrane potential in cardiac myocytes to prevent arrhythmia. Insulin is then administered to drive potassium into cells via activation of the Na-K-ATPase pump. Glucose is given simultaneously to prevent hypoglycemia. High-dose inhaled albuterol may also be administered. While these interventions stabilize cardiac cell membranes and drive potassium into cells, further treatments are needed to remove potassium from the body. These include loop diuretics, potassium binders, or dialysis in severe cases.

Following Revascularization, the Patient Develops a Swollen Leg

If ischemia–reperfusion syndrome leads to significant swelling of the extremity following revascularization, the patient can develop compartment syndrome which can have the same Ps of ALI: pain, pallor, paralysis, pulselessness, paresthesia, and poikilothermia. The major differences are that in compartment syndrome, the leg is tense (pressure), there may be pain with passive motion, and pulselessness is a *late sign*. Monitoring leg compartments is essential in order to intervene early with urgent fasciotomy.

Platelet Count Drop 5 Days After Successful Reperfusion

Patients receiving heparin should have monitoring of the platelet count as they are at risk of heparin-induced thrombocytopenia (HIT). This is a paradoxically hypercoagulable state caused by antibodies formed against heparin as it is bound to platelet factor 4. HIT should be suspected if the platelet count drops by >50%, classically on day 5 of heparin exposure. HIT can cause a clot to form leading to recurrence of ALI. In the operating room, a clot from HIT will appear white, compared to the red clot from embolus. Heparin should immediately be stopped, and the patient switched to a direct thrombin inhibitor, such as argatroban.

Acute Limb Ischemia (Fig. 59.1)

Summary of Essentials

History and Physical

- Sudden onset of a cold painful pulseless extremity is suggestive of ALI
- Ask about cardiac history (atrial fibrillation, recent MI) as these suggest cardioembolic source
- Ask about claudication as this suggests thrombotic etiology from underlying atherosclerosis
- Examine the heart for irregularly irregular rhythm (new atrial fibrillation)
- Examine for Ps (pain, paresthesia, pallor, paralysis, pulselessness, and poikilothermia):
- Pain is often the presenting symptom of ALI
- Paralysis portends the worst prognosis
- Examine contralateral nonischemic limb
- Signs of chronic peripheral arterial disease suggest a thrombotic cause
- Normal vascular exam suggests an embolic cause

Pathophysiology

- Injury of skeletal muscle tissue begins at three hours and may be irreversible at 6 h

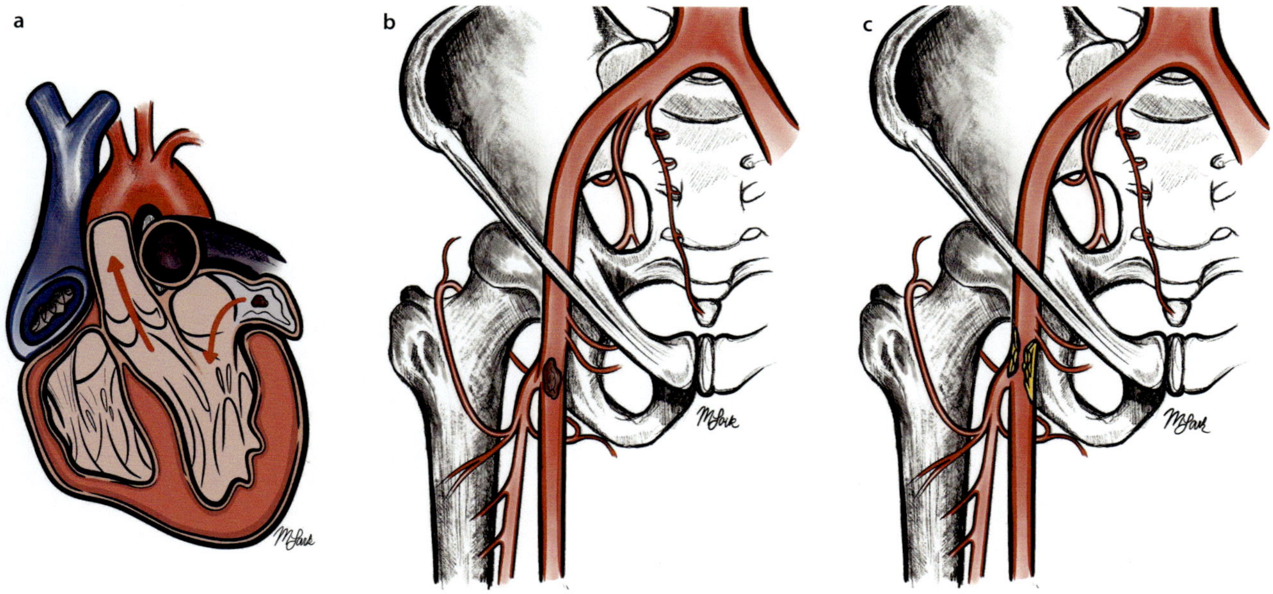

Fig. 59.1 This compares two major causes of acute limb ischemia: embolism versus atherosclerotic plaque. An embolus typically originates from the heart (**a**) or large arteries and can travel through the bloodstream, causing sudden blockage of blood flow and leading to acute onset of limb ischemia (**b**). In contrast, atherosclerotic plaque results in gradual narrowing of an arterial lumen over time leading to plaque formation and stasis, which can lead to in-situ thrombosis (**c**)

Diagnosis

- ALI is associated with motor/sensory deficits; it can easily be confused with a primary neurologic etiology
- Doppler ultrasound establishes diagnosis; CTA is a gold standard, is fast, and provides more information
- The severity of ALI is determined by physical exam, primarily by the motor and sensory exam

Management

- Immediately begin IV heparin and IV fluids, and place limb in a dependent position
- Definitive treatment: catheter-directed thrombolysis or open surgical intervention
- Intervention is time sensitive
- Catheter-directed thrombolysis can take 24–48 h to complete
- Surgical revascularization is immediate
- Amputation for irreversible disease (complete anesthesia and paralysis)

Complications

- Reperfusion syndrome with hyperkalemia, acidosis, rhabdomyolysis, acute renal failure, and compartment syndrome

Areas Where You Can Get into Trouble

- Monitoring for elevated serum CPK and myoglobinuria is essential in order to prevent acute renal failure secondary to rhabdomyolysis after revascularization

Suggested Reading

Björck M, Earnshaw JJ, Acosta S, et al. Editor's choice – European Society for Vascular Surgery (ESVS) 2020 Clinical Practice Guidelines on the Management of Acute Limb Ischaemia. Eur J Vasc Endovasc Surg 2020;59(2):173–218. doi:https://doi.org/10.1016/j.ejvs.2019.09.006

Campbell W, Ridler B, Szymanska T. Current management of acute leg ischaemia: results of an audit by the Vascular Surgical Society of Great Britain and Ireland. Br J Surg. 1998;85:1498–503.

Norgren L, Hiatt WR, Dormandy JA, Nehler MR, Harris KA, Fowkes FG, Rutherford RB, TASC II Working Group. Inter-society consensus for the management of peripheral arterial disease. Int Angiol 2007;26(2):81–157. Review. PubMed PMID: 17489079.

Vascular

Question Set: Vascular

Questions

1. A 76-year-old woman presents to the emergency department with sudden onset of severe abdominal pain. The pain began 4 h ago and is constant, located around her umbilicus. She says the pain is "excruciating" and rates it a 10/10, yet on examination her abdomen is soft and only mildly tender without guarding or rebound. She has a history of atrial fibrillation and takes warfarin. Her temperature is 37.3 °C, blood pressure is 108/68 mmHg, pulse is 118/min and irregular, and respirations are 20/min. Bowel sounds are decreased. Laboratory studies show:
White blood cell (WBC) count: 17,500/mm^3, Lactate: 6.1 mmol/L (normal: 0.5–2.2 mmol/L), Serum amylase: 180 U/L (normal: 25–125 U/L), Serum phosphate: 6.3 mg/dL (normal: 2.5–4.5 mg/dL). What is the most appropriate next step in management?
(A) Emergent exploratory laparotomy
(B) Abdominal plain film
(C) CT angiography of the abdomen
(D) Mesenteric doppler ultrasound
(E) Intravenous fluids and serial abdominal exams

2. A 71-year-old man comes in to the physician, along with his wife, and reports a 4-month history of increasing left calf pain with exercise. He works as a grocery store manager and describes having the pain every morning after he walks from his car in the parking lot to the grocery store. The pain disappears once he is able to sit down. He has smoked one pack per day for the past 50 years. His pulse is 88/min, respirations are 18/min, and blood pressure is 156/96 mmHg. His total cholesterol is 300 mg/dL. His right ankle–brachial index (ABI) is 0.7. His wife is very worried and asks the physician what his prognosis is. In patients with this condition, the 5-year survival is:
(A) The same as that of age- and gender-matched controls without claudication
(B) Reduced primarily due to the risk of limb gangrene
(C) Reduced primarily due to lung cancer
(D) Reduced primarily due to coronary artery disease
(E) Reduced primarily due to stroke

3. A 61-year-old patient with coronary artery disease, diabetes, and hypertension presents to the emergency department with difficulty speaking and right-sided hemiparesis. His wife reports that he had multiple episodes a few days ago where he had difficulty speaking but they only lasted a few minutes. A CT scan of the head without contrast did not identify any hemorrhage in the brain. His systolic blood pressure is found to be 230 mmHg, and heart rate is 102/min. What is the most appropriate next step in management?
(A) Labetalol
(B) Nimodipine
(C) Nitroglycerin
(D) Nitroprusside
(E) Hydralazine

4. A 65-year-old male carpenter states that his left arm gets tired when he uses it at work, forcing him to stop and rest. In addition, he notes that when using his left arm, he

experiences dizziness and vertigo. He has a long-standing history of smoking. Physical examination reveals normal brachial and radial pulses on the right but markedly decreased brachial and radial pulses on the left. In addition, there is an audible bruit just above his left clavicle. Which of the following is true about this condition?

(A) The dizziness and vertigo are due to blood being diverted from the anterior brain circulation
(B) Stenting of the left subclavian artery may be helpful
(C) Systolic blood pressure measurements in right and left arms are likely to be the same
(D) It is most likely due to an inflammatory arteritis
(E) It more commonly affects the right arm

5. A 63-year-old male comes to the physician's office for a non-healing ulcer on his right great toe and intermittent calf pain. His calf pain is brought on by walking for 10 min and relieved by rest. He wakes up at night with pain in his great toe and has to get up to relieve it. He has a past medical history significant for hypertension, hyperlipidemia, and diabetes. He has a 30-pack-year smoking history. On physical exam, his temperature is 37.8 °C, pulse is 80/min, blood pressure is 139/82, and respirations are 16/min. His low-density lipoprotein (LDL) level is 70 mg/dL. Exam is significant for absent dorsalis pedis and popliteal pulses on the right. The ulcer appears dull gray without purulence. He has diminished sensation to light palpation in both feet. Ankle–brachial index (ABI) is 0.3 on the right and 0.7 on the left. What is the most appropriate next step in management?

(A) Diabetic shoe to off-load pressure
(B) Angiography of the lower extremities
(C) Tight glucose control
(D) Start oral antibiotics
(E) Start heparin

6. A 62-year-old man presents to the physician with swelling in both legs that has been going on for several months. He has a past medical history significant for hypertension and hyperlipidemia. He states that the swelling becomes progressively worse throughout the day. He denies any pain associated with the swelling. Physical exam reveals a temperature of 37.7 °C, blood pressure of 125/72 mmHg, pulse of 77/min, and respiratory rate of 16/min. The heart is in regular rate and rhythm with no murmurs. Jugular venous pressure (JVP) is 7 cm. The lungs are clear to auscultation. On extremity exam, there are strong posterior tibialis and dorsalis pedis pulses bilaterally. The legs are edematous up to the knee with a small patch of eczematous, erythematous-brown scaling skin rash located on the medial malleolus of the right ankle. Which of the following is the most likely cause of his edema?

(A) Peripheral artery disease
(B) Acute deep venous thrombosis (DVT)
(C) Renal protein loss
(D) Reduced cardiac output
(E) Valve incompetence

7. Which of the following patients should undergo carotid endarterectomy (CEA)?

(A) A 70-year-old male with a history of transient painless right eye vision loss and 75% stenosis of the right internal carotid artery (ICA)
(B) A 70-year-old male with a history of transient painless right eye loss and 100% occlusion of the right ICA
(C) A 65-year-old female who sustained a stroke one week ago, is aphasic, has no motor function in her right arm or leg, and has 80% left ICA stenosis
(D) A 68-year-old male became acutely dizzy and passed out 4 days ago with 60% right ICA stenosis
(E) A 72-year-old male with an irregularly irregular rhythm who presents with left-sided weakness for the last several hours and has a 40% right ICA stenosis

8. A 70-year-old male presents with right calf pain after walking three blocks, forcing him to stop and rest. He denies pain at rest in his foot. He smokes one pack per day. His pulse is 74/min, respiratory rate is 16/min, and blood pressure is 136/86 mmHg. Physical examination reveals diminished pulses in his right foot. The ankle–brachial index (ABI) on the right leg is 0.7. The next step in the management is:
   (A) Smoking cessation
   (B) CT angiogram
   (C) MR angiogram
   (D) Formal angiogram
   (E) Stenting of iliac artery

9. A 55-year-old male comes to the physician complaining of bilateral leg pain with walking that is relieved by rest. He has a history of hypertension, hyperlipidemia, chronic obstructive pulmonary disease, and a 30-pack-year smoking history. On physical exam, his blood pressure is 139/79 mmHg, temperature is 37.8 °C, pulse is 89/min, and respirations are 16/min. Present behind both knees are pulsatile masses. What is most strongly associated with this finding?
   (A) Aortic dissection
   (B) Hypercoagulable state
   (C) Degenerative joint disease (DJD)
   (D) Abdominal aortic aneurysm (AAA)
   (E) Thoracic aortic aneurysm

10. A 68-year-old male comes to the physician's office for a non-healing ulcer in his medial malleolus that has been present for several months. He has a past medical history significant for diabetes and hyperlipidemia. On physical exam, his temperature is 37.8 °C, pulse is 70/min, blood pressure is 133/79 mmHg, and respirations are 16/min. Physical exam is significant for pitting right leg edema up to the knee. The leg is warm, and the skin is shiny and has a reddish–brown appearance with several enlarged surface veins. The ulcer has granulation tissue without purulence. Dorsalis pedis pulses are 2+ bilaterally. He notes that the swelling is mild when waking up in the morning but worsens throughout the day. Which of the following is most likely to assist in healing the ulcer?
   (A) A compressive dressing impregnated with zinc oxide
   (B) Diuretics
   (C) A custom-fitted diabetic shoe
   (D) Heparin
   (E) Oral antibiotics

11. At a follow-up appointment two weeks after undergoing left carotid endarterectomy (CEA), it is observed that the patient's tongue deviates to the left when he is asked to stick his tongue out. Which of the following is the most likely explanation?
   (A) Perioperative stroke of the medulla
   (B) Hematoma compressing the musculature of the oropharynx
   (C) Injury to cranial nerve VII
   (D) Injury of cranial nerve X
   (E) Injury of cranial nerve XII

12. A 61-year-old man comes to the physician with an 8-month history of increasing bilateral calf pain during his morning walks. The pain disappears with rest. He reports that the last time he saw a doctor was 20 years ago. He has a 30-pack-year smoking history, but recently quit. His pulse is 68/min, respirations are 18/min, and blood pressure is 126/76 mmHg. His total cholesterol is 320 mg/dL. His doctor recommends that the patient starts a statin and aspirin to reduce the risk of adverse cardiac events. In addition, he recommends that the patient begins an exercise walking program. Which of the following is true about a walking program for his condition?
   (A) It will improve his overall cardiac health but will not improve his walking distance
   (B) It would be expected to result in an increase in his ankle–brachial index (ABI)
   (C) It is less effective than administering a vasodilator
   (D) It can result in a doubling of his walking distance
   (E) It is contraindicated

23. A 65-year-old male presents with new onset claudication. An ankle–brachial index (ABI) confirms that he has peripheral arterial disease (PAD). Which of the following would provide the least amount of benefit to the patient?
(A) Warfarin
(B) Aspirin
(C) Statin
(D) Cilostazol
(E) Clopidogrel

24. A 65-year-old male comes to the physician for a routine physical exam. He has a past medical history significant for hypertension and hyperlipidemia. He is on hydrochlorothiazide, aspirin, and a statin. He has a ten-pack-year smoking history but quit over 30 years ago. Which of the following screening tests is appropriate for this male?
(A) CT scan of the abdomen
(B) Duplex scan of the carotid arteries
(C) Abdominal ultrasonography
(D) Pulmonary spirometry
(E) Ankle–brachial index (ABI)

25. A 52-year-old male is seen at the emergency department for the acute onset of swelling in his right leg that began 6 h ago. He has a past medical history significant for hypertension and colon cancer being treated with chemotherapy in the outpatient setting. Physical exam reveals a temperature of 37.9 °C, blood pressure of 125/72 mmHg, pulse of 77/min, and respiratory rate of 16/min. On extremity exam, there are 2+ posterior tibialis and dorsalis pedis pulses bilaterally. The right leg is edematous, warm, and markedly more swollen than the left leg. What is the best initial study in the workup?
(A) Ankle–brachial index (ABI)
(B) Venous duplex scan
(C) CT angiogram of lower extremities
(D) CT of the head
(E) Measurement of compartment pressures

26. A 69-year-old man comes into the hospital with a 2-day history of severe pain in his left calf. He took Vicodin that a neighbor gave him with only minimal relief. Over the last day, he has lost sensation and movement in his left foot, which prompted him to finally come to the hospital. He has had no medical care and has no past medical history. Physical exam reveals a temperature of 37.8 °C, blood pressure of 147/79 mmHg, heart rate of 85/min, and respiratory rate of 16/min. On extremity exam, there are absent popliteal, posterior tibialis, and dorsalis pedis pulses on the left. Sensation to pinprick is absent in the left, and he cannot plantar- or dorsiflex his foot. The skin of the foot appears to be mottled. Doppler of the foot vessels reveals no audible signals. What is the definitive treatment?
(A) Catheter-assisted thrombolysis
(B) Open surgical intervention
(C) Amputation
(D) Aspirin
(E) Intravenous heparin

Answers

1. Answer C
This patient presents with acute mesenteric ischemia, a life-threatening condition characterized by sudden, severe abdominal pain out of proportion to exam findings, decreased bowel sounds, and evidence of metabolic acidosis (elevated lactate, phosphate, leukocytosis). Risk factors include atrial fibrillation (suggesting a cardioembolic etiology), which is present in this patient. Initial imaging of choice is CT angiography or

MR angiography to confirm the diagnosis and localize the site of vascular compromise. Emergent exploratory laparotomy is indicated only if there are signs of peritonitis or bowel perforation. This patient does not have guarding, rebound, or hemodynamic instability. Imaging should be obtained first (A). Abdominal plain film has low sensitivity for mesenteric ischemia and is not diagnostic. It may show nonspecific signs like ileus or pneumatosis if infarction is advanced (B). Mesenteric Doppler ultrasound may assess for chronic mesenteric ischemia but is not sensitive for acute cases and is operator-dependent (D). Intravenous fluids and serial abdominal exams are appropriate for unclear or nonsurgical causes of abdominal pain, such as nonspecific abdominal pain or early gastroenteritis. However, this patient has clear signs of a vascular emergency (pain out of proportion to exam, metabolic acidosis, risk factors), and delaying imaging would be dangerous (E).

2. Answer D
Although claudication is associated with a very low 5-year risk of limb loss (2–5%), it is associated with a significantly reduced 5-year survival (70%) as compared to matched controls without claudication (A). This is primarily due to the associated coronary artery disease and risk of myocardial infarction (B–C, E). Patients with claudication also have an increased risk of carotid stenosis and, as such, an increased risk of stroke, but stroke is not the primary cause of death in these patients.

3. Answer A
This patient is suffering from an ischemic stroke. Permissive hypertension is considered beneficial following an ischemic stroke so as to maximize cerebral perfusion pressure (CPP). For ischemic strokes, do not use antihypertensive medications to lower blood pressure unless diastolic is greater than 120 mmHg or systolic is greater than 220 mmHg, to ensure proper cerebral perfusion. If it is due to a hemorrhage, keep systolic blood pressure less than 150 mmHg. In both cases, avoid nitroglycerin or nitroprusside, which can serve as potent vasodilators in the cerebral arteries and veins, increasing intracranial pressure (ICP) (C–D). Recall that increasing ICP can further compromise CPP (CPP = mean arterial pressure – ICP). Labetalol can be used safely. In the case of hemorrhage, administer nimodipine to avoid cerebral vasospasms related to irritants in blood. Hydralazine is typically reserved for pregnant patients (E). In addition, hydralazine should be avoided in patients with tachycardia as this medication has high risk for reflex tachycardia after administration.

4. Answer B
Subclavian steal syndrome is due to an atherosclerotic stenosis or occlusion of the subclavian artery, most commonly on the left side (D–E). This leads to claudication symptoms of the affected arm and can be detected on physical examination based on diminished pulses, a significant (>20 mmHg) difference in arm blood pressure, and often a bruit above the clavicle (C). In addition, as the patient exercises, the arteries in the affected arm dilate, lowering resistance, so as to receive more blood. Since the occluded subclavian artery cannot increase blood flow, blood instead travels in a reverse fashion from the vertebral artery (the first branch off the subclavian) down to the arm, essentially stealing blood from the posterior brain circulation, leading to simultaneous symptoms of dizziness and vertigo (A).

5. Answer B
This patient has ischemic rest pain and a non-healing ulcer, both of which are manifestations of critical peripheral artery disease (PAD) that are considered limb threatening. The patient will likely progress to an amputation unless blood flow is improved. As such, the next step is to obtain arterial imaging of the lower extremities. This can be done by either CT angiography (most commonly), MR angiography, or formal transfemoral arteriography in anticipation of either balloon angioplasty, stenting, or an arterial bypass. Tight glucose control will not help in achieving healing of an ischemic ulcer (C). Diabetic shoes are useful for ulcers that form over bony prominences in the setting

of neuropathy (A). Although the patient has evidence of neuropathy, the location of the ulcer (distal toe), its appearance (lack of granulation tissue), absent pulse, and low ABI indicate that the ulcer is from arterial insufficiency. Oral antibiotics are not indicated as there is no evidence of infection (D). Heparin is helpful for acute limb ischemia (ALI) but not for chronic PAD (E).

6. Answer E
Chronic venous insufficiency caused by valve incompetence is the most common cause of lower extremity edema. The presence of hemosiderin-laden skin and ulceration at the medial malleolus is highly characteristic. Edema secondary to valve incompetence is worse when the affected extremity is in the dependent position and improves with extremity elevation (recumbent position). Insufficient venous return causes blood to pool in dependent areas and results in increased capillary pressure causing fluid and red cells to leak out of the capillaries. The skin turns reddish-brown due to hemosiderin deposition. Peripheral artery disease causes atrophy of the affected muscles, decreased pulses, decreased hair growth, shiny skin, and claudication (A). Acute DVT causes sudden onset of pain and swelling of the affected limb (B). Renal protein loss, most commonly caused by nephrotic syndrome, leads to decreased oncotic pressure (C). In the setting of decreased oncotic pressure, there is leakage of fluid into the interstitial space. Nephrotic syndromes would present with hypertension and widespread edema. Reduced cardiac output would present with respiratory symptoms, crackles, and elevated JVP (D).

7. Answer A
The best indication for CEA is a symptomatic high-grade (70–99%) ICA stenosis. Symptoms include ipsilateral arm/leg weakness or contralateral amaurosis fugax. Option A fits that description. Since strokes from ICA stenosis are characteristically embolic, once the artery completely occludes, there is no longer any embolic risk and thus no benefit from CEA (B). Patients who have had massive strokes and have no significant neurologic function to preserve should not undergo CEA (as the goal is to prevent further damage to the motor cortex) (C). Dizziness and syncope are not symptoms of ICA stenosis (D). The patient in answer E likely sustained a stroke secondary to his atrial fibrillation, as opposed to carotid artery embolism.

8. Answer A
The patient has PAD, manifested by claudication, which is not immediately limb threatening. The diagnosis is confirmed by the ABI <0.9. Further testing is not necessary at this time to confirm the diagnosis. Additional imaging should be reserved for patients in whom an intervention is being planned (B–D). Initial management of claudication includes smoking cessation, a walking program, and modification of risk factors (lipid-lowering agents, hypertension control). Stenting is a treatment option (after failed medical management), but one must first obtain imaging to properly plan a possible intervention.

9. Answer D
The clinical scenario is consistent with a popliteal artery aneurysm. Popliteal artery aneurysms are the most common type of peripheral aneurysms. Risk factors for popliteal aneurysm include smoking, hypertension, male sex, and older age. Patients with a popliteal artery aneurysm have a high risk for aneurysm in the contralateral popliteal artery, femoral arteries, and abdominal aorta. Therefore, patients found to have a popliteal artery aneurysm should be screened with ultrasound for aneurysms at these locations. Hypercoagulable state is associated with deep vein thrombosis (B). DJD is associated with popliteal (Baker's) cysts (C). Popliteal aneurysms are not directly associated with thoracic aortic aneurysms or aortic dissection (A, E).

10. Answer A
The patient presents with a classic case of a venous stasis ulcer. These ulcers develop as a result of chronic venous insufficiency, due to vein valve incompetence. Most patients report swelling that worsens throughout the day and improves after lying in bed (recumbent position). Such valve incompetence can be inherited or be the result of a prior deep vein thrombosis (DVT) that scars and damages valves, rendering them incompetent. The ensuing venous hypertension results in increased capillary pressure causing fluid and red and white blood cells to leak out of the capillaries. When the red cells break and lyse, they release the iron-containing hemosiderin and lead to the classic reddish-brown discoloration seen in stasis dermatitis. The pooling of blood leads to capillary damage and activation of an inflammatory process. The exact cause of ulceration in venous stasis is unclear but is likely a combination of leukocyte activation, endothelial damage, and intracellular edema. The cornerstone of treatment of venous stasis ulcers is compression therapy (A). The Unna boot is a compressive gauze that contains zinc oxide and calamine to promote wound healing. Diuretics do not benefit venous insufficiency (B). Diabetic shoes would be appropriate for a neuropathic ulcer, which would typically be located over a bony prominence (C). Heparin would be indicated for a DVT but not for chronic venous stasis (D). Venous stasis ulcers can become infected and require antibiotics; however, their routine use is not recommended (E).

11. Answer E
Cranial nerve deficits occur in about 8% of patients after CEA. In 80–90%, the deficit resolves within 6 months as the injury is due to nerve irritation from retraction and inflammation. In this case, the patient's tongue deviates to the left on protrusion, suggesting an injury to the left cranial nerve XII. This is the most common neuropathy following CEA. Hypoglossal nerve lies lateral to the carotid artery and is vulnerable to traction injury during CEA. Perioperative stroke of the medulla would present with a larger constellation of symptoms (A). Hematoma is a concern in the immediate postoperative period and would be more likely to compromise the airway than a specific cranial nerve (B). Injury to the marginal mandibular branch of cranial nerve VII would cause a droop at the corner of the mouth (C). Cranial nerve X (D) transection would lead to voice hoarseness (D).

12. Answer D
The best medical management for sustained improvement in claudication is a walking program, which can double the walking distance (A, E). A supervised walking program, consisting of 40–50 min of walking 4 days per week is more effective than a non-supervised program. Contrary to common perception, a walking program does not appear to increase collateral blood flow nor does it reliably increase the ABI (B). The exact mechanism by which it improves claudication is not known, but possible mechanisms include improvements in endothelial function, skeletal muscle metabolism, and blood viscosity and a reduction in systemic inflammation. In response to peripheral arterial disease, the distal arterial bed undergoes significant vasodilation. As such, administering pure vasodilators are of no benefit (C).

13. Answer A
This patient is presenting with bowel ischemia secondary to compromised blood flow during open surgical repair of the rAAA. This is most common at the splenic flexure and rectosigmoid junction due to watershed zones. During aortic grafting, the inferior mesenteric artery is usually intentionally ligated, which rarely leads to inadequate colonic blood flow. The incidence of colonic ischemia is 7–27% for open repair of rAAA and 1–13% for elective AAA repair. C. difficile colitis presents with abdominal pain, fever, and watery diarrhea, typically following antibiotic use (B). Diverticulitis presents with abdominal pain and fever but not bloody diarrhea (C). IBD presents with bloody diarrhea, constipation, fecal incontinence, joint pain, and rash but is more chronic in nature (D). Colon cancer presents as occult gastrointestinal bleeding, weight loss, and a change in bowel habits (E).

14. Answer A

The most likely etiology of her neurologic deficits is transection of the common peroneal nerve at the fibular head. The most common presentation of peroneal nerve injury at the fibular neck is acute foot drop (difficulty dorsiflexing the foot against resistance or gravity) along with numbness of the dorsum of the foot. Compartment syndrome presents with the "six Ps": pain (on passive motion), pallor, paresthesias, paralysis, poikilothermia, and pulselessness (late sign) following trauma (B). However, this patient is warm and well perfused and is not complaining of any pain. Arterial thrombosis can occur after trauma; however, the patient has normal distal pulses (C). Fracture of the fibular head would not typically cause injury to the deep peroneal nerve (D). Pain at the fracture site should not cause such a profound motor deficit nor would it cause a sensory deficit (E).

15. Answer B

Jaw pain with chewing, or jaw claudication, is suggestive of giant cell arteritis, also called temporal arteritis, which is managed with steroids. Giant cell arteritis affects the temporal artery, not the carotid artery (A). CT angiogram showing 80% stenosis confirms the diagnosis of carotid stenosis (C). Left-hand weakness may be found in patients with middle cerebral artery stroke which may or may not be due to carotid emboli (D). An atrial mass on echocardiogram may be an intracardiac tumor, such as atrial myxoma, that will need to be resected surgically (E).

16. Answer A

Claudication alone, in the absence of ischemic rest pain or tissue loss, is a relatively benign condition that rarely leads to amputation. The risk of amputation is only about 2–5% (B-E). Thus, medical management can safely be utilized as the first step in its management. Five-year mortality in claudicants, however, is significantly increased as compared to non-claudicants. This is predominantly due to an increased risk of myocardial infarction and to a lesser degree stroke.

17. Answer A

The triad of Leriche syndrome is (1) buttock and thigh claudication, (2) erectile dysfunction, and (3) absent femoral pulses. It is due to chronic progressive atherosclerosis of the distal aorta and proximal common iliac arteries (not the superficial femoral artery) that eventually occludes the aorta (B–C). Since the occlusion is gradual, collaterals have had a chance to enlarge and refill (reconstitute) the femoral arteries distally. Important collaterals come from the superior mesenteric artery, inferior mesenteric artery (superior hemorrhoidal), lumbar arteries, median sacral artery, and internal mammary (via epigastric arteries). Because the aorta and common iliac arteries are occluded, the blood supply to the buttocks (through the internal iliac arteries) is compromised, as is the blood supply to the penis (via the internal pudendal artery, a branch of the internal iliac artery). Thus, the patients endorse buttock claudication, as well as erectile dysfunction. Because of the rich collateral supply around the distal aorta and the chronic nature of the occlusion, the ABI typically drops by only 30% (to about 0.7). Thus, toe gangrene is rare. Patients with diabetes typically develop atherosclerosis more distally in the leg, in the superficial femoral and tibial arteries (not in the aorta). Acute aortic occlusion is a devastating, severe acute ischemia of both lower legs, which manifests by rapid onset of motor and sensory loss. It is seen following a large embolus from atrial fibrillation lodging at the distal aorta. The sudden onset does not permit adequate collateral enlargement. Untreated, it results in limb loss, massive acidosis, and death. Spinal stenosis compresses nerve roots, leading to generalized weakness of both legs that is worse with walking (D). Unlike claudication, it is usually relieved by leaning forward (such as over a shopping cart). Bilateral hip osteoarthritis more commonly affects older women and presents with tenderness on palpation of the hips (E).

18. Answer D
PAD is defined as an ABI <0.9. The normal ABI ranges from 1 to 1.2. Symptomatic PAD can readily be diagnosed via history and physical examination, and in fact the classic history, combined with physical exam evidence of diminished pulses, is highly specific, but not sufficiently sensitive (C). Early PAD can be asymptomatic and is best detected by ABI. Arteriography is invasive and is thus reserved for patients who are to undergo an interventional procedure (E). The pulse exam is very subjective and cannot alone be relied upon to establish a diagnosis of PAD (B). History of pain in legs with exertion is not specific to PAD (A).

19. Answer C
Buerger's disease, also known as thromboangiitis obliterans, is a non-atherosclerotic vascular occlusive disease seen in young (<40 years), mostly male smokers. It predominantly involves the arteries in the leg below the knee (popliteal and tibial arteries) as well as hands. It also causes venous thrombosis. The cause is unknown. Stenting and surgical bypass (A–B) are ineffective as the occlusions involve the most distal arteries. The only effective treatment is smoking cessation. It is associated with high rates of amputation, especially if the patient continues smoking. The remaining answer choices (D–E) are not used in the management of Buerger's disease.

20. Answer B
This patient is presenting with a ruptured abdominal aortic aneurysm (AAA). Hemodynamically unstable patients presenting with classic symptoms and signs of aortic rupture such as hypotension, flank pain, and a pulsatile mass should be taken emergently to the operating room (OR) for immediate control of hemorrhage. Surgical intervention should not be delayed waiting for CT scan of the abdomen or transfusion of packed red blood cells (A, C). In fact, permissive hypotension is preferable to aggressive fluid resuscitation prior to the OR, as excessive fluids prior to aortic control may lead to more bleeding. In patients who are hemodynamically stable, CT scan of the abdomen should be obtained to assess for feasibility of endovascular repair. For patients who are unstable and are not previously known to have AAA, ultrasound may be performed quickly prior to abdominal laparotomy, to confirm the presence of AAA, but cannot determine rupture (D). Intubation should be performed in the OR, as it can trigger worsening hypotension (E).

21. Answer C
This patient is presenting with acute limb ischemia (ALI) given the pain, pulselessness, and paresthesias (recall the "Ps").The etiology of ALI includes thrombus formation (most likely due to long-standing peripheral arterial disease in the legs), embolization (most often from the heart), and trauma. Lack of claudication history and normal contralateral limb exam supports embolic etiology. The most common cause of ALI is a cardiac source, most often due to atrial fibrillation. Arterial thrombosis is another cause of ALI (A). Such patients often have a history of claudication and decreased pulses in the nonischemic leg. Peripheral neuropathy is an important cause of numbness in diabetic patients and would cause decreased sensation in a stocking glove pattern starting on the dorsum of the foot but would not account for the acute onset and absent pulses (B). Aortic aneurysms rarely cause embolization. (D). Paradoxical embolism from a deep venous thrombosis crossing a patent foramen ovale is another cause of ALI but is very rare (E).

22. Answer C
Patients who present with symptoms concerning for stroke should undergo a non-contrast CT scan of the brain to rule out intracranial hemorrhage. Once hemorrhage has been ruled out, consideration should be given for thrombolytic therapy for an ischemic stroke (intravenous if within 3 h of symptom onset, intra-arterial if within 6 h of onset). Doppler of the carotid artery, echocardiogram, ECG, or CT angiogram may be performed to evaluate for the cause of the stroke (carotid plaque vs. cardioembolic), but they are not part of the acute management of this patient (A–B, D–E).

23. Answer A

Warfarin is useful for the prevention of embolic events associated with atrial fibrillation and for the prevention of venous thrombotic events (such as deep venous thrombosis and pulmonary embolus). Since PAD is due to atherosclerosis and not due to embolus/thrombus, there is no evidence that warfarin benefits patients with PAD. Clopidogrel inhibits platelet aggregation by blocking activation of the glycoprotein IIb/IIIa pathway. In patients with PAD, it has been shown to reduce the combined endpoint of stroke, myocardial infarction, and acute limb ischemia (E). Given its high costs, its routine use in PAD is not recommended. Cilostazol is a quinolinone derivative that inhibits cellular phosphodiesterase. It inhibits platelet aggregation and is a direct arterial dilator. It inhibits vascular smooth muscle proliferation and improves the lipid profile (D). The exact mechanism by which it improves walking distance in patients with claudication is unclear. Aspirin does not directly improve claudication but is effective in reducing the risks of stroke and acute coronary events, which are common in PAD patients (B). Statins also do not directly improve walking distance but are beneficial in PAD patients via their lipid-lowering and anti-inflammatory (atherosclerotic plaque stabilizing) properties (C).

24. Answer C

The United States Preventive Services Task Force (USPSTF) recommends a one-time screening for abdominal aortic aneurysm (AAA) by ultrasonography in men aged 65–75 that have any smoking history. Screening is not recommended for women, even those who have smoked, unless they have additional risk factors such as a strong family history of aneurysm. CT of the abdomen is not appropriate for AAA screening (A). Screening for carotid artery stenosis is not recommended nor is screening adults for chronic obstructive pulmonary disease using spirometry or screening for peripheral artery disease with an ABI (B, D–E).

25. Answer B

The most likely etiology is a deep vein thrombosis (DVT) given the swelling and history of colon cancer (hypercoagulability). The best diagnostic test is a venous duplex scan. An ABI is appropriate for suspected peripheral arterial disease (PAD), however, that would not cause swelling (A). CT angiogram would be a useful follow-up study for PAD prior to a planned intervention (C). CT of the head would be useful for a suspected stroke (D). Compartment pressure measurements are sometimes used to rule out compartment syndrome when suspicion is low to moderate; however, it presents with pain with passive motion as well as the other "six Ps": pain, pallor, paresthesias, paralysis, poikilothermia, and pulselessness (late sign) (E). It classically presents after trauma or after ischemia reperfusion.

26. Answer C

The patient presents with irreversible acute limb ischemia. Muscle begins to become damaged after 3 h of ischemia, whereas irreversible ischemia sets in after 6 h. Exam findings that support irreversible ischemia include the 48-h duration of ischemia, profound sensory loss, paralysis of the muscles, mottling of the skin, and inaudible Doppler signals. When acute limb ischemia progresses to irreversible tissue damage, as in the case presented, primary amputation should be performed (A-B, D-E). Attempting to revascularize an irreversibly ischemic limb (besides not helping the limb) puts the patient at risk of developing reperfusion syndrome, which manifests with severe hyperkalemia, acidosis, and rhabdomyolysis that can lead to renal failure due to acute tubular necrosis.

Supplementary Information

C. de Virgilio, A. Grigorian (eds.), *Surgery*, https://doi.org/10.1007/978-3-032-09799-6

Index

A

B

D

E

F

G

H

I

J

K

L

M

N

O

P

Q

R

S

T

U

V

W

X

Z